Imaging of the Pediatric Head, Neck, and Spine

Imaging of the Pediatric Head, Neck, and Spine

Mauricio Castillo, M.D.
Associate Professor of Radiology
Chief, Section of Neuroradiology
Department of Radiology
University of North Carolina School of Medicine
Chapel Hill, North Carolina

Suresh K. Mukherji, M.D.
Assistant Professor of Radiology and Head and Neck Surgery
Chief, Head and Neck Radiology, Section of Neuroradiology
Department of Radiology
University of North Carolina School of Medicine
Chapel Hill, North Carolina

All illustrations by Mauricio Castillo, M.D.

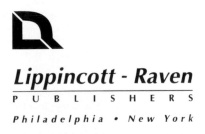

Lippincott - Raven
PUBLISHERS
Philadelphia • New York

Acquisitions Editor: James D. Ryan
Sponsoring Editor: Susan Skand
Production Editor: Virginia Barishek
Interior Designer: Arlene Putterman
Cover Designer: Becky Baxendell
Production: P.M. Gordon Associates, Inc.
Indexer: Roger Wall
Compositor/Prepress: Maryland Composition Company
Printer/Binder: Quebecor/Kingsport

Library of Congress Cataloging-in-Publication Data

Castillo, Mauricio.
    Imaging of the pediatric head, neck, and spine / Mauricio
Castillo, Suresh K. Mukherji ; all illustrations by Mauricio
Castillo.
        p.   cm.
    Includes bibliographical references and index.
    ISBN 0–397–51577–4 (alk. paper)
    1. Pediatric neurology.   2. Pediatric diagnostic imaging.
3. Skull—Imaging.   4. Spine—Imaging.   5. Neck—Imaging.
6. Central Nervous System Diseases—diagnosis—atlases.
I. Mukherji, Suresh K.   II. Title.
    [DNLM: 1. Central Nervous System Diseases—in infancy & childhood—
atlases.   2. Diagnostic Imaging—in infancy & childhood—atlases.
3. Brain—pathology—atlases.   4. Head—pathology—atlases.
5. Neck—pathology—atlases.   6. Spine—pathology—atlases.   WL 17 C3521   1996]
RJ488.5.R33C37   1998
618.92′8—dc20
DNLM/DLC   95–44623
for Library of Congress   CIP

The material contained in this volume was submitted as previously unpublished material,
except in the instances in which credit has been given to the source from which some of the
illustrative material was derived.

Great care has been taken to maintain the accuracy of the information contained in the
volume. However, neither Lippincott-Raven Publishers nor the editors can be held responsible for
errors or for any consequences arising from the use of the information herein.

The authors and publisher have exerted every effort to ensure that drug selection and dosage
set forth in this text are in accord with current recommendations and practice at the time of
publication. However, in view of ongoing research, changes in government regulations, and the
constant flow of information relating to drug therapy and drug reactions, the reader is urged to
check the package insert for each drug for any change in indications and dosage and for added
warnings and precautions. This is particularly important when the recommended agent is a new
or infrequently employed drug.

Materials appearing in this book prepared by individuals as part of their official duties as U.S.
Government employees are not covered by the above-mentioned copyright.

9 8 7 6 5 4 3 2 1

To Michelle, patient wife, and a good friend.
To the memory of my father, with love.

MC

To my wife Rita, for all her love and understanding.
To my parents Chandra and Phatick Mukherji, MD,
for their love and encouragement.

SKM

"Ultimately, encompassing
compassion is the
commitment to devote
oneself to the discipline
and to the child as if every
patient were one's own
child, whose happiness and
continued health depended
solely on your skill. The
rewards for such devotion
make the commitment
a joy."

T.P. NAIDICH

Foreword

Pediatric neuroradiology today encompasses not only imaging of the brain, but all other relevant structures that are functionally related to the central nervous system. Thus, it is appropriate that a new book in this field should address the head, neck, and spine. This, the authors have admirably done.

While a book foreword is not a book review, the thought processes of the writer are not dissimilar. Does this book provide a new and worthwhile contribution to the medical literature? Will I want this on my bookshelf? Will I use it? Happily, the answer to all of these questions is "Yes." The field of pediatric neuroradiology is represented by several recent texts, none of which encompasses the entire field as does this one. Drs. Castillo and Mukherji have carried out an outstanding task in making this a worthwhile and significant contribution to the field. Not surprisingly, both authors have been highly prolific in their publications in the recent medical literature, encompassing the field of pediatric neuroradiology inclusive of pediatric head and neck.

The purpose of this text by Drs. Castillo and Mukherji is to convey as much information as possible in the most reasonable space, giving, at the same time, a comprehensive overview of pediatric neuroradiology. The information given will apply to all interested disciplines, including not only pediatric neuroradiology but also those practicing pediatric specialties of neurology, neurosurgery, pediatric oncology, and ENT. All physicians who occasionally encounter the pediatric patient for diagnostic imaging studies will also find this text highly valuable. The organization and presentation of the book provide accessibility to both the commonly and less commonly encountered entities. The references are appropriate and recent, and are from journals that most medical libraries will have. The text is well illustrated, with captions concise and to the point.

ROBERT A. ZIMMERMAN, MD
Department of Radiology, Neuroradiology
Children's Hospital of Philadelphia
Philadelphia, Pennsylvania

Preface

A rapid glance at the current radiology literature readily shows that pediatric neuroradiology has become a mature discipline. Other books available on this topic concentrate on the evaluation of the brain and the spine. Our book provides coverage of all aspects of brain, neck, and spine imaging that pediatric neuroradiologists, pediatric radiologists, and general radiologists may come across. Therefore, this book has a substantial portion dealing with imaging of the face, orbits, temporal bones, paranasal sinuses, airway, and neck. In preparing this book, we realize how little of the clinical aspects of the disorders here addressed is available in other imaging books. Consequently, this book includes discussions on the epidemiologic and clinical features of each entity. We have been careful to place equal emphasis on the clinical and imaging features of each disorder; and thus, believe this book will not only be useful to radiologists, but to some primary care clinicians as well. The illustrations portray common and unusual manifestations of the entities addressed. Rather than providing an extensive bibliography, we have listed the titles of a few of the references that we found particularly useful while writing the text. Furthermore, many of the observations made here are our own. Each chapter begins with a short discussion on embryology as it applies to the pathology thereafter dealt with. All illustrations are simple line diagrams intended to facilitate understanding of a complex topic. We hope that this book will be useful to all who deal with imaging of children with disorders of the head, neck, and spine.

MAURICIO CASTILLO, MD
SURESH K. MUKHERJI, MD

Acknowledgments

MC wishes to acknowledge:

Ms. Della Williams for her secretarial work. Our colleagues at the Neuro-radiology Section here at UNC. At Lippincott-Raven, Jim Ryan continues his enthusiastic support of our ideas. Many physicians have contributed with il-lustrations and I have carefully tried to acknowledge their help. I apologize for any unintended omissions.

SKM wishes to acknowledge:

My former mentors, Joseph Sanfillopo, M.D., C. V. Rao, Ph.D., George Padi-lla, Ph.D., Vladimir Petrov, Ph.D., John Harbert, M.D., and Anthony Man-cuso, M.D., for giving me the opportunity to make this possible. My parents for instilling in me the belief that no hard work goes unrewarded.

Both authors acknowledge:

Support and encouragement from Joseph K. T. Lee, M.D., and Bo Strain for photography.

Contents

Imaging of the Pediatric Head, Neck, and Spine
by Mauricio Castillo and Suresh K. Mukherji,
Lippincott-Raven Publishing, Philadelphia © 1996.

1

Imaging Considerations

1.0 *Computed Tomography*

Computed tomography (CT) continues to be the examination of choice for patients with acute trauma (suspected acute intracranial hemorrhage), bone abnormalities (including the skull and spine), intracranial abnormalities suspected to harbor calcifications, paranasal sinus disease, facial bone abnormalities, for follow-up studies in patients with treated hydrocephalus, and for initial evaluation of neck abnormalities. Helical CT offers an alternative to conventional CT when the latter is not possible because of motion artifacts related to the length of the examination. Helical CT, however, is lower in signal-to-noise ratio and therefore results in images of lesser quality than conventional CT. We use helical CT as an alternative to conventional CT especially if the suspected abnormality involves the bones. Helical CT does not produce adequate soft tissue resolution unless the abnormality is large (eg, epidural hematoma). When helical CT is used, a pitch of 1 is preferred. The need to perform contrast-enhanced CT studies should also be less if magnetic resonance (MR) imaging is available. We believe, if a contrast CT is needed, the patient is better served by being studied with MR imaging. If contrast-enhanced CT is to be performed, we administer 3 ml/kg (up to a total of 120 ml) of nonionic contrast (300 mg/ml concentration). This dose is given as a single hand-pushed bolus. The slice thickness may be varied according to the age of the patient (which is reflected in the size of the head). Patients younger than 5 years of age are studied using 3-mm thick contiguous slices (no gap between slices) from the base of the skull to the vertex. Patients older than 5 years of age are studied using contiguous 5-mm slices through the posterior fossa and 5-mm contiguous slices supratentorially (identical to CT studies for adults). For follow-up of hydrocephalus studies (ie, rule out shunt malfunction), 10-mm slices throughout the entire brain usually suffice. We recommend the following basic protocols for CT studies:

I. Routine Brain
A. Conventional CT:
> 5 Years of age: 5-mm thick contiguous slices through posterior fossa, 5-mm thick contiguous slices through cerebral hemispheres
< 5 Years of age: 3-mm thick contiguous slices throughout entire head
B. Helical CT:
All ages: acquire at 5-mm slice thickness and reconstruct at 5- or 3-mm thickness, pitch = 1
NOTE: Identical protocols to be performed before and after contrast media administration. Both bone and soft tissue window settings are needed. In cases of trauma, intermediate window settings are suggested.

II. Craniosynostosis
A. Conventional CT:
Three-millimeter contiguous slices from base of skull to vertex, bone windows using the high-resolution bone (edge enhancement) filter
B. Helical CT:
Acquire at 3-mm slice thickness and reconstruct at 3-mm slice thickness, pitch = 1, three-dimensional reformations may be performed
NOTE: All studies need bone and brain window setting images.

III. Orbits
    A. Conventional CT:

        Precontrast: 3-mm axial contiguous slices

        Postcontrast: 3-mm axial and coronal contiguous slices

    B. Helical CT:

        Precontrast: acquire axial slices at 5 mm and reconstruct at 3-mm slice thickness, pitch = 1

        Postcontrast: acquire axial and coronal views at 3-mm slice thickness and reconstruct at 3-mm slice thickness, pitch = 1

        NOTE: All studies need bone and soft tissue window setting images.

IV. Paranasal Sinuses
    A. Conventional CT:

        Three-millimeter contiguous coronal slices

    B. Helical CT:

        Acquire coronal views at 3-mm slice thickness and reconstruct at 3-mm slice thickness, pitch = 1

        NOTE: For screening only, coronal views may suffice. No contrast is needed. Coronal views need to be processed with high-resolution bone (edge enhancement) filter.

V. Temporal Bones
    A. Conventional CT:

        One- to 1.0–1.5-mm thick contiguous slices in both coronal and axial projection

    B. Helical CT:

        Acquire at 2-mm thick slices and reconstruct at 2-mm slice thickness, pitch = 1

        NOTE: All studies acquired prospectively with high-resolution (edge enhancement) bone filter. No contrast needed. Each side magnified independently.

VI. Neck
    A. Conventional CT:

        Three-millimeter contiguous slices from the base of the skull through the thoracic inlet

    B. Helical CT:

        Acquire 3–5-mm slices and reconstruct at 3-mm slice thickness

        NOTE: All studies done immediately after intravenous contrast administration.

VII. Spine
    A. Conventional CT:

        Three-millimeter contiguous slices through region of interest

    B. Helical CT:

        Acquire 3-mm slices through region of interest and reconstruct at 3-mm slice thickness

        NOTE: No intravenous contrast is needed. Same protocol applies for CT studies after myelography. If findings are questionable, then 1.5-mm thick slices may be performed through the region of interest.

1.01 *Magnetic Resonance*

MR IMAGING

Magnetic resonance (MR) is the imaging modality of choice in most disorders that affect the pediatric brain. Exceptions (as in adults) include the presence of subarachnoid hemorrhage, acute trauma, and detailed evaluation of bony abnormalities. In head and neck imaging, MR plays important roles in the evaluation of orbital disease and disorders located in the upper portion (the nasopharynx) of the aerodigestive tract. In the evaluation of spinal disorders, MR is the imaging modality of choice except when the vertebrae need to be visualized in detail. Intracranial ferromagnetic vascular clips are not to be imaged unless there is no optional imaging method and the manufacturer has stated their safety. Other metallic components usually found in children that may interfere with MR imaging include Harrington (or other spinal) rods and dental braces (which may produce enough artifact to obscure the base of the skull).

Magnetic resonance contrast may be safely administered except in the presence of obvious contraindications, such as prior allergic reaction or sickle cell disease (contrast may induce further hemolysis). Written consent is needed from the parents/guardian in patients younger than 2 years of age. As of this writing, only gadolinium-DTPA is approved for use in children. The dose, 0.1 mmol/kg, is similar to that used in adults. Sedation, which will keep the patient still, is critical if good-quality images are desired. As a general rule, we sedate all patients older than 6 months of age and younger than 10 years of age. Young infants (< 6 months) usually fall asleep in the unit. Children older than 10 years usually cooperate if gently coached. We usually begin with the mildest form of sedation, which is oral chloral hydrate. If the patient fails the chloral hydrate, other forms of sedation (generally parenteral) or general anesthesia are planned. Sedation protocols often vary greatly from one institution to another. (See Sedation and Post Sedation Section)

All brain examinations are done in a dedicated head MR coil. If the patient is extremely small, such as a premature baby, the head may be placed in the knee coil. Imaging of the spine should always be obtained with a surface coil (preferably the "license plate" coil), using a small field of view (FOV), and several placements. If the child is very small, adequate spine examinations may be obtained using the head coil.

I. Routine Brain

A. Younger than 12 months of age:
Sagittal and axial T1-weighted images (echo time [TE]: 15, repetition time [TR]: 600, NEX: 1, FOV: 220 mm, slices: 5 mm)
Axial fast spin echo T2-weighted images (TE: 19/93, TR: 3500–4000, NEX: 1, FOV: 200 mm, slices: 5 mm)

B. Older than 12 months of age:
Sagittal T1-weighted images (TE: 15, TR: 600, NEX: 1, FOV: 240 mm, slices: 5 mm)
Axial and coronal fast spin echo T2-weighted images (TE: 19/93, TR: 3500–4000, NEX: 1, FOV: 230 mm, slices: 5 mm)

NOTE: If contrast material is administered, axial and coronal T1-weighted images are added. If a posterior fossa tumor is present, postcontrast sagittal T1-weighted images are generally useful to the neurosurgeon.

All studies are performed with rectangular matrix (192 × 256).

If the study is being done for partial complex seizures, high-resolution fast T2 spin echo and/or inversion recovery imaging of the hippocampi may be done as follows:

Angle slices perpendicular to the long axis of the temporal horn of the lateral ventricle, initiate coronal slices on the midline sagittal pilot view at the level of the mamillary bodies. For fast spin echo: (TE: 90, TR: 4600, NEX: 2–4, FOV: 200–220 mm, slices: 3 mm, resolution [with rectangular matrix]: 288 × 512) For inversion recovery: TE: 20, TR: 3500, NEX: 1, FOV: 230 mm, slices: 3 mm, resolution: 192 × 256, inversion time: 300 msec.

II. Routine Orbits

Precontrast imaging:
Sagittal brain T1-weighted images (TE: 16, TR: 600, NEX: 1, FOV: 220–240 mm, slices: 5 mm)
Axial brain fast spin echo T2-weighted images (TE: 19/93, TR: 3550, NEX: 1, FOV: 230 mm, slices: 5 mm)
Axial orbits T1-weighted images (TE: 15, TR: 500, NEX: 4, FOV: 200 mm, slices: 3 mm)
Postcontrast imaging:
Axial orbits T1-weighted images (TE: 15, TR: 650, NEX: 4, FOV: 160–200 mm, slices: 4 mm, fat saturation pulse: 230–250)
Coronal orbits T1-weighted images (TE: 15, TR: 650, NEX: 4, FOV: 160–200 mm, slices: 4 mm, fat saturation pulse: 230–250)

NOTE: Fat saturation pulse may need individual shimming.

III. Sella and Parasellar Regions

Sagittal brain T1-weighted images (TE: 16, TR: 600, NEX: 1, FOV: 220 mm, slices: 5 mm)
Axial fast spin echo T2-weighted images (TE: 19/93, TR: 3500, NEX: 1, FOV: 230 mm, slices: 5 mm)
Coronal precontrast sella T1-weighted images (TE: 15, TR: 500, NEX: 4, FOV: 200 mm, slices: 3 mm if a small abnormality was seen in brain images, 5 mm if a large abnormality was seen on brain images)
Coronal and sagittal postcontrast sella T1-weighted images (same protocol as coronal precontrast T1-weighted images)

IV. Cervical and Thoracic Spine

Sagittal T1-weighted images (TE: 15, TR: 500, NEX: 2, FOV: 150–220 mm, slices: 4 mm)
Sagittal fast spin echo T2-weighted images (TE: 19/93, TR: 3500–4000, NEX: 1, FOV: 150–220 mm, slices: 4 mm)
Axial gradient echo T2-weighted images (TE: 20, TR: 650, NEX: 2–4, FOV: 150–200 mm, slices: 4 mm, flip angle: 25–30 degrees)

V. Lumbar Spine

Sagittal T1-weighted images (TE: 16, TR: 600, NEX: 2, FOV: 180–240 mm, slices: 4 mm)
Sagittal fast spin echo T2-weighted images (TE: 19–93, TR: 3500–4000, NEX: 1, slices: 4 mm)
Axial T1-weighted images (TE: 20, TR: 650, NEX: 2–4, FOV: 150–200 mm, slices: 4 mm)

NOTE: If contrast material is administered, axial and sagittal sequences (same protocols as described above) are repeated.

VI. Suspected Spinal Dysraphism without Scoliosis

1. Sagittal T1-weighted image of lumbar spine:
   I. If normal, stop
   II. If dysraphism or low conus medullaris are present, continue with:
2. Sagittal fast spin echo T2-weighted images
3. Axial T1-weighted images extending from T11 to tip of sacrum
4. Sagittal T1-weighted images of the thoracic and cervical spinal cord,
   I. If normal, stop
   II. If syrinx is found, do axial T1-weighted images through abnormality
   III. If diastematomyelia is found, do coronal T1-weighted images and axial T2-weighted gradient echo sequences at level of abnormality

NOTE: No contrast material administration is needed for spinal dysraphism studies unless superimposed infection is a clinical consideration.

VII. Childhood Scoliosis

A. Occult dysraphism (patients with a fatty mass, hairy patch, hemangioma, dermal sinus): Do sagittal and coronal T1-weighted images extending from T11 to tip of sacrum and axial T1-weighted images (5 mm thick) spaced throughout same region. Axial T2-weighted images may be needed if an epidermoid is suspected.
B. Open myelomeningocele repaired at birth (Chiari II patients): Same protocol as described above for suspected dysraphism (item VI).
C. Congenital vertebral anomalies: Sagittal and coronal T1-weighted images of lumbar spine (check for tethering of conus medullaris), axial and coronal T1-weighted images of abnormality; if diastematomyelia is suspected, do axial T2-weighted gradient echoes at level of abnormality.
D. None of the above: Do sagittal T1-weighted images of the lumbar spine (to confirm the position of the conus medullaris) and if normal, do sagittal, coronal, and axial T1-weighted images (precontrast and postcontrast) through curvature to exclude either an intramedullary tumor or nerve sheath tumor. If no tumor is found, then do sagittal T1-weighted images of cervical spine (including the foramen magnum) to exclude a Chiari type I malformation.

MR SPECTROSCOPY In our experience, the clinical use of MR spectroscopy (MRS) is limited to the diagnosis of tumors, determination of tumor versus radiation necrosis, and use in some metabolic and destructive disorders such as Canavan disease and infarctions. Hydrogen MR spectroscopy is more commonly used, although phosphorus MRS provides important information when ischemia is suspected. We performed most of our studies using single-volume techniques with either PRESS or, preferably, STEAM (which allows for shorter TEs). The first large peak seen to the left in a hydrogen spectrum corresponds to choline at approximately 3.21 parts per million (ppm). Choline is an important basic component for the phospholipids that constitute cell membranes, and in the brain also reflects the structure and integrity of the myelin sheaths. It is increased in processes in which there is active cell growth and duplication, such as tumors. The second most obvious peak is that of creatinine, which occurs at 3.03 ppm. It reflects the concentration of phosphocreatine, which is critical in the energy systems of cells. *N*-acetyl aspartate (NAA) is the largest peak seen at 2.01 ppm. Although its exact function is uncertain, it is considered by most to be a neuronal marker. Therefore, in adults gray matter has a higher NAA concentration than white matter. In children, both gray and white matter contain similar concentrations of NAA. Lactate, which usually occurs with anaerobic metabolism, is seen at 1.4 ppm. It may be normal in premature babies but is not present after a term gestation.

1.02 *Sonography (including Doppler)*

The main advantage of ultrasonography continues to be its portability and therefore its ability to produce bedside images. For most neonatal brains, a 5-MHz transducer produces adequate images. The surface of the brain may be imaged with 7.5- or 10-MHz transducers. Stand-off pads may be needed for these transducers. Lower-frequency transducers have been advocated if penetration through bone or almost closed fontanelles is desired. Examinations are usually performed through the anterior fontanelle. The posterior fontanelle offers an alternative window when the bregma is not available, and is especially useful in the evaluation of posterior fossa abnormalities. The lateral fontanelle may be used to view the upper brain stem. Scanning through the coronal suture or thin temporal squama allows for identification of extraaxial fluid collections and visualization of the circle of Willis.

Duplex Doppler sonograms of the circle of Willis and its major branches are easily obtained via the anterior fontanelle. Through this approach, the angle of insonation of the anterior cerebral arteries is close to 0 degrees and correct sampling is easily performed. Evaluation of the velocities in the middle and posterior cerebral arteries may be underestimated if the anterior fontanelle is used as a window because of a high insonation angle. The normal Doppler pattern always consists of sharp systolic upstroke, gentle downstroke, and the presence of diastolic flow. Absence of inversion of diastolic flow is always abnormal. With age, arterial velocities increase and cerebrovascular resistance decreases (reflected by a decrease in the resistive index).

The main indications for brain sonography include suspected intracranial hemorrhage in the newborn, screening for hydrocephalus, visualization of the circle of Willis after carotid ligation for extracorporeal membrane oxygenation (ECMO), history of perinatal hypoxia/ischemia, and screening for vascular malformations such as vein of Galen malformations.

Sonography of the spine produces much less accurate images than does MR imaging. Five- or 10-MHz transducers may be used. The patient is placed prone with a pillow under the abdomen to separate the spinous processes (which improves the acoustic window). Linear-array transducers are preferred because they cover wider regions. The tip of the conus medullaris should always be identified. Its location may be determined by remembering that L4 is at the level of the superior aspect of the iliac crests. The main value of spinal sonography continues to be its ability to guide the surgeon when performed intraoperatively through a laminectomy.

SONOGRAPHY PROTOCOLS

I. **Brain**

    A. Coronal sections level:
       Frontal horns anterior to foramina of Monroe
       Foramina of Monroe
       Posterior third ventricle through thalami
       Quadrigeminal plate cistern
       Trigones of lateral ventricles
    B. Sagittal sections level:
       Midline

Caudothalamic notch
Body of lateral ventricles
Sylvian fissures

II. Duplex Doppler

Circle of Willis:
Midsagittal view for insonation of proximal anterior cerebral arteries
Coronal view for insonation of proximal middle cerebral artery (insonation angle: 10–30 degrees) and for proximal posterior cerebral artery (insonation angle: 45–65 degrees)

III. Spinal Sonogram

Several midsagittal longitudinal and parasagittal projections
Several axial views from lower thoracic spine to sacrum

1.03 Angiography

Indications for cerebral angiography in children are few. These mainly include the evaluation of aneurysms (which are very rare in the pediatric population); defining the architecture of arteriovenous malformations, vasculopathies (such as Moya-Moya), and arterial dissections; and as mapping before interventional procedures. Childhood infarction may also need to be evaluated with catheter angiography. Screening (and follow-up, if required) for most vascular disorders may be successfully performed with MR angiography for most of the aforementioned problems. Indeed, the use of MR angiography has markedly decreased the use of conventional catheter angiography at our institution. For angiography, we routinely schedule patients younger than 12 years of age under general anesthesia. For older patients, the need for general anesthesia needs to be determined on an individual basis. Verbal and written consent needs to be obtained from the parents/guardian before the procedure. The risks of cerebral angiography include:

> Bleeding, groin hematoma, damage to vessels leading to arterial thrombosis and ischemia of the involved extremity, damage to nerves, damage to the arteries in the neck or head leading to transient or permanent neurologic deficits, allergic reaction, and death.

Consent for anesthesia is usually obtained independently from the consent for angiography. If a prior documented allergic reaction to iodinated contrast media has occurred, anesthesia will be present during the procedure and generally there is no need for premedication (as in adults).

ANGIOGRAPHY LABORATORY STUDIES

a. Blood urea nitrogen and serum creatinine
b. Prothrombin time and partial thromboplastin time
c. Hemoglobin, hematocrit, and platelet count

A note should be placed in the patient's chart. This note should include the following:

a. Reason for performing the angiogram
b. Pertinent findings in other imaging studies
c. Past medical history
d. Allergies
e. Results of laboratory values (if these are not yet available, they need to be ordered)
f. A statement that the procedure was fully explained to the parents/guardian and that their oral and written consent has been given

---

In adolescent girls it is always wise to check for the possibility of pregnancy. Contrary to the case with adults, the radiologist need not always write preangiography orders because these are usually written by the anesthesiologist.

As a general rule, we use a 4-Fr system in patients younger than 5 years of age. In patients older than 5 years, a 5-Fr system (identical to that used in adults) may easily be used. In our experience, the easiest catheter to use in pediatric patients is the H1H. Because the studies are not being done for athero-sclerotic disease, we do not routinely obtain an aortic arch angiogram. Exceptions to this rule include cases of vasculopathies that involve large vessels, such as Takayasu disease. Similarly, unless the extracranial circulation is suspected of being involved (eg, trauma leading to dissection) views of the neck are not performed. Frontal and lateral magnified views of the head are indispensable. Coned down views of the posterior fossa are also helpful when disease involving the vertebrobasilar circulation is suspected. Oblique views are done on an "as needed" basis. If the intracranial flow is extremely fast, the anesthesiologist can be asked to hyperventilate the patient just before the angiography run to try to slow the intracranial circulation and get higher-quality films. This is seldom required if the angiographic system is capable of deliver-

TABLE 1.03-1. *Angiographic Filming Rates*

Vessel Injected	Films per Second*
Aortic arch	1/3/3/3/1/1/1/1
Common carotid artery	1/2/2/2/1/0/1/0/1/0/1
Internal carotid and vertebral arteries	1/3/3/3/1/1/1/1/1
External carotid artery	1/2/2/2/1/0/1/0/1/0/1

*With digital subtraction equipment we use 4–8 frames/sec in all vessels.

ing two to three films per second. Filming rates are given in Table 1.03-1, but if circulation is extremely fast, rates may need to be increased.

The amounts of contrast material injected vary according to the weight of the patient, as suggested in Table 1.03-2.

TABLE 1.03-2. *Amounts of Angiographic Contrast Media*

Vessel Injected	Amount of Contrast (mL) per Patient's Weight*			
	> 10 kg	10–20 kg	20–40 kg	> 40 kg
Internal carotid artery	2–3	4–6	6–7	8
External carotid artery	1	2–3	3–4	5–7
Common carotid artery	4–5	5–7	6–8	8–10
Vertebral artery	1–3	3–4	4–5	5–6

*Amounts of contrast are given as a *total* dosage, and need to be given in an injection of 2 to 3 seconds' duration. Doses may also need to be tailored because some children have very dynamic flow and may require slightly greater amounts of contrast.

After finishing the angiogram, hemostasis is achieved by holding the groin in the standard fashion. However, a lighter pressure is needed to avoid thrombosis of the punctured artery. A practical way to avoid overpressure while holding the artery is to make sure that the pulses in the corresponding foot (dorsalis pedis and tibialis posterior) are strongly felt. If the pulses cannot be felt, then the amount of pressure being exerted is probably too much. Although many femoral arteries in children undergo thrombosis after an angiogram, they are rapidly recanalized with no complications. After hemostasis is achieved, a note should be placed in the patient's chart that includes the following:

1. Procedure performed
2. Preliminary findings
3. Complications, if any
4. Status of the patient's peripheral pulses (it is always a good idea to mark them with a permanent marker so that the nurse on the floor can easily find and check them)

Postangiogram orders may already be preprinted or written on the chart. They should include:

1. Strict bed rest with leg (right or left) straight for 6 hours
2. Bed rest with bathroom privileges for the next 6 hours
3. If no anesthesia was given, normal diet and encourage fluids PO; if anesthesia was given, the diet is as ordered by that service
4. Vital signs, check groin (right or left) for bleeding/hematoma and pulses, and peripheral pulses (as marked) q15 minutes for 4 hours, then q30 minutes for 4 hours, and afterward only routine vital signs

In our experience, the rate of complications in children is less than that observed in adults, which is generally 1% for all complications and 0.5% or less for permanent neurologic deficits.

Only on very few occasions is myelography indicated in the pediatric patient because most clinical problems may be solved with MR imaging. These rare indications include the patient with excessive orthopedic hardware in whom MR imaging is not possible because of multiple artifacts, determination of a diastem that is not appreciated by MR imaging, severe scoliosis, and when the diagnosis of either leptomeningeal metastases or abnormal vessels on the spinal cord surface (seen in arteriovenous malformations) is unclear from the MR study. We have also performed myelography in trauma patients in whom the life support system does not permit them to be placed in the MR unit. Like angiography, we choose to perform myelography under general anesthesia if the patients are 12 years of age or younger. All myelographic studies are followed by CT scanning of the region of interest. Despite the presence of metallic hardware, the bone windows of the CT study usually allow for some visualization of the spinal canal contents, which provides useful information.

The great majority of pediatric myelograms are scheduled well ahead of the actual date of the procedure. The parents/guardian need to be informed of the risks.

PEDIATRIC MYELOGRAM RISKS

Postprocedure headaches and occasional chronic CSF leakage (which may or may not require treatment such as an epidural blood patch), bleeding, infection, seizures, nausea, vomiting, damage to nerves, paralysis, bowel, bladder, and muscle dysfunction, allergic reaction to the contrast media, and death.

A signed consent form should be placed on the patient's chart. Consent for anesthesia is obtained separately by that service. If the patient does not have a systemic disorder (eg, a coagulopathy), we usually do not obtain routine laboratory values. A short note is placed in the patient's chart indicating the reason for the study and that verbal and written consent was obtained from the parents/guardian.

With the patient in a prone position, under general anesthesia, prepared and draped, a 22-gauge needle is inserted at the L2–L3 space. There usually is no need to use a spinal needle. In most pediatric patients, a 1- to 1.5-inch needle will suffice. If tethering of the spinal cord is suspected, a small amount of 30% iodinated contrast is gently injected and the position of the contrast confirmed with fluoroscopy or a cross-table lateral radiograph of the region. Sometimes, puncturing or injecting into the tethered segment of spinal cord may not be avoided. If this occurs, the needle is repositioned. There is no set amount of contrast in pediatric myelography. In general, we inject enough to visualize the upper lumbar spinal canal. After the injection is finished, *the needle and its attachments should be left in place to avoid escape of contrast through the puncture site.* Spot radiographs generally include a frontal, and shallow and steep obliques. The technician takes one or more cross-table lateral views, and then the patient's head may be gently tilted down and a fluoroscopically guided spot film of the region of the conus medullaris taken. After these radiographs have been taken, *the needle is removed.* While the patient is still under general anesthesia, he or she is taken to the CT suite. The CT study is performed using 1.5- to 3-mm contiguous thick sections through the area of interest. If the entire spinal cord is to be studied, we perform 5-mm sections, either contiguous or equally spaced. If the position of the conus medullaris was not determined on the conventional myelogram, 5-mm sections from T11–L1 are helpful in assessing its position. After the procedure is complete, a short note should be placed in the patient's chart that includes a preliminary impression and any complications that occurred. The postmyelogram orders may be preprinted, but in their absence the following orders should be placed in the patient's chart.

POSTMYELOGRAM ORDERS

1. Seizure precautions for 8 hours
2. Keep head elevated 45 degrees for 8 hours
3. Diet and intravenous fluids as per Anesthesia Service
4. Discharge as per Admitting Service

After myelography, pediatric patients are usually taken to the recovery room by the Anesthesia Service.

Cervical spine punctures (C1–C2) are not discussed because they almost never are needed in the pediatric patient.

1.05 *Sedation and Postsedation Guidelines*

Sedation protocols for the pediatric patient vary widely. All sedations are administered by a physician, registered nurse, or nurse anesthetist. Patients are usually monitored with a pulse oximeter. Normal values are: adequate O_2 saturation, $> 95\%$; O_2 desaturation (significant), $< 80\%$.

At some institutions, oxygen is routinely administered during all sedations. The following sedation protocols are suggested:

Oral:
a. Chloral hydrate: 75–100 mg/kg, up to maximum dose of 2000 mg (in children who weigh more than 20 kg, the maximum dose may be increased to 2500 mg). Sleep deprivation is helpful.
OR
b. Diazepam: 0.3 mg/kg (especially useful in older children and adolescents).

Parenteral:
a. Demerol cocktail: meperidine (25 mL/kg), chlorpromazine (6.25 mL/kg), and promethazine (6.25 mL/kg) given IM for a maximum dose of 2 mL.
OR
b. Nembutal: 2.5–6.0 mg/kg (average dose: 4 mg/kg) administered IV (give ½ of total dose and wait 30 seconds; if needed, give ¼ of total dose and wait 30–60 seconds; if needed, repeat ¼ of total dose. Absolute maximum dose is 200 mg IV).
OR
c. Propofol: induction dose of 2.5 mg/kg

Rectal:
a. Thiopental sodium: 25 mg/kg initially; if needed, repeat dose of 15 mg/kg may be given 15–20 minutes after initial dose

Intranasal:
a. Midazolam: 0.1–0.3 mg/kg for a maximum dose of 14 mg

We recommend the use of postsedation guidelines for the parents or guardians. These are provided when the sedation was not administered by the Anesthesia Department.

1. Your child _____ has been given the medication _____ today so that an imaging examination could be obtained. Although most of it is quickly excreted from the body, some may remain and produce loss of sense of balance, dizziness, awkward or clumsy movements, and sleepiness. For the next 8 hours, follow these instructions.
2. Provide a safe environment for your child. Keep the child inside and under the supervision of adults.
3. Despite sleepiness, you should be able to wake up the child by gently touching him or her or calling his or her name. The child will usually go back to sleep.

4. Give only clear liquids until he or she returns to normal. If the child is nauseated or is vomiting, stay on clear liquids and soft food for the rest of the day. Normal diet can be resumed if the child has been feeling well for 2 hours.
5. Be sure to secure your child in your car for the trip home.
6. If any questions arise, please call the radiology nurse or the radiologist.

PART ONE
BRAIN

Imaging of the Pediatric Head, Neck, and Spine
by Mauricio Castillo and Suresh K. Mukherji,
Lippincott-Raven Publishing, Philadelphia © 1996.

2

Developmental Anomalies, Supratentorial

2.0 *Applied Embryology*

Approximately 75% of fetal deaths and 40% of infant deaths are associated with congenital malformations of the central nervous system (CNS). These malformations are also present in 7% of stillborn children and in approximately 3% of live births. The malformation is determined by the time of the insult rather than its type.

Step 1: Primary Neurulation

Induction of the CNS occurs during the 4 weeks that follow conception. The CNS begins as a plate or disc in the dorsal aspect of the embryo (Fig. 2.0-1). This disc contains a shallow longitudinal depression called the "neural groove." Flanking the neural groove are two (one on each side) slightly raised bridges of tissue called the "neural folds." By the middle of the third week of life, this disc is composed of three basic elements: ectoderm, mesoderm, and endoderm. The notochord lies ventral to the neural groove and induces it to become deeper. As the neural groove deepens, the neural folds become prominent and protrude further dorsally (Fig. 2.0-2). Each neural fold contains the elements that later become one half of the neural crest. The outside margins of the neural folds invaginate and fuse with each other, establishing the closure of the neural tube (Fig. 2.0-3). The closure of the neural tube begins at 24 days of age at the cephalic end of the embryo and progresses caudally. Closure of the caudal end of the neural tube occurs between 26 to 28 days of life. The neural tube is now complete and lies deep to the newly fused neural folds. Between the neural tube and fused neural folds (surface ectoderm) lie the cells of the neural crest. During this same period, the cells that form the dorsal root ganglia, sensory ganglia of the cranial nerves, and autonomic ganglia are also formed. At this time the "primary neurulation" stage of dorsal induction is completed. The disorders of primary neurulation include cranioschisis (anencephaly and some cephaloceles), rachischisis (myelocele, myelomeningocele), Chiari malformations types II and III, and hydromyelia.

Step 2: Secondary Neurulation

The next process in the development of the CNS is the closure of the distal end of the neural tube, which is called "secondary neurulation." A group of cells located in the caudal neural tube aggregate and coalesce with one another. They close the distal neuropore, and the previous communication between the central canal and the amniotic cavity is obliterated. The formation of the distal spinal cord involves two important mechanisms, retrogressive differentiation and canalization. Disorders of secondary neurulation include myelocystocele, diastematomyelia, diplomyelia, meningocele, lipomeningocele, intraspinal lipoma, dermal sinus, tight filum terminale syndrome, neuroenteric anomalies, and caudal regression syndrome.

Step 3: Ventral Induction

The next step in the development of the CNS is termed "ventral induction." During the fourth to seventh weeks of life, the cephalic portion of the neural tube expands to form the lamina terminalis, which marks the cephalic end of the notochord. This end of the neural tube will give rise to the three segments that develop into the brain. These segments are the rhombencephalon (hindbrain), the mesencephalon (midbrain), and the prosencephalon (forebrain). The prosencephalon divides into the diencephalon (thalami and hypothalamus) and the telencephalon (which will form the cerebral hemispheres). During this same period, the cephalic notochord induces the formation of the cephalic mesoderm (which forms the face) and the optic vesicles (which form the eyes). Therefore, abnormalities in the development of the telencephalon produce a combination of brain, face, and eye anomalies. Abnormal development of the rhombencephalon produces cerebellar anomalies. The disorders of ventral induction include holoprosencephaly, septooptic dysplasia, cerebral hemiatrophy, dysgenesis of the cerebellar hemispheres and vermis, Dandy-Walker complex, craniosynostosis, and diencephalic cyst.

Step 4: Cellular Proliferation and Differentiation

Once the previous steps are completed, the CNS is formed. The next steps are those of cellular proliferation and differentiation, which begin during the third month of intrauterine life. The periphery of the ventricular system is lined by thickened areas of cellular proliferation called the germinal matrix. The primitive cells in these regions become the neuroblasts, which are destined to migrate in a radial fashion and establish the cerebral/cerebellar cortex (Fig. 2.0-4). Before neuronal migration, the radial glial fibers (which will guide the traveling neurons) need to be established. Destruction of the germinal matrix, migrating neurons, or the radial glial fibers may result in the following disorders: micrencephalia vera, megalencephaly, hemimegalencephaly, some types of aqueductal stenosis, colpocephaly, porencephaly, some types of cystic malacia, and hydranencephaly.

Anomalies at this stage may also involve the formation of the CNS vasculature, the subarachnoid spaces, and the persistence of primitive cellular elements in the brain. Insults at this stage result in disorders of histogenesis, which include neurocutaneous syndromes, vascular malformations, malformative tumors, and disorders of the subarachnoid space (lipomas and cysts).

Step 5: Cellular Migration and Involution

At the beginning of the second trimester, the neuroblasts residing in the germinal matrix lose their ability to multiply and begin migrating laterally along the radial glial fibers. There is a one-to-one correspondence between the site of origin and eventual resting place within the cortex for these neurons. After the deepest layer of neurons has been established, the younger neurons migrate close to the pial surface of the brain and then reverse their pattern, so that the more recent arrivals are located in the deeper layers of the cortex. As the cortex thickens, the intracranial space becomes relatively small for the developing brain, which has to undergo a series of convolutions to accommodate within the skull. At the end of the second trimester, the radial glial fibers begin to involute. They will eventually transform into astrocytes. However, lesser waves of neuronal migration probably continue until birth. Insults during this step result in anomalies of neuronal migration and sulcation, which include lissencephaly (agyria), pachygyria, neuronal heterotopias, dysgenesis of the corpus callosum, and open-lip schizencephaly.

Vascular insults (usually ischemia) to the formed cortex affect its middle layers and result in polymicrogyria (nonlissencephalic cortical dysplasia) and closed-lip schizencephaly.

Step 6: Insults to the Formed Brain

Insults to the formed brain usually occur during the third trimester and are almost always secondary to ischemia. They include hydranencephaly, porencephaly, some types of multicystic malacia, some types of aqueductal stenosis, hemorrhage, and infarction.

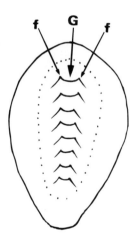

FIGURE 2.0-1.

The dorsal surface of the embryo. The CNS begins as a disc *(dotted line)* and contains two parallel ridges called the neural folds (f) that flank a depression called the neural groove (G).

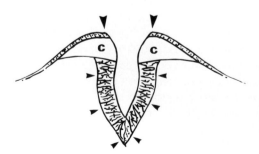

FIGURE 2.0-2.

Transverse section through the dorsal surface of the embryo. The neural groove is deep *(small arrowheads)*, and dorsal to it are the neural folds *(large arrowheads)* that contain the neural crests (c).

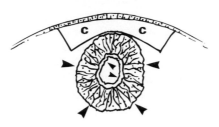

FIGURE 2.0-3.

At approximately 1 month of life, the neural groove has folded upon itself and is closed in the form of a cylinder called the neural tube *(large arrowheads).* Inside the neural tube is a cavity lined by a thin layer of ependyma *(small arrowheads).* The neural crest (c) has formed a single structure posterior to the neural tube, and will give origin to dorsal root ganglia, sensory ganglia of the cranial nerves, and autonomic ganglia. The skin now covers these structures completely and the neural folds have disappeared.

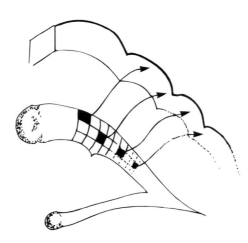

FIGURE 2.0-4.

During the second trimester, neuroblasts migrate from the germinal matrix *(checkerboard)* along the radial glial fibers to the cortex. There is a one-to-one correspondence between their site of origin and their eventual resting place *(arrows).*

2.01 *Normal Maturation of White and Gray Matter*

Myelination starts during the middle portion of the second trimester of intrauterine life. It begins in the brain stem and the cranial nerves. At birth, the medulla, medial cerebellar structures, brain stem, dorsal midbrain, and the ventral thalami exhibit myelin. Supratentorially, the single most important marker of adequate brain maturation at birth is the presence of myelin in the posterior limb of the internal capsules. The optic tracts and calcarine regions are also myelinated at birth. By 3 months of age, the precentral and postcentral gyri, the central and posterior aspects of the centra semiovale, and the cerebellum are mature. At 4 months of age, the anterior limbs of the internal capsule show mature myelin. The corpus callosum myelinates from back to front and, as such, myelin is present in the splenium by 3 months and in the genu by 6 months. The corpus callosum should have a normal appearance (similar to that of the adult) by 8 months of age. By 7 to 9 months of age, the hemispheric white matter begins to acquire its "arborized" pattern. The frontal lobes show myelin at 12 to 14 months, and the brain should have an "adult" appearance at 2 years of age. The only zones that normally may remain "unmyelinated" are the peritrigonal white matter (so-called areas of terminal association). As a general rule, myelination progresses from inferior to superior and posterior to anterior.

Gray matter structures also follow a definite pattern of maturation. At birth, low T_2 signal intensity is present in the gray matter lining the central sulci, calcarine cortices, and insulae. By 4 months of age, these differences become less obvious, and by 10 months of age, the cerebral gray matter is all of the same signal intensity. The basal ganglia and thalami are of low T_2 signal intensity at 3 months of age, but become isointense to other gray matter by the 10th month of extrauterine life. In our experience, expected patterns of maturation involving both the gray and white matter are disrupted by perinatal insults. Deep gray matter structures also change in their signal intensity because of deposition of iron. Low signal intensity in the globus pallidi and the substantia nigra due to iron deposition becomes obvious at about 10 years of age and is present in 90% of teenagers 15 years of age or older. Iron deposition in the dentate nuclei begins around 15 years of age and is seen in up to one third of subjects 25 years of age. Iron deposition is readily seen in T2-weighted gradient echo or spin echo sequences. Fast spin echo T2-weighted images are less sensitive to the magnetic susceptibility effects caused by iron.

Magnetic resonance (MR) is the imaging method of choice to assess brain maturation. Before 6 months of age, T1-weighted images allow for rapid characterization of the mature portions of the brain (Fig. 2.01-1). With this sequence, myelin is of relatively high signal intensity compared to "unmyelinated" portions of the brain. Magnetization transfer contrast may be added to this sequence, resulting in a drop in measured signal intensity in regions of mature myelin because of transfer of energy from the macromolecules (in myelin) to less myelinated brain regions (which contain relatively more water). Therefore, mature myelin, or residual myelinated regions in the setting of destruction of white matter, appear bright on T1-weighted images with magnetization transfer added. At our institution, fast spin echo images are routinely used in all children. These sequences are especially helpful to evaluate maturation of myelin after 6 months of age. Fast spin echo imaging allows for a long TR (3500–4500 msec) and therefore produce heavily T2-weighted images (Fig. 2.01-2).

The relationship between MR signal intensity and the structure of myelin is not understood completely. The MR signal intensity changes reflect differences between the proportion of free and bound water with respect to the amount of cholesterol and glycolipids that are present in oligodendrocytes and are needed to form myelin. The relatively high T1 signal intensity of mature myelin is believed to reflect displaced water as a result of accumulation of cholesterol/glycolipids, which are hydrophobic. As myelin continues to mature, the sheath structure "tightens" and there are changes in the protein conformation and in the saturation of its polyunsaturated fatty acids. This increases the displacement of free water and results in lower signal intensity on T2-weighted images.

We believe that MR imaging is useful in patients with gross alteration of brain maturation. However, in patients with minor alterations, the changes may be subtle and not definite. If a patient exhibits MR imaging changes believed to represent an alteration of myelin maturation, we routinely reimage that patient 8 to 12 months after the initial study before labeling him or her as having delayed brain maturation. In cases of gross alterations, the diagnosis may be confidently made on a single MR imaging study.

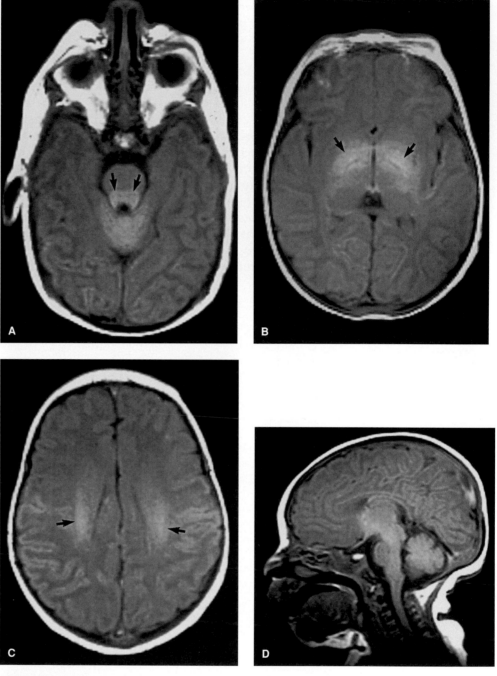

FIGURE 2.01-1.

Normal myelination at term birth. **A.** Axial magnetic resonance (MR) T1-weighted image in a normal newborn shows increased signal intensity (mature myelin) from the medial cerebellum and the dorsal midbrain *(arrows)*. **B.** Axial MR T1-weighted image shows increased signal intensity (mature myelin) in the posterior limb of both internal capsules *(arrows)*. This normal finding should be present in all term newborns. **C.** Axial MR T1-weighted image shows high signal intensity (mature myelin) in the mid portion *(arrows)* of both centra semiovale. **D.** Midsagittal MR T1-weighted image shows increased signal intensity (mature myelin) in medulla, dorsal half of brain stem, and the midbrain. The pituitary is bright and normal for a newborn. The corpus callosum is not yet myelinated.

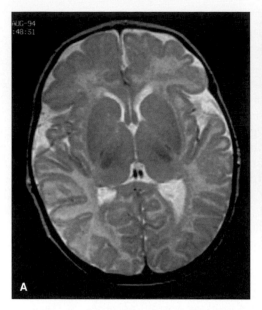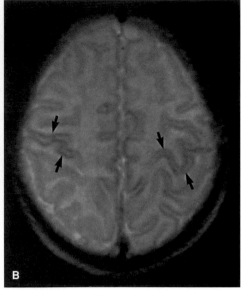

FIGURE 2.01-2.

Mature myelin and gray matter on T2-weighted magnetic resonance (MR) images.
A. Axial MR T2-weighted image in a newborn shows relatively decreased signal intensity from the posterior limb of the internal capsules and lateral thalami, related to mature myelin. Also note decreased signal intensity from the calcarine and insular cortex, which is normal and may be related to myelinated fibers coursing through these regions. **B.** Axial MR T2-weighted image shows subtle but definite decreased signal intensity from the cortex lining the central sulci *(arrows)*. This is a normal finding in newborns.

SUGGESTED READINGS

1. Barkovich AJ. Normal development of the neonatal and infant brain, skull, and spine. In: Pediatric Neuroimaging. New York: Raven Press, 1995:9.
2. Barkovich AJ, Wimberger DM. Magnetic resonance of brain development. In: Kucharczyk J, Mosely M, Barkovich AJ, eds. Magnetic Resonance Neuroimaging. Boca Raton, FL: CRC Press, 1994:167.
3. Castillo M, Smith JK, Mukherji SK. MR appearance of cerebral cortex in children with and without a history of perinatal anoxia. AJR 1995;164:1481.

2.02 *Dysgenesis of Corpus Callosum*

EPIDEMIOLOGY

The corpus callosum may be totally absent, hypoplastic, or partially absent. Agenesis of the corpus callosum is found in 1 to 3:1000 live births. Although it is more commonly a spontaneous malformation, it is found in approximately 25 genetic syndromes, inborn errors of metabolism, and the fetal alcohol syndrome. Maternal cocaine use may also be a predisposing factor. It is generally accepted that the corpus callosum forms from front to back and myelinates from back to front. Therefore, segmental agenesis is always expected to involve the body and splenium of the corpus callosum. Isolated agenesis of the rostral portion of the corpus callosum is almost always related to holoprosencephalies, frontal schizencephalies, and insults of the frontal white matter. Agenesis of the mid-portion of the corpus callosum with presence of the genu and splenium may be seen in rare variants of holoprosencephaly.

CLINICAL FEATURES

This condition is usually associated with profound developmental delay, but rarely, normal or near-normal patients are found. Patients with dysgenesis of the corpus callosum commonly have seizures, which may be the result partly of an increased incidence of gray matter heterotopias found in these patients. Asynchronous sleep spindles, hypsarrhythmia, and burst suppression may be seen on electroencephalography (EEG). One cerebral hemisphere may show EEG activity that appears independent of that seen in the contralateral hemisphere. Regardless of whether the condition is found by in utero sonography or later in life, many authors recommend chromosomal analysis in all patients.

IMAGING FEATURES

In cases of agenesis, midline sagittal images (magnetic resonance [MR], sonograms, or both) show complete absence of the corpus callosum (Fig. 2.02-1A). The gyri and sulci of the medial surface of the cerebral hemispheres radiate toward the center in a "spoked wheel" or "sunburst" fashion (Fig. 2.02-1B). The cingulate sulcus is absent. The third ventricle may be large or small, but is always high riding and the massa intermedia may be prominent. On coronal MR images, the frontal horns of the lateral ventricles acquire a "crescentic" or "steer horns" configuration (Fig. 2.02-1C). The medial and superior borders of the frontal horns are formed by the bundles of Probst (which, if fused, form the normal corpus callosum). Over the most medial aspect of the frontal horns, shallow cingulate sulci may be seen, and cephalad to them the cingulate gyri are everted. At times, the hippocampal commissure (connecting the fornices) may become enlarged and simulate a thin corpus callosum on sagittal images. On axial images, the lateral ventricles lose their normal medial concavity and assume a parallel configuration (Fig. 2.02-1D). The atria and occipital horns may be dilated out of proportion to the degree of dilation of the remaining ventricular system (Fig. 2.02-1E). This is termed "colpocephaly," and is believed to occur secondary to abnormal formation of the white matter in the dorsal regions of the cerebral hemispheres. The interhemispheric fissure is deep and may be contiguous with lateral ventricles. The third ventricle may project between the lateral ventricles and appear cyst-like. Occasionally a true interhemispheric cerebrospinal fluid-filled cyst may be present, and is more often encountered in the dorsal portion of the brain (Fig. 2.02-2). This cyst often communicates with the third or lateral ventricles, and may be unilocular or multilocular. Lipomas are also quite commonly seen in association with dysgenesis of the corpus callosum, and are usually midline in location. These lipomas may have internal or shell-like calcifications. The temporal horns of the lateral ventricles are everted (probably secondary to abnormal formation of the mesial temporal lobe structures) and prominent. The anterior cerebral arteries have a meandering course. The anterior and posterior commissures may appear enlarged in patients with agenesis of the corpus callosum. Common associated anomalies include the Chiari II malformation, Dandy-Walker complex, and cephaloceles. The rostrum of the corpus callosum may be absent (Fig. 2.02-3).

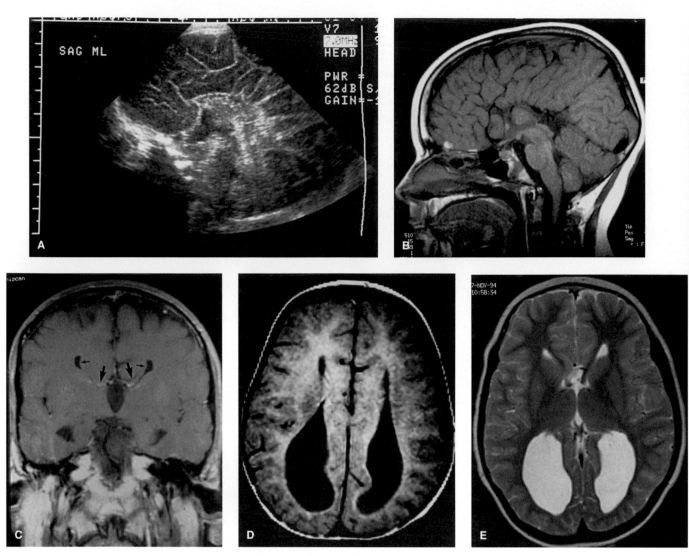

FIGURE 2.02-1.

Complete agenesis of the corpus callosum. **A.** Midline sagittal sonogram shows complete absence of the corpus callosum. The medial sulci radiate outward in a "spoked wheel" pattern. The massa intermedia is prominent. **B.** Midsagittal magnetic resonance (MR) T1-weighted image shows complete absence of the corpus callosum in a different patient. Note the "spoked wheel" pattern of radiating sulci and the prominent massa intermedia. **C.** Coronal MR T1-weighted image shows "steer horn" configuration of the lateral ventricles. The medial indentation *(small arrows)* is caused by the bundles of Probst, and the cingulate gyri are everted *(large arrows).* The temporal horns are prominent despite absence of hydrocephalus secondary to hypoplasia of the hippocampi. **D.** Axial MR T1-weighted image shows that the lateral ventricles lie parallel to each other. The posterior body and atria are dilated (colpocephaly). The amount of white matter in the occipitoparietal regions is diminished. **E.** Axial MR T2-weighted image in a different patient with agenesis of the corpus callosum shows colpocephaly.

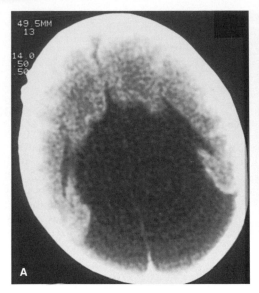

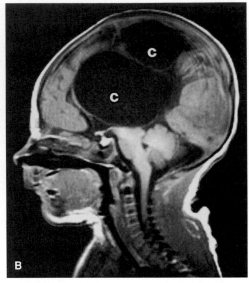

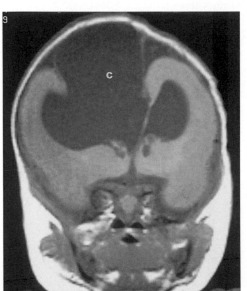

FIGURE 2.02-2.

Agenesis of the corpus callosum with dorsal interhemispheric cyst. A. Axial computed tomography shows absence of corpus callosum and a large dorsal cerebrospinal fluid-filled interhemispheric cyst. Note lateral ventricles splayed by the cyst and anterior interhemispheric fissure contiguous with cyst. **B.** Midsagittal magnetic resonance (MR) T1-weighted image in a different case of absent corpus callosum shows large, septated, and mostly dorsal interhemispheric cyst (c) that is separate from the third ventricle. The pituitary gland is bright, a normal finding in newborns. **C.** Coronal MR T1-weighted image in a different patient shows agenesis of the corpus callosum and a midline interhemispheric cyst (c). Note lissencephaly (smooth brain) involving both cerebral hemispheres. The association between lissencephaly and dysgenesis of the corpus callosum is well known.

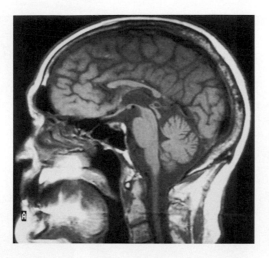

FIGURE 2.02-3.

Hypogenesis of the corpus callosum.
Midsagittal MR T1-weighted image shows small corpus callosum with absent rostrum. The rostrum is the last portion of the corpus callosum to form, and therefore it may be absent in the presence of relatively normal genu, body, and splenium.

SUGGESTED READINGS

1. Barkovich AJ. Congenital malformations of the brain and skull. In: Pediatric Neuroimaging. New York, Raven Press, 1995:180.
2. Baker L, Barkovich AJ. The large temporal horn: MR analysis in developmental brain anomalies versus hydrocephalus. AJNR 1992;13:115.
3. Georgy BA, Hesselink JR, Jernigan TL. MR imaging of the corpus callosum. AJR 1993;160:949.

2.03 *Disorders of Ventral Induction: Holoprosencephaly*

EPIDEMIOLOGY

Holoprosencephalies comprise a spectrum of abnormalities involving the face and forebrain that range from the mild type (lobar) to an intermediate type (semilobar) to the most severe type (alobar). Differentiation between them may not be clear. One variant of septooptic dysplasia is considered by some as the mildest form of lobar holoprosencephaly. It is found in approximately 1:16,000 live births, more often in the offspring of diabetic mothers, dizygotic twinning, bleeding during early pregnancy, and several chromosomal abnormalities (trisomies 13 and 15, 13q syndrome, deletion of the short arm of chromosome 18, and Meckel and Kallman syndromes). It may also be seen in association with intrauterine toxoplasmosis, syphilis, and fetal alcohol and cocaine exposure.

CLINICAL FEATURES

Median facial defects are seen in the alobar and semilobar types (Fig. 2.03-1A). In alobar holoprosencephaly, there are abnormalities of the premaxillary segment (hypotelorism, flat nose, single nostril, central frontal proboscis). Cyclopia is rare (most patients with this abnormality are stillborn). Microcephaly is always present. Cleft lip is not always present; colobomas may be present. These infants show failure to thrive, developmental delay, poor temperature control, seizures, and/or spastic quadraparesis. Most infants die before reaching 1 year of age. In patients with semilobar holoprosencephaly, the most typical facial abnormalities are cleft upper lip and palate, flat nose, hypotelorism, and microcephaly. Patients usually have profound developmental delay and occasionally live beyond infancy. In the lobar type, the facial malformations may be subtle and include cleft lip, single central incisor, trigonocephaly, and microcephaly. Severe mental retardation is common.

IMAGING FEATURES

In alobar holoprosencephaly, the brain is small, with the lateral ventricles fused into a single horseshoe-shaped monoventricle devoid of a septum pellucidum (Fig. 2.03-1B–D). The corpus callosum is absent and there is continuation of the gray and white matter across the midline. The interhemispheric fissure and falx cerebri are absent. The thalami are fused and the olfactory nerves absent. The anterior cerebral artery is single (azygous) and the deep venous system is malformed. The venous sinuses may be absent or ectopic (Fig. 2.03-1E). The choroid plexus may also be fused.

In semilobar holoprosencephaly, the brain has a slightly greater degree of differentiation. Rudimentary atria and occipital horns of the lateral ventricles may be present (Fig. 2.03-2). The septum pellucidum is absent. The posterior interhemispheric fissure and dorsal falx cerebri may be recognizable. A small third ventricle is seen. The posterior aspect of the corpus callosum may be formed.

In lobar holoprosencephaly, the brain may be almost normal. The lateral ventricles show malformed temporal, occipital, and frontal horns. The septum pellucidum is absent (Fig. 2.03-3). The third ventricle is small and the thalami may be partially fused. The anterior aspect of the corpus callosum may be deficient. Some patients with septooptic dysplasia fit into the category of lobar holoprosencephaly.

Middle interhemispheric fusion is an unusual variant of holoprosencephaly. In this anomaly, there is absence of the mid-body of the corpus callosum with fusion of the hemispheres at that level with a segmentally absent interhemispheric fusion. The genu and splenium of the corpus callosum are present. This type of anomaly is discordant with the traditional explanation for the formation of the corpus callosum.

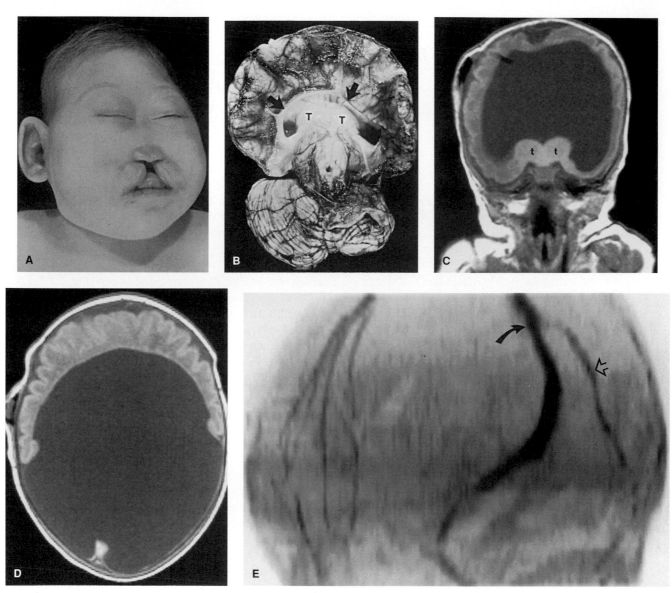

FIGURE 2.03-1.

Alobar holoprosencephaly. **A.** Photograph of stillborn child with alobar holoprosencephaly shows low midline facial cleft, hypotelorism, and microcephaly. **B.** Photograph of fixed brain of same child shows a monoventricle *(arrows)* and fused thalami (T). There is no interhemispheric fissure or corpus callosum. **C.** Coronal magnetic resonance (MR) T1-weighted image showing horseshoe-shaped monoventricle with fused thalami (t). The corpus callosum is absent and there is continuation of gray and white matter across the midline. The interhemispheric fissure is rudimentary and the falx is absent. (With permission from Castillo M. Neuroradiology Companion. Philadelphia, JB Lippincott, 1995.) **D.** Axial MR T1-weighted image in a different patient shows monoventricle and majority of residual cerebral tissues to be located rostrally. The interhemispheric fissure and falx are absent. There is a large dorsal midline cyst that is contiguous with the ventricle. **E.** Oblique posterior view of MR venogram in a different patient shows high location of torcular *(curved arrow)* and hypoplasia of left transverse *(open arrow)* and sigmoid sinuses. Deep venous system is not seen. Localizing the veins is of importance to the neurosurgeon before insertion of a ventricular shunt. (With permission from Castillo M, Scatliff JH, Bouldin T, Suzuki K. Alobar holoprosencephaly. AJNR 1993;14:1151.)

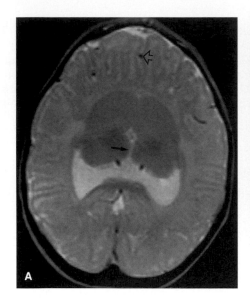 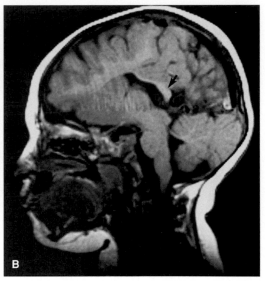

FIGURE 2.03-2.

Semilobar holoprosencephaly. **A.** Axial magnetic resonance (MR) T2-weighted image shows some differentiation of lateral ventricles. There are rudimentary occipital horns and atria. A tiny third ventricle is present *(arrow)*. The posterior interhemispheric fissure and falx cerebri are seen. The anterior aspect of the brain shows midline fusion. There is an azygous anterior cerebral artery *(open arrow)*. **B.** Midline sagittal MR T1-weighted image in same patient shows presence of splenium of corpus callosum *(arrow)*. (With permission from Castillo M, Scatliff JH, Bouldin T, Suzuki K. Alobar holoprosencephaly. AJNR 1993;14:1151.)

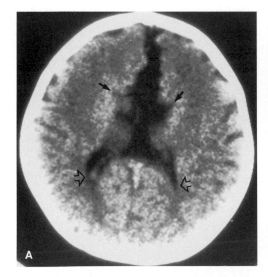 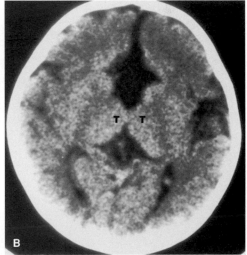

FIGURE 2.03-3.

Lobar holoprosencephaly. **A.** Axial computed tomography (CT) shows that the lateral ventricles have better-formed occipital horns *(open arrows)* and rudimentary frontal horns *(arrows)*. The septum pellucidum is absent. The interhemispheric fissure is present but the anterior falx is absent. **B.** Lower axial CT shows fusion of thalami (T) and absent septum pellucidum. The occipital horns are again well visualized.

SUGGESTED
READINGS

1. Castillo M, Bouldin TW, Scatliff JH, Suzuki K. Alobar holoprosencephaly. AJNR 1993;14:1151.
2. Barkovich AJ, Quint DJ. Middle interhemispheric fusion: an unusual variant of holoprosencephaly. AJNR 1993;14:431.
3. Barkovich AJ. Apparent atypical callosal dysgenesis: analysis of MR findings in six cases and their relationship to holoprosencephaly. AJNR 1990;11:333.

2.04 Disorders of Ventral Induction: Septo-optic Dysplasia

EPIDEMIOLOGY

The incidence of this rare disorder is unknown. Cases can be genetic (autosomal recessive or dominant), but most occur sporadically. It is more common in firstborn children, and it is also associated with maternal ingestion of quinidine, antiseizure medications, cocaine use, and maternal diabetes. Infection of the fetus by cytomegalovirus may also play a role. Most cases probably represent a mild form of lobar holoprosencephaly, but it may also be found in patients with schizencephalies.

CLINICAL FEATURES

The clinical triad comprises agenesis of the septum pellucidum, congenital optic nerve dysplasia, and multiple neuroendocrine defects. The complete triad does not need to be present; some patients have only the optic nerve dysplasia and hypothalamic–pituitary dysfunction. The diagnosis is initially suspected when optic nerve head hypoplasia is found on fundoscopy. Patients are usually hypotonic and have a wandering nystagmus if they are blind. Other clinical manifestations include color blindness, spasticity, microcephaly, and anosmia or hyposmia. There may be an association between septo-optic dysplasia and Kallman syndrome. The most common neuroendocrine abnormalities are deficient growth hormone secretion, followed by low adrenocorticotropic hormone (ACTH) and thyroid-stimulating hormone secretion. Diabetes insipidus may also be found. Hypersecretion of prolactin and ACTH may occur. Precocious puberty is rare but may also be seen. Overall, the most common clinical picture is that of panhypopituitarism. However, antidiuretic hormone secretion is usually normal. Management consists mainly of replacement therapy.

IMAGING FEATURES

Patients with septo-optic dysplasia may be broadly categorized into those who also have a schizencephaly or other neuronal migration anomalies (50%; Fig. 2.04-1), those who do not (50%), and a small percentage in whom the only other anomaly is translocation of the posterior pituitary lobe to the hypothalamus (Fig. 2.04-2). In patients with isolated septo-optic dysplasia, the septum pellucidum is typically absent. The lateral ventricles are mildly prominent. The frontal horns show a flattened roof ("box-like" configuration) and inferior pointing. The suprasellar cistern is large, and the optic chiasm and nerves are small. The fornices may be thin and the corpus callosum may also be dysgenetic. The pituitary infundibulum is thin or absent. The adenohypophysis is small or absent. The posterior pituitary lobe may be translocated to the inferior hypothalamus (this is predominantly seen in patients with growth hormone deficiency).

Patients with schizencephaly usually have normal or close-to-normal neuroendocrine function, but almost always have seizures. We have seen patients with septo-optic dysplasia in whom there is absence or dysgenesis of the olfactory nerves and bulbs, a malformed inferior surface of the frontal lobes, and ectopia of the posterior pituitary lobe. These patients are probably better classified as having a combination of type III septo-optic dysplasia and Kallman syndrome.

Isolated absence of the septum pellucidum may occur, but it is a very rare anomaly. In these patients, isolated septal agenesis is a diagnosis of exclusion to be considered only after the brain has been examined in detail with magnetic resonance imaging.

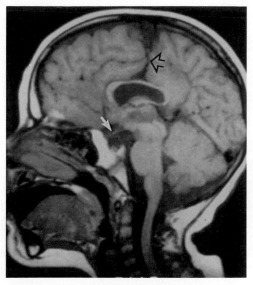

FIGURE 2.04-1.

Type 1 septo-optic dysplasia. Midsagittal magnetic resonance T1-weighted image in a patient with hypoplastic optic discs and seizures shows hypoplastic optic chiasm *(arrows)*, dysgenesis of the corpus callosum with posterior forniceal continuation, and a schizencephaly *(open arrow)*.

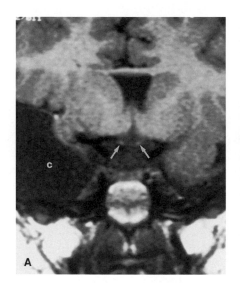 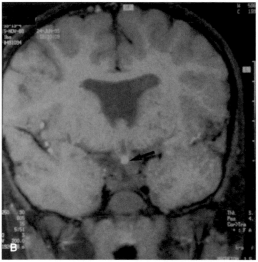

FIGURE 2.04-2.

Type 2 septo-optic dysplasia. **A.** Coronal magnetic resonance (MR) T1-weighted image shows extreme hypoplasia of the optic nerves *(arrows)*. The septum pellucidum is absent and the roofs of the frontal horns of the lateral ventricles are flat, giving them their "box-like" appearance. There is an arachnoid cyst (c) in the right middle cranial fossa. No schizencephaly or neuronal migration anomaly was present; thus, this is a type II septo-optic dysplasia. (With permission from Castillo M, Scatliff JH, Bouldin T, Suzuki K. Alobar holoprosencephaly. AJNR 1993;14:1151.) **B.** Coronal post-contrast MR T1-weighted image shows absent septum pellucidum. The roofs of the lateral ventricles are flat, and they also point down inferiorly. In this patient, the size of the optic chiasm is probably normal. The ectopic posterior pituitary lobe *(arrow)* enhances. **C.** Axial MR T1-weighted image with fat suppressed shows very thin optic nerves *(arrowheads)*. **D.** In the same patient, midsagittal MR T1-weighted image shows absent pituitary stalk, translocated posterior lobe *(arrow)*, and tiny optic chiasm *(arrowhead)*. (With permission from Castillo M. Neuroradiology Companion. Philadelphia: JB Lippincott, 1995.)

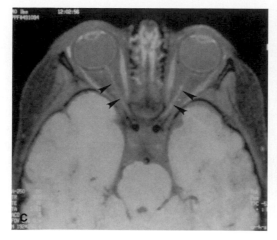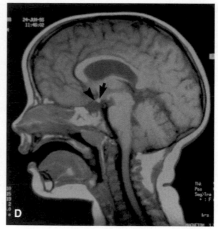

FIGURE 2.04-2.

(continued)

SUGGESTED
READING

1. Barkovich AJ, Fram EK, Norman D. MR of septooptic dysplasia. Radiology 1989;
   171:189.

2.05 *Disorders of Ventral Induction: Craniosynostosis*

EPIDEMIOLOGY

Craniosynostosis refers to bony or fibrous fusion of a cranial suture. The fusion may involve the entire length of the suture or only a part of it. It occurs in a 0.05% to 0.1% of live births, and although almost all cases are sporadic, 10% of patients have a family history of craniosynostosis. It is also found in association with craniofacial syndromes such as Apert, Carpenter, and Crouzon. When a craniofacial syndrome is present, craniosynostosis most commonly involves the coronal and basal sutures. Cerebral abnormalities are also associated with craniosynostosis, and include holoprosencephaly, dysgenesis of the corpus callosum, and the Chiari II malformation.

CLINICAL FEATURES

Premature fusion of a suture may begin during intrauterine life. A defect in the mesenchymal layer of the ossification centers of the skull may be the responsible mechanism. Alterations in the shape of the base of the skull leading to abnormal tension at sites of dural insertion (suture lines) is also proposed as an explanation. Regardless of its etiology, skull growth, which is normally perpendicular to sutures, is arrested. As a result, compensatory growth occurs perpendicular to the remaining normal sutures. At birth, the deformity of the head is usually mild, but it becomes more obvious with growth. The most important clinical problems include cosmetic abnormalities, restricted growth of the brain (craniosynostosis may result in or from microcephaly), elevation of intracranial pressure, and restriction of the growth of the orbits and temporal bones. The diagnosis may be clinically confirmed if a sutural bridge is palpable.

IMAGING FEATURES

Synostosis of the sagittal suture is the most common (60%) type of craniosynostosis. Most patients are boys. The skull in these patients grows perpendicular to the coronal and lambdoid sutures, resulting in elongation of the anteroposterior diameter of the head (dolichocephaly or scaphocephaly; Fig. 2.05-1). In premature infants, head molding may simulate craniosynostosis.

The second most common type of craniosynostosis involves the coronal suture (20%–30%; Fig. 2.05-2). It is more commonly seen in female patients. The skull is short in its anteroposterior diameter, widened in its lateral diameter, and may also be tall. Growth occurs perpendicular to the sagittal suture, resulting in brachycephaly. Orbital problems (proptosis and optic nerve atrophy) are common with coronal craniosynostosis.

The third most common type of sutural stenosis is segmental craniosynostosis (plagiocephaly; 5%–10%). It most commonly involves one side of either the coronal and lambdoid sutures (Fig. 2.05-3). This results in elevation of the structures underlying the stenotic suture. With coronal suture involvement, the ipsilateral orbit is displaced upward; with lambdoid involvement, the ipsilateral ear is displaced upward. The latter may result in torticollis.

The fourth most common type of craniosynostosis involves the metopic suture (1%–2%), and it results in an anteriorly pointed head (trigonocephaly; Fig. 2.05-4). There usually is hypotelorism, and it may be associated with midline facial and cerebral abnormalities.

Multiple stenoses result in a high and narrow skull (oxycephaly or turricephaly; Figs. 2.05-5 and 2.05-6). If untreated, this abnormality results in severe brain, orbit, and temporal bone problems.

In any patient with craniosynostosis, treatment is aimed at ensuring adequate growth of the brain, avoiding orbital and temporal complications, and correcting the cosmetic defect. Imaging is best performed using thin (3-mm) computed tomography sections. Skull views should be processed with the high-resolution (edge-enhancement) filter. Brain windows should also be filmed. These patients often show prominent subarachnoid spaces, particularly in the frontal regions. The lateral ventricles may have an unusual shape and be mildly prominent. The significance of these findings is uncertain; they may be related to slower cerebrospinal fluid resorption (external hydrocephalus?). These intracranial findings slowly resolve after correction of the craniosynostosis. Craniosynostosis may be only partial or be fibrous. In some cases the skull is flattened but the corresponding suture remains open; this has been referred to as a "sticky" suture, and is probably related to delayed growth of the perisutural bone (Fig. 2.05-7). Sutural overlapping suggests postural flattening rather than true synostosis.

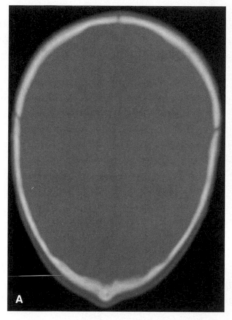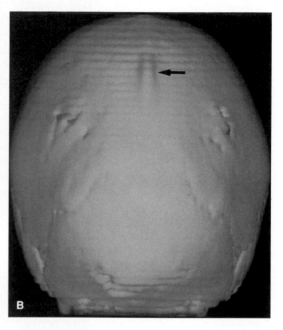

FIGURE 2.05-1.

Sagittal synostosis.   **A.** Axial computed tomography (CT) shows prominent bone ridge in a case of synostosis of the posterior aspect of the sagittal suture. There is mild dolichocephaly. Coronal and metopic sutures are open. **B.** Posterior three-dimensional CT view shows prominent bone ridge *(arrow)* in a case of synostosis involving the posterior aspect of the sagittal suture.

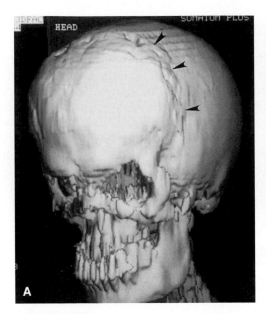 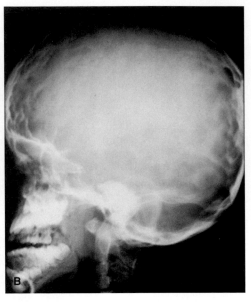

FIGURE 2.05-2.

Coronal synostosis. **A.** Anterior oblique three-dimensional computed tomography view in a patient with Apert syndrome and prominent synostosis *(arrowheads)* involving the left coronal suture. Note the midface hypoplasia characteristic of this syndrome. **B.** Lateral radiograph in a different patient with Apert syndrome shows synostosis of coronal and lambdoid sutures. The cranium has a diminished anteroposterior diameter and there are convolutional markings secondary to chronic intracranial hypertension. Midface is also hypoplastic.

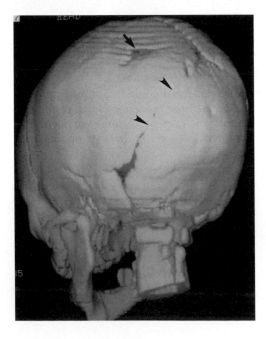

FIGURE 2.05-3.

Lambdoid synostosis. Oblique posterior three-dimensional computed tomography view shows synostosis of the superior portion *(arrowheads)* of the right lambdoid suture. The lateral and posterior fontanelles are open. Persistent parietal foramen *(arrow)* is seen.

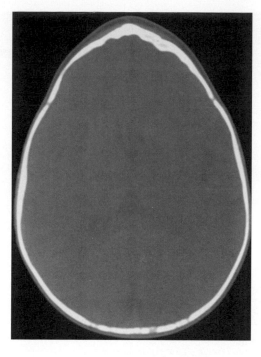

FIGURE 2.05-4.

Trigonocephaly. Axial computed tomography shows skull pointed anteriorly due to metopic suture synostosis.

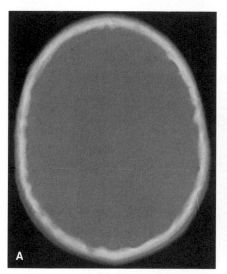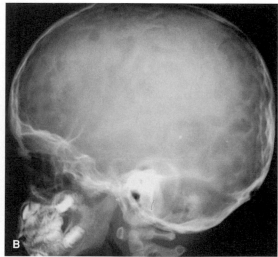

FIGURE 2.05-5.

Multiple synostoses. **A.** Axial computed tomography, bone windows, shows no coronal, lambdoid, or sagittal sutures. **B.** Lateral skull radiograph in the same patient shows oxycephaly (tower-like head), which is typical of multiple sutural synostoses.

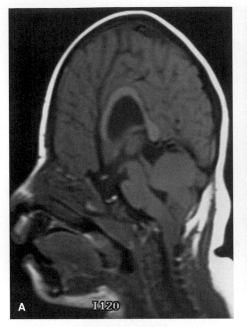 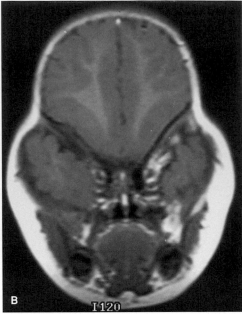

FIGURE 2.05-6.

Oxycephaly.   A. Midsagittal magnetic resonance (MR) T1-weighted image shows tower-shaped head secondary to premature universal suture synostosis. Note Chiari I malformation. **B.** Coronal MR T1-weighted image in same patient shows that the skull has assumed an almost clover-leaf shape. (Case courtesy of L. Fordham, University of North Carolina, Chapel Hill, NC.)

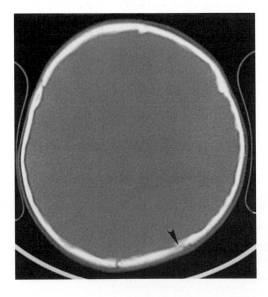

FIGURE 2.05-7.

"Sticky" suture versus fibrous synostosis.   Axial computed tomography, bone windows, in a different patient show flattening of left posterior skull with open suture *(arrowhead).* There was no partial synostosis. This skull deformity may be caused by fibrous synostosis or a "sticky" suture.

SUGGESTED READINGS

1. Jinkins JR. CT findings in complete premature craniosynostosis. Neuroradiology 1987;29:216.
2. David DJ, Poswillo DE, Simpson DA. The Craniosynostoses: Causes, Natural History, and Management. New York: Springer-Verlag, 1982.

2.06 *Disorders of Neuronal Migration: Lissencephaly/Pachygyria*

EPIDEMIOLOGY

The exact incidence of this rare anomaly is unknown; however, the overall rate of recurrence varies from 5% to 50%. This rate is lowest in patients with isolated lissencephaly and highest in patients with X-linked lissencephaly and microphallus. Maternal cytomegalovirus inclusion disease and in utero hypoperfusion have been implicated in all neuronal migration disorders. Genetic counseling is always indicated for families of lissencephalic children.

CLINICAL FEATURES

In lissencephaly (agyria), the brain retains the appearance of the fetal brain before 25 weeks of gestation. The insult, which probably occurs between 10 to 14 weeks of life, leads to arrest of neuronal migration and formation of an abnormally thickened, four-layered cortex with sparse cell populations. Lissencephaly involves the entire brain, but tends to be particularly severe in the parietooccipital regions. There are no cortical sulci and the Sylvian fissures are not formed or are very shallow. This leads to the so-called "figure-eight" appearance of the agyric brain. A lissencephalic brain weighing less than 100 g is referred to as micrencephaly vera (Fig. 2.06-1). In lissencephaly type I, the patients usually have a prominent forehead and occiput, bitemporal hollowing, and mandibular hypoplasia.

Lissencephaly type I is associated with the Miller-Dieker and Norman-Roberts syndromes. Patients with this disorder are associated with polyhidramnios, and show immediate and severe failure to thrive after birth. Poor feeding, hypotonia, and seizures develop very early in life. Spastic quadriplegia eventually develops, and most patients require placement of a gastrostomy tube because of poor nutrition and repeated aspirations.

Lissencephaly type II is a complex anomaly harboring different neuronal migration disorders. The cortex is severely disorganized with no recognizable neuronal layering. Fibroglial bands are found in the subarachnoid spaces, and may produce hydrocephalus. Lissencephaly type II is associated with Fukuyama congenital muscular dystrophy and the Walker-Warburg syndrome (which includes eye abnormalities and Dandy-Walker complex). Clinical manifestations are similar to those found in lissencephaly type I.

Type III lissencephaly comprises those patients with true micrencephaly. The brain is small and smooth, probably as a result of the premature exhaustion of the germinal matrix. Type IV lissencephaly is referred to as a radial microbrain. The size of the brain is markedly reduced despite maintaining its normal (or near-normal) sulcation and gyration. Despite this normal appearance, the neuronal population is decreased. Type V lissencephaly refers to diffuse polymicrogyria, probably caused by cytomegalovirus infection.

Pachyria is a lesser form of cortical dysplasia that is usually localized, segmental, or diffuse. When diffuse, it is usually a combination of agyria and pachygyria. These patients have clinical symptoms similar to those of patients with lissencephaly, but in addition may have pseudobulbar palsy.

IMAGING FEATURES

In lissencephaly type I, there are no cortical sulci and the cortex is markedly thickened (see Fig. 2.06-1). Under the superficial cortex, a thin, hyperintense band may be seen on T2-weighted magnetic resonance images. This band is believed to be related to a "sparse" layer of neurons. Because the Sylvian fissures are not formed or are shallow, the middle cerebral arteries course on the surface of the brain. The white matter is devoid of its normal "arborization." The cerebellum may also be dysplastic. Other associated brain abnormalities include callosal agenesis or dysgenesis, colpocephaly, neuronal heterotopias, cerebellar vermian hypoplasia, and hydrocephalus (Fig. 2.06-2). The brain stem may be hypoplastic, presumably because of incomplete formation of the corticospinal and corticobulbar tracts.

In the type II lissencephaly, the cortical sulci are absent but the cortex is thin. Microophthalmos and hydrocephalus are prominent. The white matter is devoid of "arborization" and is hypomyelinated. Neuronal heterotopias are common. Other associated brain abnormalities include Dandy-Walker complex, brain stem hypoplasia, thickened meninges, dysgenesis of the corpus callosum, and occasionally an occipital encephalocele.

Pachygyria tends preferentially to involve the frontotemporal regions and spare the posterior aspects of the brain (Fig. 2.06-3). In these patients, the occipitoparietal regions harbor some cortical sulci. In reality, most patients have a combination of both lissencephaly and pachygyria, hence the name "agyria/pachyria" complex.

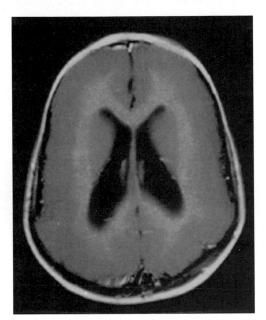

FIGURE 2.06-1.

Type 1 lissencephaly. Axial magnetic resonance T1-weighted image shows complete lack of cortical sulci, thickening of the cortex, lack of arborization of the white matter, and prominent occipital horns/atria of the lateral ventricles (colpocephaly). All findings are compatible with lissencephaly (agyria). (With permission from Castillo M. Neuroradiology Companion. Philadelphia: JB Lippincott, 1995.)

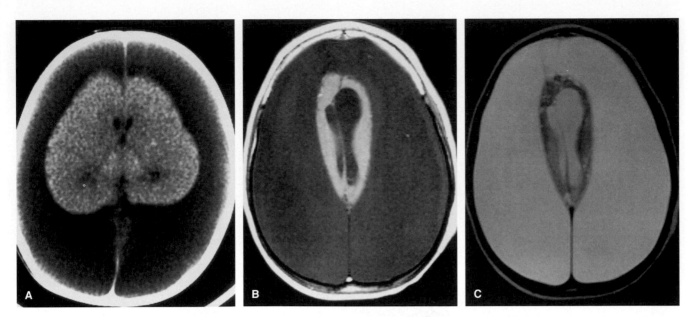

FIGURE 2.06-2.

Micrencephalia vera, type III lissencephaly. **A.** Axial computed tomography section showing very small and smooth brain. There is abundant cerebrospinal fluid in the wide extraaxial spaces. The findings are suggestive of micrencephalia vera, probably as a result of exhaustion of the germinal matrix by agents such as cytomegalovirus inclusion infection. This anomaly may be classified as lissencephaly type III. A similar appearance may be seen in chronic large bilateral subdural hematomas. (With permission from Castillo M. CT of micrencephalia vera. AJR 1992;159:905.) **B.** Axial magnetic resonance (MR) T1-weighted image shows minute, smooth brain surrounded by fluid. The ventricles are large for the size of the brain. **C.** Corresponding MR T2-weighted image shows that brain parenchyma contains scattered areas of high signal intensity, probably related to gliosis.

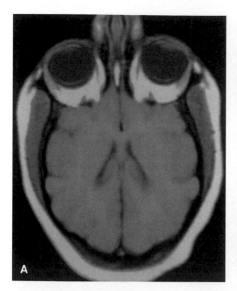 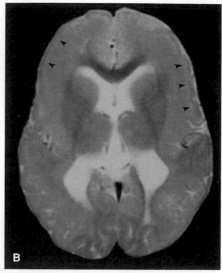 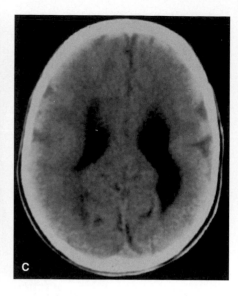

FIGURE 2.06-3.

Pachyria. **A.** Axial magnetic resonance (MR) T1-weighted image in a patient with severe microcephaly and few normal cortical sulci and gyri compatible with pachyria. The cortex is moderately thickened. This appearance is somewhat similar to radial microbrain (lissencephaly type IV), with the exception that in that entity sulcation is normal or near normal. **B.** Axial MR T2-weighted image shows absent sulci and gyri in the frontotemporal regions but presence of some sulcation and gyration in the occipitoparietal regions. Note the thin linear band *(arrowheads)* of hyperintensity underlying the superficial cortex, believed to represent a "sparse" neuron layer. The distribution of the smooth regions is a typical feature of pachyria, which preferentially involves the more rostral brain. The ventricles are prominent. **C.** Axial computed tomography shows thickened cortex with few cortical sulci and prominent lateral ventricles (especially posteriorly) in a patient with pachyria. (With permission from Castillo M. Neuroradiology Companion. Philadelphia: JB Lippincott, 1995.)

SUGGESTED READING

1. Barkovich AJ, Chuang SH, Norman D. MR of neuronal migration anomalies. AJNR 1987;8:1009.

2.07 *Disorders of Neuronal Migration: Heterotopias*

EPIDEMIOLOGY

Heterotopias are collections of gray matter located within the white matter, distal to the cerebral cortex, that are the result of errors in radial migration. However, heterotopic gray matter may also be found outside of the brain (subpial heterotopias). Their exact incidence is unknown, but they may be present in 5% to 10% of patients with intractable seizures. Possible factors contributing to their formation include genetic abnormalities (ie, trisomy 13), vascular abnormalities (ischemia?), environmental causes (eg, methyl mercury poisoning), radiation, myotonic dystrophy, neurofibromatosis, Duchenne muscular dystrophy, and fetal alcohol syndrome.

CLINICAL FEATURES

Most patients have mixed seizures and are intellectually impaired. Partial complex seizures (and other types of focal seizures), tonic–clonic seizures, and dyslexia may also be encountered. It is not clear whether behavioral problems observed in some patients are caused by the presence of heterotopias. Some patients may benefit from surgical resection of the heterotopias.

IMAGING FEATURES

Heterotopic gray matter may have different imaging features, and as such, several classification schemes have been proposed. The mildest forms of the abnormality are focal subependymal heterotopias (Fig. 2.07-1). These patients have mild clinical symptoms, many not presenting until well into the second decade of life. If the subependymal collections of gray matter are large, the severity of the symptoms increases. Subependymal heterotopias are clearly depicted by magnetic resonance (MR) imaging. They are round, smooth masses adjacent to the outer and inner walls of the lateral ventricles. They are isointense to the cortex in all MR sequences, and show no contrast enhancement. The main differential diagnosis in these cases is that of tuberous sclerosis. When subependymal heterotopias are large, the overlying cortex may be slightly thinned.

Focal subcortical heterotopias represent gray matter within the substance of the white matter (Fig. 2.07-2). Occasionally, these heterotopias may be extremely large. Because they may exert a mass effect and contain large vessels (draining veins?) and trapped cerebrospinal fluid spaces within them, it is possible initially to confuse them with true tumors. Although these dysplastic masses are heterogenous, the signal intensity of their components always parallels that of normal parenchyma in all MR imaging sequences. They do not enhance. Hydrogen MR spectroscopy may demonstrate spectra that are similar to those of normal brain. The cerebral hemisphere that contains these heterotopias may be small or large. In patients harboring these heterotopias, the clinical symptoms tend to be more severe than in those with only isolated subependymal heterotopias.

The third form of heterotopic gray matter is the so-called "band" heterotopia (also called double cortex or laminar heterotopia; Fig. 2.07-3). In these patients, there is a circumferential band of gray matter sandwiched between the superficial and deep white matter. The outer white matter stripe has a normal appearance. The cerebral cortex may be normal, thin, or pachygyric. These children have a poor prognosis and the severity of the clinical symptoms appears to be related to the thickness of the band heterotopia. Because of this, band heterotopias may be classified as a form of lissencephaly, in which the mental handicap also is related to the thickness of the dysplastic cortex.

By positron emission tomography (PET) imaging with deoxyfluoroglucose and single-photon emission computed tomography (SPECT) imaging with Tc 99m-HMPAO, the heterotopic brain shows decreased uptake reflecting decreased metabolism and perfusion, respectively. However, interictal scans show increased uptake with both techniques.

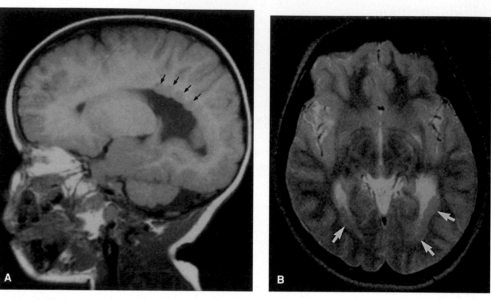

FIGURE 2.07-1.

Nodular heterotopias.   **A.** Parasagittal magnetic resonance (MR) T1-weighted image shows multiple nodular gray matter heterotopias *(arrows)* along the superoposterior border of the lateral ventricle. The signal intensity of these heterotopias is identical to that of cortex. **B.** Axial MR T2-weighted image shows multiple nodular gray matter heterotopias *(arrows)* in the outer walls of both occipital horns of the lateral ventricles. (With permission from Castillo M. Neuroradiology Companion. Philadelphia: JB Lippincott, 1995.)

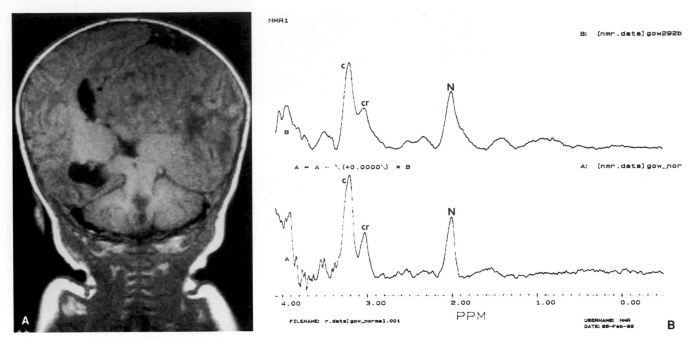

FIGURE 2.07-2.

Mass-like heterotopia (hamartoma).   **A.** Coronal magnetic resonance (MR) T1-weighted image shows a large left parietal mass-like heterotopia with mass effect. This type of heterotopia may be confused with tumor, particularly ganglioglioma, even histologically. **B.** MR hydrogen spectroscopy of large left heterotopia *(top spectra)* and of normal appearing right cerebral hemisphere *(bottom spectra)*. Both spectra are extremely similar. c, choline; cr, creatinine; N, *N*-acetyl-aspartate. (With permission from Castillo M, Kwock L, Scatliff JH, Gudeman SK, Greenwood R. Proton MR spectroscopic characteristics of a presumed giant subcortical heterotopia. AJNR 1993;14: 426.)

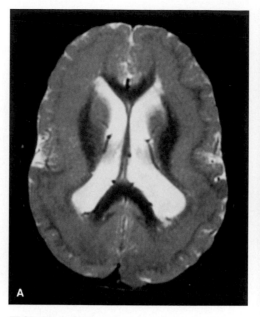 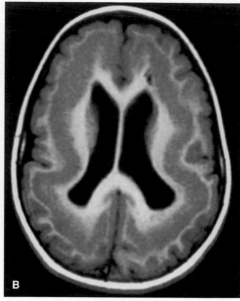

FIGURE 2.07-3.

Band heterotopia. **A.** Axial magnetic resonance (MR) T2-weighted image showing bilateral band heterotopias. The cortex is thin and pachygyric. There is white matter lateral and medial to the band of ectopic gray matter. The ventricles are enlarged. The appearance is similar to pachyria with an underlying sparse neuronal cell layer, but in older children with band heterotopia, the outer white matter layer is hypointense. In newborns, however, both entities are difficult to separate from each other. **B.** Corresponding MR T1-weighted image clearly shows the circumferential nature of the heterotopia ("double cortex" sign). (Case courtesy of S. Birchansky and N. Altman, Miami Children's Hospital, Miami, FL.)

SUGGESTED READINGS

1. Barkovich AJ, Gressens P, Evrard P. Formation, maturation, and disorders of the brain neocortex. AJNR 1992;13:423.
2. Barkovich AJ, Kjos B. Gray matter heterotopias: MR characteristics and correlation with developmental and neurological manisfestations. Radiology 1992;182:483.
3. Barkovich AJ, Jackson JDE, Boyer RS. Band heterotopias: a newly recognized neuronal migration anomaly. Radiology 1989;171:455.

2.08   *Disorders of Neuronal Migration: Megalencephaly*

EPIDEMIOLOGY

Megalencephaly refers to brain weight exceeding the mean by two or more standard deviations. It may be anatomic or metabolic; the former may be bilateral or unilateral. It is debatable whether increased venous pressure and slow cerebrospinal fluid resorption may lead to so-called hydrodynamic megalencephaly. Approximately 2.5% of the population has megalencephaly. This almost always corresponds to asymptomatic familial anatomic megalencephaly and is generally considered an anatomic variant. Table 2.08-1 addresses the most common differential diagnoses of megalencephaly.

TABLE 2.08-1.   *Differential Diagnoses for Megalencephaly*

	Focal	Unilateral	Bilateral
Anatomic megalencephaly	Oekonamakis malformation, Lhermitte-Duclos	With and without somatic hypertrophy, Klippel-Trenauny-Webber Syndrome, hamartomatous hemisphere, epidermal nevus syndrome	Asymptomatic familial type, symptomatic familial type, gigantism, Sotos syndrome, pituitary, arachnodactyly, adiposogigantism, Weaver-Smith Syndrome, achondroplasia, thanatotrophic dwarfs, Robinow Syndrome, multiple endocrinopathy, neurocutaneous syndromes, Klinefelter Syndrome
Metabolic megalencephaly			Lysosomal disorders, Canavan's, Alexander's

CLINICAL FEATURES

Patients with asymptomatic familial anatomic megalencephaly show no signs of increased intracranial pressure, have normal development and neurologic examination, have parents or siblings who also have large heads, and have no evidence of metabolic or lysosomal disorders. Patients with symptomatic familial megalencephaly have mild learning disabilities, hypothermia, or both. Patients with focal or unilateral megalencephaly (hemimegalencephaly) may have seizures, which generally ensue during the first year of life. These patients may benefit from hemispherectomy. In the case of metabolic megalencephalies, the brain is initially large, but with progression of the disease it undergoes atrophy. These patients may manifest progressive regression of developmental milestones. In most cases the clinical manifestations are related to the underlying disorder rather than to the megalencephaly.

IMAGING FEATURES

In most cases of generalized megalencephaly the brain is normal by magnetic resonance, which is the imaging method of choice in these patients. When a leukodystrophy is responsible, the findings are those of the specific disease.

Hemimegalencephaly may be secondary to hamartomatous overgrowth of one cerebral hemisphere (Fig. 2.08-1). The hemisphere usually is pachygyric and contains gray matter heterotopias. The white matter may show increased

T2 signal intensity, probably related to gliosis associated with polymicrogyria. The cortex is thick and the gray–white junction may be indistinct. The corresponding lateral ventricle and subarachnoid spaces are large, and its frontal horn appears compressed and points anterolateral. It should be noted that the imaging findings in hemimegalencephaly appear to be time related. If the patient is imaged early in life, the typical enlarged cerebral hemisphere is seen. If the patient undergoes imaging later in life, the affected hemisphere may appear smaller because of atrophy and the continued growth of the contralateral normal cerebral hemisphere.

Focal forms of megalencephaly may be isolated or related to Lhermitte-Duclos disorder (dysplastic gangliocytoma), which occurs in the cerebellum (Fig. 2.08-2). In these cases, the enlarged cerebellum is hypointense on T1-weighted images and of similar signal intensity to normal cerebellum in T2-weighted images. The thickened folia give rise to a "corduroy" appearance. Mass effect is produced. After contrast administration, the surface of the abnormality may enhance. Unilateral or bilateral thickening of the insular cortex (bilateral opercular syndrome) may be considered as a type of focal megalencephaly.

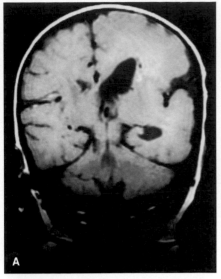

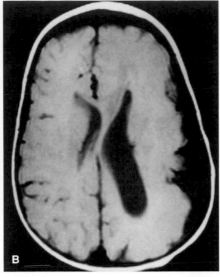

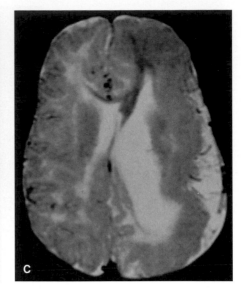

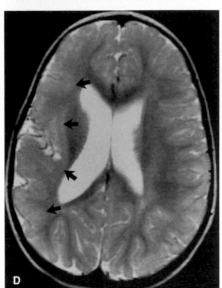

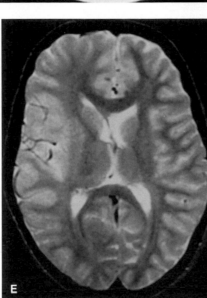

FIGURE 2.08-1.

Hemimegalencephaly. A. Coronal magnetic resonance (MR) T1-weighted image shows enlarged left cerebral hemisphere. The cerebrospinal fluid (CSF)-containing spaces are also large. The surface is smooth, compatible with pachygyria. **B.** Axial MR T1-weighted image shows the enlarged left cerebral hemisphere, which is pachyric and contains large CSF spaces. (With permission from Castillo M. Neuroradiology Companion. Philadelphia: JB Lippincott, 1995.) **C.** Axial MR T2-weighted image shows thickening of the cortex, indistinct gray–white junction, and multiple hyperintensities (gliosis?) in the white matter of the enlarged hemisphere. The left lateral ventricle is large but its frontal horn appears "compressed" and points anteriorly. **D.** Axial MR T2-weighted image in a different case shows mild enlargement of the right cerebral hemisphere with a thick and pachyric cortex *(arrows)*. The right lateral ventricle is also large. (With permission from Castillo M. Neuroradiology Companion. Philadelphia: JB Lippincott, 1995.) **E.** Axial MR T2-weighted image in a different and more subtle case of right hemispheric megalencephaly. The frontal horn of the right lateral ventricle is displaced forward and medially. The cortex in the right occipitotemporal region is mildly thickened and contains fewer sulci than the contralateral side.

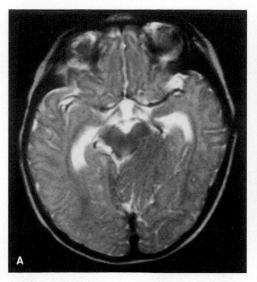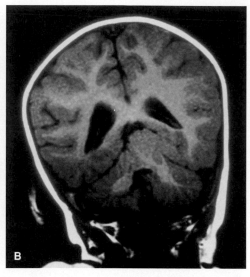

FIGURE 2.08-2.

Focal megalencephaly, Lhermitte-Duclos disease.   **A.** Axial magnetic resonance (MR) T2-weighted image in a case of Lhermitte-Duclos disease in the left cerebellar hemisphere and vermis. Note that the signal intensity of this abnormality is similar to that of normal brain and that it has a "corduroy" appearance. **B.** Coronal MR T1-weighted image in the same patient shows dysplasia of the medial left cerebellar hemisphere and vermis. At this level the cortex is thickened. There was no contrast enhancement in this case.

SUGGESTED READINGS

1. Kalifa GL, Chiron C, Sellier N, et al. Hemimegalencephaly: MR imaging in five children. Radiology 1987;165:29.
2. DeMyer W. Microcephaly, micrencephaly, megalocephaly, megalencephaly. In: Swaiman KF, ed. Pediatric Neurology, 2nd ed. St. Louis: CV Mosby, 1994:205.
3. Townsend JL, Nielsen SL, Malamud N. Unilateral megalencephaly: hamartoma or neoplasm? Neurology 1975;25:448.
4. Wolpert SM, Cohen A, Libenson MH. Hemimegalencephaly: a longitudinal MR study. AJNR 1994;15:1479.

2.09 *Disorders of Neuronal Migration: Kallmann Syndrome*

EPIDEMIOLOGY   Kallmann syndrome is an X-linked inherited disorder. The defect has been linked to the Xp22.3 portion of the short arm of the X chromosome. Some cases, however, are sporadic, autosomal dominant, or autosomal recessive. It occurs in 1:10,000 boys and in 1:50,000 girls, approximately. It is the only syndrome in which isolated and complete agenesis of one or both olfactory bulbs or nerves occurs.

CLINICAL FEATURES   Kallmann syndrome is characterized by anosmia/hyposmia and hypogonadism. Other associated abnormalities include diaphragmatic eventration, cleft palate, atrial septal defect, mitral valve prolapse, right-sided aortic arch, cryptorchism, osteopenia, hearing loss, color blindness, renal agenesis, obesity, and abnormalities of the fingers (clinodactyly and campodactyly). Secretion of luteinizing and follicle-stimulating hormones is markedly decreased or absent. It is believed to be caused by a failure of genetic expression of protein cell markers that guide the migration of cells in charge of producing luteinizing hormone-releasing hormone. These cells do not migrate (as they normally should) from the olfactory placode to the hypothalamus, and stimulation of the adenohypophysis is decreased, resulting in hypogonadism. Laboratory investigation reveals low serum testosterone and gonadotropin levels. Other pituitary hormones are normal. Treatment consists of sex hormone replacement or human chorionic gonadotropin administration (subcutaneous route). The goal of this treatment is induction of puberty, maintenance of sexual maturation, and fertility.

IMAGING FEATURES   Magnetic resonance (MR) is the imaging modality of choice. Coronal images show the olfactory bulbs and tracts to be absent or hypoplastic, either bilaterally or present in only one side (Fig. 2.09-1A,B). The olfactory bulbs may also be dysplastic and have a tangled appearance (so-called "neuromatous masses"). Because the formation of the inferior surface of the frontal lobes parallels the development of the olfactory placode, the olfactory sulci (which normally divide the gyrus rectus from the medial orbitofrontal gyrus) may be shallow or absent. If the olfactory sulci are absent, the gyrus rectus and medial orbitofrontal gyrus are fused into single broad gyrus. Despite the absence of the anterior aspect of the olfactory sulci, their posterior extension is almost always present. The anterior pituitary lobe may be normal, hypoplastic, or absent. The neurohypophysis may be translocated to the inferior hypothalamus (Fig. 2.09-1C). In most patients, the hypothalamus has a normal MR imaging appearance. Despite the absence of hypoplasia of the anterior olfactory apparatus, the amygdalae and hippocampi have a normal appearance by MR imaging.

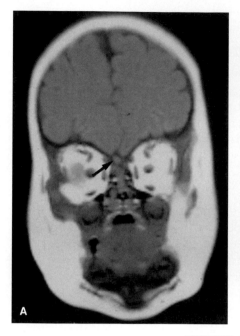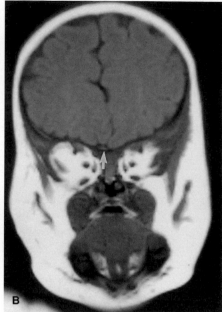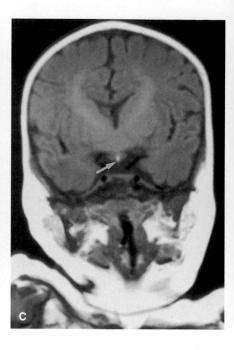

FIGURE 2.09-1.

Kallmann syndrome.   **A.** Coronal magnetic resonance (MR) T1-weighted image in a child with hypogonadism shows dysplastic neuromatous mass *(arrow)* in place of two olfactory bulbs. (With permission from Castillo M. Normal anatomy and imaging of the olfactory apparatus. MRI Decisions 1993;7:27.) **B.** Coronal MR T1-weighted image posterior to (A) shows normal-appearing right olfactory bulb *(arrow)* but absent left bulb. Note presence of olfactory sulcus in normal side and its absence in abnormal side. **C.** Coronal MR T1-weighted image shows hypoplastic pituitary gland and translocated neurohypophysis *(arrow).* The septum pellucidum is absent.

SUGGESTED READINGS

1. Truwit CL, Barkovich AJ, Grumbach MM, Martini JJ. MR imaging of Kallmann syndrome, a genetic disorder of neuronal migration affecting the olfactory and genital systems. AJNR 1993;14:827.
2. Yousem DM, Turner WJD, Li C, Snyder PL, Doty RL. Kallmann syndrome: MR evaluation of olfactory system. AJNR 1993;14:839.
3. Knorr JR, Ragland RL, Brown RS, Gelber N. Kallmann syndrome: MR findings. AJNR 1993;14:845.

2.10 Disorders of the Subarachnoid Space: Subarachnoid Cysts

EPIDEMIOLOGY

The incidence of these nonneoplastic, noninflammatory leptomeningeal cysts is not known, but they probably account for less than 1% of intracranial masses. Over three fourths of them are found in children, particularly boys. The most common locations for arachnoid cysts are given in Table 2.10-1.

TABLE 2.10-1. Locations of Arachnoid Cysts

Location of Arachnoid Cyst	Percentage
Middle cranial fossa	50%
Cerebellopontine angle cistern and cisterna magna	10%–12%
Quadrigeminal plate cistern	10%
Superior cerebellar cistern	8%
Parasellar regions	8%
Interhemispheric fissure	5%
Cerebral convexities	4%
Pontine cistern	3%

CLINICAL FEATURES

Arachnoid cysts probably originate from maldevelopment of the subarachnoid spaces. When they originate in the middle cranial fossa, it is unclear if the accompanying temporal lobe hypoplasia is the effect or the cause of the arachnoid cyst. Middle cranial fossa arachnoid cysts may produce seizures, headaches, and, occasionally, hemiparesis. Most (> 80%) arachnoid cysts are asymptomatic and are found incidentally. The most common clinical symptom is headaches. When compression of brain parenchyma occurs, seizures and focal neurologic signs may be present. Compression of cerebrospinal fluid (CSF) pathways may result in hydrocephalus. Arachnoid cysts originating in the region of the quadrigeminal plate commonly produce hydrocephalus. Most arachnoid cysts remain stable in size throughout the life of the patient, but some occasionally enlarge (ball-valve mechanism with trapping of CSF?). Enlarging cysts may produce skull abnormalities and result in developmental delay. Suprasellar arachnoid cysts may compress the optic chiasm, leading to visual field deficits, or compress the hypothalamus and the pituitary gland, producing endocrine abnormalities (including adipsia and precocious puberty). Other symptoms associated with suprasellar arachnoid cysts include craniomegaly, developmental delay, and the bobble-head doll syndrome. Arachnoid cysts are common in patients with Marfan syndrome. Treatment with surgical or endoscopic fenestration or insertion of a shunt catheter may be needed for symptomatic arachnoid cysts.

IMAGING FEATURES

Computed tomography shows a smooth CSF-density mass usually producing little or no mass effect (Fig. 2.10-1A). Arachnoid cysts do not contain calcifications and do not enhance after contrast administration. Deformity of the adjacent bones (particularly the greater wing of the sphenoid in patients with middle cranial fossa cysts) and scalloping of the inner table of the skull may be seen. Approximately one fifth of middle cranial fossa arachnoid cysts are small and have no mass effect. One half of middle cranial fossa arachnoid cysts are of moderate size and extend to the lateral aspect of the Sylvian fissure, where they open the operculae. One third of middle cranial fossa arachnoid cysts are large and produce a significant mass effect (Fig. 2.10-1B,C). By magnetic resonance (MR) imaging, arachnoid cysts are usually of equal signal intensity to CSF in all sequences. Although they lack internal architecture, flow artifacts may make them inhomogeneous. Occasionally, arachnoid cysts are of higher T1 signal intensity than CSF, a finding related to increased protein or blood within the cyst. The differential diagnosis includes an epidermoid (especially at the cerebellopontine angle cistern), a cystic tumor, and a loculated subdural effusion or hygroma.

Diffusion MR imaging holds promise in the differentiation of arachnoid cysts from solid but cystic-appearing masses. Hydrocephalus is present in up to two thirds of all patients with arachnoid cysts and in almost all children with cysts located in the posterior fossa. Posterior fossa arachnoid cysts commonly measure more than 5 cm in diameter.

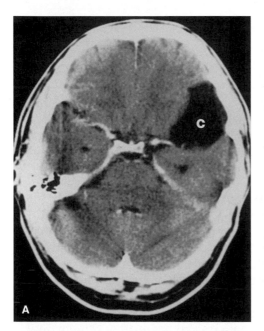
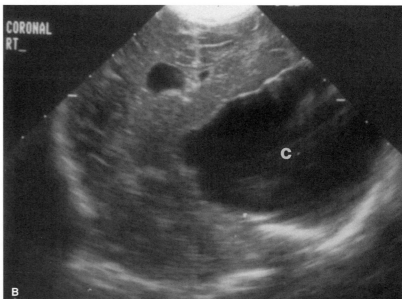
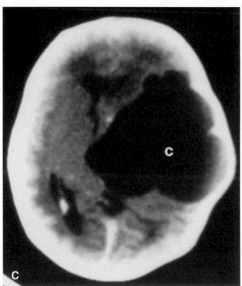

FIGURE 2.10-1.

Arachnoid cyst. **A.** Axial postcontrast computed tomography (CT) in adolescent with headaches shows cerebrospinal fluid-filled cyst (c) in left middle cerebral artery cistern. Note lack of enhancement and relatively little mass effect. **B.** Coronal sonogram in newborn with a bulge in left side of head shows fluid-filled cyst (c) occupying almost all of the left cranial cavity. Note mass effect on midline structures and dilation of the right lateral ventricle. **C.** Axial postcontrast CT image in same case shows very large left arachnoid cyst (c) displacing overlying bone laterally. There is mass effect on the third ventricle and dilation of the right lateral ventricle. This cyst was shunted.

SUGGESTED READINGS

1. Robertson SJ, Wolpert WM, Runge VM. MR imaging of middle cranial fossa arachnoid cysts: temporal lobe agenesis syndrome revisited. AJNR 1989;10:1007.
2. Wester K. Gender distribution and sidedness of middle fossa arachnoid cysts: a review of cases diagnosed with computed imaging. Neurosurgery 1992;31:940.
3. Ciricillo SF, Cogen PH, Harsh GR, Edwards MSB. Intracranial arachnoid cyst in children: a comparison of the effects of fenestration and shunting. J Neurosurgery 1991;74:230.
4. Tien RD, MacFall J, Heinz ER. Evaluation of complex cystic masses of the brain: value of steady-state–free-precession MR imaging. AJR 1992;159:1049.

2.11 *Subarachnoid Intracranial Lipomas*

EPIDEMIOLOGY

Subarachnoid intracranial lipomas are rare congenital malformations arising from faulty development of the primitive subarachnoid space cells (meninx primitiva). They comprise less than 1% of all intracranial masses and occur with equal frequency in boys and girls. Approximately 50% of patients harboring intracranial lipomas have adjacent brain malformations, particularly dysgenesis of the corpus callosum. The most common locations for intracranial lipomas include the midline (> 80%) and the basilar cisterns (suprasellar, cerebellopontine angle, quadrigeminal plate, interpeduncular, and Sylvian cisterns).

CLINICAL FEATURES

Isolated lipomas are usually asymptomatic and incidentally found. When symptomatic, the cause of the symptoms is usually a neighboring brain malformation rather than the lipoma itself. When they arise in the cisterns surrounding the brain stem, they may produce cranial neuropathies particularly involving cranial nerves VI, VII, and VIII. When lipomas arise in the quadrigeminal plate cistern, hydrocephalus may be present. Multiple intracranial lipomas may be found in patients with encephalocutaneous lipomatosis. Patients with this rare syndrome are mentally retarded and have seizures caused by multiple brain abnormalities. Patients with hypersecretion of adrenocorticotropic hormone may have fat deposits in the cavernous sinuses; these, however, may also be seen in normal individuals. If symptomatic, treatment of intracranial lipomas is aimed at producing relief of complaints with minimal decompression of the lesion.

IMAGING FEATURES

Midline lipomas may be divided into tubulonodular and curvilinear types (Fig. 2.11-1). The former are mass-like and almost always are associated with dysgenesis of the corpus callosum (Fig. 2.11-2). In these patients, the frontal lobes may be abnormal and cephaloceles may also be present. Curvilinear lipomas are usually thin and sit on a normal (or minimally dysgenetic) corpus callosum at the level of the callosal sulcus. Lipomas account for more than 50% of all masses involving the corpus callosum. All lipomas occur at levels of brain infolding where primitive subarachnoid space elements may become trapped (Fig. 2.11-3). Lipomas have little mass effect with respect to their size, and may occasionally be hemorrhagic. Rarely, midline lipomas may be associated with scalp lipomas or protrude through a cranium bifidum occultum.

On computed tomography, lipomas show low density (−50 to −100 HU). They contain peripheral shell-like or amorphous internal calcifications. After contrast administration they do not enhance. On magnetic resonance imaging, they are hyperintense on T1-weighted images, relatively hypointense on conventional spin echo T2-weighted images, and bright on fast spin echo T2-weighted images. Chemical shift artifact along the frequency encoding direction is seen in their margins. Their signal intensity may be suppressed with fat suppression techniques. Lipomas contain linear areas of low signal intensity because they are crossed by cranial nerves and vessels (Fig. 2.11-4). Remember that because lipomas represent an aberration of the development of the subarachnoid space, they tend to develop around and engulf structures coursing through the subarachnoid spaces, rather than displacing or invading them.

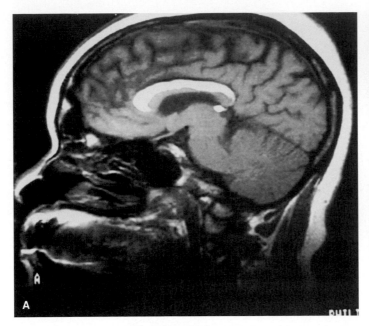
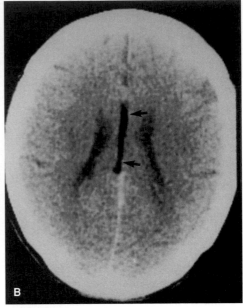

FIGURE 2.11-1.

Curvilinear lipoma. **A.** Midline sagittal magnetic resonance T1-weighted image in an adolescent with headaches shows a thin, hyperintense lipoma following the superior margin of the corpus callosum (curvilinear type). The corpus callosum is completely formed but somewhat thin. A second small lipoma is present in the superior aspect of the quadrigeminal plate cistern. Most midline lipomas are associated with dysgenesis of the corpus callosum. **B.** Axial postcontrast computed tomography in a different patient shows typical interhemispheric curvilinear lipoma *(arrows)*.

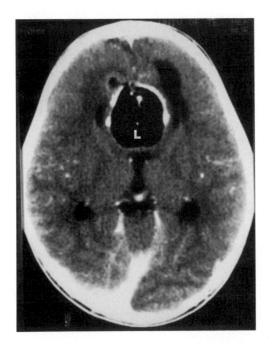

FIGURE 2.11-2.

Nodular lipoma. Axial postcontrast computed tomography in a case of dysgenesis of the corpus callosum shows large anterior interhemispheric lipoma (L) with calcified margins. Some calcifications are also present inside the lipoma.

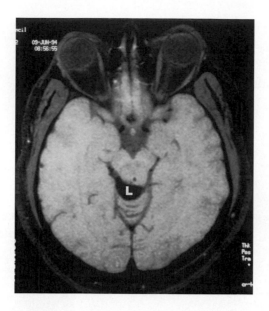

FIGURE 2.11-3.

Quadrigeminal cistern lipoma. Axial magnetic resonance T1-weighted image shows a lipoma (L) in the quadrigeminal plate cistern that has become very dark with application of fat suppression technique. Note excellent suppression of any signal intensity from other fatty structures.

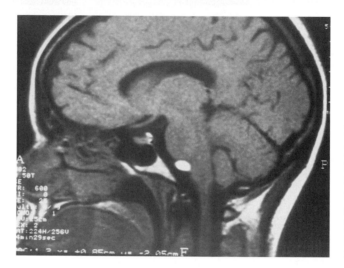

FIGURE 2.11-4.

Lipoma producing cranial neuropathy. Parasagittal noncontrast magnetic resonance T1-weighted image shows a round lipoma at the pontomedullary junction in patient with a palsy of cranial nerve VI.

SUGGESTED READING

1. Truwit CL, Barkovich AJ. Pathogenesis of intracranial lipoma: an MR study in 42 patients. AJNR 1990;11:665.

2.12 *Basal Encephaloceles*

EPIDEMIOLOGY
The term "basal encephaloceles" refers to herniations of the brain and meninges through defects in the bones forming the anterior and middle cranial fossae. Encephaloceles, in general, occur in approximately 0.8 to 3:10,000 births. Sincipital and basal encephaloceles tend to occur with greater frequency in Asia, Africa, Australia, and Latin America, and tend to be slightly more common in boys. They tend to be isolated anomalies, but occasionally are associated to the low median cleft syndrome (Sedano B). Transalar sphenoidal encephaloceles are also seen with neurofibromatosis type I. Although most are congenital defects, basal encephaloceles may be secondary to infection, surgery, or trauma. Elevated α-fetoprotein and sonography aid in the prenatal diagnosis of all encephaloceles.

CLINICAL FEATURES
Basal encephaloceles may be divided into transphenoidal (through the body or alae of the sphenoid into the nasopharynx or infratemporal fossae), sphenoorbital (through the superior orbital fissure into the orbit), transethmoidal (through the cribriform plate into the anterior nasal cavity), and sphenomaxillary (through the inferior orbital fissure into the pterygopalatine fossae). Strictly temporal encephaloceles, in which the brain herniates into the middle ear, also exist. The clinical symptoms are related to the size of the encephalocele but mainly to the configuration of the remaining intracranial brain parenchyma. Small encephaloceles are usually asymptomatic (particularly transalar types), but some patients may have seizures. Airway obstruction or chronic cerebrospinal fluid leakage may also occur. Developmental delay and dysgenesis of the corpus callosum may be present, but these are more common with occipital encephaloceles. If the pituitary gland and hypothalamus are contained within the sac, endocrine dysfunction may present. Hydrocephalus may be present. Basal encephaloceles may escape discovery until late in life; management usually consists of resection and closure of small encephaloceles. Treatment may be ineffective in large encephaloceles. Resection of the encephalocele does not alter intellectual prognosis because the tissues contained within it are usually nonfunctioning.

IMAGING FEATURES
Magnetic resonance (MR) imaging usually shows the bone defect and the contents of the sac. The tissues contained within the herniated sac may be of similar signal intensity to brain or be slightly hyperintense on T2-weighted sequences (Fig. 2.12-1). The latter may be related to gliosis. The meninges of the sac may be thickened and nodular because of the presence of fibrosis and heterotopias, respectively. The head may be small (microcephaly). MR angiography eloquently demonstrates the course of the anterior cerebral arteries, which may be contained within large encephaloceles (Fig. 2.12-2). Computed tomography is helpful in outlining the bone defect. If untreated, continued growth of the sac may cause infarction of its walls secondary to stretching. If this occurs, ulceration, infection, and rupture of the encephalocele may ensue.

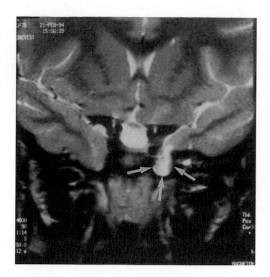

FIGURE 2.12-1.

Lateral sphenoidal encephalocele. Coronal magnetic resonance T2-weighted image in a patient with neurofibromatosis type I shows small medial right transphenoidal encephalocele *(arrows)* containing tissue of very high signal intensity, which is probably related to a combination of cerebrospinal fluid and gliosis.

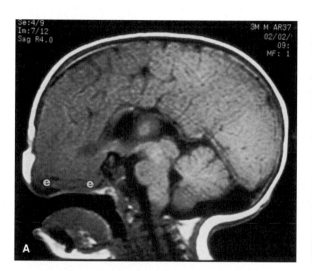

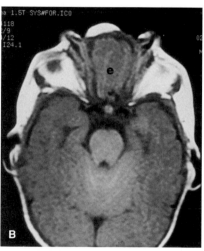

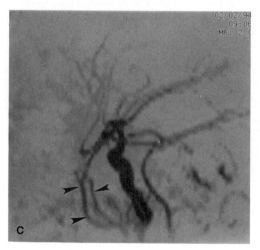

FIGURE 2.12-2.

Frontobasal encephalocele. A. Midsagittal magnetic resonance (MR) T1-weighted image shows large frontal-ethmoidal-sphenoidal encephalocele (e) in this newborn with HARD+E syndrome. **B.** Axial MR T1-weighted image shows contents of the encephalocele (e) to be of equal signal intensity to intracranial brain. **C.** Lateral view of MR three-dimensional time-of-flight angiogram shows that the encephalocele contains both anterior cerebral arteries *(arrowheads).* (Case courtesy of Rafael Rojas, M.D., ABC Hospital, Mexico City, Mexico.)

SUGGESTED READINGS

1. Elster AD, Branch CL. Transalar sphenoidal encephaloceles: clinical and radiology findings. Radiology 1989;170:245.
2. Naidich TP, Altman NR, Braffman BH, McLone DG, Zimmerman RA. Cephaloceles and related malformations. AJNR 1992;13:655.

Imaging of the Pediatric Head, Neck, and Spine
by Mauricio Castillo and Suresh K. Mukherji,
Lippincott-Raven Publishing, Philadelphia © 1996.

3

Developmental Anomalies, Infratentorial

3.0 *Applied Embryology*

According to the stage of development, the cerebellum may be divided into three portions. The most primitive portion is the "archicerebellum," which contains the vestibular nuclei. The "paleocerebellum" develops later and includes the flocculi and the vermis. The "neocerebellum" designates the hemispheres (with the exception of the flocculi).

Step 1: The Rhombencephalon Divides

At the end of the third week of gestation, and before the rostral neural tube closes, the rhombencephalon (hindbrain) divides into two portions: the metencephalon (future pons and cerebellum) and the myelencephalon (future medulla; Fig. 3.0-1A). Insults at this stage may result in cerebellar aplasia, which is very rare.

Step 2: The Rhombencephalon Enlarges

Between the fourth to seventh weeks of life, the lateral aspects of the rhombencephalon enlarge to form the alar plates (Fig. 3.0-1B). The anlagen for cranial nerves V to X develop. Neuronal migration produces thickening of the lateral aspects of the alar plates. The fourth ventricle, choroid plexus, and superior cerebellar peduncles also form during this time (Fig. 3.0-1C).

Step 3: The Hemispheres Fuse and the Vermis Appears

Approximately during the ninth week of gestation, the cerebellar hemispheres fuse in their midline. Fusion begins superiorly and progresses inferiorly. The vermis arises from this fusion and is completely formed by the 15th week of life. The flocculi, the superior cerebellar peduncles, and dentate and olivary nuclei also form during this period. The fourth ventricle assumes its typical shape, and its choroid plexus matures. Although the growth of the cerebellar hemispheres lags behind that of the vermis, they soon catch up and obscure the vermis. The foramina of Luschka appear at approximately the fourth month of life. The time of appearance of the foramen of Magendie is uncertain. During this period of development the formation of the paleocerebellum is completed. Disorders arising from insults at this stage include the Dandy-Walker complex, Joubert syndrome, rhombencephalosynapsis, and tectocerebellar dysraphia. Because the subarachnoid space is being formed simultaneously, arachnoid cysts also originate during this time.

Step 4: Insults to the Developing Hemispheres

The developing and maturing cerebellar hemispheres constitute the neocerebellum. Insults to them may result in aplasia, hypoplasia, or dysplasia of one or both hemispheres. Disorders affecting the neocerebellum may also affect the paleocerebellum (vermis). A typical example of this is the full Dandy-Walker complex anomaly. Insults during this period may also inhibit or produce disorganization of neuronal migration, and may result in cortical dysplasias such as the Lhermitte-Duclos disease.

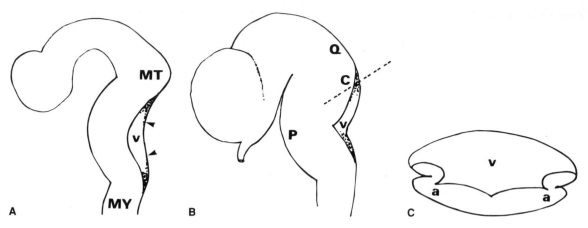

FIGURE 3.0-1.

Normal development of the cerebellum.   **A.** The rostral end of the neural tube is closed by the end of the third week of life and begins to fold on itself. The protuberances are seen posteriorly; the superiorly located one represents the metencephalon (MT), which gives origin to the pons and cerebellum. The inferior protuberance represents the myelencephalon (MY), which gives origin to the medulla. The fourth ventricle (v) exists in a rudimentary form and is covered dorsally by a thin tela *(arrowheads)*. **B.** The rostral neural tube continues to fold and the pons (P), quadrigeminal plate (Q), future cerebellum (C), and fourth ventricle (v) are present by the end of the seventh week of gestation (*dotted line* represents level of [C]). **C.** Diagram at the level of the dotted line in (B) shows the alar plates (a), which will form the cerebellar hemispheres, located dorsally to the large fourth ventricle (v).

3.01 *Occipital Encephaloceles*

EPIDEMIOLOGY

Encephaloceles occur in approximately 0.8 to 3:10,000 births. Occipital encephaloceles are more common in North America and in Europe. Girls are more commonly affected than boys. Occipital encephaloceles are associated with defects of neural tube closure and with the Chiari type II malformation. They are also closely associated with Meckel syndrome, which comprises occipital encephalocele, holoprosencephaly, facial clefts, microphthalmia, retinal dysplasia, polydactyly, polycystic kidneys, heart anomalies, and ambiguous genitalia.

CLINICAL FEATURES

Occipital encephaloceles are large (45% are larger than 10 cm in diameter) but almost always covered by intact skin. Microcephaly is proportional to the size of the encephalocele. If unresected, most encephaloceles show some growth over time. Most contain portions of cerebellum, occipital and parietal lobes, basilar cisterns, arteries, and venous sinuses. The parenchyma contained within the sac is dysplastic and nonfunctioning. Occasionally, there is also herniation of the brain stem into the sac. By location, occipital encephaloceles may be divided into those located under the venous torcular, above the torcular, and, less commonly, those involving both compartments. Encephaloceles below the venous torcular are usually accompanied by dysraphism of the upper cervical spine with absence of the posterior elements of C1 and C2. They are confluent with the foramen magnum. In supratorcular encephaloceles, there is a bone defect, which usually is small, located in or off the midline of the occipital bones. These encephaloceles contain occipital and parietal lobes. Anomalies of the venous system (hypoplastic, absent, or aberrant sinuses) are common. The superior sagittal sinus may be split by the encephalocele. The hippocampus is abnormally formed in all cases of encephaloceles and may account for intractable seizures in these patients. Surgical correction is usually aimed at easing the care of these children.

IMAGING FEATURES

Sagittal magnetic resonance (MR) T1-weighted images readily show the relationship of the encephalocele to the venous torcular (Fig. 3.01-1A). They also are helpful in demonstrating the presence of aqueductal stenosis, which may lead to noncommunicating hydrocephalus. The intracranial brain is often malformed and may harbor multiple areas of cortical dysplasia. The corpus callosum is often dysgenetic and myelination may lag behind normal. The posterior aspect of the falx cerebri is absent or hypoplastic in most supratorcular and mixed encephaloceles. The tentorium is also malformed. Occasionally, these patients have intracranial findings similar to those present in the Chiari type II malformation, and some authors have applied the term "Chiari III malformation" to these patients. Some occipital encephaloceles contain cerebrospinal fluid-filled cysts that are in communication with the fourth ventricle (Fig. 3.01-1B). These "ventriculoceles" may belong to the Dandy-Walker complex. In some cases, the encephaloceles contain an extremely hypoplastic cerebellum and are referred to as inverse cerebellum with encephalocele, or tecto-cerebellar dysraphia with occipital encephalocele (Fig. 3.01-1C,D). MR angiography helps to delineate the course of arteries arising from the vertebrobasilar system. MR venography may demonstrate important venous structures inside the sac, or other anomalies such as hypoplasia, fenestration, absence, or ectopia of the venous sinuses.

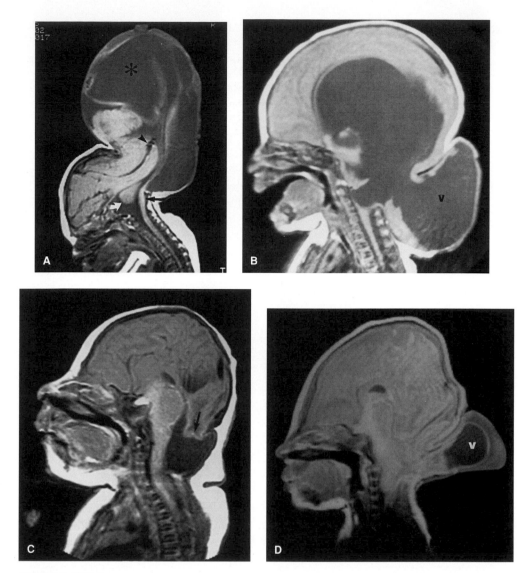

FIGURE 3.01-1.

Occipital encephaloceles. **A.** Midline sagittal magnetic resonance (MR) T1-weighted image shows extremely large supratorcular and infratorcular encephalocele containing cerebrospinal fluid (CSF) spaces *(asterisk)*, dysplastic brain, venous sinuses *(arrowhead)*, and a portion of the medulla *(arrow)* and pons *(curved white arrow)*. There is microcephaly, and the residual intracranial contents are markedly disorganized. The corpus callosum is not seen. **B.** Midline sagittal MR T1-weighted image shows infratorcular encephalocele containing a markedly enlarged fourth ventricle (V). The posterior elements of C1–C3 are absent. Pronounced hydrocephalus is present and produces marked thinning of the corpus callosum. These findings could be categorized as Dandy-Walker complex with encephalocele. **C.** Midline sagittal MR T1-weighted image shows infratorcular cephalocele containing mostly CSF (fourth ventricle vs. cisterna magna) due to aplasia of the cerebellum (tectocerebellar dysraphia). There is inferior herniation of the occipital lobes *(arrow)* secondary to a malformed tentorium. The posterior elements of C1–C4 are absent. Microcephaly is present and the corpus callosum is not clearly seen. **D.** Midsagittal MR T1-weighted image shows infratorcular encephalocele containing cerebellum and possibly a dilated fourth ventricle (v). Posterior elements of C1 and C2 are absent. (All figures with permission from Castillo M, Quencer RM, Dominguez R. Chiari III malformation: imaging features. AJNR 1992;13:107.)

SUGGESTED READINGS

1. Naidich TP, Altman NR, Braffman BH, McLone DG, Zimmerman RA. Cephaloceles and related malformations. AJNR 1992;13:655.
2. Diebles CD, Dulac O. Cephaloceles: clinical and neuroradiology appearance. Neuroradiology 1983;25:199.
3. Leong ASY, Shaw CM. The pathology of occipital encephalocele and a discussion of the pathogenesis. Pathology 1979;11:223.
4. Castillo M, Quencer RM, Dominguez R. Chiari III malformation: imaging features. AJNR 1992;13:107.

3.02 *Chiari Type I Malformation*

EPIDEMIOLOGY

Chiari I malformation refers to a simple anomaly characterized by displacement of the cerebellar tonsils inferior to the foramen magnum. The general incidence of this malformation is unknown, but it can be seen 0.5% to 1% of all magnetic resonance (MR) imaging studies of the brain. It is often an incidental and asymptomatic finding. Chiari I malformation is more common in female than in male patients.

CLINICAL FEATURES

Clinical symptoms are directly proportional to the degree of cerebellar tonsillar herniation. Clinical manifestations may take decades to develop. The most common symptoms include recurrent occipital and frontal headaches, neck pain, gait abnormalities, progressive ataxia, and difficulty swallowing. Many abnormalities result from dysfunction involving cranial nerves IX to XII. Downbeat nystagmus and periodic alternating nystagmus are typical of Chiari I malformation and of other anomalies of the craniovertebral junction. Myelopathy signs may also be found. Hydrocephalus may develop. Treatment is aimed at relieving pressure from the tonsils via a suboccipital craniotomy with extension into the foramen magnum (to enlarge it) and lysis of multiple dural bands located posterior to the tonsils. Hydrocephalus necessitates shunting, and spinal cord fluid cysts may need decompression.

IMAGING FEATURES

Cerebellar tonsils extending 3 mm or less below the foramen magnum may be considered a normal variant (benign cerebellar tonsillar ectopia). Cerebellar tonsils extending between 3 to 6 mm below the foramen magnum are of uncertain significance. Some of these patients may be asymptomatic, whereas others may have mild symptoms. Herniation of the cerebellar tonsils by more than 6 mm below the foramen magnum may be considered a Chiari type I malformation (Fig. 3.02-1). The severity of the clinical symptoms correlates well with the degree of tonsillar displacement. Patients with herniations 12 mm or larger are almost always symptomatic, whereas only 5% to 30% of patients with herniations ranging between 6 to 10 mm show symptoms. Abnormalities of the craniovertebral junction (ie, Klippel-Feil syndrome) may produce tonsillar herniation. Acquired malformations of the foramen magnum leading to tonsillar herniation have been misclassified as Chiari type I malformations. Overall, skeletal anomalies are present in 20% to 40% of Chiari I patients and mainly include basilar invagination and atlantooccipital assimilation. Occasionally one encounters a patient with cerebellar tonsillar herniation only and with an open dysraphism in the lower spine. Although this combination of abnormalities has been categorized as a subgroup of Chiari I malformations, it is better classified as a type II Chiari anomaly because of its similar surgical management. In patients with Chiari I malformation, the tonsils are typically triangular with their apex pointing down. The foramen magnum is small and appears crowded, leading to neural and vascular compression. The posterior dural bands (typically encountered during surgery) that contribute to tonsillar compression are not identifiable by MR imaging. A spinal cord cyst may be seen in 20% to 40% of Chiari I patients (Fig. 3.02-2). These spinal cord cysts occur more commonly in the high cervical region. We have seen one case of an incidental Chiari I malformation that resolved in time with the growth of the patient (Fig. 3.02-3).

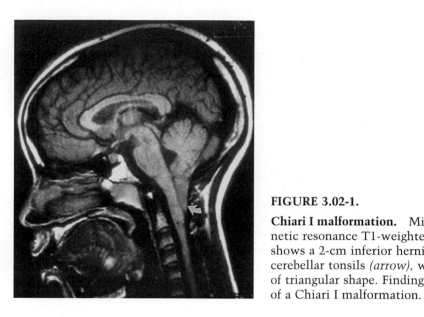

FIGURE 3.02-1.

Chiari I malformation. Midsagittal magnetic resonance T1-weighted image shows a 2-cm inferior herniation of the cerebellar tonsils *(arrow),* which are also of triangular shape. Findings are typical of a Chiari I malformation.

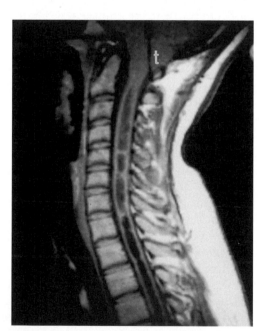

FIGURE 3.02-2.

Spinal cord cyst in Chiari I malformation. Midsagittal magnetic resonance T1-weighted image shows a multiseptated, fluid-filled cyst within the lower cervical and thoracic spinal cord of this patient with a Chiari I malformation. Note low position of tonsils (t). (With permission from Castillo M. Neuroradiology Companion. Philadelphia: JB Lippincott, 1995.)

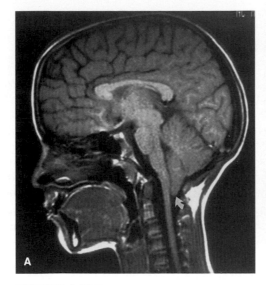 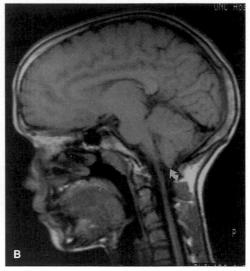

FIGURE 3.02-3.

Spontaneously resolving Chiari I malformation. **A.** Midsagittal magnetic resonance (MR) T1-weighted image shows the cerebellar tonsils *(arrow)* projecting approximately 1 cm below the foramen magnum. The tonsils also point down. This patient had a history of seizures, and this finding was thought to be incidental. There was no history of recent seizures or lumbar puncture at the time of this study. **B.** Midsagittal MR T1-weighted image (slightly tilted) in same patient 3 years after initial study shows normal position of cerebellar tonsils *(arrow)*. (With permission from Castillo M., Wilson D. Spontaneous resolution of a Chiari I malformation. AJNR, 1995;16:1158.)

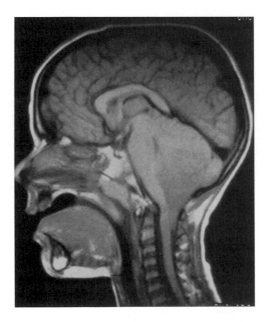

FIGURE 3.02-4.

Pseudo Chiari I malformation, basilar artery thrombosis. Midsagittal magnetic resonance T1-weighted image shows herniation of the cerebellar tonsils inferior to foramen magnum but also swelling of the cerebellum, effacement of the fourth ventricle, and flattening of the belly of the pons. This "pseudo Chiari I" appearance is caused by thrombosis of the basilar artery.

SUGGESTED READINGS

1. Elster AD, Chen MYM. Chiari I malformations: clinical and radiology reappraisal. Radiology 1992;183:347.
2. Barkovich AJ, Wippold FJ, Sherman JL, Citrin CM. Significance of cerebellar tonsillar postion on MR. AJNR 1986;7:795.

3.03 *Chiari Type II Malformation*

EPIDEMIOLOGY

Chiari II malformation is a complex anomaly involving the brain and skull. The hallmarks of this anomaly are deformity of the hindbrain and presence of a myelomeningocele. It probably results from a failure of primary neurulation that leaves a dorsal opening through which chronic drainage of cerebrospinal fluid occurs, and which also produces downward traction of the cerebellum and collapse of the brain vesicles. The exact incidence of the Chiari II malformation is not known, but is probably similar to that of myelomeningocele, which occurs in 2 to 3:1000 births. The risk of recurrence for myelomeningocele in subsequent siblings varies from 4% to 8%. Genetic counseling is therefore indicated. Lipomyelomeningoceles are not typically associated with the Chiari II malformation.

CLINICAL FEATURES

The diagnosis of myelomeningocele may be made in utero by sonography or elevated α-fetoprotein in amniotic fluid. Most myelomeningoceles occur in the lumbosacral area, followed by the thoracic and cervical regions, and are present in almost 100% of patients with the Chiari II malformation. Hydrocephalus is present in 25% of patients at birth but eventually develops in up 90% of Chiari II patients. Spinal cord fluid-filled cysts are found in 50% to 90% of patients. Diastematomyelia probably occurs in 1% to 5% of patients with this malformation. Some patients are developmentally delayed and may have seizures, but others are intellectually normal. Apnea may be present and is probably secondary to hypoplasia of brain stem nuclei. Varying degrees of lower extremity paresis and sphincter dysfunction are present. Urinary retention may lead to infections and renal failure. Congenital hip dislocation and deformities of the feet are present. Early management is aimed at reducing the size of the dysraphism and covering it. Hydrocephalus requires shunting.

IMAGING FEATURES

Magnetic resonance is the imaging modality of choice in these patients (Fig. 3.03-1). Computed tomography may be used to follow ventricular size. Herniation of the lower vermis into the spinal canal is a classic finding. Occasionally, the herniated vermis extends down to the lower cervical region, but more often stops at the C3 level. The choroid plexus may also be displaced inferiorly. The medulla is displaced caudally and "kinks" at the level where it is attached to the spinal canal by the dentate ligaments (70% of patients). The foramen magnum is large, but the posterior fossa is small. The cerebellum compensates for this relative lack of space by protruding superiorly ("towering") through an incompetent tentorial incisura. On axial images, this superiorly displaced cerebellum assumes a "heart" shape. The cerebellar hemispheres wrap around the brain stem and should not be mistaken for true cerebellopontine angle cistern masses. The fourth ventricle is not seen if the patient has been adequately shunted and has no hydrocephalus. A normal-appearing fourth ventricle in Chiari II patients should raise the suspicion of shunt failure. Occasionally a very small cerebellum is seen, which is presumed to represent atrophy due to pressure necrosis as a result of herniation through the foramen magnum. It is possible that in the past this anomaly was erroneously labeled as Chiari type IV malformation. The posterior surfaces of the petrous bones and clivus are scalloped. Midbrain anomalies include fusion of the colliculi ("tectal beaking") and aqueductal stenosis. Supratentorially, there may be hydrocephalus and the corpus callosum may be dysgenetic in up to 90% of patients. Colpocephaly may be present. The third ventricle is relatively small and the massa intermedia appears large. Neuronal heterotopias are not unusual. The falx cerebri may be fenestrated, hypoplastic, or absent, leading to interdigitation (in a zipper-like fashion) of the gyri located in the medial surface of the cerebral hemispheres. The interhemispheric fissure is wide. The gyri in the occipital and parietal regions are normally formed but appear to be numerous and slightly small (stenogyria). The medial occipital lobes are dysplastic and may have a bizarre configuration, particularly after ventricular shunting.

In the spine, segmentation anomalies of the high cervical spine (particularly the posterior arch of C1) are present in 10% of patients. Spinal cord abnormalities include syringomyelia, diastematomyelia, and diplomyelia. Imaging of the craniocervical junction in patients with Chiari II malformations helps in identifying stenosis of the foramen magnum and postsurgical trapped fourth ventricle.

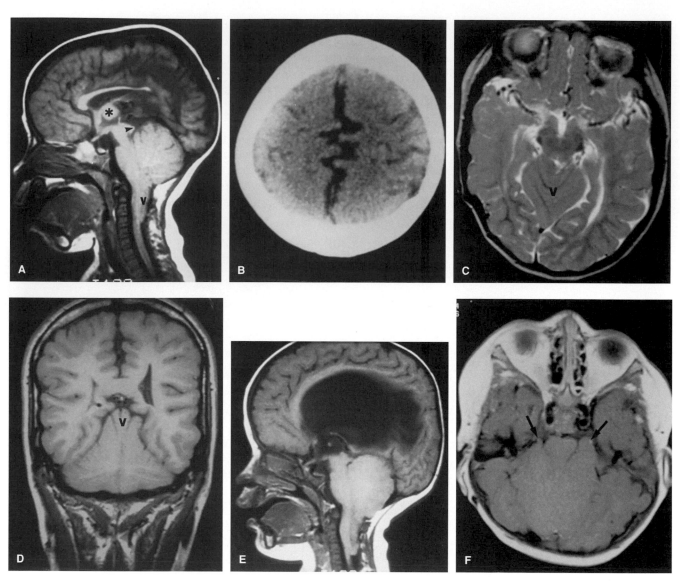

FIGURE 3.03-1.

Chiari II malformation. **A.** Midsagittal magnetic resonance (MR) T1-weighted image shows nonvisualized fourth ventricle, herniation of cerebellar vermis (V) to C4 level, smooth cerebellar vermis, beaked tectum *(arrowhead),* small third ventricle, enlarged massa intermedia *(asterisk),* and dysplastic corpus callosum. (With permission from Castillo M. Neuroradiology Companion. Philadelphia: JB Lippincott, 1995.) **B.** Axial computed tomography shows absence of the mid-portion of the falx cerebri with interdigitation in a zipper-like fashion of the cortical sulci of both medial cerebral hemispheres. (With permission from Castillo M, Dominguez R. Imaging of congenital abnormalities of the brain and spine. Clinical Imaging 1992;16:73.) **C.** Axial MR T2-weighted image shows heart-shaped superior herniation of the cerebellar vermis (V) and medial hemispheres due to hypoplasia of the tentorium and an incompetent incisura. **D.** Coronal MR T1-weighted image in a different case shows that the upward herniation of the cerebellum (V) has a "tower-like" configuration. The number of gyri is increased (stenogyria). **E.** Midsagittal MR T1-weighted image shows obstruction of the aqueduct of Sylvius, resulting in massive hydrocephalus in this child with Chiari II malformation. Note nonvisualized fourth ventricle, inferiorly herniated vermis (to level of C4), smooth vermis, and beaked tectum. **F.** Axial MR T1-weighted image shows cerebellopontine angle "pseudomasses" (left greater than right; *arrows)* secondary to overgrowth of the cerebellar hemispheres anteriorly to the brain stem.

SUGGESTED READINGS

1. Wolpert SM, Anderson M, Scott RM, Kwan ESK, Runge VM. Chiari II malformation: MR imaging evaluation. AJNR 1987;8:783.
2. El Gammal T, Mark EK, Brooks BS. MR imaging of Chiari II malformation. AJR 1988;150:163.
3. McClone DG, Knepper PA. The cause of Chiari II malformation: a unified theory. Pediatr Neurosci 1989;15:1.

3.04 *Chiari Type III Malformation*

EPIDEMIOLOGY

This controversial anomaly refers to the presence of an occipital encephalocele in combination with several of the intracranial features seen in the Chiari II malformation. Its incidence is unknown, but it probably is very rare. In our experience with 13 such cases, there were no associated systemic abnormalities or syndromes.

CLINICAL FEATURES

The etiology of Chiari III malformations is probably similar to that of the type II Chiari anomaly. A defect in primary neurulation produces a high cervical/occipital dysraphic state through which, or into which, cerebrospinal fluid leaks chronically. This produces downward displacement of the cerebellum and collapse of the brain vesicles. As such, Chiari malformations types II and III are related, but are different from the type I anomaly. Treatment is aimed toward reduction of the size of the encephalocele and shunting if hydrocephalus coexists.

IMAGING FEATURES

Magnetic resonance (MR) is the imaging method of choice. It allows for identification of the exact site of herniation, which may be supratorcular, infratorcular, in the high (C1–C2) cervical spine, or a combination of all these (Fig. 3.04-1A). MR also serves to identify the presence of vascular structures within the cephalocele (see section 3.01, Occipital Encephaloceles). The presence of venous sinuses within the sac may represent a contraindication to surgery because their ligation results in intracranial hypertension. Occasionally, the brain stem is contained within the sac. Similar to Chiari II malformations, there are multiple mesodermal defects, including scalloping of the posterior surface of the petrous bones and clivus, incompetent tentorial incisura, and absent posterior falx cerebri and falx cerebelli. Medial overgrowth of the cerebellar hemispheres into the cerebellopontine angle cisterns, superior towering of the cerebellum, and inferior herniation of tonsils/vermis may be seen (Fig. 3.04-1B,C). The dorsal midbrain is either deformed or not clearly seen. The corpus callosum may be dysgenetic and there may be hydrocephalus. Spinal cord fluid-filled cysts may be found.

As stated earlier, many investigators do not recognize this constellation of findings as a type of Chiari malformation, but prefer to group these patients as part of the Dandy-Walker complex or as simple occipital encephaloceles.

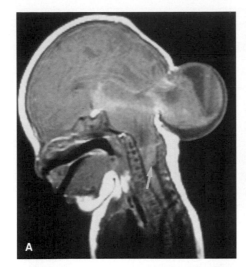

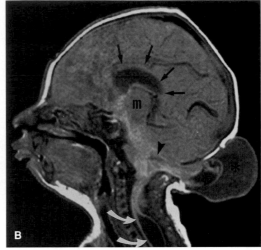

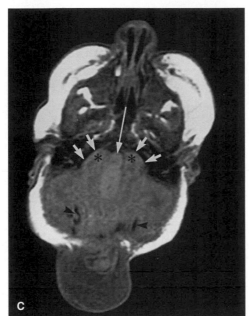

FIGURE 3.04-1.

Chiari III malformation. **A.** Midsagittal magnetic resonance (MR) T1-weighted image shows infratorcular occipital cephalocele with agenesis of posterior elements of upper cervical vertebrae. The sac contains mostly cerebellum and some cerebrospinal fluid (CSF) spaces. Residual cerebellar vermis *(arrow)* is herniated down through the foramen magnum to the C5 level. The fourth ventricle is not seen. The clivus is scalloped. The corpus callosum and tectum are not well seen. The pituitary gland is bright, a normal finding in the newborn. **B.** Midsagittal MR T1-weighted image shows a small, high cervical, low occipital encephalocele containing a small amount of cerebellum and large CSF spaces *(asterisk;* cisterna magna?). The fourth ventricle *(arrowhead)* is probably inside the cranium. The tectum is distorted and the massa intermedia (m) is large. The corpus callosum *(arrows)* is probably present, but not clearly seen. A cervical cord fluid-filled cyst *(curved arrows)* is present. **C.** Axial MR T1-weighted image in the same case shows anterior "overgrowth" of the cerebellar hemispheres *(asterisk)*, which wrap around and project anteriorly to the brain stem *(long white arrow)*. There is scalloping *(short white arrows)* of the posterior surface of the petrous bones. Anomalous venous sinuses *(arrowheads)* are located in the cerebellum at the mouth of the encephalocele. (B and C with permission from Castillo M, Quencer RM, Dominguez R. Chiari III malformation: imaging features. AJNR 1992;13:107.)

SUGGESTED READING

1. Castillo M, Quencer RM, Dominguez R. Chiari III malformation: imaging features. AJNR 1992;13:107.

3.05 *Dandy-Walker Complex*

EPIDEMIOLOGY

The Dandy-Walker complex consists of a spectrum of malformations ranging from a mega cisterna magna to atresia of the outlet foramina of the fourth ventricle. It occurs in approximately 1:30,000 live births. Most cases are sporadic, but a familial form with autosomal recessive inheritance is known to exist. In this form, the Dandy-Walker complex is accompanied by polycystic kidneys, cataracts, retinal abnormalities, and posterior coloboma. It has been found in offspring of mothers exposed to isotretinoin during the first trimester of pregnancy. It is associated with encephaloceles.

CLINICAL FEATURES

The exact etiology of these anomalies is probably related to a combination of failure of development of the anterior medullary velum, atresia of the outlet foramina of the fourth ventricle, and delayed opening of the foramen of Magendie. An insult isolated to the fourth ventricle results in a mega cisterna magna. A more severe insult involving the developing cerebellar hemispheres may produce the Dandy-Walker variant. The most severe insult, which involves the cerebellar hemispheres, vermis, and the fourth ventricle, produces the full syndrome. Because all three anomalies appear to be different points on a spectrum, the term "Dandy-Walker complex" is appropriate for all of them. Associated abnormalities include dysgenesis of the corpus callosum (30%) with or without a dorsal interhemispheric cyst, neuronal heterotopias and other migration disorders (10%–15%), occipital encephaloceles (10%), aqueductal stenosis, hamartomas of the pituitary stalk, Klippel-Feil syndrome, and anomalous lumbar vertebrae. Clinically, the patients are developmentally delayed and may have hydrocephalus, nystagmus, spasticity, titubation, and apnea. Rarely, the intellect is normal. Treatment is directed toward decompression of the dilated fourth ventricle, hydrocephalus, and interhemispheric cyst. Hydrocephalus is present in approximately 75% of these patients at birth, but eventually develops in over 90% of them.

IMAGING FEATURES

In the complete syndrome, the fourth ventricle is markedly dilated (Fig. 3.05-1). The inferior vermis is hypoplastic or agenetic. The residual vermis rotates up because of compression by the large fourth ventricle. The posterior fossa is large and the occipital bones balloon out. The tentorium inserts high and the venous torcular may be located above the lambdoid (lambdoid–torcular inversion). The brain stem may be hypoplastic. The aqueduct of Sylvius may be stenotic, resulting in hydrocephalus. The corpus callosum is dysgenetic in 30% of patients, and there may be a dorsal interhemispheric cyst. Magnetic resonance (MR), which is the imaging modality of choice, also readily demonstrates other associated anomalies (Fig. 3.05-2).

The Dandy-Walker variant represents the midpoint in the complex (Fig. 3.05-3). In these patients there is mild hypoplasia of the inferior vermis. A prominent cisterna magna communicates through an enlarged vallecula with a moderately dilated fourth ventricle. Supratentorially, only hydrocephalus appears to be a constant anomaly.

The mildest form of Dandy-Walker complex is the mega cisterna magna. In these cases, the vermis and fourth ventricle are normal (Fig. 3.05-4). The cisterna magna is larger than usual and may extend superior to the vermis, flatten the dorsal vermis slightly, and scallop the inner table of the occipital bone. It should be differentiated from an arachnoid cyst, with which there is deformity and compression of the fourth ventricle (Figs. 3.05-5–3.05–7). Also, the mega cisterna magna is usually crossed by linear areas of low signal intensity on MR imaging. These represent veins and the falx cerebelli, and they are not present with arachnoid cysts.

All three anomalies may be grouped under the heading of "Dandy-Walker complex" because the prognosis of the patients is not related to the posterior fossa malformations, but rather to the supratentorial anomalies and the control of hydrocephalus.

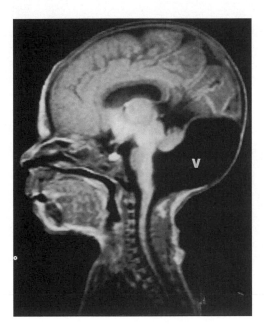

FIGURE 3.05-1.

Dandy-Walker complex, full spectrum.
Midsagittal magnetic resonance T1-weighted image in a newborn shows a markedly dilated fourth ventricle (v) that balloons out of the posterior fossa. Only the superior-most portions of the cerebellar vermis are present and are rotated anteriorly and superiorly. The venous torcular inserts high. The corpus callosum appears to be intact and there is mild hydrocephalus. The pituitary gland is bright, a normal finding at this age.

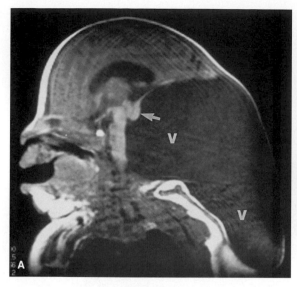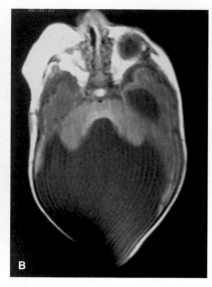

FIGURE 3.05-2.

Dandy-Walker complex and encephalocele. **A.** Midsagittal magnetic resonance (MR) T1-weighted image shows that the dilated fourth ventricle (v) is herniated posteriorly and inferiorly through a cephalocele. Note hypoplastic and upwardly rotated vermis *(arrow).* **B.** Axial MR T1-weighted image shows the posterior cerebrospinal fluid collection to be contiguous with a large fourth ventricle. The cerebellar hemispheres are hypoplastic. The temporal tip of the left lateral ventricle is dilated. This encephalocele was resected and its interior was found to be lined by ependyma, confirming that it is the fourth ventricle.

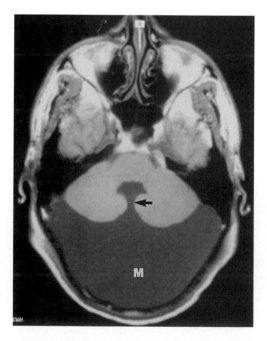

FIGURE 3.05-3.

Dandy-Walker complex, moderate anomalies (previously known as Dandy-Walker variant). Axial magnetic resonance T1-weighted image shows very large posterior cerebrospinal fluid collection (M) (possibly the cisterna magna) that communicates through an enlarged vallecula *(arrow)* with the fourth ventricle. The cerebellar hemispheres are small.

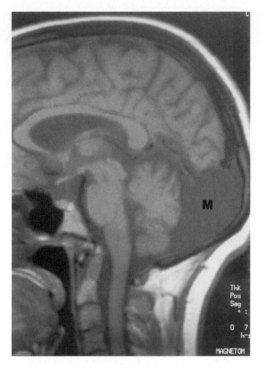

FIGURE 3.05-4.

Mega cisterna magna. Midsagittal magnetic resonance T1-weighted image shows large retrovermian cerebrospinal fluid collection (M) scalloping the occipital bone and mildly flattening the dorsal vermis. There is no mass effect on the fourth ventricle and no hydrocephalus. The vermis is well formed. The anomaly is presumed to be a mega cisterna magna rather than a true arachnoid cyst.

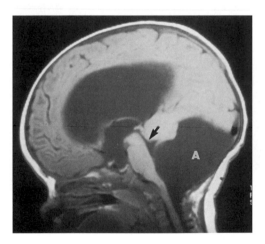

FIGURE 3.05-5.

Arachnoid cyst simulating Dandy-Walker complex. Midsagittal magnetic resonance T1-weighted image shows a very large arachnoid cyst (A) in the posterior fossa simulating Dandy-Walker complex. Note intact fourth ventricle *(arrow)* and cerebellar vermis pushed superiorly by the cyst. There is marked hydrocephalus with intrasellar herniation of the third ventricle and dilation of the lateral ventricles.

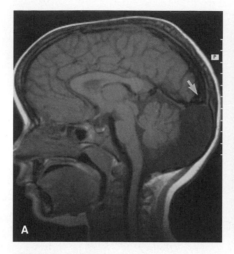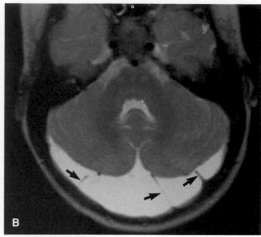

FIGURE 3.05-6.

Mild Dandy-Walker versus mega cisterna magna. **A.** Midsagittal magnetic resonance (MR) T1-weighted image shows large cerebrospinal fluid collection posterior to a well formed cerebellar vermis. Note high position of venous torcular *(arrow)*. **B.** Axial MR T2-weighted image in same patient shows subarachnoid septations *(arrows)* crossing the cisterna magna. If this were an arachnoid cyst, these septations would be displaced.

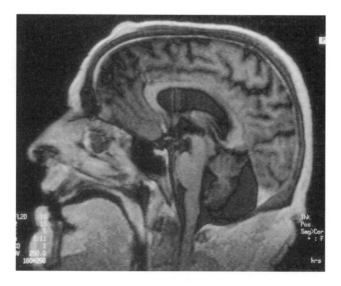

FIGURE 3.05-7.

Autism. Midsagittal magnetic resonance T1-weighted gradient echo image shows agenesis of the posterior lobules of the cerebellum in a patient with autism. The cisterna magna is therefore large. Note the normally shaped fourth ventricle.

SUGGESTED READINGS

1. Barkovich AJ, Kjos BO, Edwards MS. Revised classification of posterior fossa cysts and cystlike malformations based on the results of multiplanar MR imaging. AJNR 1989;10:977.
2. Altman NR, Naidich TP, Braffman BH. Posterior fossa malformations. AJNR 1992; 13:691.
3. Kollias SS, Ball WS, Prenger EC. Cystic malformations of the posterior fossa: differential diagnosis clarified through embryologic analysis. RadioGraphics 1993;13: 1211.
4. deSouza N, Chaudhuri R, Cox BT. MRI in cerebellar hypoplasia. Neuroradiology 1994;36:148.

3.06 *Joubert Syndrome*

EPIDEMIOLOGY

Joubert syndrome is an anomaly pathologically characterized by agenesis of the cerebellar vermis. The incidence of this syndrome is unknown, but it appears to be very rare. Its mode of inheritance is autosomal recessive. Boys are affected more often than girls. Isolated, nonhereditable vermian agenesis may be asymptomatic and is not considered as Joubert syndrome. Joubert syndrome may occur in association with the Dandy-Walker complex, occipital cephaloceles, or both. The cerebellar hypoplasia seen in Werdnig-Hoffman disease may be related to Joubert syndrome.

CLINICAL FEATURES

The typical clinical presentation of Joubert syndrome includes neonatal hyperpnea alternating with apnea, abnormal eye movements, ataxia, and developmental delay. Other clinical manisfestations include hypotonia, decreased deep tendon reflexes, incoordination, tremor, truncal ataxia, hemifacial spasms, syndactyly, reduced visual acuity, retinal abnormalities, and multicystic kidneys. Clinically, these children may fall into the category of oculomotor apraxia. The typical eye findings are dysmetric saccades, impairment of smooth pursuit, and optokinetic nystagmus. These symptoms are probably related to abnormalities in the vermis and brain stem nuclei. No treatment is available.

IMAGING FEATURES

Magnetic resonance imaging demonstrates the abnormality well. The cerebellar vermis may be completely absent or partially agenetic (particularly its posterior lobules). On axial images, the posterior surface of the cerebellar hemispheres is medially indented and communicates with a prominent vallecula (Fig. 3.06-1). The cerebellar hemispheres may be smooth secondary to dysplasia of the cerebellar cortex. The fourth ventricle is high riding, prominent, and indented posteriorly by the medial cerebellar hemispheres. It has a "batwing" appearance. The superior cerebellar peduncles are elongated, thin, and project straight back. They also appear parallel with each other. Contrary to normal children, the superior cerebellar peduncles are easily seen in children with Joubert syndrome. The inferior cerebellar peduncles are very small. Hydrocephalus is not present. On sagittal images, the roof of the fourth ventricle is superiorly convex. The inferior aspect of the aqueduct of Sylvius is stretched. The vermian folia are absent or hypoplastic. An occipital meningocele or meningoencephalocele may be present. A mega cisterna magna or full Dandy-Walker complex may occasionally be seen. Other findings include dysgenesis of the corpus callosum and cerebral atrophy.

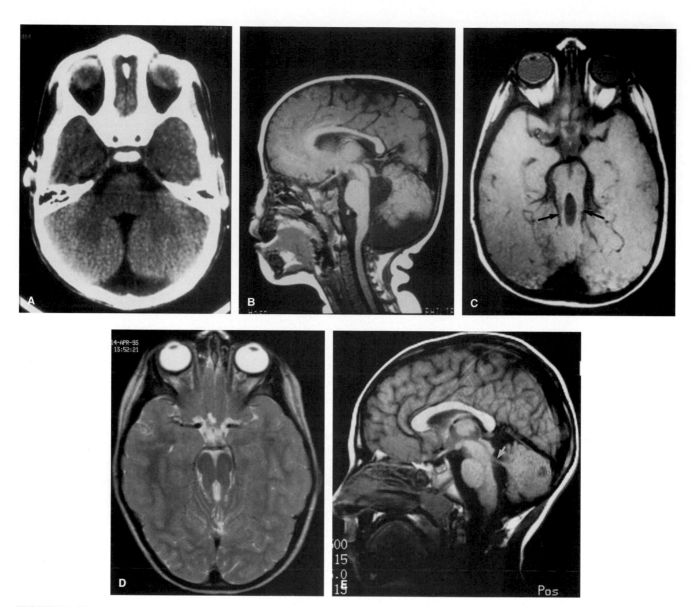

FIGURE 3.06-1.

Joubert syndrome.   **A.** Axial computed tomography shows abnormally shaped fourth ventricle that communicates with a large vallecula. The cisterna magna is slightly prominent and the dorsomedial borders of the cerebellar hemispheres are rounded. The vermis is not present. **B.** Midsagittal magnetic resonance (MR) T1-weighted image shows absent cerebellar vermis with a superiorly placed and enlarged fourth ventricle. The rostral fourth ventricle is convex superiorly. The brain stem is somewhat small. **C.** Axial MR T1-weighted image in a different patient shows elongation of the superior fourth ventricle and straightening of the superior cerebellar peduncles *(arrows)*, which are parallel to each other. No vermis is present. **D.** Axial MR T2-weighted image in a different patient again shows small and parallel superior cerebellar peduncles. The superior aspect of the fourth ventricle is elongated. The cerebral peduncles are small. Note midline approximation of the cerebellar hemispheres due to lack of vermis. **E.** Midsagittal MR T1-weighted image shows absent cerebellar vermis with a mildly prominent fourth ventricle that has a convex upper border. The superior cerebellar peduncles *(arrow)* are thin and long. All of these findings are encountered in patients with oculomotor apraxia, which anatomically may be a variant of Joubert syndrome. (With permission from Witzel E, Castillo M, D'Cruz O. Congenital oculomotor apraxia: MR imaging. AJNR, 1995;16:831.)

SUGGESTED READING

1. Altman NR, Naidich TP, Braffman BH. Posterior fossa malformations. AJNR 1992; 13:691.

3.07 *Rhombencephalosynapsis*

EPIDEMIOLOGY

Rhombencephalosynapsis is a malformation characterized by agenesis of the cerebellar vermis and midline fusion of the hemispheres. Its incidence is unknown, but it is a very rare abnormality. It is not known to be associated with any specific syndromes. In one case, an anomaly involving chromosome 2q was found.

CLINICAL FEATURES

Most patients present with developmental delay, abnormal equilibrium, and seizures. Other symptoms include convergent strabismus, optic nerve atrophy, spastic quadriparesis, behavioral disorders, dysarthria, and apraxia. Most cases are encountered early in life, but some may also be found in older (30–40 years of age) patients. Life expectancy is variable, but most patients die in infancy or childhood.

IMAGING FEATURES

Magnetic resonance (MR) is the imaging modality that best demonstrates this anomaly. The cerebellar vermis is completely absent and there is midline fusion of hemispheres (Fig. 3.07-1). The dentate nuclei are also fused. On axial MR images, the folia and sulci are continuous across the entire width of the cerebellum, producing a characteristic appearance. The size of the fourth ventricle is variable and axial images usually show it to have a "keyhole" shape. This appearance is the result of dorsal and rostral convergence of the dentate nuclei, cerebellar peduncles, and the inferior colliculi. The tectum is deformed and often fused. On sagittal images, the fourth ventricle is located higher than usual and has a convex upper border. The brain stem may appear small. The tentorial incisura is wide. Supratentorially, abnormalities of sulcation, fusion of the cerebral peduncles, and fusion of the thalami may be found. The corpus callosum is often dysgenetic and thin and may be contiguous with the fornices, which also may be fused (Fig. 3.07-2). The hippocampi are hypoplastic and may produce enlargement of the temporal horns of the lateral ventricles, even in the absence of hydrocephalus. However, hydrocephalus is also a prominent finding in patients with rhombencephalosynapsis. Because the septum pellucidum is often absent and the optic chiasm may be hypoplastic, some investigators have associated rhombencephalosynapsis with septooptic dysplasia.

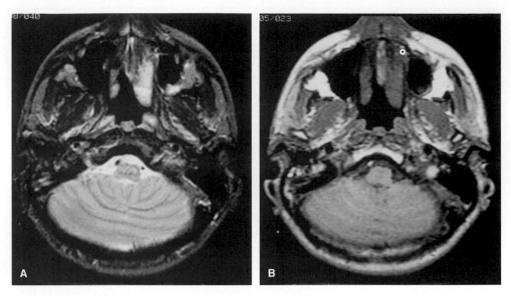

FIGURE 3.07-1.

Rhombencephalosynapsis. **A.** Axial magnetic resonance (MR) T2-weighted image shows absent vermis and midline fusion of the cerebellar hemispheres with continuation of the sulci and folia. **B.** Axial MR T1-weighted image in the same patient shows the absent vermis and vallecula. No supratentorial abnormalities were present in this case. (Case courtesy of Robert Tien, M.D., Duke University Medical Center, Durham, NC.)

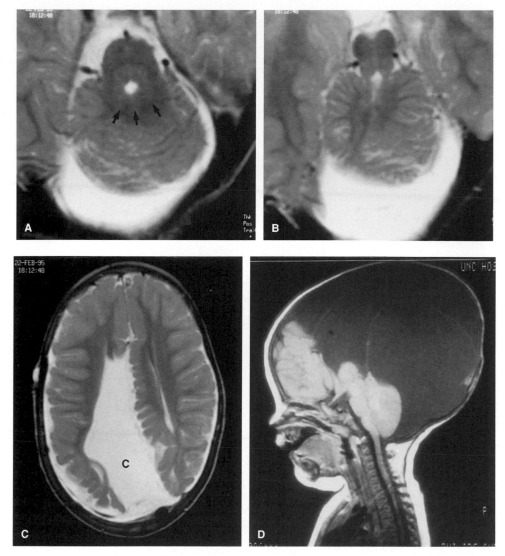

FIGURE 3.07-2.

Rhombencephalosynapsis with agenesis of the corpus callosum. **A.** Axial magnetic resonance (MR) T2-weighted image at mid-cerebellar level shows midline fusion of hemispheres and of the dentate nuclei *(arrow)*. **B.** Axial MR T2-weighted image in same patient, superior to (A), shows absent vermis, midline fusion, and small cerebellar size with large cerebrospinal fluid spaces. **C.** Axial MR T2-weighted image in same patient shows agenesis of corpus callosum and dorsal midline interhemispheric cyst (c). **D.** In the same patient, midsagittal MR T1-weighted image shows abnormally small cerebellum with absent vermis and fourth ventricle, agenesis of corpus callosum, and large interhemispheric cyst.

SUGGESTED READINGS

1. Truwit CL, Barkovich AJ, Shanahan R, Maroldo TV. MR imaging of rhobencephalosynapsis: report of three cases and review of the literature. AJNR 1991;12:957.
2. Simmons G, Damiano TR, Truwit CL. MRI and clinical findings in rhombencephalosynapsis. J Comput Assist Tomogr 1993;17:211.

Imaging of the Pediatric Head, Neck, and Spine
by Mauricio Castillo and Suresh K. Mukherji,
Lippincott-Raven Publishing, Philadelphia © 1996.

4

Metabolic and Degenerative Disorders

4.0 Congenital Disorders of the Pituitary Gland

EPIDEMIOLOGY

Congenital disorders of the pituitary gland may result from hypoplasia or agenesis of the pituitary gland, or ectopia of the posterior pituitary lobe. A familial form of central diabetes insipidus is known to exist. Table 4.0-1 lists the most common congenital disorders of the pituitary gland.

TABLE 4.0-1. **Common Congenital Disorders of the Pituitary Gland**

Disorder	Associated Anomalies
Absence or Hypoplasia	Agenesis of corpus callosum
	Anencephaly
	Sphenoidal cephalocele
	Septo-optic dysplasia
	Kallmann syndrome
	Hall-Pallister syndrome
	Polan syndrome
	Radiation injury
	CHARGE syndrome
	Holoprosencephaly
	Perinatal anoxia/ischemia
Ectopic Posterior Lobe	Median facial cleft syndrome
	Congenital hypopituitarism
	Poland syndrome
	Septo-optic dysplasia
	Holoprosencephaly
	Perinatal anoxia/ischemia

The pituitary gland may also be damaged during difficult breech deliveries or forceps extraction. Rare congenital sellar tumors such as teratoma, craniopharyngioma, Rathke's cleft cyst, and histiocytosis of Langerhans may compress and destroy the gland.

CLINICAL FEATURES

The most common symptoms of decreased pituitary function include hypothyroidism, hypogonadism, and hypoadrenalism (anterior lobe); and diabetes insipidus and growth hormone deficiency (posterior lobe).

Diabetes insipidus is characterized by excretion of large volumes of dilute urine. Approximately half of the cases of diabetes insipidus are congenital, and the remainder are the result of injury or surgery.

Pituitary dwarfism is characterized by short stature, slow growth, poor dentition, and delayed skeletal maturation. Males are affected more often than females. Up to 50% of these patients have a history of difficult delivery. In addition to involvement of the neurohypophysis, the anterior lobe may be defective in these patients.

IMAGING FEATURES

Magnetic resonance (MR) imaging is the ideal method to evaluate the hypofunctioning gland in the pediatric patient (Fig. 4.0-1A). The posterior lobe is seen as an area of increased T1 signal intensity in up to 90% of normal patients.

The bright posterior lobe is absent in all cases of central diabetes insipidus

(Fig. 4.0-1B,C). If a patient presents with polydipsia and polyuria but has a normal bright posterior lobe on MR imaging, the nephrogenic type of the disease should be suspected. Patients with primary polydipsia also have a normal bright posterior lobe on MR imaging. Very rarely, patients with defects in the hypothalamic osmoreceptors may have central diabetes insipidus with a normal-appearing gland by MR imaging. The ectopic posterior lobe may compensate completely for hormonal production, and some of these patients may be endocrinologically normal.

Patients with pituitary dwarfism have a hypoplastic sella, an absent or very small anterior lobe, hypoplasia or partial absence of the stalk, and an ectopic posterior lobe. All of the above findings are seen in almost 50% of patients with pituitary dwarfism. Birth trauma is an important predisposing factor. In some patients, the pituitary gland has a normal MR appearance. The pituitary gland can also be abnormal in some systemic disorders such as hemochromatosis (Fig. 4.0-2).

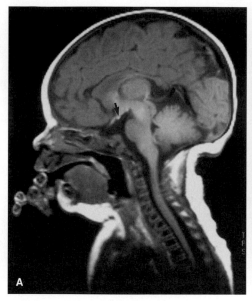

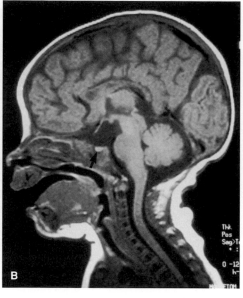

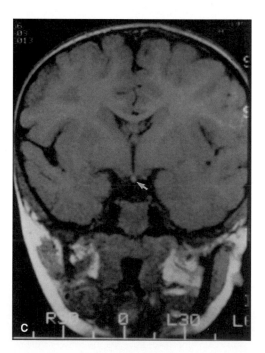

FIGURE 4.0-1.

Congenital absence of the pituitary stalk. **A.** Midsagittal magnetic resonance (MR) T1-weighted image in a patient born via breech delivery and with panhypopituitarism but no diabetes insipidus. The intrasellar portion of the gland and stalk is absent. The posterior lobe *(arrow)* is translocated to the lower hypothalamus. The possible responsible mechanism is infarction of the stalk. **B.** Midsagittal MR T1-weighted image in a newborn via breech delivery shows absent stalk, presence of the adenohypophysis (which is bright, *arrow*), and absence of the posterior lobe. This patient had diabetes insipidus. In newborns, the anterior pituitary lobe may be normally bright on T1-weighted images presumably due to increased hormone production. **C.** Coronal MR T1-weighted image in a patient with panhypopituitarism but no history of trauma. The adenohypophysis is absent and the neurohypophysis *(arrow)* is translocated. The septum pellucidum is present, excluding septo-optic dysplasia.

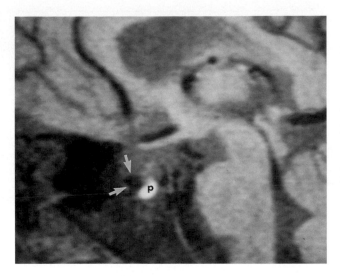

FIGURE 4.0-2.

Hemochromatosis of the pituitary gland. Midsagittal magnetic resonance T1-weighted image in a young patient with sickle cell anemia; note very dark signal intensity in the adenohypophysis *(arrows)* due to hemochromatosis. The posterior lobe (p) is present. This patient had hormonal deficiencies involving those secreted by the anterior lobe.

SUGGESTED READINGS

1. Abrahams JJ, Trefelner E, Boulware SD. Idiopathic growth hormone deficiency: MR findings in 35 patients. AJNR 1991;12:155.
2. Kuroiwa T, Okabe Y, Hasuo K, Yasumori K, Mizushima A, Masuda K. MR imaging of pituitary dwarfism. AJNR 1991;12:161.
3. Sato N, Ishizaka H, Yagi H, Matsumoto M, Endo K. Posterior lobe of the pituitary in diabetes insipidus: dynamic MR imaging. Radiology 1993;186:357.
4. Fujisawa I, Kikuchi K, Nishimura K, et al. Transection of the pituitary stalk: development of an ectopic posterior lobe assessed with MR imaging. Radiology 1987;165:487.
5. Detrich RB, Lis LE, Greensite FS, Pitt D. Normal MR appearance of the pituitary gland in the first 2 years of life. AJNR 1995;16:1413.

4.01 *Amino Acid Disorders*

EPIDEMIOLOGY

Amino acid disorders may arise from either a deficiency of an enzyme or a defect in their transport, usually at the level of the bowel or kidneys. Table 4.01-1 describes the genetic characteristics of the most common aminoacidopathies.

CLINICAL AND IMAGING FEATURES

Table 4.01-2 lists the clinical and imaging features of the more common aminoacidopathies.

TABLE 4.01-1. Genetic Characteristics of Aminoacidopathies

Disorder	Genetics	Deficiency
Phenylketonuria	1:14,000 Newborns, greater incidence in blacks and Jews, mutation in chromosome 12	Phenylalanine hydroxylase, dihydropteridine reductase, coenzyme tetrahydrobiopterin
Tyrosinemia	Rare, autosomal recessive	p-Hydroxyphenylpyruvic acid oxydase
Maple syrup urine disease	1:500,000 Newborns, autosomal recessive	Block in catabolic pathways involving alpha-keto-isovalerate (valine), alpha-keto-beta-methylvalerate (isoleucine), and alpha-keto-isocaproate (leucine)
Homocystinuria	Rare, autosomal recessive	Mostly due to deficiency of cystathionine beta-synthase
Methylmalonic acidemia	Unknown	Methylmalonyl-CoA mutase
Glutaric acidemia	Unknown	Glutaryl-CoA dehydrogenase (type 1) and acyl-CoA dehydrogenases (type 2)
Leigh disease	Unknown	Cytochrome c oxidase, ?thiamine pyrophosphate-ATP* phosphoryl transferase
Lesch-Nyhan disease	X-linked	Hypoxanthine-guanine phosphoribosyltransferase
Hartnup disease	Very rare, autosomal recessive	Error in transport of monoaminomonocarboxylic amino acids affecting renal tubular resorption and intestinal absorption
Lowe (oculocerebrorenal) syndrome	X-linked recessive (Xq25–q26)	Unknown

* ATP, adenosine triphosphate.

TABLE 4.01-2. Clinical and Imaging Features of Aminoacidopathies

Disorder	Clinical Features	Imaging Features
Phenylketonuria	Normal at birth, irritability, developmental delay (esp. language), vomiting, eczema, seizures, spasticity, tremor	Microcephaly, white matter abnormalities, atrophy (Fig. 4.01-1)
Tyrosinemia	Mental retardation, diarrhea, vomiting, polyneuropathy, liver failure	No specific findings
Maple syrup urine disease	Somnolence, seizures, spasticity, hypoglycemia, developmental delay	Heterotopias, cortical dysplasias, white matter abnormalities, high T2 signal intensity in occipital white matter, posterior limb internal capsule, dorsal brain stem, and cerebellum
Homocystinuria	Osteoporosis, scoliosis, pes planus, arachnodactyly, glaucoma, cataracts, retinal degeneration, thromboembolic events, myocardial infarcts, mental retardation	Arterial and/or venous thrombosis with infarcts
Methylmalonic acidemia	Vomiting, hypotonia, altered consciousness, lactic acidosis, pancytopenia	Atrophy, delayed myelination, abnormally high T2 signal in globus pallidus (identical findings are seen in propionic acidemia)
Glutaric acidemia	Mental retardation, dystonia, choreoathetosis, acidosis, seizures, ketoacidosis	Atrophy, severe underdevelopment of temporal operculae, involvement of U-fibers
Leigh disease	Swallowing and feeding difficulties, hypotonia, weakness, ataxia, peripheral neuropathy, external ophthalmoplegia, loss of vision, hearing loss, seizures	Abnormally high T2 signal intensity in putamen, caudate and dentate nuclei, tectum, tegmentum, medullary olives, and cerebral white matter (Fig. 4.01-2)
Lesch-Nyhan disease	Hyperuricemia, mental retardation, choreoathetosis, compulsive self-mutilation	Atrophy
Hartnup disease	Ataxia, double vision, tremor, spasticity, nystagmus, dystonia, headaches, mood instabilities	Atrophy (esp. occipital), white matter abnormalities (Fig. 4.01-3)
Lowe (oculocerebrorenal) syndrome	Frontal bossing, hypotonia, microcephaly, cataracts, blindness, nystagmus, rickets	Periventricular white matter cystic abnormalities

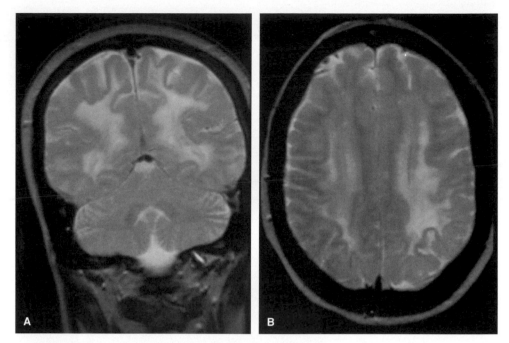

FIGURE 4.01-1.

Phenylketonuria. **A.** Coronal magnetic resonance (MR) T1-weighted image in a young patient with phenylketonuria that was not recognized at birth (no screening done) shows hyperintensities in the white matter and mild cortical atrophy. **B.** Axial MR T2-weighted image shows white matter hyperintensities in the centrum semiovale bilaterally. (With permission from Castillo M. Neuroradiology Companion. Philadelphia: JB Lippincott, 1995.)

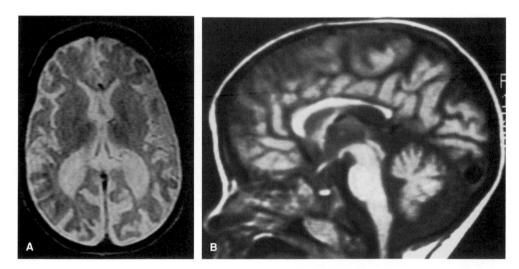

FIGURE 4.01-2.

Hartnup disease. **A.** Axial magnetic resonance (MR) T2-weighted image in a patient with Hartnup disease shows significant atrophy that is somewhat more prominent in the occipital regions. Myelination is delayed. **B.** Midsaggital MR T1-weighted image shows diffuse atrophy that is more pronounced in the occipital lobes, and thinning of the posterior aspects of the corpus callosum. (With permission from Erly W, Castillo M, Foosaner D, Bonmatic C. Hartnup's disease: MR findings. AJNR 1992;12:1026.)

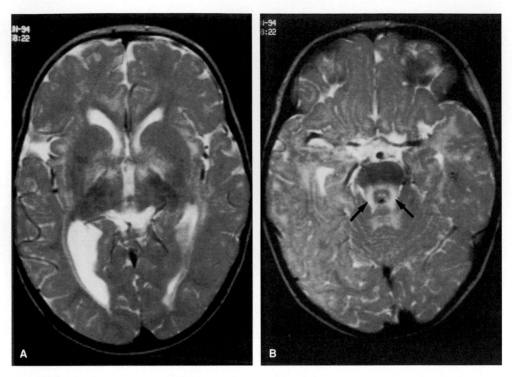

FIGURE 4.01-3.

Leigh disease. **A.** Axial magnetic resonance (MR) T2-weighted image in a patient with Leigh disease shows abnormal hyperintensity in the globus pallidi, genu of internal capsules–thalami, and in the subinsular regions. The cerebrospinal fluid spaces are prominent. **B.** Axial MR T2-weighted image shows abnormally high signal intensity in the dorsal midbrain *(arrows)*.

SUGGESTED READINGS

1. van der Knaap MS, Ross B, Valk J. Uses of MR in inborn errors of metabolism. In: Kucharczyk J, Moseley M, Barkovich AJ, eds. Magnetic Resonance Neuroimaging. Boca Raton, FL: CRC Press, 1994:245.
2. Brismar J, Ozand PT. CT and MR of the brain in disorders of the propionate and methylmalonate metabolism. AJNR 1994;15:1459.
3. Swaiman KF. Aminoacidopathies or organic acidemias resulting from deficiency of enzyme activity. In: Swaiman KF, ed. Pediatric Neurology, 2nd ed. St. Louis: Mosby, 1994:1195.
4. Swaiman KF. Diseases resulting from amino acid transport defects. In: Swaiman KF, ed. Pediatric Neurology, 2nd ed. St. Louis: Mosby, 1994:1243.
5. Andreula CF, DeBlai R, Carella A. CT and MR studies of methylmalonic acidemia. AJNR 1991;12:410.
6. Brismar J, Ozand P. CT and MR of the brain in glutaric acidemia type I: a review of 59 published cases and a report of 5 new patients. AJNR 1995;16:675.

4.02 *Lysosomal Disorders*

EPIDEMIOLOGY

Lysosomal disorders are characterized by abnormal accumulation of normal substrates (lipids, mucopolysaccharides, glycoproteins, and glycogen) and their metabolites inside the lysosomes. Tables 4.02-1 through 4.02-3 summarize the genetics and deficiencies responsible for the most common lysosomal disorders.

TABLE 4.02-1. *Genetics and Deficiencies of the GM_2 Gangliosidoses*

Disorder	Genetics	Deficiency
Tay-Sachs disease	Autosomal recessive, 80% of patients have Jewish ancestry	Accumulation of GM_2 ganglioside due to deficiency of hexosaminidase A
Juvenile (partial) GM_2 gangliosidosis	Unknown	Hexosaminidase A
Adult-onset GM_2 gangliosidosis	Familial disorder, more common in Jews	Deficient or absent hexosaminidase A
Sandhoff disease	Familial disorder, more common in Jews, Mexicans, and Central Americans	Abnormal storage of GM_2, asialo GM_2, and globoside due to deficiency of hexosaminidase A and B

TABLE 4.02-2. *Genetics and Deficiencies of Other Gangliosidoses*

Disorder	Genetics	Deficiency
GM_1 gangliosidosis	Probably familial	GM_1 beta-galactosidase
GM_3 gangliosidosis	Unknown	GM_1, GM_2, and N-acetylgalactosaminyl transferase
Fabry disease	Defect in long arm of X chromosome	Gamma-galactosidase A impairing final cleavage of galactose
Niemann-Pick disease	All four types are autosomal recessive	Group A: sphingomyelinase Groups B, C, D, and E: sphingomyelinase is normal or almost normal, exact deficiency is uncertain
Krabbe disease	Autosomal recessive, defect probably in chromosome 14	Galactocerebroside beta-galactosidase
Gaucher disease	Autosomal recessive, more common in Ashkenazi Jews	Glucocerebrosidase
Metachromatic leukodystrophy	Autosomal recessive, probable abnormality in chromosome 22	Arylsulfatase-A

TABLE 4.02-3. Genetics and Deficiencies of the Mucopolysaccharidoses

Disorder	Genetics	Deficiency
Hurler syndrome (MPS₁)*	Autosomal recessive	Alpha-L-iduronidase, dermatan and heparan sulfates are stored
Scheie syndrome (MPS₁)	Autosomal recessive	Alpha-L-iduronidase, dermatan and heparan sulfates are stored
Hunter syndrome (MPS₂)*	X-linked (long arm of X chromosome)	Iduronate-2-sulfatase, dermatan and heparan sulfates are stored
Sanfilippo syndrome	Autosomal recessive	Group A: heparan-*N*-sulfate Group B: *N*-acetyl-alpha-D-glucosamide Group C: Acetyl-CoA-alpha-glucosaminide-*N*-acetyl transferase Group D: *N*-acetyl-alpha-D-glucosamine-6-sulfatase, in all heparan sulfate is stored
Morquio syndrome	Autosomal recessive	Group A: *N*-acetyl-galactosamine-6-sulfatase and galactose-6-sulfate sulfatase, keratan and chondroitin sulfates are stored Group B: beta-galactosidase, keratan sulfate is stored

* Most common mucopolysaccharidoses.
Other mucopolysaccharidoses, such as MPS₄ and MPS₇, multiple sulfatase deficiency, Maroteaux-Lamy syndrome, beta-glucoronidase deficiency, and the mucolipidoses are not reviewed here because they are extremely rare.

TABLE 4.02-4. Clinical and Imaging Features of the GM₂ Gangliosidoses

Disorder	Clinical Features	Imaging Features
Tay-Sachs disease	Exquisite sensitivity to noise, hypotonia, blindness (cherry spot in macula), seizures	Megalencephaly, involvement of basal ganglia (esp. head of caudate nuclei), calcification in thalami, white matter abnormalities
Juvenile (partial) GM₂ gangliosidosis	Seizures, progressive dementia, dystonia, visual abnormalities	Macrocephaly, demyelination, gliosis, late atrophy
Adult-onset GM₂ gangliosidosis	Ataxia, spasticity, dystonia, muscular atrophy, behavioral problems, choreoathetosis	Atrophy (esp. cerebellar)
Sandhoff disease	Cherry spot in macula, decerebrated rigidity, cardiomyopathy, ataxia, megalencephaly, slurred speech, intellectual impairment, spasticity	Atrophy

CLINICAL AND IMAGING FEATURES

Severe impairment of the hydrolytic enzymatic system (residual function less than 10%) is needed before patients become overtly symptomatic. Tables 4.02-4 through 4.02-6 summarize the clinical and imaging features of the most common lysosomal disorders.

TABLE 4.02-5. Clinical and Imaging Features of Other Gangliosidoses

Disorder	Clinical Features	Imaging Features
GM$_1$ gangliosidosis	Edema and hypertrophy of soft tissues, corneal opacities, developmental delay, kyphoscoliosis, seizures, blindness, deafness, spasticity, decerebrated rigidity	Macrocephaly, white matter abnormalities (Fig. 4.02-1)
GM$_3$ gangliosidosis	Seizures, thickened soft tissues	Macrocephaly, white matter abnormalities, delayed myelination
Fabry disease	Cutaneous lesions (angiokeratoma corporis diffusum universale), lens opacities, blindness, burning pain in extremities, myocardial infarction, aortic stenosis, mitral insufficiency, thrombotic central nervous system events, renal failure	Infarctions in white matter, basal ganglia, and thalami, white matter may be diffuse and confluent, atrophy
Niemann-Pick disease	Organomegaly, progressive intellectual and motor deterioration, seizures, peripheral neuropathy, severe hepatic disease	Demyelination and gliosis, atrophy
Krabbe disease	Irritability, vomiting, seizures, increased muscular tone, opisthotonos, blindness, deafness	Macrocephaly, by CT high density in thalami, cerebellum, corona radiata, brain stem, and head of caudate nuclei; white matter abnormalities (esp. parietal), atrophy abnormalities in cerebellum, optic nerve hypertrophy, CT may be normal initially
Gaucher disease	Strabismus, increased muscle tone, dysphagia, motor retardation, seizures, splenohepatomegaly, anemia, thrombocytopenia, leukopenia	Focal infarctions, focal hemorrhages, atrophy
Metachromatic leukodystrophy	Painful polyneuropathy, ataxia, spastic tetraparesis, progressive retardation, dementia	Symmetric white matter abnormalities with sparing of subcortical U-fibers, atrophy (Fig. 4.02-2)

CT, computed tomography.

TABLE 4.02-6. *Clinical and Imaging Features of the Mucopolysaccharidoses*

Disorder	Clinical Features	Imaging Features
Hurler syndrome (MPS₁)	Coarse facial features, glaucoma, gait abnormalities, lumbar lordosis, thoracic kyphosis, contractures of knees/elbows, deafness, heart valve disease, hepatosplenomegaly, dwarfism	Macrocrania, dilated perivascular spaces, thick dura and skull, communicating hydrocephalus, dolicocephalic appearance (Fig. 4.02-3A,B)
Scheie syndrome (MPS₁)	Restriction of joint movement, hirsutism, deafness, corneal opacity, retinitis pigmentosa, aortic insufficiency, carpal tunnel syndrome	Same as Hurler and Hunter syndromes, arachnoid cysts
Hunter syndrome (MPS₂)	Same as Hurler syndrome but less mental retardation, carpal tunnel syndrome	Same as Hurler syndrome, in the spine dural thickening may produce myelopathy (Fig. 4.02-3C)
Sanfilippo syndrome	Progressive intellectual deterioration, mild body abnormalities	Marked cortical atrophy, abnormal white matter, ?communicating hydrocephalus
Morquio syndrome	Deafness, mild corneal opacities, atlantoaxial subluxation and other ligamentous laxities, possible mental retardation	Hypoplasia or absent dens, thickened spinal dura producing cord compression, white matter abnormalities, widening of all cerebrospinal fluid spaces

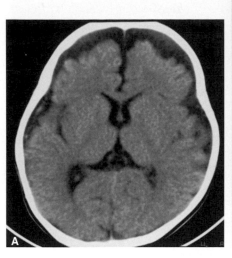
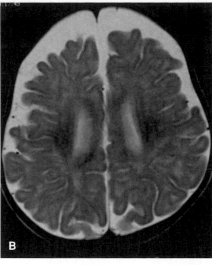
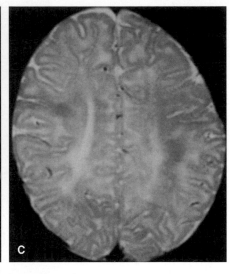

FIGURE 4.02-1.

Gangliosidosis. **A.** Axial noncontrast computed tomography scan in a patient with GM$_1$ disease shows atrophy and prominent cerebrospinal fluid spaces. Note thick meninges in right temporal region. **B.** Axial magnetic resonance (MR) T2-weighted image in a different patient with GM$_1$ disease shows diffusely increased signal intensity from the white matter (changes are more prominent in the posterior periventricular areas). **C.** Axial MR T2-weighted image in a different patient with GM$_1$ disease shows pronounced atrophy and abnormally increased signal intensity in white matter other than in the mid-portion of the centrum semiovale. The findings may be related to delayed myelination.

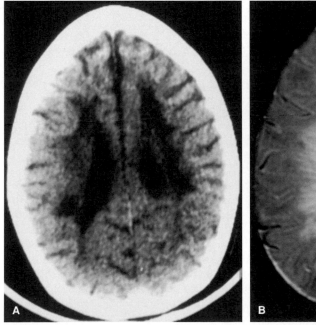
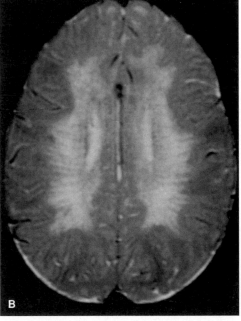

FIGURE 4.02-2.

Metachromatic leukodystrophy. **A.** Axial noncontrast computed tomography scan in a patient with metachromatic leukodystrophy shows symmetric low density in both centra semiovale. The abnormality does not extend to the subcortical white matter. **B.** Axial magnetic resonance T2-weighted image in a different patient with metachromatic leukodystrophy shows abnormal hyperintensity in white matter of both corona radiata and sparing of the subcortical U-fibers.

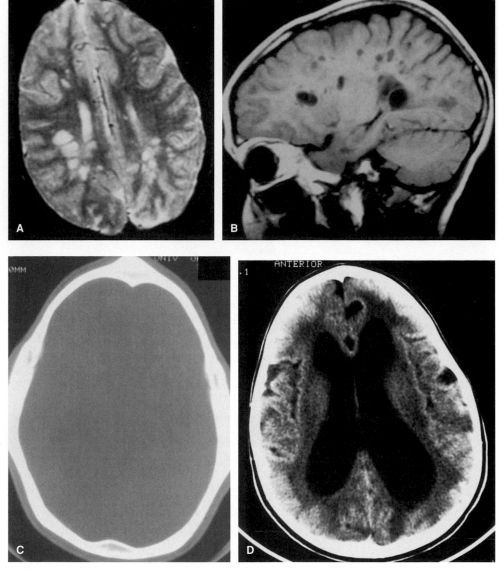

FIGURE 4.02-3.

Mucopolysaccharidosis. **A.** Axial magnetic resonance (MR) T2-weighted image in a patient with Hurler syndrome shows cystic areas in the periventricular white matter, especially posteriorly. These cysts are "radially" oriented with respect to the ventricles, following the course of the medullary veins. **B.** Parasagittal MR T1-weighted image in a different case of Hurler syndrome shows multiple white matter cysts. **C.** Axial computed tomography (CT) scan, bone windows, shows thick skull, absent diploic space, dolicocephaly, and frontal beak in this patient with Hunter syndrome. (With permission from Castillo M. Neuroradiology Companion. Philadelphia: JB Lippincott, 1995.) **D.** Axial CT scan in patient with MPS$_6$ shows mild dolicocephaly, hydrocephalus, diffuse white matter hypodensities, and prominent cortical sulci.

SUGGESTED READINGS

1. Kendall BE. Disorders of lysosomes, peroxisomes, and mitochondria. AJNR 1992;13: 621.
2. Hittmair K, Wimberger D, Wiesbauer P, Zehetmayer M, Budka H. Early infantile form of Krabbe disease with optic hypertrophy: serial MR examinations and autopsy correlation. AJNR 1994;15:1454.
3. Demaerel P, Wilms G, Verdu P, Caron H, Baert AL. MR findings in globoid cell leukodystrophy. Neuroradiology 1990;32:520.
4. Swaiman KF. Lysosomal diseases. In: Swaiman KF, ed. Pediatric Neurology, 2nd ed. St. Louis: Mosby, 1994:1275.
5. Finelli DA, Tarr RW, Sawyer RN, Horwitz SJ. Deceptively normal MR in early infantile Krabbe disease. AJNR 1994;15:167.

4.03 *Peroxisomal Disorders*

These disorders may be caused by a lack of normal development of the peroxisome or lack of function of its enzymes. Peroxisomal enzymes are found in abundance in the brain during myelinogenesis. The overall incidence of these disorders (as a group) is approximately 1:25,000 newborns. Tables 4.03-1 through 4.03-3 summarize the genetics and deficiencies associated with these disorders:

TABLE 4.03-1. Genetics and Deficiencies of Disorders Due to Abnormal Formation of Peroxisomes

Disorder	Genetics	Deficiency
Zellweger syndrome	Autosomal recessive, 1:30,000 live births	Uncertain
Neonatal ALD (NALD)	Autosomal recessive	Fatty acyl-CoA oxidase
Infantile Refsum disease	Autosomal recessive	Phytanic acid alpha-hydroxylase, resulting in accumulation of C20 branched-chain fatty acid (phytanic acid)
Hyperpipecolic acidemia	Autosomal recessive	Probably related to generalized peroxisomal dysfunction

ALD, adrenoleukodystrophy.

TABLE 4.03-2. **Genetics and Deficiencies Associated with Defects of Single Peroxisomal Enzymes**

Disorder	Genetics	Deficiency
X-linked ALD	X-linked (Xq28)	Excess of saturated unbranched VLCFA (C22–C30)
Acyl-CoA oxidase deficiency	Unknown, very rare	Peroxisomal beta-oxidation enzyme, leading to excretion of VLCFA
Bifunctional enzyme deficiency	Unknown, very rare	Probable deficiency of enoyl-CoA hydratase, leading to accumulation of VLCFA and bile acid intermediates
Thiolase deficiency	Unknown, very rare	3-Oxoacyl-CoA thiolase, leading to accumulation of VLCFA and bile acid intermediates
Acatalasemia	Probable defect in chromosome 11p13, more common in Japanese and Swiss	Catalase
Hyperoxaluria type 1	Autosomal recessive, 1–5 per 15 million newborns	Alanine glyoxylate aminotransferase, leading to increased urinary excretion of oxalate, glycolate, and glyoxyalate
Glutaryl-CoA oxidase deficiency	Unknown, very rare	Glutaryl-CoA oxidase, leading to accumulation of glutaric acid

ADL, adrenoleukodystrophy; VLCFA, very long-chain fatty acids.

TABLE 4.03-3. **Genetics and Deficiencies Associated with Multiple Peroxisomal Defects**

Disorder	Genetics	Deficiency
Rhizomelic chondrodysplasia punctata	Autosomal recessive, 1:84,000 live births	Impaired plasmologen synthesis, increased levels of phytanic acid, and presence of 3-oxoacyl-CoA thiolase in precursor form

CLINICAL AND IMAGING FEATURES

Tables 4.03-4 through 4.03-6 summarize the most common clinical and imaging features of these peroxisomal disorders.

TABLE 4.03-4. ***Clinical and Imaging Features of Disorders Due to Abnormal Formation of Peroxisomes***

Disorder	*Clinical Features*	*Imaging Features*
Zellweger syndrome	Mental retardation, weakness, hypotonia, renal cysts, liver insufficiency	Cortical dysplasias, pachyria, neuronal heterotopias, delayed myelination, gliosis, stippling of cartilages
Neonatal ALD (NALD)	Dysmorphism, hypotonia, poor feeding, enlarged liver, deafness, retinal pigmentary degeneration	Pachygyria, polymicrogyra, diffuse demyelination (may enhance), cerebellar atrophy and/or neuronal migration anomalies
Infantile Refsum disease	Peripheral neuropathy, abnormal myelination, skeletal dysplasia	Abnormal white matter, affected nerves may be enlarged
Hyperpipecolic acidemia	Progressive neurologic disease, hepatomegaly, retinopathy	Absent or delayed myelination

ADL, adrenoleukodystrophy.

TABLE 4.03-5. *Clinical and Imaging Features Associated with Defects of Single Peroxisomal Enzyme*

Disorder	Clinical Features	Imaging Features
X-linked ALD (and variants such as adrenomyeloneuropathy)	Boys, disorders of behavior, vision, and hearing; difficulty swallowing, seizures, fulminant in childhood, spastic paraparesis, impaired vibratory sense, bladder dysfunction	White matter abnormalities in peritrigonal regions, splenium of corpus callosum, medial and lateral geniculate ganglia, pyramidal tracts, atrophy of spinal cord (Fig. 4.03-1)
Acyl-CoA oxidase deficiency	Dysmorphism, hypotonia, feeding difficulties, neonatal seizures	Unknown
Bifunctional enzyme deficiency	Hypotonia, neonatal seizures	Cortical dysplasias, neuronal heterotopias
Thiolase deficiency	Liver cirrhosis, renal cysts, progressive neurologic disease, seizures	Demyelination, gliosis, neuronal heterotopias in cerebellum
Acatalasemia	Oral ulcers, aniridia, Wilms tumor, gonadoblastoma	Unknown
Hyperoxaluria type 1	Ataxia, peripheral neuropathy, urolithiasis, renal failure	No known brain findings, but possible increased bone density, renal stones, nephrocalcinosis

ADL, adrenoleukodystrophy.

TABLE 4.03-6. *Clinical and Imaging Features Associated with Multiple Peroxisomal Defects*

Disorder	Clinical Features	Imaging Features
Rhizomelic chondrodysplasia punctata	Midface hypoplasia, severe shortening of proximal limbs, icthyosis	Delayed myelination, demyelination (esp. occipital regions), progressive atrophy, coronal clefts in vertebral bodies, stippled epiphyses

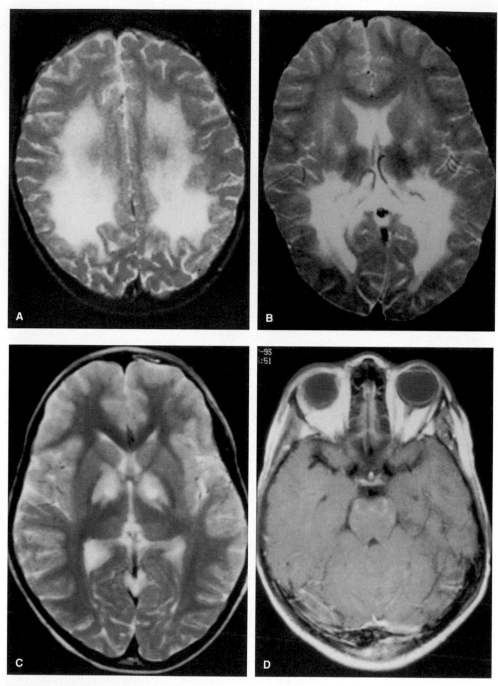

FIGURE 4.03-1.

Adrenoleukodystrophy.   **A.** Axial magnetic resonance (MR) T2-weighted image in a patient with advanced X-linked adrenoleukodystrophy shows marked hyperintensities in both centra semiovale, more prominent posteriorly. The abnormalities extend to the subcortical white matter. **B.** Axial MR T2-weighted image shows hyperintensities in the white matter of both occipitotemporal regions and in the genu of the internal capsules. (With permission from Castillo M. Neuroradiology Companion. Philadelphia: JB Lippincott, 1995.) **C.** Axial MR T2-weighted image in a patient with early X-linked adrenoleukodystrophy shows hyperintensities in the globus pallidus and internal capsules. These findings are usually present in the early disease. **D.** Axial postcontrast MR T1-weighted image in different patient with early X-linked adrenoleukodystrophy shows enhancement in the ventral superior pons in the region of the corticospinal tracts. This was the only abnormality in this patient with very early disease.

SUGGESTED READINGS

1. Naidu S, Moser H. Value of neuroimaging in metabolic disease affecting the CNS. AJNR 1991;12:413.
2. Kendall BE. Disorders of lysosomes, peroxisomes, and mitochondria. AJNR 1992;13:621.
3. Becker LE. Lysosomes, peroxisomes and mitochondria: function and disorder. AJNR 1992;13:609.
4. Naidu S, Moser H. Peroxisomal disorders. In: Swaiman KF, ed. Pediatric Neurology, 2nd ed. St. Louis: Mosby, 1994:1357.

4.04 Oxidative and Carbohydrate Metabolism Disorders

OXIDATIVE
METABOLISM
DISORDERS:
EPIDEMIOLOGY

Most cellular energy requirements are generated by oxidation of pyruvate, fatty acid, or ketone bodies via the citric acid cycle. Disorders involving this pathway result in metabolic acidosis, lactic acidemia, hypoglycemia, and hyperammonemia. The incidence of these disorders is not known.

CLINICAL FEATURES

Table 4.04-1 summarizes the clinical features of the most common oxidative metabolism disorders.

TABLE 4.04-1. *Symptoms of Oxidative Metabolism Disorders*

Disorder	Symptoms
Substrate transport defects (carnitine)	Myalgia, myoglobinuria, encephalopathy, cardiomyopathy, hypoglycemia, hypotonia
Pyruvate dehydrogenase complex deficiencies	Metabolic acidosis, lactic acidemia, ataxia, encephalopathy, Leigh syndrome, hypotonia, facial dysmorphism, developmental delay
Beta oxidation defects	Sudden infant death, Reye syndrome, hypoglycemia, hyperuricemia, vomiting, developmental delay, encephalopathy, cardiomyopathy, hyperammonemia, facial dysmorphism, polycystic kidneys
Glucogenesis defects	Metabolic acidosis, lactic acidemia, developmental delay, hepatomegaly, hyperammonemia, citrulinemia, hyperlysinemia, hypotonia, hyperlipidemia, epistaxis, granulocytopenia, recurrent infections
Multiple carboxylase deficiencies	Metabolic acidosis, lactic acidemia, alopecia, immunodeficiency
Citric acid cycle defects	Lactic acidemia, hypotonia, developmental delay
Respiratory chain abnormalities	Metabolic acidosis, lactic acidemia, Leigh syndrome, encephalopathy, hypotonia, myalgia, exercise intolerance, weakness, cardiomyopathy, renal tubulopathy, hepatopathy, ataxia, epilepsy

IMAGING FEATURES

Most oxidative metabolic disorders show cerebral edema, which may be generalized or focal. Infarctions may also occur. Areas of low attenuation (computed tomography) or abnormal hyperintensities (magnetic resonance [MR] T2-weighted images) in the basal ganglia, particularly the putamina, are not uncommon. Only one-fourth of patients will have positive imaging findings. Hydrogen MR spectroscopy may show elevated lactic acid (Fig. 4.04-1).

CARBOHYDRATE
METABOLISM
DISORDERS:
EPIDEMIOLOGY

The modes of inheritance and defects for the most common disorders of carbohydrate metabolism are summarized in Table 4.04-2.

TABLE 4.04-2. *Genetics and Deficiencies Associated with Disorders of Carbohydrate Metabolism*

Disorder	Genetics	Deficiency
Galactosemia	Autosomal recessive	Galactose-1-phosphate uridyltransferase
Fructose intolerance	Autosomal recessive, 1:20,000 newborns	Fructose-1-phosphate aldolase
Von Gierke disease	Autosomal recessive	Glucose-6-phosphatase
Pompe disease	Autosomal recessive, chromosome 17 (q21–q23)	Acid maltase
Forbes disease	Autosomal recessive (infantile type)	Debranching enzyme
Brancher enzyme deficiency disease	Autosomal recessive	Brancher enzyme
McArdle disease	Autosomal recessive	Myophosphorylase
Hers disease	Autosomal recessive, chromosome 14	Hepatophosphorylase
Tarui disease	Autosomal recessive	Muscle phosphofructokinase
Glycogen storage disease type IV	Autosomal recessive	Hepatic phosphorylase kinase

CLINICAL AND IMAGING FEATURES

Most of these disorders manifest similar clinical symptoms. These include mental retardation, seizures, hypotonia, weakness, growth retardation, myopathy, hyperlipidemia, hypoglycemia, cardiomegaly, hepatomegaly, cirrhosis, nephromegaly, swallowing and respiratory difficulties, and calf muscle hypertrophy.

Imaging findings are nonspecific, and often the brain is normal. Galactosemia may present with neonatal and generalized brain edema. Atrophy of the cerebral hemispheres and cerebellum as well as punctate white matter hyperintensities are noted in most patients. Diffuse high signal intensity throughout most of the hemispheric white matter is present in patients with galactosemia and no measurable transferase activity.

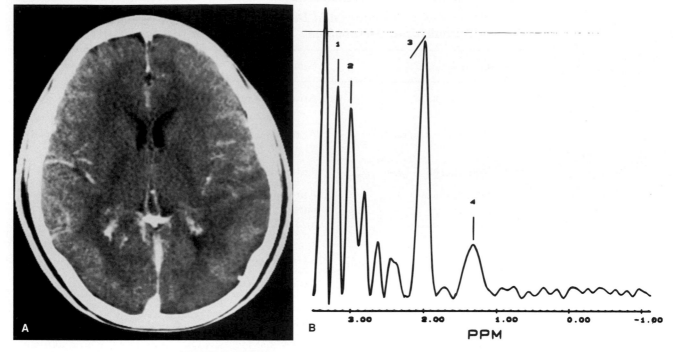

FIGURE 4.04-1.

Respiratory chain abnormality (possible MELAS [mitochondrial myopathy, encephalopathy, lactic acidosis, stroke-like episodes]). **A.** Axial postcontrast computed tomography is normal in this patient with transient ischemic attacks. **B.** Hydrogen magnetic resonance single-volume spectrum shows increased lactate (4) in left posterior temporal region (1, choline; 2, creatinine; 3, *n*-acetyl-aspartate).

SUGGESTED READINGS

1. Breningstall GN. Oxidative metabolism disorders. In: Swaiman KF, ed. Pediatric Neurology, 2nd ed. St. Louis: Mosby, 1994:309.
2. Swaiman KF. Diseases associated with primary abnormalities in carbohydrate metabolism. In: Swaiman KF, ed. Pediatric Neurology, 2nd ed. St. Louis: Mosby, 1994: 1249.
3. Spar JA, Lewine JD, Orrison WW. Neonatal hypoglycemia: CT and MR findings. AJNR 1994;15:1477.
4. Nelson MD, Wolff JA, Cross CA, Donnell GN, Kaufman FR. Galactosemia: evaluation with MR imaging. Radiology 1992;184:255.

4.05   *Mitochondrial Disorders*

EPIDEMIOLOGY

In mitochondrial disorders, enzymes involved in the respiratory chain, pyruvate metabolism and fatty acid oxidation are deficient. Table 4.05-1 summarizes the genetics and deficiencies found in the most most common mitochondrial disorders:

TABLE 4.05-1.   *Genetics and Deficiencies in Mitochondrial Disorders*

Disorder	Genetics	Deficiency
MELAS	Unknown, few familial cases reported	Specific mutation in mitochondrial tRNA
MERRF	Unknown	
Leigh syndrome	Autosomal recessive	Pyruvate dehydrogenase complex, pyruvate carboxylase, cytochrome C oxidase
Kearns-Sayre syndrome	Autosomal dominant	Elevated serum pyruvate
Alper disease	Unknown, some cases autosomal recessive	Cytochrome C oxidase, pyruvate cocarboxylase

MELAS, mitochondrial myopathy, encephalopathy, lactic acidosis, stroke-like episodes; MERRF, myoclonus, epilepsy, ragged red fibers.

Both clinical and imaging features for all of these disorders tend to overlap. Table 4.05-2 summarizes the most common clinical and imaging features for these disorders.

TABLE 4.05-2. *Clinical and Imaging Features of Mitochondrial Disorders*

Disorder	Clinical Features	Imaging Features
MELAS	Stroke-like episodes, strokes, lactic acidosis, migraines, vomiting, short stature, seizures	Areas of edema resolving spontaneously, infarcts, basal ganglia infarcts with calcifications, atrophy, hydrogen magnetic resonance (MR) spectroscopy (Fig. 4.05-1) may show lactate
MERRF	Myoclonic epilepsy, muscle weakness, short stature, cardiac conduction defects, endocrine deficiencies	Abnormalities of white matter, atrophy, multiple cortical and basal ganglia infarcts
Leigh syndrome	Ophthalmoplegia, extrapyramidal and cerebellar signs, spasticity, bulbar palsy	Abnormal MR T2 hyperintensity in globus pallidi, putamen, caudate, thalamus, periventricular and periaqueductal gray matter (Fig. 4.01-3)
Kearns-Sayre syndrome	Chronic progressive external ophthalmoplegia, pigementary retinal degeneration, heart block, limb weakness, elevated serum pyruvate	Diffuse abnormalities in white matter (including cerebellum and brain stem) and deep gray matter nuclei (Fig. 4.05-2)
Alper disease	Seizures, mental retardation, spasticity, liver failure, microcephaly	White matter abnormalities in occipitoparietal regions, with atrophy (Fig. 4.06-1)

MELAS, mitochondrial myopathy, encephalopathy, lactic acidosis, stroke-like episodes; MERRF, myoclonus, epilepsy, ragged red fibers.

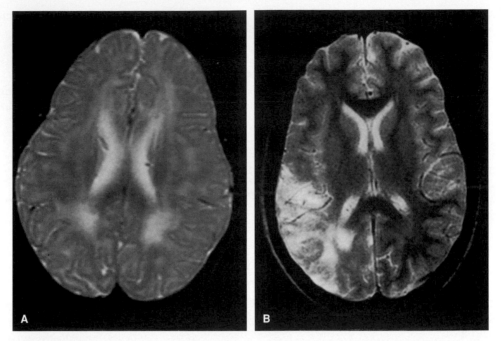

FIGURE 4.05-1.

MELAS. A. Axial magnetic resonance (MR) T2-weighted image in a patient with MELAS shows patchy periventricular white matter hyperintensities. **B.** Axial MR T2-weighted image in a different patient with MELAS shows a right posterior temporal occipital infarction. (With permission from Castillo M, Kwock L, Green C. MELAS syndrome: imaging and proton MR spectroscopic findings. AJNR 1995;16:233.)

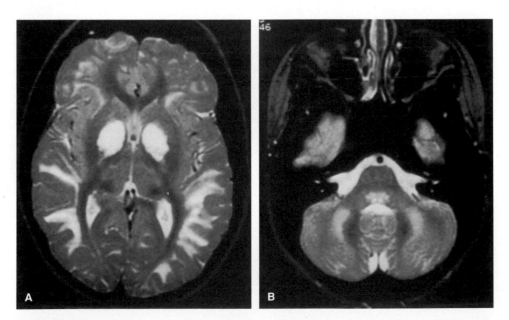

FIGURE 4.05-2.

Kearns-Sayre syndrome. A. Axial magnetic resonance (MR) T2-weighted image shows increased signal intensity in the globus pallidi and white matter (especially the posterior temporal and occipital regions). **B.** Axial MR T2-weighted image shows abnormal hyperintensities in the dorsal brain stem and the cerebellar white matter. There is mild cerebellar atrophy.

SUGGESTED READINGS

1. Davis PC, Hoffman JC, Braun IF, et al. MR of Leigh's disease (subacute necrotizing encephalomyelopathy). AJNR 1987;8:71.
2. Allard JC, Tilak S, Carter AP. CT and MR of MELAS syndrome. AJNR 1988;9:1234.
3. Demange P, Gia HP, Kalifa G, Sellier N. MR of Kearns-Sayre syndrome. AJNR 1989;10(S):91.
4. Barkovich AJ, Good WV, Koch TK, Berg BO. Mitochondrial disorders: analysis of their clinical and imaging characteristics. AJNR 1993;14:1119.

4.06 *Deep Gray Matter Nuclei Disorders: Alper Disease*

EPIDEMIOLOGY

Alper disease is also known as progressive neuronal degeneration of childhood or progressive infantile poliodystrophy. Its genetics are uncertain, but in some cases a matrilineal mode of inheritance has been described. Other cases are the result of an autosomal recessive trait. It is a very rare disorder (approximately 70 cases reported in the literature).

CLINICAL FEATURES

Alper disease is secondary to defects in cytochrome C oxidase, pyruvate cocarboxylase, and other deficiencies involving the mitochondrial electron transport chain. From animal experiments, a possible infectious cause (similar to that of Creutzfeldt-Jacob disease) has been suggested. The initial clinical presentation is seizures commencing during the first year of life. Mental deterioration and motor abnormalities become obvious soon thereafter. Flaccidity, hemiplegia, or spastic quadriparesis characterize the final stages of the disease. Death occurs within 3 years after the onset. Most patients show evidence of liver failure, but it has been suggested that hepatic abnormalities are not necessary to make the diagnosis of Alper disease. Cerebrospinal fluid is normal and the electroencephalogram (EEG) shows slow, high-amplitude activity mixed with low-amplitude polyspikes. Over 75% of patients show this EEG pattern, but in some cases it may be transient. Visual evoked potentials become progressively extinguished. On autopsy there is generalized atrophy with spongy degeneration of the cortex and neuronal loss particularly involving layers three and five. Necrosis of the hippocampi, lateral geniculate bodies, and the substantia nigra is present. The cerebellum and brain stem may be atrophic.

IMAGING FEATURES

Computed tomography shows areas of low density involving gray and white matter, especially in the parietooccipital regions. There is diffuse atrophy. On magnetic resonance (MR) imaging, the parieto-occipital regions may show a diminished amount of white matter, delayed myelination, and thinning of the cortex (Fig. 4.06-1). In our experience, disproportionate atrophy involving the occipital lobes is usually present. MR T2-weighted images also show abnormal hyperintensities in the caudate nuclei and the thalami (similar to mitochondrial disorders).

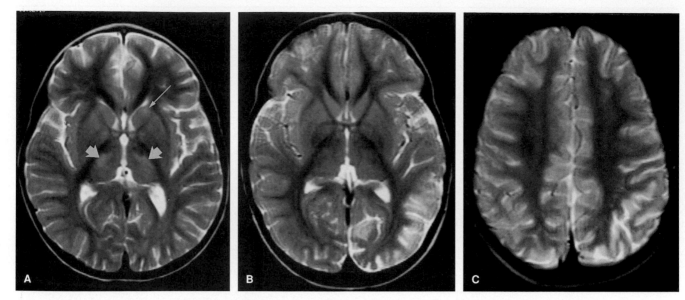

FIGURE 4.06-1.

Alper disease.   **A.** Axial magnetic resonance (MR) T2-weighted image shows focal hyperintensities in the head of the left caudate nucleus *(long arrow)* and in the lateral thalami *(short arrows)* in a patient with Alper disease. There is mild atrophy. **B.** Axial MR T2-weighted image in a different patient with Alper disease shows atrophy in the left occipital lobe. In this region, the cortex is abnormally bright. **C.** Axial MR T2-weighted image in same patient shows bilateral posterior parietal atrophy (left more than right) and hyperintensity in left posterior parietal white matter.

SUGGESTED
READINGS

1. Harding BN. Progressive neuronal degeneration of childhood with liver disease (Alpers-Huttenlocher syndrome): a personal review. J Child Neurol 1990;5:273.
2. Barkovich AJ, Good WV, Koch TK, Berg BO. Mitochondrial disorders: analysis of their clinical and imaging characteristics. AJNR 1993;14:1119.

4.07 Deep Gray Matter Nuclei Disorders: Congenital Disorders of the Basal Ganglia

EPIDEMIOLOGY AND CLINICAL FEATURES

Congenital disorders of the basal ganglia are characterized by tremor (rhythmic regular movements). Tremors may occur at rest or during motion, or can be related to posture. These disorders may also be associated with dystonia (torsion posturing of the trunk and extremities). Abnormalities in the basal ganglia also produce myoclonus and chorea. Table 4.07-1 summarizes the most common of these disorders:

TABLE 4.07-1. Genetics and Clinical Features of Congenital Disorders of the Basal Ganglia

Disorder	Genetics	Clinical Features
Juvenile Parkinson disease	Autosomal dominant with incomplete penetrance	Tremor, rigidity, bradykinesia, impaired postural stability, dystonia
Hallervorden-Spatz syndrome	Some cases are autosomal recessive with an increased familial incidence	Dystonia, rigidity, choreoathetosis, progressive intellectual deficits, retinitis pigmentosa, septic atrophy, seizures
Myoclonic encephalopathy	Unknown	Bizarre eye movements extending to trunk and extremities, associated with neuroblastoma, viral disease and immunizations, aseptic meningitis
Tourette syndrome	Autosomal dominant	Tic-like movements of eyes and face, vocalizations, hyperactivity, sleep and learning disorders
Menkes kinky-hair syndrome	X-linked, 1:250,000 live newborns	Motor seizures, hypothermia, coarse hair, intellectual delay, hypotonia, blindness
Sydenham chorea	None, postinfectious disorder	Choreic movements, emotional lability, hypotonia, poststreptococcal, associated with rheumatic fever
Huntington chorea	Autosomal dominant, 1:24,000 live births	Dementia, rigidity, seizures, choreoathetosis, ataxia
Wilson disease	Autosomal recessive, chromosome 13 (13q14.1–14.2), 1:1,000,000 individuals, higher in European Jews, southern Italians, Taiwanese, and Japanese	Liver failure, tremor, drooling, dysarthria, Kayser-Fleischer rings, dementia, speech abnormalities
Fahr disease	X-linked	Seizures, dementia, rigidity

IMAGING FEATURES   There are no characteristic imaging features for juvenile Parkinson disease. In Hallervorden-Spatz syndrome, computed tomography (CT) shows high density in the globus pallidi (Fig. 4.07-1A). Magnetic resonance (MR) T2-weighted images show marked hyperintensity in the globus pallidi surrounded by a rim of hypointensity ("eye of tiger" appearance; Fig. 4.07-1B–D). The hypointensity may be related to iron deposition, and the hyperintensity is probably related to gliosis. In some cases, the rim of T2 hypointensity is also surrounded by a second rim of marked hyperintensity.

In myoclonic encephalopathy, there are no specific imaging findings. Tourette syndrome is another entity in which no specific imaging features usually are found. In one series, reduced volume of the basal ganglia was found, and in an isolated case, a porencephalic cyst involving the basal ganglia was found.

In Menkes kinky-hair syndrome, MR imaging and cerebral angiography reveal increased diameter, elongation, and tortuosity of the intracranial arteries. By angiography, stenoses and occlusions may also be seen. Infarctions may occur. Cerebral and cerebellar atrophy are often present.

Enhancing lesions accompanied by mild mass effects involving the head of the caudate nuclei may be seen in Sydenham chorea. The abnormality may extend to involve the adjacent putamen. In Huntington chorea, the most common finding is that of atrophy of the head of the caudate nuclei (similar to the findings in adults). In Wilson disease, CT shows low density in the basal ganglia bilaterally. MR T2-weighted images show abnormal hyperintensity in the basal ganglia and subinsular regions, accompanied by diffuse mild atrophy (Fig. 4.07-2). The most striking signal intensity alterations are in the peripheral portion of the putamina. The thalami and dentate nuclei also are occasionally abnormal. In Fahr disease, CT shows symmetric calcification in the basal ganglia and, less commonly, in the dentate nuclei (Fig. 4.07-3). However, calcification in other parts of the brain may occur, including the white matter (centrum semiovale).

Kernicterus is an abnormality in which there is macroscopic staining of the basal ganglia with bilirubin in cases of neonatal hyperbilirubinemia. It is uncommon because of the widespread use of phototherapy. We have seen one case in which the basal ganglia were bright on T1- and T2-weighted images, a phenomenon similar to that seen in adults with chronic liver failure (Fig. 4.07-4). Chronic changes include delayed myelination, diffuse atrophy, and high T2 signal intensity in the subthalamic nuclei and globi pallidi.

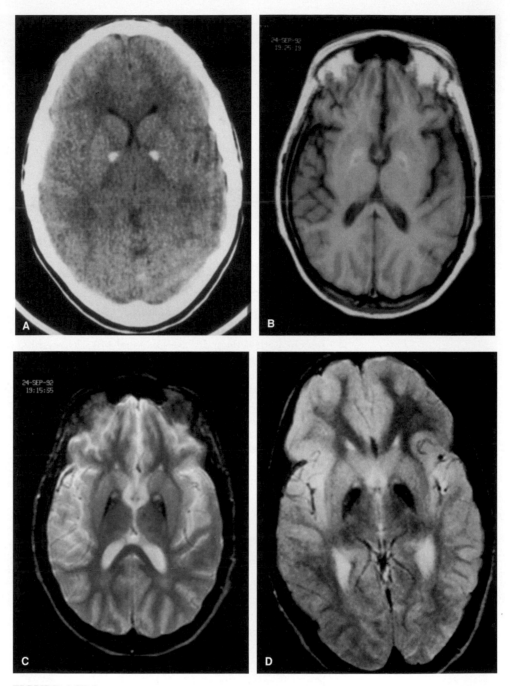

FIGURE 4.07-1.

Hallervorden-Spatz syndrome. **A.** Axial noncontrast computed tomography (CT) shows calcification in the medial globus pallidi. **B.** Axial magnetic resonance (MR) T1-weighted image in the same patient shows subtle increased signal intensity surrounding the regions of calcification seen on CT. The calcifications are slightly hypointense. **C.** Axial MR T2-weighted image shows the calcifications are bright and surrounded by a hypointense region, producing the so-called "eye-of-the-tiger" appearance. **D.** Axial MR T2-weighted image in a different patient with Hallervorden-Spatz syndrome shows typical "eye-of-the-tiger" abnormality. (With permission from Castillo M. Neuroradiology Companion. Philadelphia: JB Lippincott, 1995.)

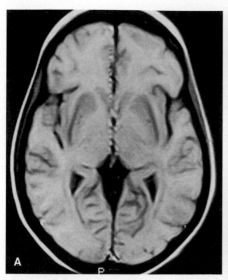 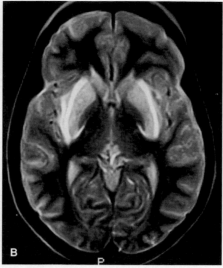 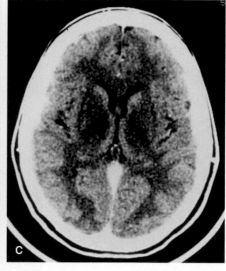

FIGURE 4.07-2.

Wilson disease. **A.** Axial magnetic resonance (MR) T1-weighted image shows low intensity in both basal ganglia (particularly in the outer zone of the putamina) in an adolescent with Wilson disease. **B.** Axial MR T2-weighted image in the same patient shows abnormal hyperintensities in the putamina (more pronounced in their outer zones) and the heads of both caudate nuclei. Both globus pallidi show small areas of increased signal intensity dorsally. **C.** Axial noncontrast computed tomography in a different patient with Wilson disease shows hypodensity in the lentiform nuclei, particularly in the outer aspect of the putamina. Portions of the thalami are also of abnormally low density. (With permission from Castillo M. Neuroradiology Companion. Philadelphia: JB Lippincott, 1995.)

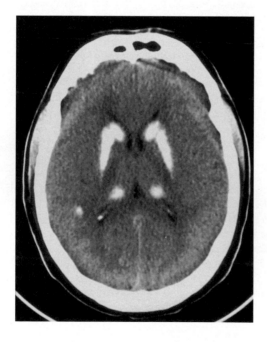

FIGURE 4.07-3.

Fahr disease. Axial noncontrast computed tomography shows calcification in head of caudate nuclei, putamina, thalami, and posterior right temporal white matter.

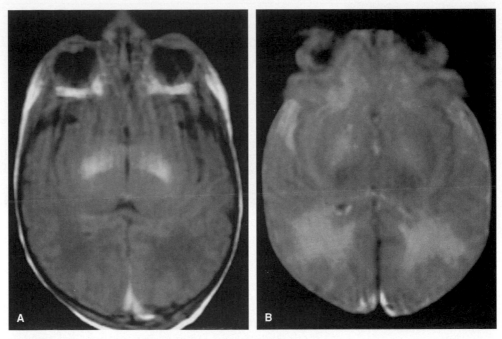

FIGURE 4.07-4.

Kernicterus. **A.** Axial magnetic resonance T1-weighted image obtained during acute phase of kernicterus shows increased signal intensity in globus pallidi. **B.** Corresponding T2-weighted image also shows increased signal intensity in these regions.

SUGGESTED READINGS

1. Savoiardo M, Halliday WC, Nardocci N, et al. Hallervorden-Spatz disease: MR and pathologic findings. AJNR 1993;14:155.
2. Kienzle GD, Breger RK, Chun RWM, Zupanc ML, Sackett JF. Sydenham chorea: MR manifestations in two cases. AJNR 1991;12:73.
3. Nazer H, Brismar J, Al-Kawi MZ, et al. Magnetic resonance imaging of the brain in Wilson's disorder. Neuroradiology 1993;35:130.
4. Swaiman KF. Disorders of the basal ganglia. In: Swaiman KF, ed. Pediatric Neurology, 2nd ed. St. Louis: Mosby, 1994:1071.
5. Magalhaes ACA, Caramelli P, Menezes JR, et al. Wilson's disease: MRI with clinical correlation. Neuroradiology 1994;36:97.
6. Peterson B, Riddle MA, Cohen DJ, et al. Reduced basal ganglia volumes in Tourette's syndrome using three-dimensional reconstruction techniques from magnetic resonance images. Neurology 1993;43:941.
7. Jacobs DS, Smith AS, Finelli DA, Lanzieri CF, Wiznitzer M. Menkes kinky hair disease: characteristic MR angiographic findings. AJNR 1993;14:1160.
8. Penn AA, Enzmann DR, Hahn TS, Stevenson DK. Kernicterus in a full term infant. Pediatrics 1994;93:1003.
9. Ho VB, Chuang V, Rovira MJ, Koo B. Juvenile Huntington disease: CT and MR features. AJNR 1995;16:1405.

4.08 Deep Gray Matter Nuclei Disorders: Idiopathic Disorders of the Basal Ganglia

EPIDEMIOLOGY

Ceroid lipofuscinosis is an autosomal recessive disorder in which an undetermined substance is deposited in several organs. The gene for infantile ceroid lipofuscinosis is located on chromosome 1, whereas the gene for the juvenile type is located on chromosome 16. Inheritance patterns for other forms of the disease are unknown. Cockayne syndrome is a disorder characterized by impaired DNA repair, is inherited as an autosomal recessive trait, and has been found in twins. We have seen a family in which all members were affected.

CLINICAL FEATURES

Patients with ceroid lipufuscinosis may present during early infancy (Norman-Wood type), late infancy (Jansky-Bielschowsky type), adolescence (Batten-Mayou-Spielmeyer-Vogt type, which is the most common form), or adulthood (Kufs-Hallervorden type). Biochemically, patients may be divided into those in whom the subunit C component of adenosine triphosphate is present and those in whom it is absent. The most common symptoms are seizures, mental retardation, ataxia, myoclonus, and progressive loss of vision. The diagnosis is made by discovering fingerprint, curvilinear, or granular-like cytosomal inclusions of autofluorescent lipopigment. All patients eventually succumb to the disease.

Patients with Cockayne syndrome may be classified as having a variant of Pelizaeus-Merzbacher disease. These patients are normal at birth but soon develop a photosensitive dermatitis. Other clinical features include mental retardation, microcephaly, abnormal facies, retinitis pigmentosa, optic atrophy, growth retardation, dwarfism, kyphosis, cerebellar dysfunction, and upper motor neuron signs. There are no specific laboratory findings. Pathologically, the brain is atrophied and shows islands of demyelination. Calcifications in the basal ganglia, cerebellum, and cerebral arteries are present.

IMAGING FEATURES

Ceroid lipofuscinosis shows generalized atrophy, which is more pronounced in the cerebellum. The white matter of the cerebral hemispheres may be hypodense by computed tomography and mildly hyperintense on magnetic resonance T2-weighted images.

Cockayne syndrome shows calcifications in the lentiform nuclei, dentate nuclei, thalami, and cerebral cortex (Fig. 4.08-1). Other imaging findings include a reduced size of the brain, thick calvarium, hydrocephalus (communicating type), symmetric and patchy zones of demyelination, and atrophy of the cerebellum and the brain stem.

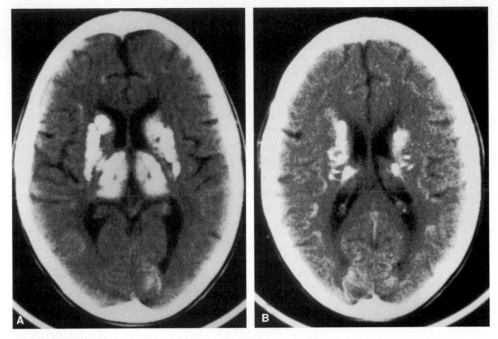

FIGURE 4.08-1.

Cockayne syndrome. **A.** Axial noncontrast computed tomography (CT) in a young patient with a family history of Cockayne syndrome. There are calcifications in the lentiform nuclei, caudate nuclei, and thalami. Small calcifications are present in the left calcarine region. **B.** Axial CT in the same patient shows calcifications involving the bodies of both caudate nuclei. Some subcortical hyperdensities suggesting calcifications are present.

SUGGESTED READINGS

1. Kendall BE. Disorders of lysosomes, peroxisomes, and mitochondria. AJNR 1992;13: 621.
2. Swaiman KF, Dyken PR. Degenerative diseases primarily of gray matter. In: Swaiman KF, ed. Pediatric Neurology, 2nd ed. St. Louis: Mosby, 1994:1030.
3. Fishman MA. Disorders primarily of white matter. In: Swaiman KF, ed. Pediatric Neurology, 2nd ed. St. Louis: Mosby, 1994:1011.

4.09 Deep Gray Matter Nuclei Disorders: Hippocampal Atrophy and Sclerosis

EPIDEMIOLOGY

Approximately 60% to 80% of children with complex partial seizures have pathologic evidence of hippocampal (mesial temporal) sclerosis. The remaining patients with this type of seizures have tumors, vascular malformations, neuronal migration anomalies, or hamartomas in this region. The etiology of hippocampal sclerosis is probably birth-related hypoxia/ischemia. Some investigators have proposed kindling of this region secondary to febrile seizures in childhood. Seizures (all types) are slightly more common in boys. Most seizures present between 1 to 4 years of age and occur in 30 to 50:100,000 individuals. A cause for the epilepsy may be identified in less than 30% of cases.

CLINICAL FEATURES

Complex partial seizures (previously called psychomotor seizures) are those that are associated with impairment of consciousness. This impairment may follow the onset of simple partial seizures or coincide with the onset of the seizure activity. They may be accompanied by automatisms and often begin in one temporal lobe. Other sites of seizure activity are the anterior or basal frontal lobes. Approximately 5% to 10% of all seizure patients become medically intractable. The histologic feature of hippocampal sclerosis consists of neuronal loss in the pyramidal cell layer of regions CA1, CA3, and CA4. Synaptic reorganization at this level induces epileptogenic electrical activity. Surgical treatment usually consists of focal resection of the hippocampus. For widespread hemispheric abnormalities, such as Sturge-Weber syndrome or Rasmussen syndrome (chronic encephalitis), a total or partial hemispherectomy may be done. After hippocampectomy, 70% to 90% of patients experience a significant reduction in their seizure frequency or become seizure free.

IMAGING FEATURES

High-resolution, thin-section, coronal T1-weighted inversion recovery and fast spin echo T2-weighted images are the sequences of choice in the evaluation of patients with suspected abnormalities of the hippocampi. The first image is obtained at the level of the amydalae and should extend to include the tail of the hippocampi. The purpose of imaging is to lateralize the abnormality before surgical resection.

The two most common findings are atrophy of the hippocampi (>80%) and increased signal intensity on T2-weighted images (60–80%) (Fig. 4.09-1). Increased signal intensity tends to be generalized but may be isolated to sectors CA1 and CA3. This abnormality may be related to gliosis. Atrophy is commonly diffuse but tends to occur preferentially in the body of the hippocampus. Volume measurements are especially helpful when bilateral abnormalities (which may be harder to visually recognize) are present. This occurs in approximately 10% of cases. Atrophy involving the ipsilateral mammillary body and the forniceal column may also be present. On T1-weighted inversion recovery images, a bright stripe (the stratum radiatum) is always present in the hippocampi. Its absence is abnormal and may imply gliosis or an infiltrating process. Atrophy of the white matter adjacent to the diseased hippocampus is the third most common MR imaging sign in these patients. Asymmetric enlargement of one temporal horn has historically been an important sign of underlying hippocampal anomalies. We believe that this is not a reliable sign, and is meaningful only in the face of the previously mentioned MR imaging findings. Loss of the gray–white demarcation in the temporal lobe is usually seen with infiltrating neoplasms of this region (Fig. 4.09-2). The least sensitive sign probably is reduction in the size of one temporal lobe. This finding may be seen as a normal variant.

Other lesions occurring in the hippocampus that also produce complex partial seizures include vascular malformations, astrocytomas, dysembryoplastic neuroepithelial tumors, cortical dysplasias, and Rasmussen encephalitis (chronic viral encephalitis). Patients in status epilepticus also demonstrate increased signal intensity in the hippocampus.

Recently described and relatively uncommon anomalies are neuronal migration errors in the perihippocampal regions. These gray matter heterotopias and cortical dysplasias are the foci of seizures and are better visualized on heavily T1-weighted images.

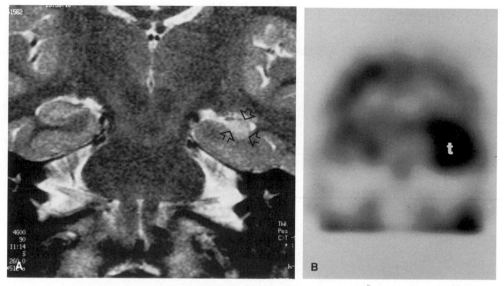

FIGURE 4.09-1.

Hippocampal sclerosis. **A.** Coronal magnetic resonance T2-weighted image shows atrophy and hyperintensity in the left hippocampus *(arrows)* compatible with hippocampal sclerosis. **B.** Coronal single photon emission computed tomography view after interictal administration of Tc-99m HMPAO in the same patient shows increased activity in the entire left temporal lobe (t).

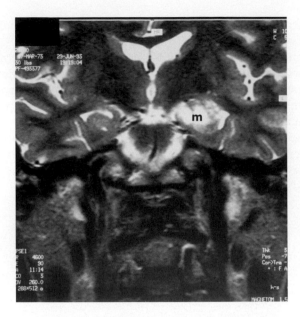

FIGURE 4.09-2.

Hippocampal low-grade astrocytoma. Coronal magnetic resonance T2-weighted image in a patient with partial complex seizures shows hyperintense mass (m) in left hippocampus.

SUGGESTED READINGS

1. Meiners LC, van Gils D, Jansen GH, et al. Temporal lobe epilepsy: the various MR appearances of histologically proven mesial temporal sclerosis. AJNR 1994;15:1547.
2. Tien RD, Felsberg GJ, Krishnan R, Heinz ER. MR imaging of diseases of the limbic system. AJR 1994;163:657.
3. Jack CR. Epilepsy: surgery and imaging. Radiology 1993;189:635.
4. Tien RD, Felsberg GJ, Campi de Castro C, et al. Complex partial seizures and mesial temporal sclerosis: evaluation with fast spin echo MR imaging. Radiology 1993; 189:835.
5. Lehericy S, Dormont D, Semah F, et al. Developmental abnormalities of the mesial temporal lobe in patients with temporal lobe epilepsy. AJNR 1995;16:617.
6. Achten E, Boon P, DePoorter J, et al. An MR protozol for presurgical evaluation of patients with complex partial seizures of temporal lobe origin. AJNR 1995;16:1201.

4.10 *Idiopathic White Matter Disorders: Alexander Disease*

EPIDEMIOLOGY

Alexander disease (also known as fibrinoid leukodystrophy) is an uncommon degenerative disorder of the central nervous system caused by dysfunction of the astrocytes. The peripheral nervous system is spared. It is probably inherited as an autosomal recessive trait, but its genetics are uncertain. However, familial cases have been reported. There is no predilection for either sex.

CLINICAL FEATURES

Most cases of Alexander disease are of the infantile form. Symptoms begin between 6 months and 2 years of age. Most patients die from the disease within 5 years of the onset. Symptoms include mental and motor retardation, megalencephaly, spasticity, and seizures. Hydrocephalus may be present.

In the juvenile form, symptoms begin between 7 to 14 years of age and include difficulty swallowing, nystagmus, ptosis, facial diplegia, and atrophy of the tongue. There is no evidence of mental retardation. The adult form of the disease is rare and is not addressed here.

No enzymatic or biochemical defects have been identified in this disease. Brain biopsy is required to establish the diagnosis. The histologic landmark is the presence of eosinophilic bodies within astrocytes. These are also found in the subpial, subependymal, and perivascular regions. The astrocytes that harbor these eosinophilic bodies are large and may be found anywhere in the brain and cerebellum (including white and gray matter). Electron microscopy reveals the presence of Rosenthal fibers. There is loss of myelin that is diffuse in children and patchy in the juvenile form of the disease. In juvenile Alexander disease, the brain stem is prominently involved. There is no treatment for the disease.

IMAGING FEATURES

Computed tomography (CT) and magnetic resonance show low attenuation and signal intensity involving the white matter of the frontal lobes (Fig. 4.10-1). These changes are symmetric. The basal ganglia may also be involved. The periventricular areas (particularly the tips of the frontal horns) and the corpus callosum may be of slightly high density on precontrast CT and enhance prominently after contrast administration. The occipital and cerebellar white matter is usually preserved. Occasionally, enhancement in the caudate nuclei and anterior columns of the fornices, and optic radiations may be seen. With progression of the disease, the areas of contrast enhancement disappear. The areas of enhancement correlate well with prominent deposition of Rosenthal fibers. In the late stages of the disease, cystic changes (particularly in the temporal lobes) and atrophy (especially of the corpus callosum) become evident (Fig. 4.10-2). The cavum vergae is commonly widened.

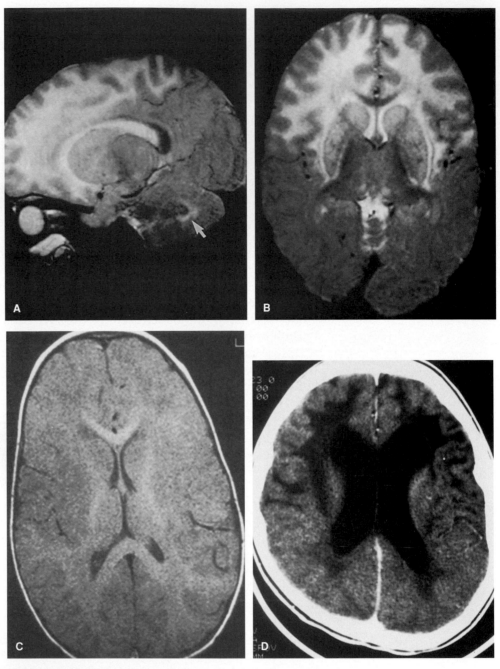

FIGURE 4.10-1.

Alexander disease. **A.** Parasagittal magnetic resonance (MR) T2-weighted image shows abnormally increased signal intensity in the frontal region in a patient with Alexander disease. Abnormal signal intensity is also present in the cerebellum *(arrow).* (With permission from Castillo M. Neuroradiology Companion. Philadelphia: JB Lippincott, 1995.) **B.** Axial MR T2-weighted image shows hyperintensity in the white matter of both frontal lobes involving the subinsular regions and the internal capsules. The basal ganglia are also abnormally bright, probably secondary to involvement of the white matter fibers that course through them. **C.** Axial noncontrast MR T1-weighted image (different patient) shows loss of normal hyperintensity of the white matter in the frontal regions. This case illustrates how the abnormalities are better seen on T2-weighted images. There is no atrophy. **D.** Axial postcontrast computed tomography in a case of juvenile Alexander disease shows low density in the matter of both frontal lobes. Note the central atrophy leading to dilatation of the lateral ventricles, especially at the frontal horns.

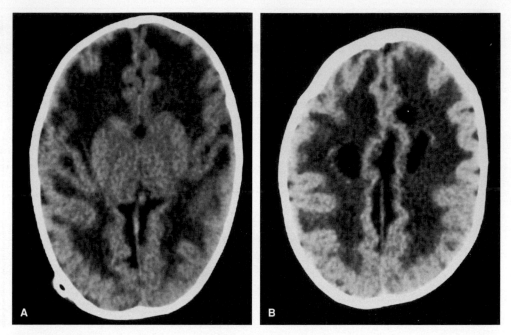

FIGURE 4.10-2.

Alexander disease (presumed) with cystic changes.   **A.** Axial computed tomography (CT) shows marked white matter hypodensity, mostly in frontal lobes but also extending posteriorly. **B.** CT shows diffuse white matter hypodensity in both centra semiovale and at least three areas of cystic changes.

SUGGESTED READINGS

1. Shah M, Ross JS. Infantile Alexander disease: MR appearance of a biopsy proven case. AJNR 1990;11:1105.
2. Clifton AG, Dendall BE, Kingsley DPE, et al. Computed tomography in Alexander's disease. Neuroradiology 1991;33:438.

4.11 *Idiopathic White Matter Disorders: Canavan Disease*

EPIDEMIOLOGY

Canavan disease (also known as spongiform degeneration) is a rare degenerative disorder associated with decreased levels of adenosine triphosphate (ATP) within astrocytes. As such, it could conceivably be classified as a mitochondrial disorder. There is no set pattern of inheritance for the neonatal and juvenile forms of the disease. However, the infantile form is an autosomal recessive trait and is more common in Jews of northeastern European background and in Saudi Arabians. Both sexes are equally affected.

CLINICAL FEATURES

The neonatal form of the disease is relatively uncommon. The symptoms are lethargy, irritability, decreased movements, difficulties swallowing and breathing, and hypotonia. Death occurs in a matter of weeks. The most common form is the infantile type, which is characterized by hypotonia, seizures, decortication, and death within 3 to 4 years of onset. Megalencephaly is common but not always present. The juvenile form begins after 5 years of age and is characterized by tremors, ataxia, ptosis, mental deterioration, dementia, and spasticity. Megalencephaly does not occur in the juvenile form of Canavan disease.

Laboratory studies show increased *N*-acetylaspartic acid in urine and plasma. This occurs secondary to a deficiency in aspartoacylase. It is unclear how deficiencies of this enzyme and of mitochondrial ATP produce the pathologic changes found in this disease. Histologically, the brain is somewhat enlarged and there are multiple, enlarged, fluid-filled vacuoles giving the brain its "spongiform" appearance. Myelin sheaths are decreased in size and are eventually lost with progression of the disease. There is no specific treatment for Canavan disease.

IMAGING FEATURES

Computed tomography (CT) shows diffuse decreased attenuation of the white matter. The subcortical U-fibers are also involved. Occasionally there is sparing of the internal capsules, corpus callosum, and the deep cerebellar white matter. In some cases, the involvement of the occipital areas is more severe than that elsewhere in the brain. There is no correlation between the severity of the imaging findings and the patient's clinical status. Involvement of the thalami and the basal ganglia has been observed. The cortex may appear thin but there usually is no significant atrophy. Magnetic resonance imaging findings mirror the CT features already mentioned (Fig. 4.11-1). Hydrogen MR spectroscopy shows increased NAA. Canavan disease is the only leukodystrophy in which MR spectroscopy offers a definitive diagnosis.

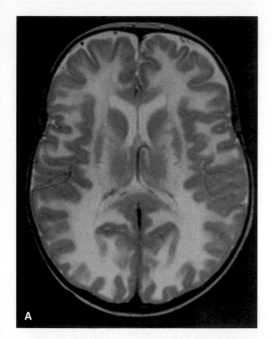
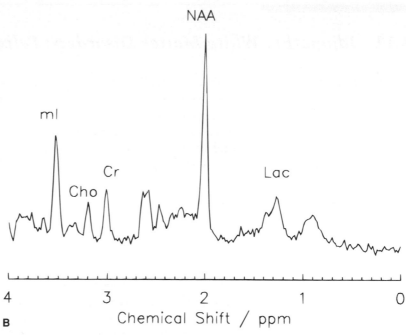

FIGURE 4.11-1.

Canavan disease. **A.** Axial magnetic resonance T2-weighted image shows diffuse abnormal hyperintensity involving all white matter (including subcortical U-fibers). The cortex is thin and there is no atrophy. (With permission from Castillo M. Neuroradiology Companion. Philadelphia: JB Lippincott, 1995.) **B.** Proton MRS shows increased n-acetyl-aspartate (NAA), which is typical for Canavan disease: ml, myoinositol; Cho, choline; Cr, creatine; Lac, lactate. (Courtesy of R. Zimmerman, Children's Hospital of Philadelphia, PA.)

SUGGESTED READING

1. Brismar J, Brismar G, Gascon G, Oznan P. Canavan disease: CT and MR imaging of the brain. AJNR 1990;11:805.

4.12 *Idiopathic White Matter Disorders: Pelizaeus-Merzbacher Disease*

EPIDEMIOLOGY

Pelizaeus-Merzbacher disease is also known as sudanophilic leukodystrophy and is characterized by breakdown of myelin. Although traditionally it has been classified as a dysmyelinating disorder, it probably is a demyelinating disorder. The classic and connatal forms are X-linked, but sporadic and autosomal recessive cases have been reported. The transitional type is sporadic, whereas the adult form is autosomal dominant.

CLINICAL FEATURES

Pelizaeus-Merzbacher disease has been divided into six subtypes. In the classic form (type 1), tremor and nystagmus occur during the first months of life. Ataxia, choreoathetosis, spasticity, and seizures also develop. The connatal form (type 2) is characterized by complete absence of mental and motor development from birth. It is the most severe form of the disease. Death occurs rapidly. Type 3 is a transitional form of the disorder (between types 1 and 2) characterized by nystagmus, tremor, spasticity, and optic atrophy. The patients are moderately mentally retarded and death occurs 5 to 7 years after the onset. In adults, the disease (type 4) takes a protracted course. Clinical symptoms include ataxia, hyperreflexia, nystagmus, seizures, and mild mental retardation. Several disorders with ill-defined clinical manifestations but similar pathologic findings have been grouped under transitional (type 5) variants. The sixth subtype is Cockayne syndrome.

There are no consistently recognizable biochemical abnormalities in patients with Pelizaeus-Merzbacher disease, but lack of proteolipid apoprotein (lipophilin) has been found in some patients. Pathologically, areas of demyelination are mixed with zones of preserved myelin, giving the brain a "tigroid" appearance. Sudanophilic material is deposited in the centra semiovale, brain stem, and cerebellum. Because no products of myelin breakdown are found, lack of myelin formation (dysmyelination) has in the past been proposed as an explanation for this disease.

IMAGING FEATURES

Computed tomography shows areas of low density in the white matter and generalized atrophy in longstanding cases. Because of its better sensitivity, magnetic resonance imaging shows the white matter abnormalities to be extensive. There is an almost total lack of normal myelination involving deep and superficial (including subcortical U-fibers) white matter (Fig. 4.12-1). The appearance of the patient's brain is that of a newborn. In some patients, focal islands of normally myelinated white matter are mixed with the abnormal white matter, giving a patchy appearance. At times, the white matter in the brain stem, cerebellum, and subcortical regions may remain intact. The basal ganglia and the thalami may appear mildly hypointense; this appearance is probably because of iron deposition in these sites.

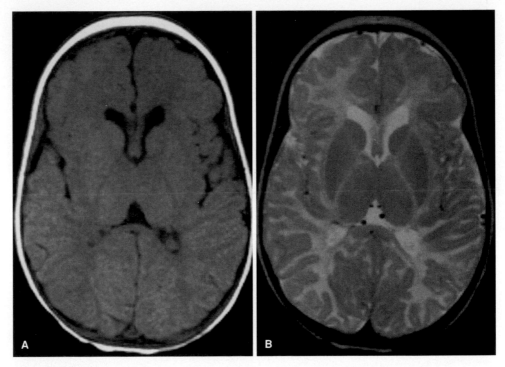

FIGURE 4.12-1.

Pelizaeus-Merzbacher disease.   A. Axial magnetic resonance T_1-weighted image shows complete absence of normal bright myelin. **B.** Corresponding T_2-weighted image confirms lack of myelin (no dark regions are present). There is no significant atrophy.

SUGGESTED
READINGS

1. van der Knaap MS, Valk J. The reflection of histology in MR imaging of Pelizaeus-Merzbacher disease. AJNR 1989;10:94.
2. Caro PA, Marks HG. Magnetic resonance imaging and computed tomography in Pelizaeus-Merzbacher disease. Magn Reson Imaging 1990;8:791.
3. Silverstein AM, Hirsh DK, Trobe JD, Gebarski SS. MR imaging of the brain in five members of a family with Pelizaeus-Merzbacher disease. AJNR 1990;11:495.

Imaging of the Pediatric Head, Neck, and Spine
by Mauricio Castillo and Suresh K. Mukherji,
Lippincott-Raven Publishing, Philadelphia © 1996.

5

Destructive, Ischemic, and Vascular Disorders

5.0 Ischemic Damage to the Glial Radial Fibers

Ischemia to the glial radial fiber unit during the second trimester results in a spectrum of abnormalities ranging from nonlissencephalic cortical dysplasias (polymicrogyria) to hydranencephaly (Figs. 5.0-1–5.0-4). Table 5.0-1 summarizes this spectrum of disorders:

TABLE 5.0-1. Disorders Resulting from Ischemic Damage to the Glial Radial Fibers

Defect Produced	Time of Insult	Severity of Insult	Clinical Handicap
Hydranencephaly	Early 2nd trimester	Marked	Severe, hemiparesis, seizures, developmental delay (Fig. 5.0-5)
Open-lip schizencephaly	Early to middle 2nd trimester	Marked	Severe, seizures, hemiparesis, developmental delay (Fig. 5.0-6)
Closed-lip schizencephaly	Middle 2nd trimester	Moderate	Moderate to severe, seizures, varying degree of muscular dysfunction in opposite side of body (Fig. 5.0-7)
Deep cleft of polymicrogyria	Middle to late 2nd trimester	Moderate to mild	Moderate to mild, seizures (Fig. 5.0-8)
Focal polymicrogyria	Late 2nd trimester	Mild	Mild, seizures (Fig. 5.0-9)

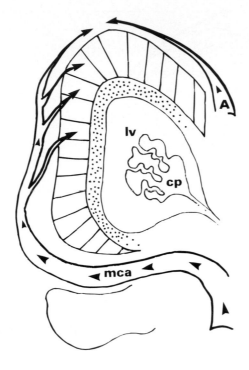

FIGURE 5.0-1.

Drawing showing the normal blood supply to the radial–glial unit *(lined area)* from the middle cerebral (mca) and anterior cerebral (A) arteries during the early second trimester. The germinal matrix *(dotted area)* is intact and found outside the lateral ventricle (lv). cp, choroid plexus.

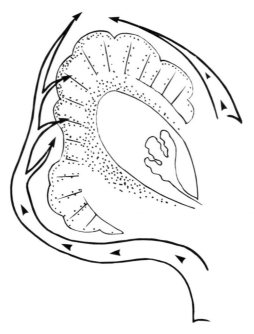

FIGURE 5.0-2.

During the second trimester, neuronal migration takes place. The neurons *(dots)* originate in the zone adjacent to the ventricle and migrate along the radial–glial fibers to their eventual resting place in the cortex.

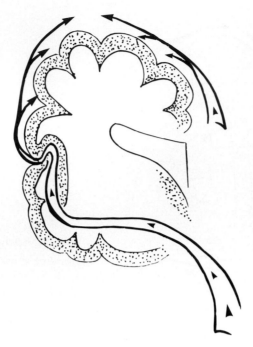

FIGURE 5.0-3.

During the third trimester, normal neuronal migration has occurred and the cortex *(dotted area)* is well formed. The radial–glial units have transformed into astrocytes and the white matter is normally arborized. Residual germinal matrix is seen along the inferior aspect of the lateral ventricle. The insula has closed and normal circulation is established.

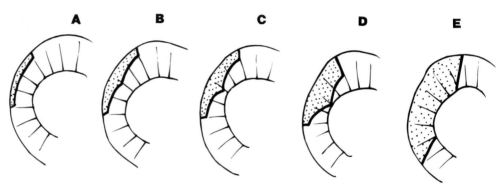

FIGURE 5.0-4.

Diagram illustrating the different degrees of insult to the radial–glial unit. **A.** superficial injury resulting in polymicrogyria; **B,C.** partial-thickness injury resulting in deep clefts of polymicrogyria; **D.** moderate-thickness injury that at one point extends into germinal matrix and ventricle, resulting in closed-lip schizencephalies; **E.** large, full-thickness injury resulting in open-lip schizencephalies (when bilateral, the result is hydranencephaly).

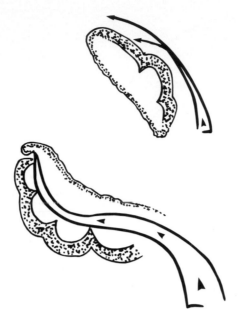

FIGURE 5.0-5.

Occlusion of the proximal middle cerebral artery, anterior cerebral artery, or supraclinoid internal carotid artery results in a large cleft. Only a small portion of the occipital, posterior temporal, or frontal lobes may be present in these cases. If bilateral, the result is hydranencephaly.

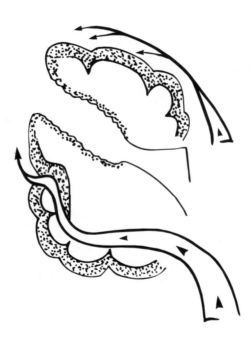

FIGURE 5.0-6.

A severe vascular occlusion occurring during the middle to late second trimester that involves the entire width of the radial–glial unit and results in a cleft communicating with the corresponding lateral ventricle. The borders of the cleft are separated and filled with cerebrospinal fluid (open-lip schizencephaly). The gray matter lining the cleft is polymicrogyric. The corresponding lateral ventricle is enlarged and the septum pellucidum is completely or partially absent.

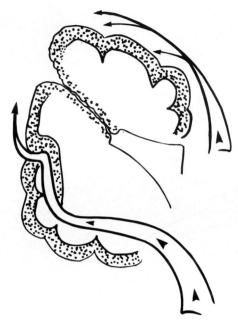

FIGURE 5.0-7.

Occlusion of distal arterial branches during the middle portion of the second trimester that involves the entire thickness of the radial–glial unit, resulting in a cleft that extends into the ventricle. The lips of the cleft touch each other (closed-lip schizencephaly) and are lined by polymicrogyria. The corresponding lateral ventricle is enlarged.

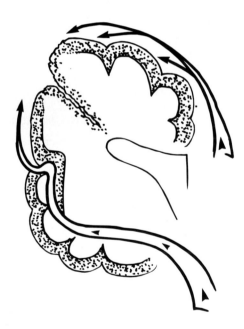

FIGURE 5.0-8.

Occlusion of the distal middle cerebral artery produces damage to the radial–glial unit, resulting in a deep cleft (which does not communicate with the ventricle) lined by dysplastic cortex (polymicrogyria). These clefts are typically located in the Sylvian or peri-Sylvian regions.

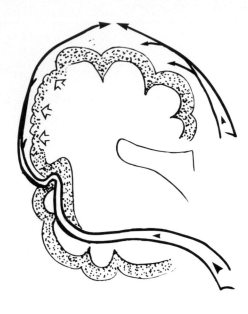

FIGURE 5.0-9.

Occlusion of some branches of the middle cerebral artery during the latter part of the second trimester leads to necrosis of deep cortical layers producing a thin cortex *(open arrows)* and lack of formation of the sulci. The surface of the dysplastic cortex is "bumpy." The findings are those of focal polymicrogyria.

SUGGESTED READING

1. Barkovich AJ, Kjos BO. Nonlissencephalic cortical dysplasias: correlation of imaging findings with clinical deficits. AJNR 1992;13:94.

5.01 *Polymicrogyria*

EPIDEMIOLOGY

The incidence of this disorder is unknown. Etiologic factors include intrauterine hypoxia or ischemia, maternal cytomegalovirus inclusion disease, fetal toxoplasmosis and syphilis, maternal carbon monoxide poisoning, and the Chiari type II malformation.

CLINICAL FEATURES

Polymicrogyria produces dysplasia of the cerebral cortex. Polymicrogyria is not a disorder of neuronal migration per se, but results from ischemia of the formed fetal cerebral cortex. Because of this, several authors endorse the term "nonlissencephalic cortical dysplasia" for this disorder. Although six layers of neurons are present in polymicrogyric cortex, there is reduced cellular proliferation in the middle layers (particularly layer 5). The presence of a six-layered cortex suggests that the insult occurs after the 20th week of gestation. The result is a region of cortex that is flat but has a wrinkled surface. These wrinkles may simulate the appearance of small gyri, hence the name polymicrogyria. These patients almost always have epilepsy (particularly infantile spasms), and at times may be developmentally delayed. Children may also be initially hypotonic but later manifest spasticity.

IMAGING FEATURES

By magnetic resonance (MR; the imaging method of choice), polymicrogyria is identical in appearance to a zone of pachygyria (Fig. 5.01-1). The minute gyri that characterize this anomaly cannot be resolved with routine brain MR imaging. Polymicrogyria tends to involve the peri-Sylvian regions but may occur anywhere in the brain (Fig. 5.01-2). Nonlissencephalic cortical dysplasias are commonly seen in the superoposterior aspect of the Sylvian fissure, which itself is usually abnormal and extends further superiorly and posteriorly than usual. The proximity of polymicrogyria to the Sylvian fissure has led some authors erroneously to label nonlissencephalic cortical dysplasias as "schizencephaly type I." In approximately one-fourth of the cases, MR T2-weighted images show areas of high signal intensity in the white matter directly under the dysplastic cortex. This probably reflects gliosis secondary to ischemia. Anomalous venous drainage is also seen in association with polymicrogyria (Fig. 5.01-3). Anomalous veins are more common where there is an infolding of dysplastic cortex. It should be recognized as such and not confused with an arteriovenous malformation. MR angiography is helpful in ruling out an arteriovenous malformation if doubt exists. Nonlissencephalic cortical dysplasias may be bilateral and located in similar regions of the cerebral hemispheres. It is possible that polymicrogyria is the mildest form of a spectrum of ischemic defects that also includes schizencephaly (moderate form, lips are usually lined by polymicrogyric cortex) and hydranencephaly, which is the most severe form (see section 5.0).

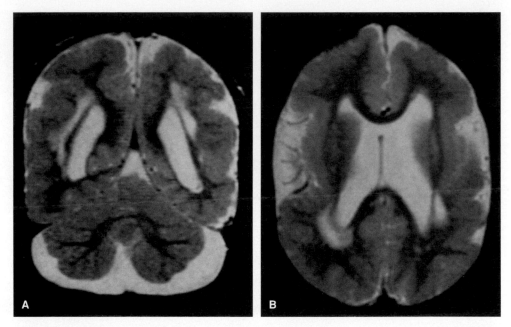

FIGURE 5.01-1.

Polymicrogyria. **A.** Coronal magnetic resonance (MR) T2-weighted image shows bilateral temporoparietal dysplastic cortex (polymicrogyria) with underlying areas of hyperintensity (gliosis) in the periventricular white matter. The cerebrospinal fluid spaces are prominent. The cerebellum is small. **B.** Axial MR T2-weighted image in same patient shows areas of hyperintensity in periatrial white matter. All of the visualized cortex is dysplastic and, despite being polymicrogyric, has an appearance identical to pachygyria. The temporal opercula are open.

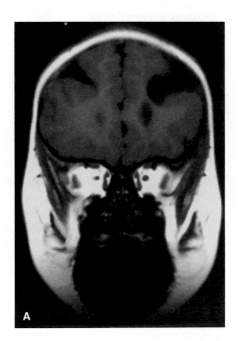

FIGURE 5.01-2.

Deep clefts of polymicorgyria. **A.** Coronal magnetic resonance (MR) T1-weighted image shows bifrontal deep clefts of polymicrogyria. Note dysplastic cortex lining the clefts and in lateral left frontal lobe. The clefts do not extend into the ventricles, and therefore may not be considered schizencephalies.

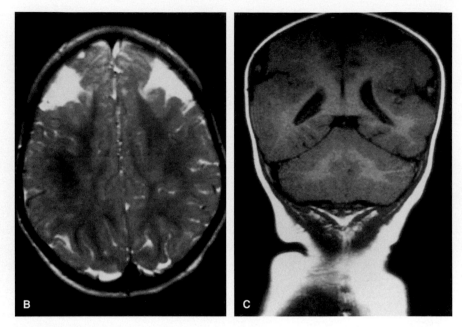

FIGURE 5.01-2. *(continued)*

B. Axial MR T2-weighted image again shows bifrontal clefts. **C.** Coronal MR T1-weighted image in a different patient shows bilateral deep clefts lined by dysplastic (polymicrogyric?) cortex extending from the posterior margin of the Sylvian fissures. This is a typical example of the deep clefts of polymicrogyria. As in the previous case, these clefts are separated from the lateral ventricles by white matter, and therefore they are not schizencephalies.

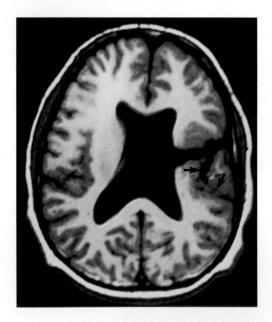

FIGURE 5.01-3.

Schizencephaly (open-lip type). Axial magnetic resonance T1-weighted image in a patient with a left-sided schizencephaly that by definition is lined by polymicrogyric cortex shows multiple vessels *(arrows)* associated with the dysplastic cortex, most likely representing anomalous venous drainage (persistent embryonic veins).

SUGGESTED READINGS

1. Barkovich AJ. Abnormal vascular drainage in anomalies of neuronal migration. AJNR 1988;9:939.
2. Barkovich AJ, Kjos BO. Nonlissencephalic cortical dysplasias: correlation of imaging findings with clinical deficits. AJNR 1992;13:95.

5.02 *Schizencephaly*

EPIDEMIOLOGY

Schizencephalies are clefts of dysplastic gray matter extending from the surface of the brain into a ventricle. Their inner margin is formed by a continuous seam of ventricular ependyma and pia matter. The exact incidence of this rare anomaly is not known. Although it typically is a sporadic occurrence, a familial form is recognized. Because the dysplastic gray matter contained in the lips of the defect is polymicrogyric, factors that are believed to induce polymicrogyria (carbon monoxide poisoning and fetal ischemia/anoxia) are also believed to be responsible for schizencephalies. Approximately 35% of schizencephalies are bilateral, and most are found in the peri-Sylvian region (similar to polymicrogyria). It is possible that schizencephalies are a more severe form of anomaly in the same pathologic spectrum as the less severe polymicrogyria.

CLINICAL FEATURES

The initial insult (presumably vascular) responsible for the formation of schizencephalies probably occurs during the 12th to 17th weeks of life. Because most clefts occur close to the Sylvian fissure, end-arterial ischemia may be responsible. The severity of the clinical symptoms is related to the size of the defect. Patients with bilateral defects usually have diffuse motor impairment, are mentally retarded, and have seizures. Some of these patients are also blind as a result of hypoplasia of the optic nerves or interruption of the optic pathways. Mental deficiencies correlate well with the presence of frontal schizencephalies. Patients with unilateral clefts have a good prognosis for intellectual development, but may have seizures. Schizencephalies that contain a cerebrospinal fluid (CSF)-filled cleft (open-lip type) produce more symptoms than those in which the lips abut each other (closed-lip type). Some patients may have visual problems that may be caused by underlying septooptic dysplasia.

IMAGING FEATURES

Open-lip schizencephalies are CSF-filled clefts extending from the surface of the brain usually into a lateral ventricle (Figs. 5.01-3 and 5.02-1). The lips of the cleft are lined by dysplastic (polymicrogyric) gray matter. As such, abnormally large vessels (probably representing anomalous venous drainage) may be present along the margins of the cleft and should not be confused with a true arteriovenous malformation. The cerebral hemisphere involved by the cleft is usually small. The adjacent lateral ventricle may be enlarged. The superficial subarachnoid spaces neighboring the cleft may also be enlarged. At times, a cyst-like structure is found overlying the schizencephaly and may produce scalloping of the inner table of the skull or enlargement of that hemicranium (presumably due to CSF pulsations). These patients may need insertion of a shunt catheter into the cyst. The septum pellucidum is absent. The optic apparatus may be atrophic, indicating that septooptic dysplasia coexists. In one-third of cases, a contralateral schizencephaly is present. It may be of the same type or of different configuration. Roughly, the location of bilateral clefts is similar.

The second form of schizencephaly is the so-called closed-lip type (Fig. 5.02-2). In this anomaly, there is a band of smooth gray matter extending from the surface of the brain into a ventricle (usually the lateral ventricles). It contains no CSF between its lips, and produces a nipple-like projection or a dimple of gray on the outer wall of the lateral ventricle that it joins. Increased T2 signal intensity from the white matter close to the lips may be seen, and may be related to gliosis (similar to that found in polymicrogyria). Closed-lip schizencephaly needs to be differentiated from a deep cleft of polymicrogyria in which the defect does not extend into the ventricle. Both types of schizencephalies may show hypoplasia of the portion of the corpus callosum located geographically close to the cleft.

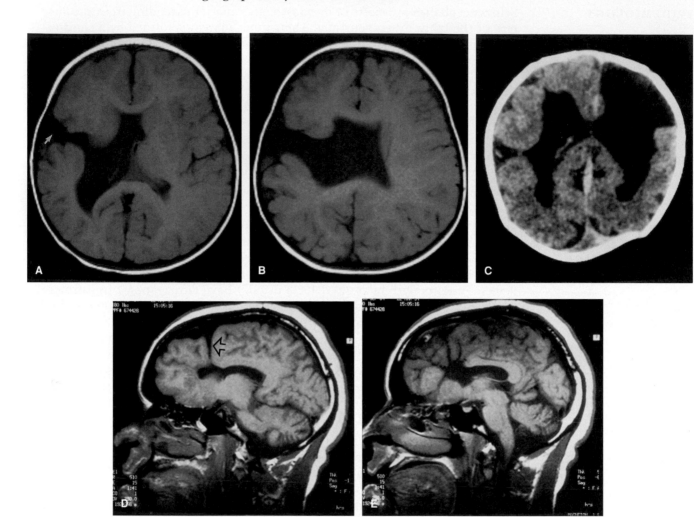

FIGURE 5.02-1.

Schizencephaly (open-lip type). **A.** Axial magnetic resonance (MR) T1-weighted image shows right temporal transcerebral cleft that contains cerebrospinal fluid (CSF) between its lips (type I schizencephaly). The CSF space (lateral cleft) contains a large vessel *(arrow)*, probably representing anomalous venous drainage due to persistence of embryonic veins. The right lateral ventricle is prominent and there is no septum pellucidum. **B.** Axial MR T1-weighted image superior to (A) shows open-lip cleft and absence of septum pellucidum. **C.** Axial noncontrast computed tomography (different patient) shows bilateral (left > right) open-lip schizencephalies. **D.** Parasagittal MR T1-weighted image shows frontal open-lip schizencephaly *(arrow)*. **E.** Midsagittal MR T1-weighted image in the same patient shows agenesis of the genu and rostrum of the corpus callosum. Similar findings may be seen in holoprosencephaly. The inferior vermian segments are also missing.

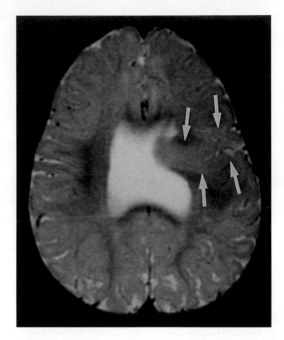

FIGURE 5.02-2.

Schizencephaly (closed-lip type).
Axial magnetic resonance T2-weighted image shows a band of thickened gray matter *(arrows)* extending from the surface of the left temporal region into the left lateral ventricle. It contains no cerebrospinal fluid, and therefore represents a closed-lip schizencephaly (type II). Note nipple-like projection (representing heterotopic gray matter) into the left lateral ventricle and absence of septum pellucidum. (With permission from Castillo M. Neuroradiology Companion. Philadelphia: JB Lippincott, 1995.)

SUGGESTED READINGS

1. Barkovich AJ, Norman D. MR of schizencephaly. AJNR 1988;9:297.
2. Barkovich AJ, Kjos BO. Schizencephaly: correlation of clinical findings with MR characteristics. AJNR 1992;13:85.
3. Castillo M. MRI of schizencephaly. MRI Decisions 1992;6:22.

5.03 *Hydranencephaly*

EPIDEMIOLOGY

Hydranencephaly is a rare, devastating malformation in which there is almost complete absence of the cerebral hemispheres. Its incidence is not known and there appears to be no gender predilection. Postnatal hydranencephaly has been shown to occur after extensive infarction, hemorrhage, and meningitis.

CLINICAL FEATURES

Although it is generally accepted that hydranencephaly is probably secondary to in utero occlusion of the internal carotid arteries, maternal cocaine use and cytomegalovirus and toxoplasma infections have also been implicated as etiologic factors. In patients with hydranencephaly, the calvarium is intact. The cranium is mostly filled with cerebrospinal fluid (CSF), but there may be residual brain tissues in the occipital, posterior temporal, and basal frontal regions. Superiorly, the CSF-filled sac is lined by leptomeninges and a very thin mantle of residual and often gliotic cortex; thus, infarction with liquefaction of the cerebral hemispheres seems an attractive explanation. The optic nerves are hypoplastic and the brain stem and cerebellum are present but small. A portion of the midbrain may also be present.

Neonates are usually normal clinically. Initially, the head circumference is normal or reduced, but it enlarges progressively. After a few weeks of life, the patients manifest myoclonic seizures and spasticity. Electroencephalography shows suppressed or absent activity. A CSF shunt may be needed to avoid massive macrocephaly and make handling of the child easier. Most patients die during the first year of life. The most important differential diagnosis is that of massive hydrocephalus. Because patients with both hydranencephaly and massive hydrocephalus may require a shunt, distinction between these entities may be of academic interest only. In patients with massive hydrocephalus, regrowth of the cortical mantle is usually evident on follow-up imaging studies.

IMAGING FEATURES

A significant number of cases are discovered by in utero sonography. Color Doppler may show absence of arterial flow above the supraclinoid portion of the internal carotid arteries, suggesting the diagnosis. Magnetic resonance is the imaging modality of choice (Fig. 5.03-1). The cerebellum and brain stem are present but atrophic. The midbrain is usually seen, and occasionally the thalami are present. A small amount of the occipital and frontal lobes usually is present. These residues are commonly dysplastic, and it is difficult to recognize normal structures within them. The falx cerebri is usually absent in its mid-portion. The posterior and anterior-most aspects of the falx may, however, be seen. Cortical branches from the anterior and middle cerebral arteries are absent. Some investigators consider hydranencephaly a similar entity to bilateral open-lip schizencephalies.

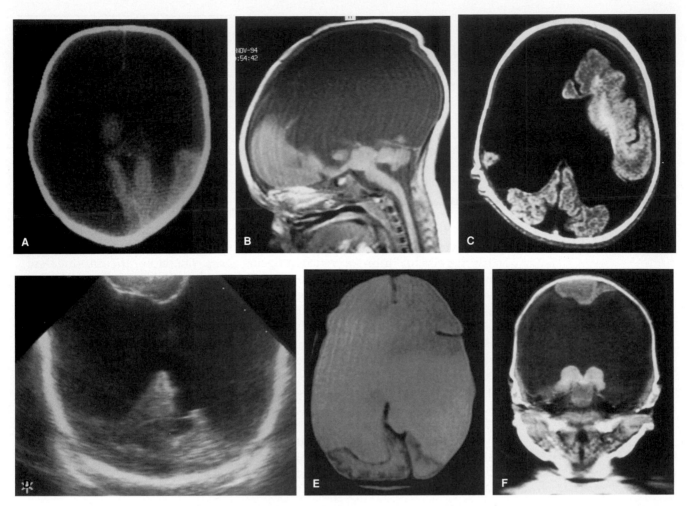

FIGURE 5.03-1.

Hydranencephaly. **A.** Axial noncontrast computed tomography in a patient with hydranencephaly shows most of the cranium to be filled with cerebrospinal fluid (CSF). Posteriorly, there are residual brain tissues that receive blood supply from the posterior circulation, which remains intact in these cases. **B.** Midsagittal magnetic resonance (MR) T1-weighted image in a different patient shows absent cerebral hemispheres. The overall size of the head is normal. Hypoplastic brain stem and cerebellar vermis are present. Residual frontobasal brain parenchyma is present. **C.** Axial MR T1-weighted image shows residual brain tissues posteriorly and in the left temporofrontal region. This appearance may be classified as hydranencephaly or large bilateral open-lip schizencephalies. **D.** Coronal sonogram (different patient) shows hydranencephaly with residual brain in the occipital region and along the superior convexity. **E.** Axial MR T2-weighted image in the same patient shows a mostly CSF-filled cranium with residual brain dorsally. The anterior aspect of the falx cerebri is present. **F.** Coronal MR T1-weighted image in the same patient shows that the thalami and upper brain stem are present but hypoplastic. This image confirms that, as was seen in the sonogram, there are residual tissues along the convexity. Note that these are dysplastic and do not contain an interhemispheric fissure. The thalami are not fused excluding holoprocencephaly.

SUGGESTED READINGS

1. Rayband C. Destructive lesions of the brain. Neuroradiology 1983;25:265.
2. Rais-Bahrami K, Naqvi M. Hydranencephaly and maternal cocaine use: a case report. Clin Pediatr (Phila) 1990;29:729.

5.04 *Periventricular Leukomalacia*

EPIDEMIOLOGY

Periventricular leukomalacia (PVL) is a hypoxic–ischemic insult to the watershed periventricular (parasagittal) white matter, resulting in coagulative necrosis. It occurs in approximately 85% of newborns weighing between 900 to 2200 g and surviving past the first week of life. Although prematurity is a predisposing factor, PVL may occur regardless of gestational age or weight.

CLINICAL FEATURES

The deep white and gray matter surrounding the ventricles receive their blood supply from deep perforating and choroidal arteries (ventriculofugal flow), whereas the superficial white matter and cortex receive their blood from penetrating vessels arising from cortical branches from the anterior, middle, and posterior cerebral arteries (ventriculopedal flow). Therefore, the intermediate (parasagittal) white matter may be considered watershed or border-zone between the two major circulations. Ischemia leading to anaerobic metabolism and possibly an endotoxin are implicated in the damage.

The clinical manifestations of PVL in the neonatal period are not well defined. Decreased tone and movement of the lower extremities are relatively common. The long-term sequelae include spastic diplegia or quadriplegia with lesser involvement of the upper extremities. Intellectual deficits and visual difficulties are also present. These findings correlate well with the location of the injury, which affects predominantly the white matter in the periatrial region and in the posterior limb of the internal capsules. These regions are also more prone to damage because they contain more myelinated fibers, are metabolically more active, and also contain a greater amount of excitatory amino acids. Other entities that may lead to damage of the periventricular white matter include meningitis, ventriculitis, metabolic disorders, and maternal cocaine use.

IMAGING FEATURES

The imaging features of PVL may be divided into those occurring in the acute period and those that are the sequelae (chronic changes) of this insult. Sonography via the anterior fontanelle is an excellent screening method, detecting up to 80% of cases. Caution is needed because PVL may be confused with the normal hyperechoic areas seen in the periventricular regions. Ultrasound is also helpful in documenting the formation of cysts in the injured regions (Fig 5.04-1A). Magnetic resonance (MR) imaging may depict the features of this disease accurately, but may be difficult to obtain in these infants. Commonly, T2-weighted images show increased signal intensity in the white matter close to the atria and occipital horns of the lateral ventricles. T1-weighted images may demonstrate focal and nodular hyperintensities, suggesting hemorrhage (Fig. 5.04-1B). Hemorrhage may be seen in 25% of patients with PVL, and rarely will be large enough to extend into the ventricles. The findings are usually bilateral. In the subacute period, there is formation of microcysts, which are better seen with ultrasound. Computed tomography is the least sensitive method for the detection of acute PVL, demonstrating positive findings in only 42% of patients with abnormalities shown by MR imaging.

In the late subacute period, the periventricular cysts coalesce. These patients invariably have symptoms. Chronic findings include a diminished amount of white matter in the posterior periventricular regions (Fig. 5.04-2). The posterior body and splenium of the corpus callosum are atrophic as a result of degeneration of transcallosal fibers. The sulci and gray matter extend almost to the lateral border of the ventricles. The lateral walls of the ventricles are wavy. In severe cases, the centrum semiovale and frontal white matter may be involved. There is increased T2 signal intensity in these regions.

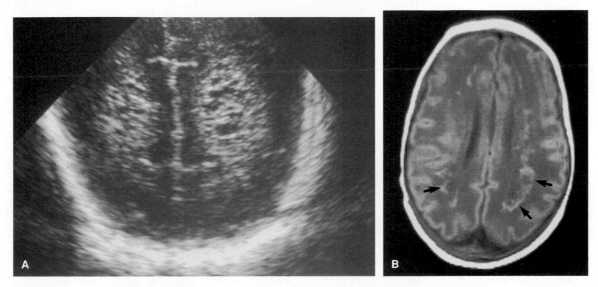

FIGURE 5.04-1.

Acute periventricular leukomalacia (PVL). **A.** Coronal sonogram shows zones of increased echogenicity bilaterally. Note that these zones contain multiple cystic areas. The findings are typical of PVL. **B.** Axial magnetic resonance T1-weighted image (different patient) shows periventricular regions of high signal intensity *(arrows)*; methemoglobin) surrounding areas of early cavitation in a case of PVL.

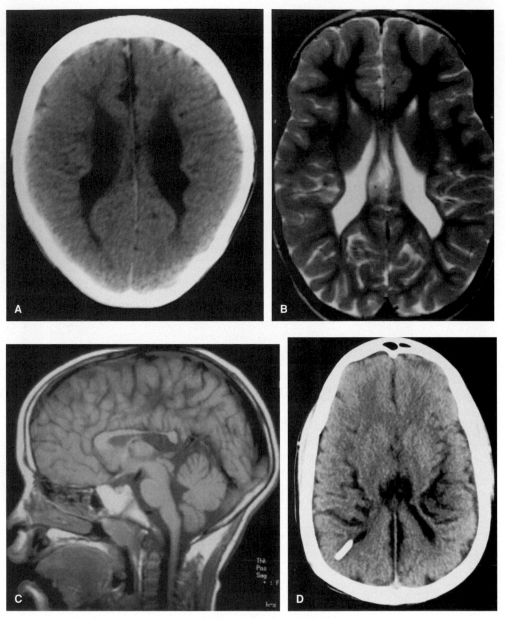

FIGURE 5.04-2.

Chronic changes from periventricular leukomalacia (PVL). **A.** Axial noncontrast computed tomography (CT) shows prominent lateral ventricles with a wavy outer border. The periventricular white matter is severely diminished and the sulci extend deep and almost to the ventricles. These findings are compatible with chronic features of the disease. Note that in this case the white matter of both the parietal and frontal regions is reduced. **B.** Axial magnetic resonance (MR) T2-weighted image in a different patient shows markedly reduced white matter in the posterior regions of the brain and enlarged lateral ventricles (posteriorly) with wavy outer borders. Findings are typical of chronic sequelae of PVL. (With permission from Castillo M. Neuroradiology Companion. Philadelphia: JB Lippincott, 1995.) **C.** Midsagittal MR T1-weighted image in the same patient shows atrophy of the posterior body and splenium of the corpus callosum, probably secondary to degeneration of white matter fibers. **D.** Axial CT in a different patient shows marked reduction of posterior white matter with medial displacement of the posterior Sylvian fissure. Note normal-appearing white matter in the frontal lobes. A right ventricular shunt is partially seen.

SUGGESTED READINGS

1. Schouman-Claeys E, Henry-Feugeas MC, Roset F, et al. Periventricular leukomalacia: correlation between MR imaging and autopsy findings during the first two months of life. Radiology 1993;189:59.
2. Baker LL, Stevenson DK, Enzmann DR. End-stage periventricular leukomalacia: MR evaluation. Radiology 1988;168:809.
3. Grant EG, Schellinger D, Richardson JD, Coffey ML, Smirniotopuolous JG. Echogenic periventricular halo: normal sonographic finding or neonatal cerebral hemorrhage. AJNR 1983;4:43.
4. DiPietro MA, Brody BA, Teele RL. Peritrigonal echogenic "blush" on cranial sonography: pathologic correlates. AJR 1986;146:1067.

5.05 *Hypoxic–Ischemic Encephalopathy*

EPIDEMIOLOGY

As used here, hypoxic–ischemic encephalopathy implies diffuse cerebral hypoxia–ischemia in infants well after birth, and not focal hypoxia–ischemia, which leads to regional infarcts. The etiology of hypoxic–ischemic encephalopathy is multifactorial and may be secondary to hemoglobinopathies, infections, radiation therapy, effects of certain medications, angiitis, drowning, cardiac arrest, hypoglycemia, and trauma.

CLINICAL FEATURES

A clear history of hypoxia–ischemia may be obtained in most patients. Unclear or questionable histories should raise suspicion of child abuse. The symptoms may be mild and include jitteriness, irritability, and increased deep tendon reflexes. Patients with these symptoms may be expected to have a good prognosis. Clinical signs of a moderate insult include lethargy, hypotonia, seizures, and decreased reflexes. Sixty to 80% of these patients have a good prognosis. Signs of severe encephalopathy include coma, hypotonia, seizures, brain stem dysfunction, and elevated intracranial pressure. Most of these patients have an unfavorable prognosis and do not survive past the acute period. In most patients, electroencephalography (EEG) shows suppression of amplitude and slowing of electrical activity interposed with high-voltage sharp and slow waves. Rapid resolution of abnormal EEG findings correlates with a favorable prognosis. Profound asphyxia may result in athetosis, long tract signs, mental retardation, and seizures. Acutely, treatment is geared toward controlling intracranial hypertension (and edema) and seizures, and maintaining adequate cerebral blood flow.

Pathologically, the following abnormalities may be identified: selective neuronal necrosis, status marmoratus of the basal ganglia and thalami, parasagittal brain injury, and diffuse cerebral necrosis. Selective neuronal necrosis involves the hippocampus (particularly sector CA 1), cerebellar cortex, thalami, and anterior horns of the spinal cord. In status marmoratus there is necrosis and gliosis of deep gray matter nuclei with hypermyelination of residual fibers. Parasagittal brain injury damages the perirolandic areas, lateral thalami, and posterior lentiform nuclei. All three types of insults are seen in premature infants or term newborns and infants. In older children, the caudate nuclei, lentiform nuclei, and cortex (other than the perirolandic areas) are damaged. In diffuse cerebral necrosis, the white matter, deep gray nuclei, and cortex are involved with relative sparing of the brain stem and cerebellum. The end-result of severe injury is multicystic malacia with or without dystrophic calcifications and atrophy.

IMAGING FEATURES

There are no obvious imaging abnormalities in the acute phase of selective neuronal necrosis. The end-result may be cerebellar atrophy or hippocampal sclerosis. In status marmoratus, magnetic resonance (MR) imaging may show high T2 signal intensity in the thalami interposed with patchy areas of lower signal intensity related to hypermyelinated fibers. Other deep gray matter structures may show similar findings. Profound asphyxia may lead to parasagittal brain injury. This occurs in newborns and infants. Acutely, MR imaging may show hyperintensity in the subinsular regions (and lateral putaminal areas), globus pallidi, and lateral thalami. In the subacute period, the hyperintensities become obvious. In the chronic stages, MR imaging may show T1 shortening in the hippocampi, posterolateral lentiform nuclei, and perirolandic cortex, and diffuse cerebral atrophy (Fig. 5.05-1). T2-weighted images show increased signal intensity in all of these regions. In older children who suffer profound asphyxia, MR imaging shows diffuse edema and hyperintensity of the cerebral cortex on proton density and T2-weighted images. Also, a subtle area of hyperintensity may be seen in the immediate subcortical areas. The deep gray nuclei are also usually hyperintense. In the chronic stage, diffuse atrophy and dystrophic basal ganglia calcifications may be present (Fig. 5.05-2). Diffuse cystic encephalomalacia is usually the sequela of marked generalized infarction. Partial profound asphyxia damages the watershed regions, which show hyperintensity on T2-weighted images. Laminar necrosis may also be present, and is seen as a stripe of T1 hyperintensity in the deep cortex. In chronic stages, the brain suffers atrophy (especially in the watershed regions). Malacia may be seen in the watershed and other regions (Fig. 5.05-3).

Severe ischemia may also lead to the formation of so-called "ulegyria." In this scenario, there is more severe involvement of the gray matter in the deep portions of the cortical sulci than in the apex of the gyri. Ischemia results in diminished volume of the base of gyri, giving them a mushroom-like appearance.

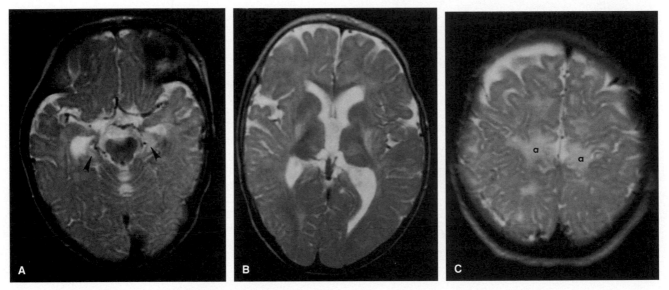

FIGURE 5.05-1.

Profound asphyxia.   **A.** Axial magnetic resonance (MR) T2-weighted image in an infant 1 year after an episode of profound asphyxia. Abnormal hyperintensity is present in the mesial temporal lobes *(arrowheads).* **B.** Axial MR T2-weighted image in the same patient shows abnormal hyperintensities in the posterior lentiform nuclei and possibly in the thalami. **C.** Axial MR T2-weighted image in the same patient shows abnormal (a) hyperintensity in the perirolandic white matter and mild cortical atrophy.

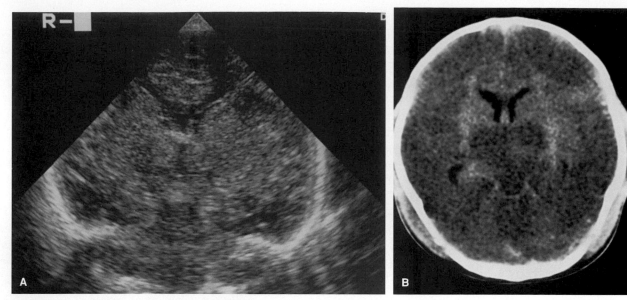

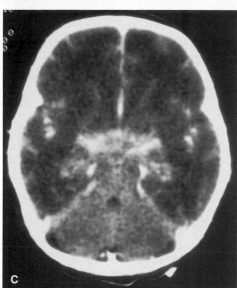

FIGURE 5.05-2.

Diffuse edema and infarctions. **A.** Coronal sonogram in a newborn with hypoxia at birth shows subtle but definite increased echogenicity throughout the brain. (With permission from Castillo M. Color duplex sonography of the neonatal brain. In: Thrall JH, ed. Current Practice in Radiology. Philadelphia: BC Decker, 1993, p 717.) **B.** Axial noncontrast computed tomography (CT) in the same patient 2 days later shows diffuse and severe hypodensity involving both cerebral hemispheres. The lentiform nuclei remain dense. This patient had perinatal asphyxia. **C.** Axial noncontrast CT in same patient 2 weeks after birth shows diffuse hemispheric malacia with residual and thin cortex. Dystrophic calcifications have been deposited in the thalami. The cerebellum is relatively normal.

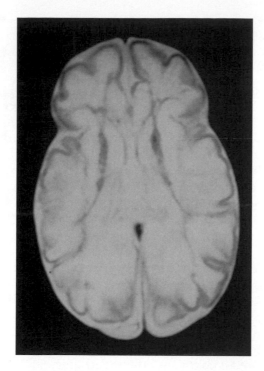

FIGURE 5.05-3.

Multicystic encephalomalacia. Axial magnetic resonance T2-weighted image in a patient 6 months after cardiac arrest shows diffuse hyperintensity throughout the entire brain secondary to postinfarction malacia. The residual cortex is well seen. The head is slightly dolichocephalic because sagittal synostosis had occurred.

SUGGESTED READINGS

1. Barkovich AJ. MR and CT evaluation of profound neonatal and infantile ischemia. AJNR 1992;13:959.
2. Hill A, Volpe JJ. Hypoxic–ischemia cerebral injury in the newborn. In: Swaiman KF, ed. Pediatric Neurology, 2nd ed. St. Louis: CV Mosby, 1994:489.

5.06 *Stroke in Childhood*

EPIDEMIOLOGY

Cerebral infarctions in childhood are rare. The overall incidence of stroke in childhood is 2.5 per 100,000 children. Predisposing factors include cardiac disease (most important cause in neonates), hemoglobinopathies (particularly sickle cell disease), disorders of thrombogenesis or thrombolysis (protein C deficiency), central nervous system (CNS) infections (meningitis), vasculitis (lupus erythematosus), trauma (child abuse), metabolic disorders (diabetes, MELAS), radiation therapy, chemotherapy, neurocutaneous syndromes, migraine, Takayasu disease, fibromuscular dysplasia, leukemia, moyamoya, and progeria. Strokes occur in almost 4% of patients with congenital heart disease.

CLINICAL FEATURES

Half of childhood strokes are hemorrhagic and half are ischemic. Clinically, it is most helpful to divide infarctions into those of arterial origin and those occurring secondary to venous thrombosis. Most embolic infarctions are secondary to congenital heart disease, mitral valve prolapse, trauma, carotid dissection, fibromuscular dysplasia, Marfan syndrome, and Takayasu and Kawasaki diseases. Most carotid dissections are secondary to trauma and preceded by penetration of an object into the mouth (Fig. 5.06-1). Hyperextension and torsion of the neck ("head banging") may also induce dissections. Patients with emboli or dissections commonly present with delayed hemiplegia. In these patients, symptoms usually begin 2 to 4 hours after the trauma. The entity "acute infantile hemiplegia" is a primary vascular disease for which no cause is found. It is a diagnosis of exclusion and should be considered only if a thorough investigation has excluded other causes. Thrombosis of vessels is usually secondary to endothelial cell damage, platelet dysfunction, meningitis, migraines, and hypercoagulable states (dehydration, protein C or S deficiencies, sickle cell disease). In sickle cell disease, only 25% of patients have other clinically referable symptoms to their underlying disease at the time of the stroke. Hemiparesis is the presenting symptom in 50% of cases, aphasia occurs in 20%, and seizures in 10%. Transient ischemic attacks preceding the actual stroke are reported in 10% of children with sickle cell disease. Arteritis may follow CNS infections, drug use, or radiation/chemotherapy, or is associated with the phakomatoses. Of the phakomatoses, Sturge-Weber disease has the highest incidence of infarctions.

Thrombosis of veins and sinuses is commonly secondary to hypercoagulability, CNS or paranasal sinus infections, meningitis, and trauma. Thrombosis of the superior sagittal sinus is usually seen in patients younger than 3 years of age. Symptoms include irritability, alteration of consciousness, seizures, and communicating hydrocephalus. In older patients, sagittal sinus thrombosis produces "pseudotumor" cerebri. Transverse sinus thrombosis is seen predominantly in cases of mastoiditis. Symptoms are those described earlier for sagittal sinus occlusion, but there may be evidence of otitis media. Cavernous sinus thrombosis usually occurs in the setting of infection of the orbits, paranasal sinuses, and oral cavity.

IMAGING FEATURES

As in adults, the role of imaging is to characterize an infarct as hemorrhagic or nonhemorrhagic and to exclude a rare underlying and unknown disease presenting in stroke-like fashion (eg, tumors, vascular malformations). In children, we prefer magnetic resonance (MR) as the initial imaging modality (Fig. 5.06-2). MR angiography detects abnormalities in up to 75% of children with strokes. Acutely, MR imaging shows hyperintense cortex (particularly on proton density images), lack of flow void in occluded or nearly occluded vessels, and intravascular enhancement after contrast administration. In the immediate subacute period, meningeal enhancement is followed by parenchymal enhancement. Chronically, there is encephalomalacia and gliosis (Fig. 5.06-3). Computed tomography, however, still plays a critical role in the initial evaluation of the stroke victims (Fig. 5.06-4).

Magnetic resonance is also the imaging method of choice to demonstrate venous thrombosis. Lack of flow void and intraluminal high signal intensity on T1-weighted images are typical findings. Although MR venography nicely portrays the abnormalities, it is not imperative to obtain it because static images are usually confirmatory. Venous thrombus (particularly in cortical veins) lyses fast, and its absence should not exclude the diagnosis if zones of edema, infarctions, or hemorrhages (especially bilateral and in the convexities) are present (Fig. 5.06-5). Approximately 25% of venous infarctions are hemorrhagic.

In cases of suspected carotid artery dissection, catheter angiography continues to be the imaging method of choice. MR angiography is also very useful. MR imaging also demonstrates the mural thrombus and residual lumen.

Systemic hypotension may produce infarctions in the watershed areas. Drowning (and other asphyxias) and some metabolic abnormalities result in diffuse cerebral edema, which can produce occipital infarction (Fig. 5.06-6).

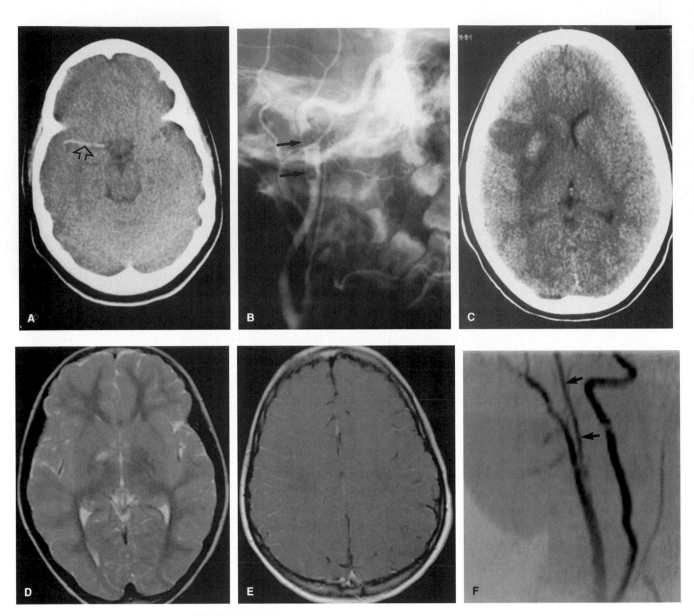

FIGURE 5.06-1.

Acute cerebral infarction. **A.** Patient sustained injury to the mouth with a pencil during a fall and presented with acute left hemiplegia. Axial noncontrast computed tomography (CT) shows hyperdense right middle cerebral artery *(arrow)*, which is a sign of acute infarction. **B.** Oblique view from catheter angiogram shows intravascular filling defect *(arrows; clot?)* in high right internal carotid artery. **C.** Noncontrast axial CT 2 days after the trauma shows well-defined and partially hemorrhagic right middle cerebral artery infarct. The patient has recovered almost all function 1 year after the event. **D.** Axial magnetic resonance (MR) T2-weighted image in a different child with left hemiplegia shows hyperintensity in genu of right internal capsule. **E.** Axial postcontrast MR T1-weighted image shows intravascular enhancement throughout right cerebral hemisphere. **F.** Lateral view from three-dimensional time-of-flight MR angiogram shows diffuse narrowing of right internal carotid artery *(arrows)*, suggesting dissection.

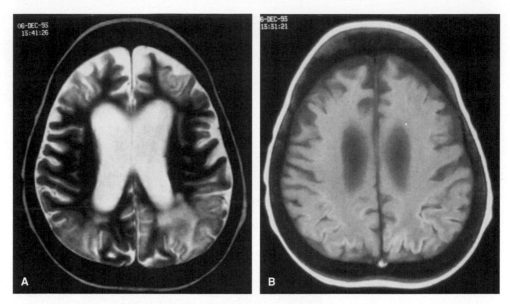

FIGURE 5.06-2.

Laminar necrosis. **A.** Axial magnetic resonance (MR) T2-weighted image in a child with thalassemia shows bilateral subacute frontal and parietal watershed infarctions. Note diffuse atrophy and thickening of the diploic space. **B.** Axial MR T1-weighted image shows subacute hemorrhage in the cortex of both parietal infarcts and, to a lesser extent, in the left frontal one. This represents laminar necrosis. (With permission from Castillo M. Neuroradiology Companion. Philadelphia: JB Lippincott, 1995.)

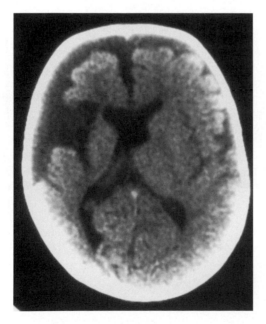

FIGURE 5.06-3.

Chronic infarction. Axial noncontrast computed tomography in patient with history of child abuse during the first week of life. There is marked atrophy of the right cerebral hemisphere, probably secondary to ischemia due to carotid artery dissection.

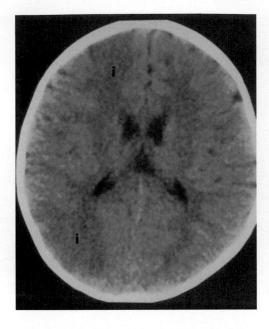

FIGURE 5.06-4.

Watershed infarcts. Axial noncontrast computed tomography in a patient after surgery for pulmonic stenosis shows watershed infarctions (i) in right frontotemporal and parieto-occipital regions.

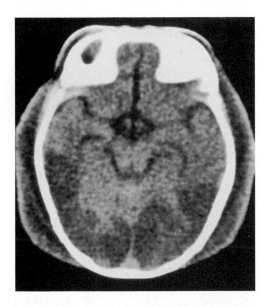

FIGURE 5.06-5.

Venous infarctions. Axial noncontrast computed tomography in a patient with nephrotic syndrome. There are bilateral posterior temporal and occipital infarctions, probably secondary to venous thrombosis. Note scalp edema secondary to hypoalbuminemia.

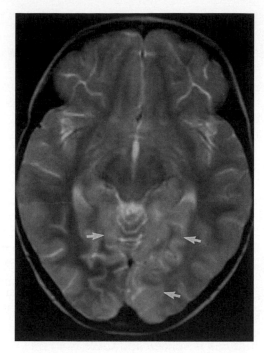

FIGURE 5.06-6.

Occipital infarctions. Axial magnetic resonance T2-weighted image after diabetic coma in a child shows bilateral occipital *(arrows)* areas of hyperintensity in the cortex, suggesting edema in early infarctions. These infarcts are presumably caused by diffuse cerebral edema with herniation and clipping of both posterior cerebral arteries.

SUGGESTED READING

1. Ball WS. Cerebrovascular occlusive disease in childhood. Neuroimaging Clinics of North America 1994;4:393.

5.07 *Intracranial Hemorrhage in Premature Newborns*

EPIDEMIOLOGY

The incidence of intracranial hemorrhage in premature newborns has decreased during the last decade. Nevertheless, intracranial hemorrhage occurs in 25% of newborns weighing less than 1500 g and in 62% of those weighing less than 700 g. Cerebral hemorrhage in term infants is rare.

CLINICAL FEATURES

The main predisposing factors for intracranial hemorrhage are low birth weight and prematurity. Other predisposing factors include low Apgar scores, vaginal delivery, blood pressure fluctuations in the baby, apnea, bradycardia, large patent ductus arteriosus, pneumothorax, β-streptococcal septicemia, and hypoxia. The roles of suctioning, benzyl alcohol and heparin in flush solutions, and indomethacin are not clear. Most hemorrhages occur before the 34th week of gestational age (after which the germinal matrix involutes). Clinically, two syndromes are seen. The "saltutory" syndrome is characterized by altered consciousness, decreased movements, hypotonia, and oculomotor abnormalities. These signs wax and wane, and the mortality is less than that associated with the "catastrophic" syndrome. In the catastrophic syndrome the onset of symptoms is sudden and there is a rapid progression to coma and death. The main symptoms in this syndrome are respiratory difficulty, extensor posturing, seizures, and brain stem dysfunction. Mortality is high in these patients. The prognosis in all intracranial hemorrhages varies mainly according to the size of the bleed and the gestational age. For patients with small hemorrhages and no hydrocephalus, the incidence of neurologic sequelae is between 10% and 30%. Patients with hydrocephalus have a 50% chance of permanent sequelae. Hydrocephalus is a complication that develops in up to 15% of all premature newborns with germinal matrix hemorrhages. In two thirds of these patients, the ventricular dilation becomes stable and nonprogressive. These patients do not require treatment. Hydrocephalus requiring shunting develops in one third of patients. Communicating hydrocephalus is secondary to an adhesive arachnoiditis. Patients with intraparenchymal hemorrhages have a 90% incidence of permanent neurologic sequelae. Small premature patients with large bleeds have a very high mortality rate. Intracranial hemorrhages in term newborns are caused by residual germinal matrix, laceration of the choroid plexuses, vascular malformations, congenital tumors, infarction, and coagulopathy. Venous thrombosis is the most common cause of thalamic bleeds. These patients have a poor prognosis.

IMAGING FEATURES

Bedside sonography continues to be the imaging method of choice in these patients. Most examinations are done through the anterior fontanelle, although imaging through the posterior fontanelle helps in identifying intraventricular hemorrhages. By sonography, germinal matrix hemorrhages may be divided into the following groups:

> Grade 1: Hemorrhage limited to the germinal matrix (subependymal germinal matrix hemorrhage; Fig. 5.07-1). This appears as a focus of echogenicity in the caudothalamic groove. The ventricles are normal in size. These small hemorrhages evolve into cysts that then collapse and eventually disappear.

Grade 2: A germinal matrix hemorrhage that has extended into the ventricles but without hydrocephalus (Fig. 5.07-2). Echogenic material is seen especially in the frontal horns of the lateral ventricles. A prominent and lumpy choroid plexus is normal and should not be confused with a bleed. The size of the ventricles is normal.

Grade 3: Intraventricular hemorrhage with hydrocephalus (Fig. 5.07-3).

Grade 4: Intraparenchymal hemorrhage (Fig. 5.07-4). Most of these bleeds are probably secondary to increased venous pressure with subsequent bleeding into the parenchyma from deep medullary veins. Large intracerebral bleeds may also be secondary to venous thrombosis induced by difficult delivery (Fig. 5.07-5).

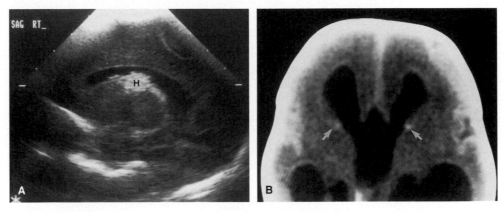

FIGURE 5.07-1.

Grade 1 hemorrhage. **A.** Parasagittal sonogram shows echogenic focus in caudothalamic notch region compatible with subependymal germinal matrix hemorrhage (H). **B.** Axial noncontrast computed tomography shows bilateral grade 1 hemorrhages *(arrows)* in a premature child with a Dandy-Walker malformation and hydrolephalus.

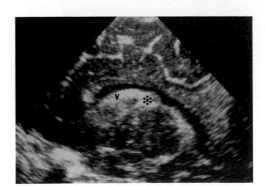

FIGURE 5.07-2.

Grade 2 hemorrhage. Parasagittal sonogram shows echogenic focus of blood in the caudothalamic notch *(asterisk)* region with extension into the adjacent frontal horn (v) of the lateral ventricle, but without ventricular dilation. (With permission from Castillo M. Neuroradiology Companion. Philadelphia: JB Lippincott, 1995.)

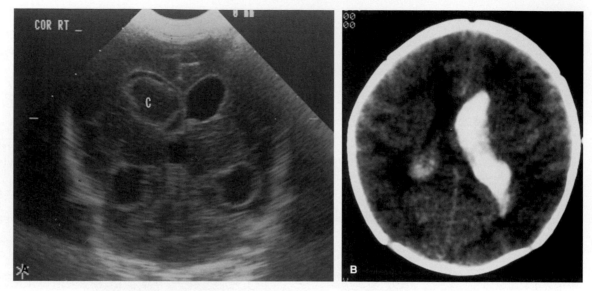

FIGURE 5.07-3.

Grade 3 hemorrhage. **A.** Coronal sonogram shows clot (C) filling most of the right lateral ventricle. There is hydrocephalus. (With permission from Castillo M. Neuroradiology Companion. Philadelphia: JB Lippincott, 1995.) **B.** Noncontrast axial computed tomography (different patient) shows acute blood in the left lateral ventricle and a small amount of blood in the right lateral ventricle. The ventricles are prominent.

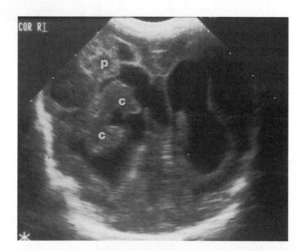

FIGURE 5.07-4.

Grade 4 hemorrhage. Coronal sonogram shows hydrocephalus and clot (c) in right lateral ventricle. Note right parenchymal hemorrhage (p).

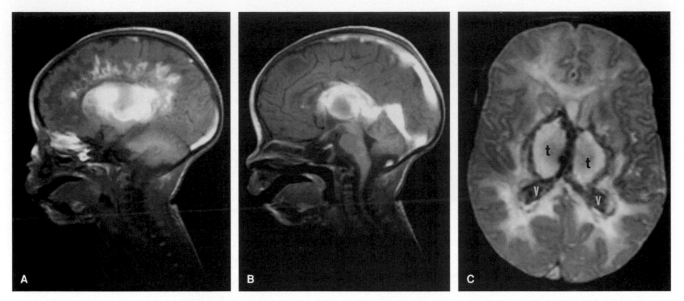

FIGURE 5.07-5.

Venous thrombosis. **A.** Parasagittal magnetic resonance (MR) T1-weighted image in a newborn after difficult delivery shows subacute hemorrhage (methemoglobin) in thalamus and basal ganglia as well as in the periventricular white matter. Note hyperintensity in cortical veins and superior sagittal sinus. This patient had thrombosis of the superficial and deep venous systems, resulting in presumed hemorrhagic infarctions. **B.** Midline sagittal MR T1-weighted image in same patient shows hyperintense clot in the superior sagittal sinus, straight sinus, torcular, vein of Galen, and internal cerebral veins. The hemorrhagic thalamic massa intermedia is well seen. **C.** Axial MR T2-weighted image shows bilateral thalamic (t) hemorrhages and blood in the atria (V) of the lateral ventricles. The white matter posteriorly is also hyperintense secondary to hemorrhage. (With permission from Castillo M. Neuroradiology Companion. Philadelphia: JB Lippincott, 1995.)

SUGGESTED READING

1. Anderson N, Alan R, Darlow B, Malpas T. Diagnosis of intraventricular hemorrhage in the newborn: value of sonography via the posterior fontanelle. AJR 1994; 163:893.

5.08 Arteriopathies

EPIDEMIOLOGY

Most arteritis in children is secondary to meningitis, encephalitis, collagen vascular disorders (especially lupus erythematosus), granulomatous angiitis, prior brain radiation, hemoglobinopathies (especially sickle cell disease), and inborn errors of metabolism and those associated with the phakomatoses. This discussion is centered on sickle cell disease-induced vasculitis and moyamoya. Approximately 8% of children with sickle cell disease will have an arteritis. Of all deaths occurring in sickle cell anemia patients, 12% are caused by cerebrovascular disease. Moyamoya is a progressive arteriopathy causing narrowing of the supraclinoid internal carotid arteries and commonly extending into other vessels. The primary disease is idiopathic and more common in Japanese patients. The secondary disease is more common in the Western world and is characterized by imaging abnormalities identical to those of the primary disease.

CLINICAL FEATURES

Strokes in children with sickle cell disease usually occur between 5 to 10 years of age. Transient ischemic attacks happen in 19% of children with sickle cell disease, aphasia in 20%, and seizures in approximately 15%. The etiology of the vascular damage in sickle cell disease patients is uncertain; injury to the vasa vasorum has not been demonstrated. Endothelial damage is more likely.

Symptoms of moyamoya are more common in girls (6:1) and include transient ischemic attacks, sudden hemiparesis, mental deterioration, and seizures (especially in the youngest patients). The symptoms may resolve, but the deficits may also become permanent. Signs indicating a poor prognosis are onset at an early age and involvement of the dominant cerebral hemisphere. Moyamoya is uncommon in children younger than 2 years of age except when associated with a phakomatosis.

Neurologic symptoms are found in up to 40% of patients with lupus erythematosus. Behavioral problems and focal deficits are the most common symptoms.

IMAGING FEATURES

Conventional angiography is still the imaging method of choice when the diagnosis of vasculitis requires confirmation. In patients with sickle cell disease, the damage may involve small or large vessels. The latter produces a "moyamoya-like" appearance. Magnetic resonance (MR) angiography is useful only in patients with large vessel abnormalities (Fig. 5.08-1). Increased velocities (> 190 cm/second) in the proximal anterior and middle cerebral arteries by Doppler sonography may identify those patients with proximal severe stenoses. These patients may be more prone to strokes. In patients with small vessel disease, angiography shows focal stenoses distal from branching points.

The diagnosis of moyamoya may be made with either catheter or MR angiography (Fig. 5.08-2). There is severe stenosis or occlusion of the supraclinoid internal carotid arteries with proliferation of deep perforating arteries. In the primary disorder, the narrowing may extend to the posterior communicating arteries and the top of the basilar artery. The proximal anterior and middle cerebral arteries may also be narrowed. The stenoses usually are smooth. On MR imaging, multiple punctate areas of flow void are present in the basal ganglia and thalami (due to hypertrophied perforating arteries), and there may absence of flow void in the distal internal carotid arteries. Multiple infarctions, both in arterial and watershed distributions, are often present.

Two important diseases that need to be emphasized are fibromuscular dysplasia and granulomatous angiitis. Fibromuscular dysplasia in children is usually seen in neurofibromatosis type I. Moyamoya may also occur in these children. In patients with granulomatous angiitis, the angiogram is usually negative because the disease involves very small vessels (< 200 μm) that are not visible by catheter angiography.

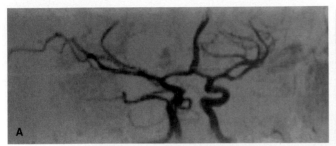
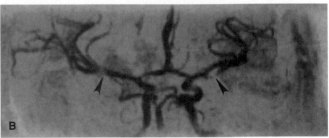

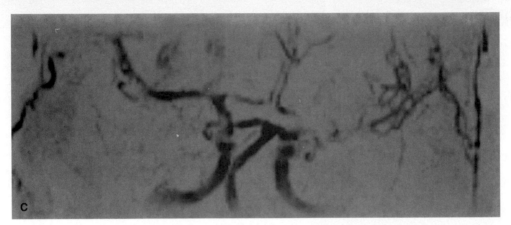

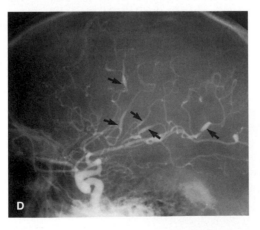

FIGURE 5.08-1.

Primary central nervous system vasculitis. **A.** Frontal view from three-dimensional time-of-flight (TOF) magnetic resonance angiography (MRA) in an adolescent with suspected cerebral vasculitis. The examination appears normal. **B.** Frontal view from three-dimensional TOF MRA enhanced with acetazolamide administration shows several defects *(arrowheads)* in large vessels in the same patient. Acetazolamide increases cerebral blood flow and "brings out" subtle abnormalities as well as enhancing visualization of peripheral vessels. **C.** In a different case of primary vasculitis, frontal view from three-dimensional TOF MRA shows multiple narrowings compatible with vasculitis. **D.** Lateral angiographic view shows multiple areas of dilation *(arrows)* in small vessels, compatible with vasculitis.

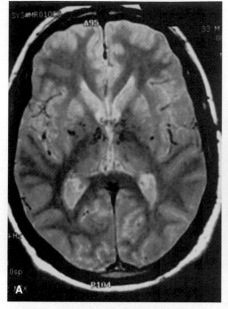

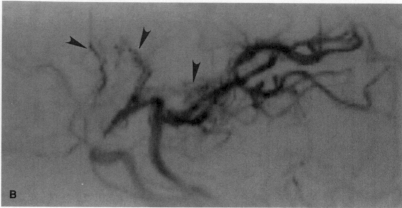

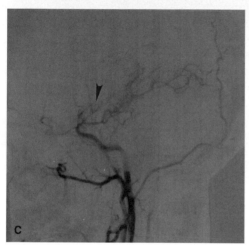

FIGURE 5.08-2.

Moyamoya phenomenon. **A.** Axial magnetic resonance (MR) T2-weighted image in a young patient with sickle cell disease and transient ischemic attacks. There are multiple punctate areas of flow void in the basal ganglia bilaterally, suggesting hypertrophy of lenticulostriate vessels. **B.** Lateral view from three-dimensional time-of-flight MR angiography in the same patient shows absent flow and supraclinoid internal carotid arteries and hypertrophy of lenticulostriate and thalamoperforating arteries *(arrowheads),* compatible with a Moyamoya phenomenon. **C.** Lateral view from catheter angiogram injection of a common carotid artery shows occluded distal internal carotid artery with patent posterior communicator and presence of hypertrophied perforating vessels *(arrowhead).*

SUGGESTED READINGS

1. Ball WS. Cerebrovascular occlusive disease in childhood. Neuroimaging Clinics of North America 1994;4:393.
2. Atlas SW. MR angiography in neurologic disease. Radiology 1994;193:1.
3. Korogi Y, Takahashi M, Mabuchi N, et al. Intracranial vascular stenosis and occlusion: diagnostic accuracy of three-dimensional, Fourier transform, time-of-flight MR angiography. Radiology 1994;193:187.

5.09 Aneurysms

EPIDEMIOLOGY

Intracranial aneurysms are rare in children younger than 10 years of age, with a peak incidence in patients younger than 2 years of age. Their incidence is approximately 0.6%. Boys are affected more commonly than girls. Infectious (previously called "mycotic") aneurysms usually are seen in the setting of congenital heart disease (particularly right-to-left shunts), rheumatic heart disease, otitis media, sinusitis, sickle cell disease, and osteomyelitis of the base of skull. Other systemic disorders that predispose to the development of aneurysm are polycystic kidney disease, collagen disorders (Marfan, Ehler-Danlos) and neurofibromatosis. Trauma may induce the development of aneurysms, especially in the anterior cerebral arteries.

CLINICAL FEATURES

The term "congenital" aneurysms is probably erroneous because aneurysms are rare in children. Most aneurysms are probably related to degenerative changes in the arterial wall rather than "congenital" weaknesses. Aneurysms in children occur most commonly in the posterior communicating artery (46%), followed by the anterior communicating artery (42%) and the internal carotid artery bifurcation (33%). The most common presentations are massive and sudden subarachnoid hemorrhage accompanied by severe headache, vomiting, and altered mental status. Focal neurologic signs are common with large (> 2.5 cm) aneurysms. Approximately 20% to 40% of all intracranial aneurysms in children are of the "giant" type. Aneurysms in children younger than 2 years of age usually are more than 1 cm in diameter. These aneurysms present with bleeds or seizures and have a greater tendency to rebleed, therefore requiring more aggressive therapy. Infectious aneurysms present as subarachnoid or intracerebral hemorrhages in 25% of patients. Cerebral infarctions may occur before these aneurysms rupture. Rupture of any intracranial aneurysm may be precipitated by use of phenylpropanolamine, amphetamine, methamphetamine, ephedrine, and crack cocaine. Surgical clipping is the treatment of choice. If unresected, 50% of childhood aneurysms eventually rebleed, often with catastrophic outcome.

In the near future, interventional neuroradiology may play an important role in the treatment of aneurysms, particularly in the acute setting. Guglielmi detachable coils (electrothermocoagulation platinum coils) may be contoured to fit the dome of large and small aneurysms with a neck. Balloon dilatation of postsubarachnoid hemorrhage vasospasm has been successfully used in adults. Approximately 69% of patients whose clinical status is deteriorating will show some improvement. Intraarterial papaverine infusion is also helpful in this setting.

IMAGING FEATURES

The imaging findings of aneurysms in children are identical to those in adults. Catheter angiography continues to be the imaging method of choice to evaluate the lumen and neck of the aneurysm. Catheter angiography also demonstrates vasospasm, which, as in adults, tends to be more pronounced between the 3 days and 3 weeks after the hemorrhage. Because of the increased incidence of giant aneurysms in children, we always obtain magnetic resonance images to evaluate intraluminal clot and determine the size of the lesion. Peripheral aneurysms in children (mostly in the middle cerebral artery territory) tend to have a more "fusiform" appearance (Figs. 5.09-1 and 5.09-2). Saccular aneurysms are seen most often in the circle of Willis.

Magnetic resonance angiography may be used to screen populations at risk. However, this technique is reliable only in demonstrating aneurysms larger than 5 mm in diameter. Smaller aneurysms may be missed. Patients with arterial fenestrations and persistent carotid-basilar primitive communications have an increased risk of aneurysms.

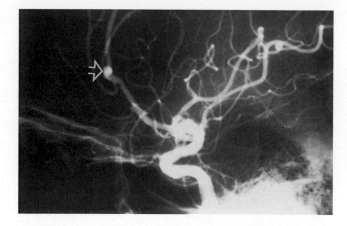

FIGURE 5.09-1.

Posttraumatic aneurysm. Oblique angiogram shows aneurysm *(arrow)* from the bifurcation of the anterior cerebral artery, presumably secondary to a motorcycle accident that occurred 10 days before this examination.

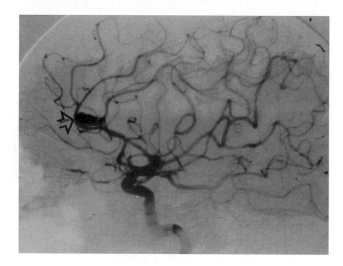

FIGURE 5.09-2.

Infectious aneurysm. Lateral view from an internal carotid artery in a patient with bacterial endocarditis shows a large, somewhat lobulated aneurysm *(arrow)* at a similar location as the posttraumatic one shown in Figure 5.09-1.

SUGGESTED READINGS

1. Meyer FB, Sundt TM, Fode NC, et al. Cerebral aneurysms in childhood and adolescence. J Neurosurg 1989;70:420.
2. Iteiskanen O, Vikki J. Intracranial arterial aneurysms in children and adolescents. Acta Neurochir 1981;59:55.
3. Matson DD. Intracranial arterial aneurysms in childhood. J Neurosurg 1965;23:578.

5.10 *Vascular Malformations*

EPIDEMIOLOGY

The exact incidence of vascular malformations in children is not known. Both genders are affected equally.

CLINICAL FEATURES

Arteriovenous malformations (AVM) are the most important type of vascular malformation in children. They represent persistence of embryologic communications (absent capillary bed) between an artery(ies) and a vein(s). One fifth of AVM become symptomatic before 20 years of age. The most common symptoms are seizures, headaches (migraines if AVM are located in the occipital lobes), progressive deficits, hydrocephalus, and intracranial hemorrhage (subarachnoid, intraparenchymal, or combined). Seizures (particularly generalized) occur in 70% of patients with cerebral AVM. Ruptured AVM are the most common causes for spontaneous intracranial bleeds in children. Up to one fifth of all strokes in childhood are associated with underlying AVM. Intraventricular rupture is unusual unless the AVM are located deep in the brain. A cranial bruit is present in 50% of children with cerebral AVM. If a cranial bruit is found in a child younger than 4 months of age, cerebral AVM should be strongly considered. There is a 10% mortality and a 50% morbidity associated with the initial hemorrhage. The risk of rebleeding is higher in children than in adults. Clinically, AVM may be classified according to their size, neurologic eloquence of adjacent brain, and pattern of venous drainage. Grade 1 and 2 lesions are small, superficial, and in noneloquent areas, and should be surgically resected. Grades 3 and 4 are intermediate lesions that should be surgically resected, especially if associated with hemorrhage or neurologic deficits (note that it is difficult to determine the course of action in grade 3 lesions). Grades 5 and 6 are large, deep, and situated in neurologically critical areas of the brain. Grade 6 AVM are considered unresectable and perhaps are better treated with a combination of embolization and irradiation. Transcatheter embolization is not uncommonly subtotal and therefore is not curative in many patients. Stereotactic radiosurgery may be useful in obliterating small (< 2.5 cm) lesions with no evidence of prior hemorrhage. Duplex Doppler sonograms offer a way to follow AVM in which multiple metallic coils have been deposited.

Cavernous angiomas are fairly common and are often incidentally discovered. They may be solitary or multiple. If multiple, they may have a familial predisposition. Some investigators classify multiple cerebral cavernous angiomas as a neurocutaneous syndrome. Most patients present with seizures, and hemorrhages tend to be subclinical. The risk of a significant bleed is increased if a prior hemorrhage has occurred. Surgical resection may be contemplated when there is associated hematoma, uncontrollable seizures, or progressive neurologic deficits, or the need for long-term anticoagulants.

Developmental venous anomalies (formerly called "venous angiomas") represent aberrant drainage of the deep medullary veins via a single dilated transcerebral vein emptying into the superficial (cortical) or deep veins. They are almost always asymptomatic. If hemorrhage occurs, it is usually because of the presence of an accompanying cavernous angioma. Some cerebellar developmental venous anomalies are said to have an increased incidence of hemorrhage. Surgery is usually performed for drainage of associated hematomas, but no attempt is made to resect the venous angioma. Capillary telangiectasias are a collection of dilated capillaries interposed with normal brain. They are more common in the pons. We have never encountered such vascular malformations in a child.

IMAGING FEATURES   As in adults, magnetic resonance (MR) imaging provides an excellent initial imaging test in patients suspected of harboring cerebral vascular malformations (Fig. 5.10-1). AVM show as serpiginous areas of flow void. MR imaging also shows perilesional hemorrhage, surrounding gliosis, and atrophy. AVM are often wedge shaped, with their apex pointing toward a ventricle. They have no preferential location. Their tendency to bleed increases in the presence of deep venous drainage, periventricular (deep) location, prior hemorrhage, and associated aneurysms. MR angiography also readily demonstrates these lesions but, in our opinion, is mostly of academic interest because all patients require catheter angiography before surgical or intravascular treatment (Fig. 5.10-2).

Cavernous angiomas appear as areas of very low signal intensity that contain speckled areas of high signal intensity (Fig. 5.10-3). A rim of hemosiderin that "blooms" on spin echo or preferentially gradient echo T2-weighted images is typical. They have no mass effect and enhance minimally. They occur anywhere in the brain, including the brain stem. Occasionally they are found in the spinal cord or the meninges.

Developmental venous anomalies appear as tubular structures containing no signal and extending from the deep white matter to the cortex or a ventricular surface. At their site of origin, a confluence of medullary veins ("medusa head") is present. As stated earlier, they may be associated with cavernous angiomas. In our experience, small developmental venous anomalies are hard to see on fast spin echo images, probably because of rephasing of their slow flow, which tends to make them isointense with surrounding tissues. Capillary telangiectasias may be seen as areas of hemosiderin on T2-weighted images or as subtle areas of hyperintensity on T1-weighted images without corresponding abnormality on the T2-weighted or postcontrast T1-weighted sequences.

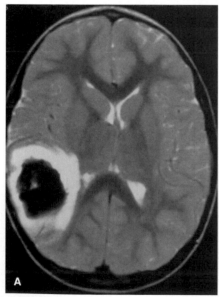 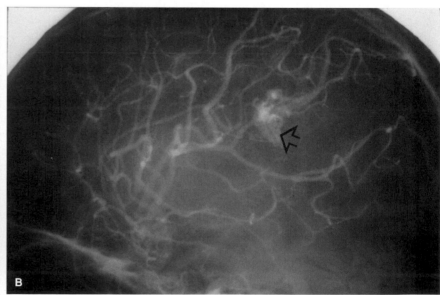

FIGURE 5.10-1.

Acute hemorrhage from arteriovenous malformation.   **A.** Axial magnetic resonance T2-weighted image in a 4-year-old boy shows right temporoparietal acute bleed. The dark area represents deoxyhemoglobin, and the rim of hyperintensity is edema. **B.** Lateral view from catheter angiogram shows arteriovenous malformation (arrow) supplied by posterior branches from right middle cerebral artery.

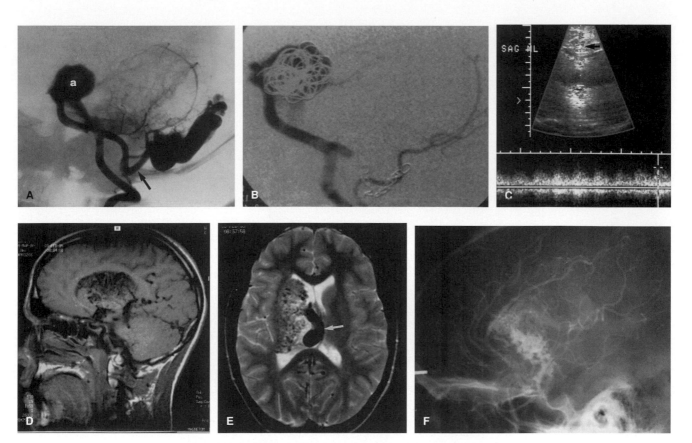

FIGURE 5.10-2.

Arteriovenous malformation (AVM). **A.** Lateral view from catheter angiogram, vertebral artery injection. There is a large arteriovenous fistula supplied by a posterior inferior cerebellar artery (PICA; *arrow*) and a large aneurysm (a) from the tip of the basilar artery, which also supplies a second arteriovenous fistula. **B.** Lateral digital subtraction view from catheter angiogram after embolization with coils in the same patient. The coils in the PICA have successfully occluded the fistula. The tip of basilar artery aneurysm is packed with coils, but there is residual lumen of the aneurysm and shunting. **C.** Coronal sonogram with Doppler probe *(arrow)* at level of basilar artery aneurysm in the same patient 2 weeks after embolization. There are turbulent spectra indicating active flow through a nonoccluded aneurysm. The patient was reembolized after this scan. Computed tomography and magnetic resonance (MR) imaging were not feasible because of the metal artifact from the coils. **D.** Parasagittal MR T1-weighted image in a 15-year-old boy with headaches shows very large AVM involving the basal ganglia. **E.** Axial MR T2-weighted image in same patient shows a myriad of vessels in right basal ganglia region forming the nidus of the malformation, and a varix of the internal cerebral vein. **F.** Lateral angiographic view in same patient shows malformation to be fed by innumerable lenticulostriate arteries. This unresectable malformation was partially embolized and then treated with stereotactic radiosurgery.

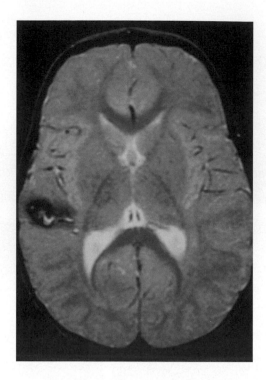

FIGURE 5.10-3.

Cavernous angioma. Axial magnetic resonance T2-weighted image in a patient with seizures shows typical right temporal cavernous angioma. Dark rim is hemosiderin and speckle areas of hyperintensity are probably related to combination of gliosis and subacute hemorrhage.

SUGGESTED READINGS

1. Yokoyama K, Asano Y, Kurakawa T, et al. Familial occurrence of arteriovenous malformation of the brain. J Neurosurg 1991;74:585.
2. Loeffler JS. Role of stereotactic radiosurgery with a linear accelerator in treatment of intracranial arteriovenous malformations and tumors in children. Pediatrics 1990;85:774.
3. Celli P, Ferrante L, Palma L, et al. Cerebral arteriovenous malformations in children: clinical features and outcome of treatment in children and in adults. Surg Neurol 1984;22:43.
4. Golfinos JG, Wascher TW, Zabramski JM, Spetzler RF. The management of unruptured intracranial vascular malformations. BNI Quarterly 1992;8:2.

5.11 *Vein of Galen Malformations*

EPIDEMIOLOGY

Vein of Galen malformations are a diverse group of vascular anomalies in which there is either shunting of arterial blood into a dilated vein of Galen or, properly, an aneurysm of this vein (only 30% of all vein of Galen malformations). The exact incidence of this anomaly is unknown, but it is very rare, with fewer than 300 cases reported in the literature. Most tertiary care institutions probably see one to two cases per year. Most are found the early neonatal period (or prenatally by sonography) or during the first year of life. However, they may present at any age, including during adulthood. Even with treatment, mortality varies from 50% to 90%, and there is significant morbidity (approximately 50%). Survival after treatment with endovascular techniques varies from 50% to 100%. Vein of Galen malformations have been found to be associated with Turner and the blue rubber bleb nevus syndromes.

CLINICAL FEATURES

Embryologically, most vein of Galen malformations are related to abnormal communications between the posterior choroidal, thalamoperforators, distal posterior cerebral, perimesencephalic, and meningeal arteries. The reason for the dilation of the vein of Galen may be related to obstruction of its distal aspect, leading to a stenosis and subsequent dilation due to the large volume of blood being shunted into it.

In the neonatal period, congestive heart failure and a cranial bruit are the most common clinical findings. The incidence of congestive heart failure is less in older patients. Other symptoms include seizures, craniomegaly, hydrocephalus, subarachnoid hemorrhage, visual problems, proptosis, hemiparesis, developmental delay, facial vein enlargement, epistaxis, and vertigo. Congestive heart failure may be associated with aortic stenosis and transposition of the great vessels, and represents the most important clinical problem in the neonate with a vein of Galen malformation. Hydrocephalus is probably secondary to an increase in venous pressure and inadequate resorption of cerebrospinal fluid.

Treatment is aimed toward controlling congestive heart failure. Surgical ligation of feeding arteries may be attempted, but is difficult and results in many complications. Endovascular therapy may be done before or after surgery or as a definite treatment. Endovascular therapy is aimed either at occlusion of feeding vessels or occlusion of the venous outflow by thrombosing the vein of Galen through a torcular approach. Rapid creation of a clot in a vein may result in thrombocytopenia and a consumptive coagulopathy, which may lead to intracranial hemorrhage. Hydrocephalus needs to be treated with insertion of a ventricular shunt. Occasionally, these malformations thrombose spontaneously.

IMAGING FEATURES

Noncontrast computed tomography (CT) shows rounded, slightly hyperdense masses located posterior to and displacing the third ventricle (Fig. 5.11-1). Hydrocephalus and intraventricular and subarachnoid hemorrhage may be present. After iodinated contrast administration, there is enhancement of this vessel and of multiple serpiginous feeding arteries. Marked hyperdensity on precontrast CT and relative lack of enhancement after contrast infusion may indicate thrombosis of the malformation (Fig. 5.11-2). Magnetic resonance (MR) imaging may show similar findings. Calcification in the wall of the "aneurysm" is present in up to 15% of cases. Calcifications in the brain parenchyma are probably dystrophic secondary to ischemia. The main benefit of

MR imaging is its demonstration of the venous outflow pattern, which may aid in planning surgery and endovascular therapies. MR angiography also demonstrates these malformations. However, turbulent and very fast flow may produce diphasing artifacts, leading to incomplete visualization of the malformation. With the use of phase-contrast MR angiography, these artifacts may be avoided. Color Doppler sonography readily estimates the size of the lesion, and baseline studies should be obtained before treatment. Color Doppler ultrasound is the ideal imaging method to follow up malformations that contain coils and in which MR imaging or CT are not helpful because of artifacts from the presence of metal.

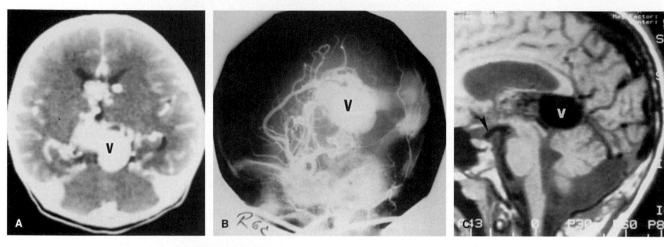

FIGURE 5.11-1.

Vein of Galen malformation. **A.** Axial contrast enhanced computed tomography (CT) shows multiple feeding vessels draining into a dilated (aneurysmal) vein of Galen (V) in a newborn. **B.** Lateral view from the catheter angiogram shows that the fistula is being supplied by branches from the anterior cerebral, middle cerebral, posterior cerebral, and perforating arteries. Note marked dilation of the vein of Galen (V). **C.** Midsagittal magnetic resonance (MR) T1-weighted image in a different patient shows dilation of the vein of Galen (V), presumably supplied by posterior perforating vessels. Note increased size of posterior communicating artery *(arrowhead)*.

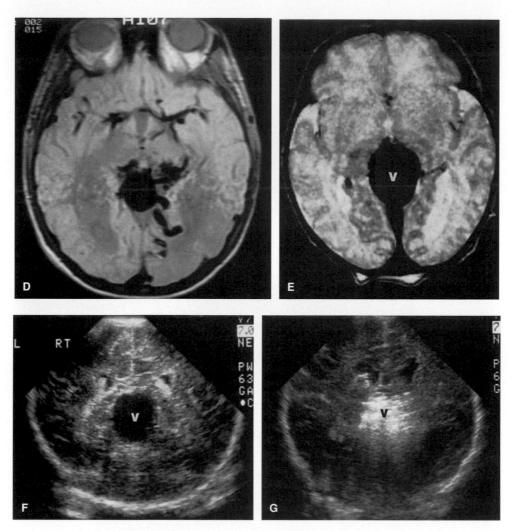

FIGURE 5.11-1. *(continued).*

D. Axial proton density MR image in the same patient shows aneurysm of vein of Galen and multiple feeders. **E.** Axial MR T2-weighted image in a different patient shows a very large vein of Galen (V). **F.** Oblique coronal sonogram in the same patient clearly shows the dilated vein of Galen (V). **G.** Oblique coronal sonogram in the same patient after embolization with coils through a torcular approach shows marked echogenicity filling the dilated vein of Galen (V). Ultrasound is very useful in following up these patients because CT and MR imaging will be degraded by artifact from the metallic coils. ([A], [B], and [D] with permission from Castillo M. Neuroradiology Companion. Philadelphia: JB Lippincott, 1995.)

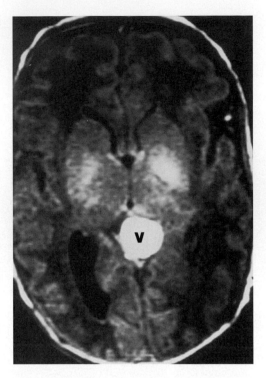

FIGURE 5.11-2.

Thrombosed vein of Galen malformation. Axial noncontrast magnetic resonance T1-weighted image in a newborn with a spontaneously thrombosed vein of Galen malformation. The vein of Galen (V) is dilated and bright because it is filled with methemoglobin. Normal myelination is present in the posterior limb of the internal capsules. A thrombosed cortical vein is present in the left Sylvian fissure.

SUGGESTED READING

1. Horowitz MB, Jungreis CA, Quuisling RG, Pollack I. Vein of Galen aneurysms: a review and current perspective. AJNR 1994;15:1486.

Imaging of the Pediatric Head, Neck, and Spine
by Mauricio Castillo and Suresh K. Mukherji,
Lippincott-Raven Publishing, Philadelphia © 1996.

6
Malignant and Benign Tumors

6.0 Posterior Fossa: Astrocytoma

EPIDEMIOLOGY

Astrocytomas in the posterior fossa may be circumscribed (juvenile pilocytic type) or diffuse (brain stem astrocytoma). Together, both types form the most common (50%) type of tumor occurring in the posterior fossa during childhood. Separately, astrocytomas in the cerebellar hemispheres comprise 30% of posterior fossa masses, whereas brain stem astrocytomas account for 15% to 20%. Most astrocytomas arising in the cerebellar hemispheres are low grade of the pilocytic type. In the brain stem, both pilocytic and diffuse fibrillary astrocytomas occur. No gender preference exists.

CLINICAL FEATURES

Most cerebellar astrocytomas occur in patients between 5 to 10 years of age. The most common clinical manifestations reflect increased intracranial pressure. Midline tumors produce truncal ataxia, whereas hemispheric tumors produce appendicular dysmetria of the ipsilateral extremities. Typical histologic features include biphasic cell pattern, tendency to microcyst formation, and presence of Rosenthal fibers. Approximately 85% of posterior fossa astrocytomas are of the pilocytic type and have a good prognosis (95% 5-year survival), whereas 15% are fibrillary and have a worse prognosis (40% 5-year survival). Leptomeningeal extension is common and is not a histologic sign of malignancy. Frank malignant transformation is uncommon, but subarachnoid space seeding may occur. We have seen some pilocytic astrocytomas with atypical behavior characterized by rapid recurrence (a matter of months) after "total" resection.

Brain stem astrocytomas may present with a triad consisting of long tract signs, cranial nerve dysfunction, and ataxia. Approximately 80% of these tumors are of the fibrillary type, and are unresectable and preferably treated with irradiation. They may undergo anaplastic transformation, and the 5-year survival rates vary from 5% to 30%. Twenty percent of brain stem astrocytomas are of the pilocytic type and have a better prognosis. Patients with symptoms of less than 6 months' duration have a poor prognosis. Focal or exophytic lesions may have a more favorable prognosis.

IMAGING FEATURES

Approximately 60% of juvenile pilocytic astrocytomas are cystic and contain one or more mural nodules (Fig. 6.0-1). Predominantly solid tumors with cystic components are seen in 30% to 40% of cases and uniformly solid tumors comprise less than 10% of cases. Tumors may be seated in the cerebellar hemisphere (10%–15%), vermis (80%), or both. The fourth ventricle is commonly obliterated, and this results in noncommunicating hydrocephalus. After contrast administration, there is intense enhancement of the mural nodule(s). The wall of the cyst usually does not enhance because it is composed of compressed normal tissue; however, tumor occasionally may extend, enhance, and form a true capsule around the cyst. On magnetic resonance (MR) T1-weighted images, the intracystic fluid tends to be slightly brighter than cerebrospinal fluid (CSF). On T2-weighted images, the intracystic fluid is bright and of equal signal intensity to CSF. Contrast (particularly iodinated if computed tomography [CT] is used) may leak into the cyst, producing a layering effect. Solid juvenile pilocytic astrocytomas enhance deeply. MR with contrast allows for identification of rare CSF seeding (Fig. 6.0-2). Although meningeal infiltration is commonly present on histology, it is not commonly seen on imaging studies. A mild degree of surrounding edema usually accompanies these tumors.

Brain stem astrocytomas are infiltrating and are better seen by MR than by

CT (Fig. 6.0-3). They are hypointense on T1-weighted images and hyperintense on T2-weighted images and enlarge the pons. They may involve cranial nerves VI and VII, encase the basilar artery, and compress the cisterns. Contrast enhancement is extremely variable. They bow the fourth ventricle and aqueduct dorsally, and therefore do not produce hydrocephalus until late in the course of the disease. In the lower brain stem they expand the medulla. We have also seen these tumors arising in the area postrema and producing intractable vomiting.

Protoplasmic astrocytomas are a rare variety of tumors that may occur in the posterior fossa. They manifest as masses with multiple microcysts that tend to infiltrate the pia. They are indistinguishable from microcystic oligodendrogliomas.

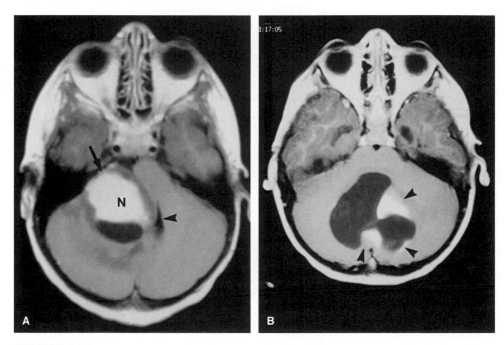

FIGURE 6.0-1.

Astrocytoma, cerebellum. **A.** Axial postcontrast magnetic resonance (MR) T1-weighted image shows typical pilocytic astrocytoma with an enhancing nodule (N) that has an exophytic component *(arrow)* protruding into the right cerebellopontine angle cistern. The tumor contains a nonenhancing cyst dorsally. The fourth ventricle *(arrowhead)* is compressed and displaced to the left. (With permission from Castillo M. Imaging and clinical features of pilocytic astrocytoma. Imaging Decisions 1994;1: 15.) **B.** Axial MR T1-weighted image after contrast in a different patient shows midline cystic pilocytic astrocytoma with three enhancing mural nodules *(arrowheads).*

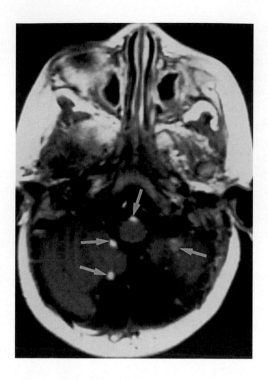

FIGURE 6.0-2.

Subarachnoid seeding from pilocytic astrocytoma. Axial postcontrast magnetic resonance T1-weighted image shows multiple metastatic nodules *(arrows)* in basilar cisterns. (With permission from Castillo M. Imaging and clinical features of pilocytic astrocytoma. Imaging Decisions 1994;1:15.)

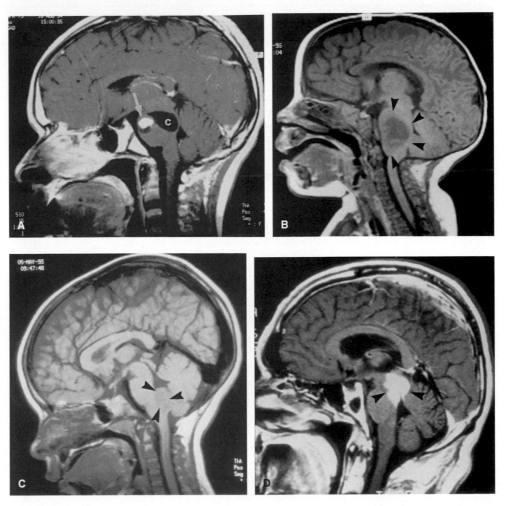

FIGURE 6.0-3.

Astrocytoma, brain stem. **A.** Midsagittal postcontrast magnetic resonance (MR) T1-weighted image in a patient with a pilocytic astrocytoma involving the brain stem. Note typical enhancing nodule *(arrow)* with a large cystic (c) component dorsally and a smaller cyst inferiorly. Despite the large size of the tumor, there is no hydrocephalus. **B.** Midsagittal noncontrast MR T1-weighted image in a 2-month-old child with a high-grade astrocytoma *(arrowheads)* of the brain stem. Note central low-intensity region, suggesting necrosis. Again, despite large size of tumor there is no hydrocephalus, a finding typical for brain stem gliomas. **C.** Midsagittal noncontrast MR T1-weighted image in a child with severe and persistent vomiting. There is a well defined mass of lower intensity *(arrowheads)* than brain in the region of the area postrema. The abnormality enhanced deeply and was a solid pilocytic astrocytoma. **D.** Midsagittal postcontrast MR T1-weighted image shows markedly enhancing astrocytoma *(arrowheads)* in the midbrain surrounding the aqueduct and producing mild hydrocephalus.

SUGGESTED
READINGS

1. Lee YY, Van Tassel P, Bruner JM, et al. Juvenile pilocytic astrocytomas: CT and MR characteristics. AJNR 1989;10:363.
2. Strong JA, Hatten HP, Brown MT, et al. Pilocytic astrocytoma: correlation between the initial imaging features and clinical aggressiveness. AJR 1993;161:369.
3. Kane AG, Robles HA, Smirniotopoulos JG, et al. Diffuse pontine astrocytoma. AJNR 1993;14:941.
4. Mishima K, Nakamura M, Nakamura H, et al. Leptomeningeal dissemination of cerebellar pilocytic astrocytoma. J Neurosurg 1992;77:788.
5. Fulham MJ, Melisi JW, Nishimiya J, Dwyer AJ, Di Chiro G. Neuroimaging of juvenile pilocytic astrocytomas: an enigma. Radiology 1993;189:221.

6.01 Posterior Fossa: Primitive Neuroectodermal Tumors—Medulloblastoma

EPIDEMIOLOGY

Medulloblastoma represents 30% of all posterior fossa tumors and therefore may be considered the most common type of neoplasia in that region. It also comprises approximately 20% of childhood brain tumors. Its peak incidence is during the first decade of life; however, during the first 2 months of life almost all posterior fossa tumors are medulloblastomas. It is more common in boys (2:1). It may occur in isolation or as part of the basal cell nevus (Gorlin) syndrome and ataxia telengiectasia.

CLINICAL FEATURES

The symptoms are nonspecific, reflect increased intracranial pressure, and are present on average for only 1 month before the diagnosis is made. Vomiting, headache, lethargy, hypotonia, decreased or absent reflexes, ataxia, and papilledema are common. Spontaneous hemorrhage with sudden onset of symptoms may be the initial presentation. At presentation, 5% to 50% of patients have subarachnoid tumor spread. Medulloblastoma is uniformly fatal if left untreated. Recurrence of tumor is always followed by death. Aggressive surgical resection is the inital and preferred modality of treatment. This is usually followed by a 5000 to 6000 cGy irradiation dose to the posterior fossa. Because all patients are assumed to have cerebrospinal fluid spread at diagnosis, 3500 cGy is usually delivered to the spinal axis. Chemotherapy is more effective when given in combination with surgery–radiation. Chemotherapy is especially helpful in children younger than 2 years of age with brain stem involvement and incomplete surgical resection. Five-year survival rates varying from 56% to 60% may be expected with combined therapies. Medulloblastoma is the most common brain tumor producing distant metastases. Metastases to the bones (sclerotic type), lungs, and lymph nodes are known to occur. Seeding of the peritoneum via shunts may occur in up to 40% of all patients.

Histologically, these tumors arise from primitive undifferentiated germinative cells located mainly in the region of the roof of the fourth ventricle. With development, these cells migrate laterally into the external granular cell layer of the cerebellar hemispheres. Medulloblastomas may be found anywhere along this path. In younger patients, these tumors are midline, whereas in older patients, a lateral position is relatively common. The tumors are hypercellular. The cells have scant cytoplasm and large nuclei. Laterally located tumors contain bands of connective tissue (desmoplastic medulloblastomas).

IMAGING FEATURES

Seventy to 90% of medulloblastomas arise in the midline, most from the roof of the fourth ventricle, but they may also arise from the floor of the fourth ventricle (Fig. 6.01-1). Occasionally, these tumors may also begin inside the fourth ventricle. Approximately 5% are located in the cerebellar hemisphere. The cerebellopontine angle is a rare site of origin. Rare instances of multicentric medulloblastomas have been described. In midline tumors, hydrocephalus may be identified in 50% to 95% of patients at presentation. Typically, medulloblastomas are rounded, homogenous, and slightly hyperdense on noncontrast computed tomography. After iodinated contrast administration, more than 95% of these tumors enhance (many show patchy enhancement). Unfortunately, the classic appearance of medulloblastoma is seen in only one third of tumors. Other common features include cyst formation and necrosis (40%), hemorrhage, calcifications (10%–20%), and absent contrast enhancement (5%–10%). Some degree of surrounding edema is commonly present (approximately 90%). Magnetic resonance (MR) imaging is the imaging modality of choice. The mass tends to be mildly hypointense on T1-weighted images and bright on T2-weighted images. The benefit of MR imaging lies in its ability to identify subarachnoid seeding. Intracranial leptomeningeal spread occurs most commonly in the vermian cisterns, ependyma of the lateral ventricles, and subfrontal regions (Fig. 6.01-2). Drop metastases to the lower thecal sac occur in 40% of patients. All patients should receive MR studies of the primary site and the spinal axis at presentation. Screening of the spinal cord after surgery may produce false-positive results because the expected surgically related hemorrhage may cause breakdown of the blood–spine barrier and of the blood–nerve barrier, resulting in areas of enhancement. If an MR study of the spine was not obtained before surgery, we prefer to wait for 6 weeks before evaluating the spinal axis. After surgery, enhancement is usually present at the resection site. These areas of enhancement tend to diminish in size progressively. Any increment in their size should be regarded as recurrent tumor until proven otherwise. Focal nodular intraaxial enhancement or enhancement along pial–ependymal surfaces is also highly suggestive of tumor. Enhancement along the meningogaleal complex is an expected postoperative finding. Delayed extraaxial hematomas at the meningogaleal complex may also occur. After treatment, particularly with a combination of intrathecal chemotherapy and irradiation, parenchymal calcifications (mineralizing micro-angiopathy) may occur throughout the brain (Fig. 6.01-3).

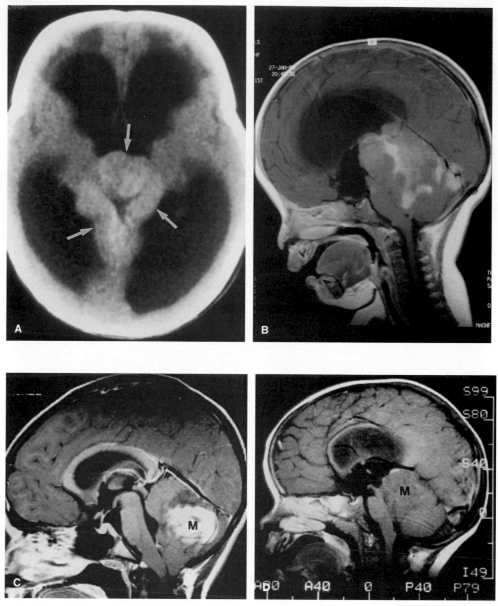

FIGURE 6.01-1.

Medulloblastoma.   A. Noncontrast axial computed tomography shows large, slightly hyperdense medulloblastoma *(arrows).* There is marked hydrocephalus. (With permission from Castillo M. Neuroradiology Companion. Philadelphia: JB Lippincott, 1995.) **B.** Midsagittal postcontrast magnetic resonance (MR) T1-weighted image in the same patient shows a large and inhomogenous tumor arising from the superior vermis. Note hydrocephalus with inferior herniation of the recesses of the third ventricle. **C.** Midsagittal postcontrast MR T1-weighted image in a different patient shows enhancing medulloblastoma (M) arising in posterior and inferior vermis. Note intact fourth ventricle and minimal herniation of the cerebellar tonsils. The ventricles are mildly prominent. **D.** Midsagittal postcontrast MR T1-weighted image shows nonenhancing medulloblastoma (M). Note hydrocephalus due to compression of the fourth ventricle, which is not seen.

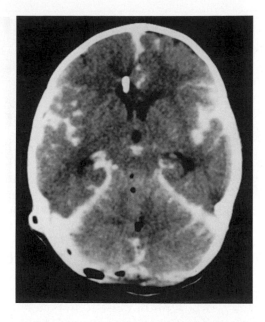

FIGURE 6.01-2.

Subarachnoid seeding from medulloblastoma. Axial postcontrast computed tomography shows extensive enhancement of the subarachnoid space in a child, with seeding from medulloblastoma. Postsurgical changes are present in the posterior fossa. Tip of shunt is in the frontal horn of the right lateral ventricle. (With permission from Castillo M. Neuroradiology Companion. Philadelphia: JB Lippincott, 1995.)

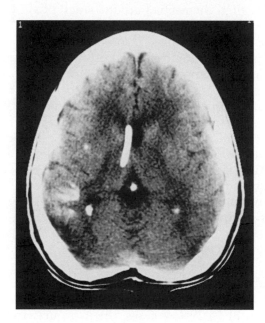

FIGURE 6.01-3.

Posttreatment changes. Axial postcontrast computed tomography in a child with prior resection of medulloblastoma (note evidence of occipital craniotomy) treated with combination radiation and chemotherapy. There are paintbrush-like calcifications at the gray–white junction of the right temporooccipital region compatible mineralizing microangiopathy. A second focus of calcification is present in the right temporal region. This complication may occur with either irradiation or chemotherapy, but is more common with a combination of both. There is a shunt in the frontal horn of the right lateral ventricle. (With permission from Castillo M. Neuroradiology Companion. Philadelphia: JB Lippincott, 1995.)

SUGGESTED READINGS

1. Meyers SP, Wildenhain S, Chess MA, Tarr RW. Postoperative evaluation for intracranial recurrence of medulloblastoma: MR findings with gadopentetate dimeglumine. AJNR 1994;15:1425.
2. Nixon KT, Hudgins PA, Davis PC, O'Brien MS, Hudgins RJ, Hoffman JC. Delayed intracranial hemorrhage in children after suboccipital craniectomy. AJR 1994;163:897.

6.02 *Posterior Fossa: Ependymoma*

EPIDEMIOLOGY

Ependymomas comprise 8% to 10% of all chidhood tumors. They represent 15% of posterior fossa tumors in children. Mean age at diagnosis is 5 to 6 years, but they may occur throughout the first decade of life. Only 4% of patients are older than 15 years of age.

CLINICAL FEATURES

Two thirds of ependymomas arise in the posterior fossa. Because they arise in the fourth ventricle and obstruct cerebrospinal fluid (CSF) flow, diagnosis is usually made within 2 months of the onset of symptoms. The most common clinical manifestations are headaches, vomiting, papilledema, cranial nerve palsies, torticollis, nystagmus, meningismus, and dysmetria. Approximately 30% to 40% of ependymomas are supratentorial. In supratentorial ependymomas, the symptoms include hemiparesis, hyperreflexia, and visual field defects. Subarachnoid spread of tumor is present in 12% of patients at diagnosis and is more common (15%–20%) in anaplastic ependymomas.

Histologically, two thirds of these tumors may be considered low grade. They arise from cells near the foramina of Luschka in the fourth ventricle. Tumor cells align themselves around small blood vessels, forming pseudorosettes, true rosettes, and canals. These cells may be well differentiated and show some mitoses and mild pleomorphism, or show high density, increased mitoses, extensive pleomorphism, and necrosis. A specific type of ependymoma is the subependymoma. These tumors arise under an ependymal lining and histologically are composed of a mixture of ependymal cells and astrocytes. In some cases, depending on the cell population that predominates, these tumors are regarded as low-grade intraventricular astrocytomas. Subependymomas also tend to occur in the obex of the fourth ventricle.

The treatment of choice is surgical resection, which, unfortunately, is not often curative. If subarachnoid metastases are present, spinal irradiation is given. At some centers, radiation therapy is given to the postoperative bed. Transient responses to chemotherapy, particularly cisplatin, have been reported. After gross total resection followed by combination therapy, a 70% 5-year survival has been reported. Metastases to bones, bone marrow, liver, lymph nodes, and lungs are known to occur.

IMAGING FEATURES

Most ependymomas arise in the floor of the fourth ventricle. They expand the fourth ventricle and CSF spaces often may be identified surrounding the mass (Fig. 6.02-1A, B). In 20% of cases, the mass may extend into the cerebellopontine angle cisterns via the foramina of Luschka or invade the adjacent cerebellum and brain stem (Fig. 6.02-1C). Ependymomas have ill-defined borders and over 50% contain calcifications. Small cysts are common, but occasionally large cysts are present. Hemorrhagic foci are found in 10% of tumors. On noncontrast computed tomography, ependymomas are usually hypodense, but occasionally they are hyperdense and difficult to differentiate from medulloblastomas. Contrast enhancement is present and is homogenous in almost half of the lesions. However, inhomogeneous (40%) or absent (10%) contrast enhancement may also be seen. On magnetic resonance (MR) imaging, ependymomas are hypointense to gray matter on T1-weighted images and hyperintense on T2-weighted images. On precontrast MR images, 40% of tumors are heterogenous and most show some degree of contrast enhancement. MR imaging is also helpful for the detection of subarachnoid and ependymal tumor seeding (Fig. 6.02-1D, E).

Approximately 30% to 40% of ependymomas are supratentorial in location. They commonly arise from ependymal rests located outside of the ventricular system and are indistinguishable from astrocytomas by imaging studies. Supratentorial ependymomas are more common in adults.

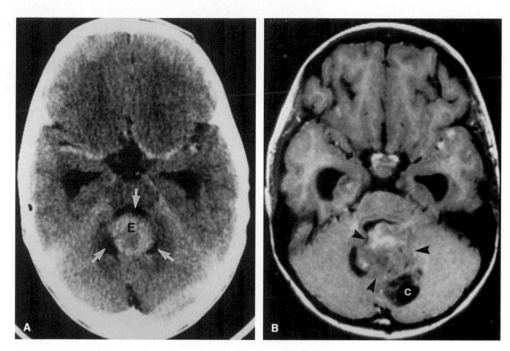

FIGURE 6.02-1.

Ependymoma. **A.** Axial postcontrast computed tomography shows enhancing ependymoma (E) in the fourth ventricle. Note fourth ventricle *(arrows)* around the tumor, confirming its intraventricular location. The temporal tips of the lateral ventricles are dilated, indicating hydrocephalus. **B.** Axial postcontrast magnetic resonance (MR) T1-weighted image in a different patient shows heterogenously enhancing ependymoma *(arrowheads)*. There is cerebrospinal fluid anterior and to the right of the tumor, confirming its intraventricular location. There is a nonenhancing tumor cyst (c) dorsally. The temporal tips are dilated, indicating hydrocephalus. Questionable tumor seeding is present in the suprasellar region. **C.** Midsagittal postcontrast MR T1-weighted image shows the mostly intraventricular location of the tumor (E), which protrudes inferiorly *(smaller arrow)* through the foramina of Luschka. Note hydrocephalus and tumor seeding in quadrigeminal plate cistern, third ventricle *(larger arrow)*, lateral ventricle, and velum interpositum. **D.** Parasagittal postcontrast MR T1-weighted image in the same patient shows to better advantage tumor seeding *(arrows)* on the surface of a dilated lateral ventricle. **E.** Axial postcontrast MR T1-weighted image (different patient) shows spread of posterior fossa ependymoma (previously partially resected) to the ependyma of the atria *(arrows)* of the lateral ventricles. Dural enhancement is either postsurgical or metastatic in nature.

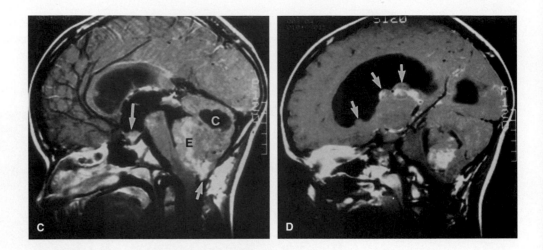

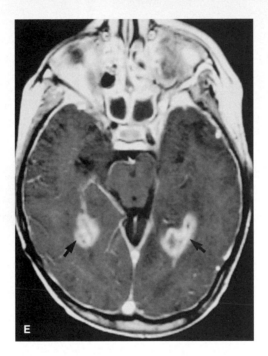

FIGURE 6.02-1.

(continued)

SUGGESTED READING

1. Spoto GP, Press GA, Hesselink JR, Solomon M. Intracranial ependymoma and sub-ependymoma: MR manifestations. AJNR 1990;11:83.

6.03 Posterior Fossa: Uncommon Tumors

EPIDEMIOLOGY AND
CLINICAL FEATURES

Tables 6.03-1 and 6.03-2 list epidemiologic data and clinical features of the less common posterior fossa tumors.

TABLE 6.03-1. Epidemiology and Clinical Features of Intraaxial Tumors

Type of Tumor	Incidence	Clinical Features
Hemangioblastoma	20% of these tumors occur in children	Most are sporadic but some are associated to Von Hippel-Lindau syndrome
Ganglioglioma	2%–3% of all intracranial tumors	Nonspecific signs of intracranial hypertension
Choroid plexus papilloma	<1% of intracranial tumors, 85% occur in children	In children, most occur in the lateral ventricles and present with headaches, prognosis is good because tumors are benign

TABLE 6.03-2. Epidemiology and Clinical Features of Extraaxial Tumors

Type of Tumor	Incidence	Clinical Features
Epidermoid	<1% of all brain tumors, very rare in children	Most occur in cerebellopontine angle cistern and fourth ventricle, and present with hydrocephalus or cerebellar signs
Dermoid	<1% of all brain tumors	Most have a sinus tract to skin, most present in fourth ventricle, vermis, or cisterna magna
Meningioma	1% of childhood tumors	Nonspecific, most are supratentorial and intraparenchymal or intraventricular
Schwannoma	Extremely rare in children	VIII, X, and IX cranial nerves more often affected, associated with neurofibromatosis type II

Tables 6.03-3 and 6.03-4 list the imaging features of the less common posterior fossa tumors.

TABLE 6.03-3. *Imaging Features of Intraaxial Tumors*

Type of Tumor	Imaging Features
Hemangioblastoma	Most are cystic with a densely enhancing mural nodule, 30% of lesions are solid, multiple tumors are more commonly solid (Fig. 6.03-1)
Ganglioglioma	May be cystic with an enhancing nodule and indistinguishable from pilocytic astrocytoma, may contain calcifications or be entirely solid (Fig. 6.03-2)
Choroid plexus papilloma	Well marginated, deeply enhancing intraventricular masses without calcifications, hydrocephalus (Fig. 6.03-3)

TABLE 6.03-4. *Imaging Features of Extraaxial Tumors*

Type of Tumor	Imaging Features
Epidermoid	Often very similar to cerebrospinal fluid or both CT and MR imaging, do not enhance, rarely they look like fat (Fig. 6.03-4)
Dermoid	Midline tumors of fatty appearance by CT and MR imaging, no enhancement unless infected
Meningioma	Intraparenchymal or intraventricular cysts, aggressive appearance, deep enhancement (often the opposite features from those seen in adults)
Schwannoma	Deeply enhancing, well marginated masses in internal auditory canal or in the region of the foramen magnum (Fig. 6.03-5)

CT, computed tomography; MR, magnetic resonance.

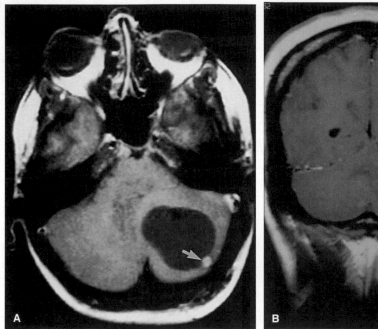
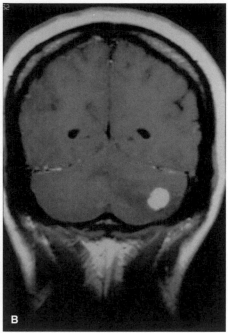

FIGURE 6.03-1.

Hemangioblastoma. **A.** Axial postcontrast magnetic resonance (MR) T1-weighted image shows large nonenhancing cyst in the left cerebellar hemisphere. A small enhancing nodule *(arrow)* is present in the left dorsolateral margin of the tumor. The nodule is pial based, a typical feature of hemangioblastoma. The fourth ventricle is compressed and effaced. (With permission from Castillo M. Contrast enhancement in primary neoplasms of the brain and spine. Neuroimaging Clinics of North America 1994;4:63.) **B.** Coronal postcontrast MR T1-weighted image shows solid hemangioblastoma in the left cerebellar hemisphere.

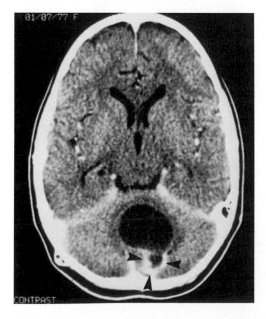

FIGURE 6.03-2.

Ganglioglioma. Axial postcontrast computed tomography shows a midline cystic lesion containing a small area of enhancement posteriorly *(arrowheads).* There is little hydrocephalus for a mass of this size. (With permission from Castillo M, Davis PC, Hoffman JC, Takei Y. Intracranial ganglioglioma: MR and CT findings. AJNR 1990;11:109.)

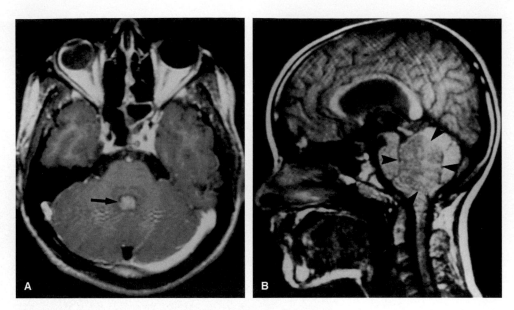

FIGURE 6.03-3.

Choroid plexus papilloma. **A.** Axial postcontrast magnetic resonance (MR) T1-weighted image in an adolescent with intermittent headaches. There is a small enhancing mass *(arrow)* in the fourth ventricle. **B.** Midsagittal noncontrast MR T1-weighted image in a young patient with a large and mostly homogenous fourth ventricular choroid plexus papilloma *(arrowheads)*. There is hydrocephalus.

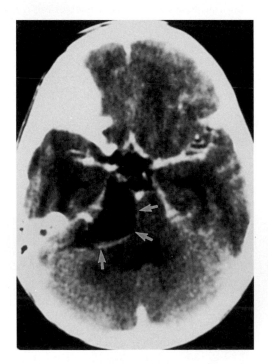

FIGURE 6.03-4.

Epidermoid. Axial postcontrast computed tomography in a patient with headaches shows a large and nonenhancing "cystic"-appearing mass *(arrows)* in the right cerebellopontine angle cistern. There is displacement of the fourth ventricle and mild prominence of the temporal tips, compatible with hydrocephalus.

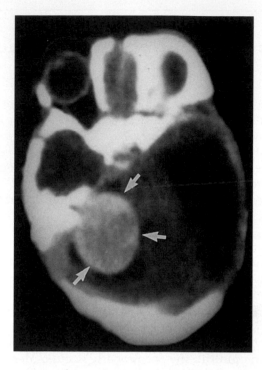

FIGURE 6.03-5.

Vestibular schwannoma. Axial postcontrast computed tomography (tilted) in a baby shows large and rounded enhancing tumor *(arrows)* in right *cerebellopontine* angle region.

SUGGESTED READING

1. Vezina LG, Packer RJ. Infratentorial brain tumors of childhood. Neuroimaging Clinics of North America 1994;4:423.

6.04 *Supratentorial: Hemispheric Astrocytoma (Including Giant Cell Astrocytoma)*

EPIDEMIOLOGY

Hemispheric astrocytomas comprise 30% to 55% of cerebral tumors in children. Both genders are equally affected. They occur throughout childhood, with a peak incidence between 7 to 8.2 years of age. Hemispheric astrocytomas are rare in patients with neurofibromatosis type I.

Giant cell astrocytomas are a unique type of glioma always seen in the context of tuberous sclerosis. These tumors occur in 1.7% to 26% of patients with tuberous sclerosis. The peak age of presentation is between 8 to 18 years of age. No gender predilection exists.

CLINICAL FEATURES

The most common presenting symptom in hemispheric astrocytoma is seizures (particularly if the tumor is located in the temporal lobes). Headaches occur in over 90% of patients. Signs of increased intracranial pressure are also common. The duration of symptoms is longer with supratentorial astrocytomas than with those arising in the posterior fossa. Most hemispheric astrocytomas are of low histologic grade (25% all pediatric brain tumors), although glioblastoma multiforme occasionally occurs. Most supratentorial astrocytomas demonstrate a fibrillary pattern on histology. Juvenile pilocytic astrocytoma is less common in the cerebral hemispheres than in the cerebellum. Surgical excision with or without radiation is the treatment of choice. Five-year survival rates vary as follows: for grade 1, 25% to 58%, and for grade 2, 13% to 32%. The role of chemotherapy is uncertain, but it seems to offer some advantages in very young patients and those with high-grade tumors.

Pleomorphic xanthoastrocytoma is a rare glioma occurring mainly in patients 7 to 25 years of age. These tumors contain cysts in 50% of cases, and all tumors show well defined contrast enhancement. These tumors involve the cortex and occur preferentially in the temporal lobes. They have a favorable prognosis, but malignant degeneration is known to occur.

Giant cell astrocytomas present with unilateral or bilateral hydrocephalus in patients with tuberous sclerosis. These tumors arise at the foramina of Monroe. It is not clear if they arise from degenerated subependymal nodules or from remnants of the germinal matrix. Occasionally, these tumors are found in the atria and temporal horns of the lateral ventricles. In general, giant cell astrocytomas are histologically benign, although anaplasia occasionally may be found. Their treatment usually consists of surgical resection. However, in patients who are devastated by their primary disorder, and because these tumors are benign and grow slowly, only ventricular shunting to relieve the hydrocephalus may be needed.

IMAGING FEATURES

The appearance of hemispheric astrocytomas is extremely variable (Fig. 6.04-1). If cysts are present, they do not enhance. Enhancement in the solid portions of the tumor is extremely variable and may be nonexistent. Their magnetic resonance (MR) imaging appearance is also variable and over 90% of high-grade tumors enhance.

Magnetic resonance is the imaging modality of choice for initial detection and follow-up of giant cell astrocytomas (Fig. 6.04-2). The tumors are hypointense to isointense on T1-weighted images and hyperintense on T2-weighted images. All enhance after contrast is given. Some subependymal nodules may also enhance, however, and therefore location and rapid growth are more important MR imaging characteristics than is enhancement. These tumors contain calcifications and abundant vascularity, which are seen as areas of signal void on MR images. Unilateral dilation of a lateral ventricle is the rule. If the tumor is large, both lateral ventricles may be dilated.

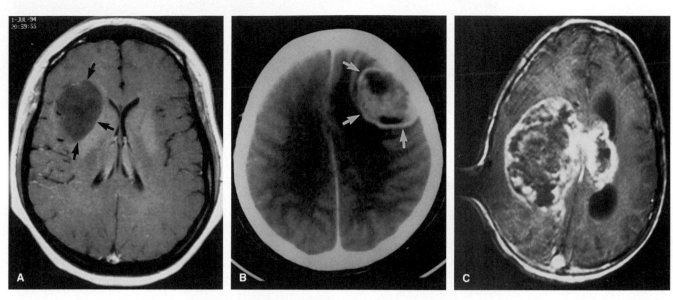

FIGURE 6.04-1.

Astrocytoma. **A.** Axial postcontrast magnetic resonance (MR) T1-weighted image in an adolescent with seizures shows nonenhancing "cystic"-appearing low-grade astrocytoma *(arrows)* in the right frontotemporal region. **B.** Axial postcontrast computed tomography shows tumor *(arrows)* in left frontal region with irregular internal enhancement and surrounding edema. The lesion was anaplastic astrocytoma. **C.** Axial postcontrast MR T1-weighted image shows large "butterfly" glioblastoma multiforme in a child. Note heterogenous enhancement, central necrosis, and a nodular rim, all of which are typical of high-grade gliomas. (With permission from Castillo M, Scatliff J, Bouldin T, Suzuki K. Intracranial astrocytoma: radiologic–pathologic correlation. AJNR 1992;13:1609. **D.** Midsagittal MR T1-weighted image before contrast administration in the same patient shows tumor with hemorrhage *(bright areas, arrows)* involving the body of the corpus callosum. Possible seeding in dependent portion of the third ventricle is noted. **E.** Axial postcontrast MR T1-weighted image shows large cystic tumor extending from the superficial gray matter to the corpus callosum. The tumor contains a septation and a laterally located enhancing nodule. The appearance is that of a pilocytic astrocytoma or a pleomorphic xanthoastrocytoma. **F.** Proton MR spectra (single volume) over high-grade astrocytoma shows typical malignant pattern with markedly increased choline (1), relatively normal creatinine (2), and a markedly reduced *N*-acetyl aspartate (3). Elevated lactate (not present in these spectra) may be seen in high-grade and necrotic intraaxial tumors. **G.** Compare (F) with these single-volume proton MR spectra obtained in a region of normal brain (1, choline; 2, creatinine; 3, *N*-acetyl aspartate).

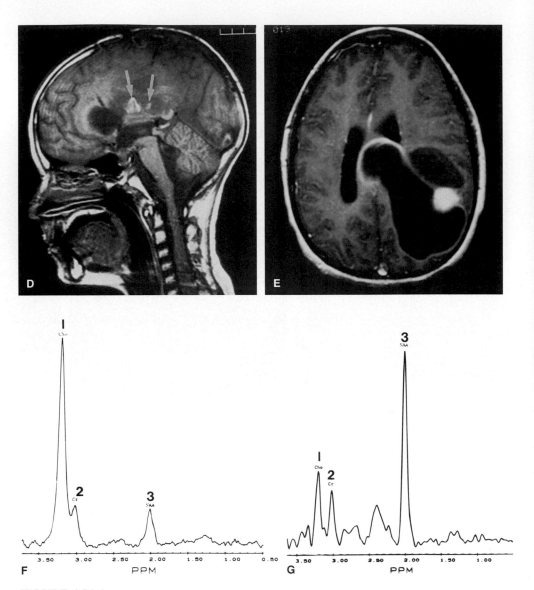

FIGURE 6.04-1.

(continued)

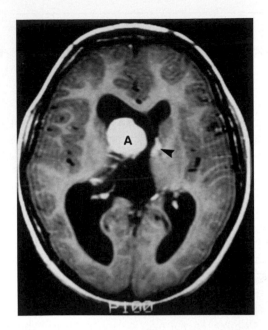

FIGURE 6.04-2.

Giant cell astrocytoma. Axial postcontrast magnetic resonance T1-weighted image in a patient with tuberous sclerosis shows a large, homogenous, rounded, and deeply enhancing giant cell astrocytoma (A) in the region of the right foramen of Monroe. There is a smaller tumor *(arrowhead)* in the left foramen of Monroe. Hydrocephalus, right greater than left, is present.

SUGGESTED READINGS

1. Braffman BH, Bilaniuk LT, Naidich TP, et al. MR imaging of tuberous sclerosis: pathogenesis of this phakomatosis, use of gadopentetate dimeglumine and literature review. Radiology 1992;183:227.
2. Lipper MH, Eberhand DA, Phillips CD, Vezina LG, Cail WS. Pleomorphic xanthoastrocytoma, a distinctive astroglial tumor: neuroradiology and pathologic studies. AJNR 1993;14:1397.

6.05 *Supratentorial: Optic Chiasm and Hypothalamic Astrocytomas*

EPIDEMIOLOGY

These tumors are discussed together because at the time of diagnosis it may be impossible to differentiate them. Optic astrocytomas represent 3% to 5% of brain tumors in childhood. The true incidence of hypothalamic astrocytomas is not known. Optic astrocytomas are mainly seen between 2 to 9 years of age. Half of the children with optic astrocytomas have neurofibromatosis type I.

CLINICAL FEATURES

Diminished visual acuity is the presenting symptom in most patients with chiasmal astrocytomas. The progression of the visual impairment is slow, and therefore up to 80% of tumors are very large when detected. Proptosis and nystagmus may also be present. Papilledema suggests hydrocephalus. Histologically, most of these tumors are classified as pilocytic astrocytomas. However, fibrillary and infiltrating varieties are not uncommon. Surgery is not possible in most patients, but irradiation may be given to symptomatic patients older than 5 years of age. In younger patients, chemotherapy has been used. The results of chemotherapy are as yet uncertain.

Hypothalamic astrocytomas are usually of the pilocytic type and therefore different from thalamic astrocytomas, which tend to be more malignant. Symptoms include failure to thrive, emaciation, loss of subcutaneous fat, serum sodium alterations, hypoglycemia, accelerated bone growth, obesity, diabetes insipidus, hypogonadism, lethargy, precocious puberty, and eventually signs of increased intracranial pressure due to hydrocephalus. The so-called "diencephalic syndrome" is seen between 18 months and 3 years of age. These patients grow and behave normally (even happily) despite being emaciated. Irradiation is the treatment of choice and survival rates are 71% and 56% for 5 and 10 years, respectively. The role of chemotherapy is not established, but it may be useful in recurrent tumors.

IMAGING FEATURES

Magnetic resonance is the imaging modality of choice in the evaluation of these tumors (Fig. 6.05-1). It permits gross determination of the extent of the neoplasia along the optic pathways. Determining the exact site of origin is difficult in most tumors and not essential because both hypothalamic and optic chiasm astrocytomas behave and are treated in similar ways (Fig. 6.05-2). Most of these tumors are hypointense on T1-weighted images and hyperintense on T2-weighted images. They are solid, lobulated, and have mostly well defined margins. Invasion of the third ventricle is not unusual. Hydrocephalus is also commonly seen. Invasion of the posterior fossa or extension along the optic apparatus is seen in 50% of patients. Most tumors show marked contrast enhancement, but occasionally little or no enhancement may be documented (Fig. 6.05-3). Extension along the meningeal surfaces and metastases to the subarachnoid space may be seen.

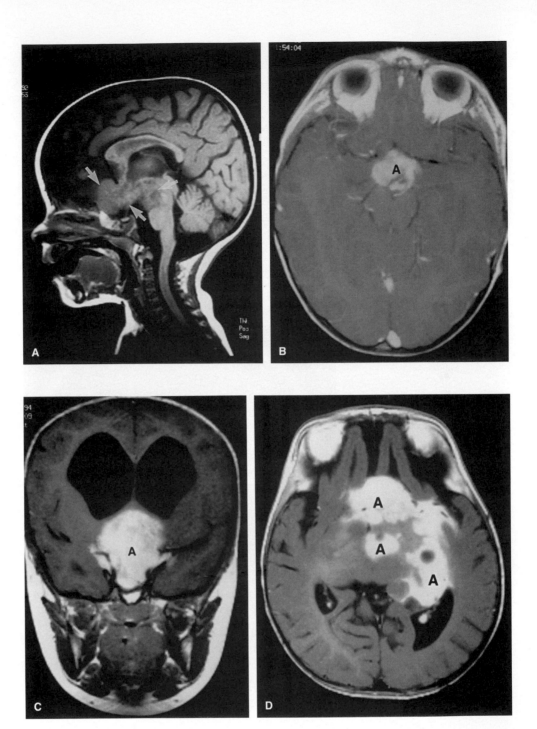

FIGURE 6.05-1.

Optic chiasm astrocytoma. **A.** Midsagittal magnetic resonance (MR) T1-weighted image before contrast administration shows large and lobulated mass *(arrows)* in the region of the optic chiasm and hypothalamus. It is not possible accurately to determine its site of origin. The third ventricle appears invaded inferiorly. There is tumor in the interpeduncular cistern. **B.** Axial postcontrast MR T1-weighted image shows marked enhancement of this suprasellar pilocytic astrocytoma (A). (With permission from Castillo M. Imaging and clinical features of pilocytic astrocytoma. Imaging Decisions 1994;1:15.) **C.** Coronal postcontrast MR T1-weighted image in a different patient shows large and deeply enhancing optic chiasm astrocytoma (A). **D.** Axial postcontrast MR T1-weighted image in the same patient shows astrocytoma (A) extending into the midbrain and posteriorly along the left optic radiation.

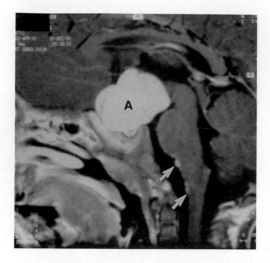

FIGURE 6.05-2.

Hypothalamic–chiasmatic astrocytoma. Midsagittal postcontrast magnetic resonance T1-weighted image shows markedly enhancing hypothalamic–chiasmatic astrocytoma (A) extending in the sella (note J-shaped sella). There are tumor deposits *(arrows)* on the ventral surface of the pons and upper medulla.

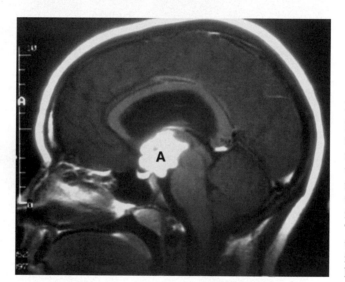

FIGURE 6.05-3.

Hypothalamic astrocytoma. Midsagittal magnetic resonance T1-weighted image shows a markedly enhancing astrocytoma (A) presumably arising from the hypothalamus. The tumor has invaded the third ventricle, which is filled with tumor, producing hydrocephalus.

SUGGESTED READING

1. Kollias SS, Barkovich AJ, Edwards MSB. Magnetic resonance analysis of suprasellar tumors in childhood. Pediatr Neurosurg 1991;17:284.

6.06 *Supratentorial: Oligodendroglioma and Ependymoma*

EPIDEMIOLOGY

Oligodendrogliomas represent less than 1% of all childhood brain tumors. Although they may occur at any age, they are slightly more common during adolescence. They are more common in boys.

Of all ependymomas (6% of childhood brain tumors), 20% to 40% are found supratentorially. Most are discovered between 1 to 5 years of age. Unlike ependymomas occurring in the posterior fossa, supratentorial ependymomas tend to arise outside the ventricular system.

CLINICAL FEATURES

For both types of tumor, the clinical signs and symptoms are nonspecific and include seizures (often refractory), headaches, focal neurologic deficits, and hydrocephalus. Other less common symptoms include hyperreflexia, hemiparesis, and visual field deficits.

In oligodendrogliomas, the treatment of choice is surgical resection. Approximately 70% of patients are alive 5 years after diagnosis. Chemotherapy and irradiation are usually reserved for recurrences. Histologically, oligodendrogliomas are commonly mixed with glioma components. Pure oligodendrogliomas are relatively uncommon. Oligodendrogliomas are characterized by monomorphic cells with a surrounding halo that imparts a "honeycomb" appearance. The presence of oligodendrocytes is said to improve the prognosis. The World Health Organization recognizes two types of oligodendrogliomas, benign and frankly malignant. When malignant degeneration occurs, it is the astrocytic component that usually undergoes the change. Therefore, mixed oligodendrogliomas have a worse prognosis than "pure" or benign ones. Malignant oligodendrogliomas may result in leptomeningeal metastases. Spontaneous and fatal hemorrhage is seen more often with oligodendroglioma than with any other kind of glioma.

Ependymomas in the supratentorial compartment are histologically similar to infratentorial ones. A regular cellular pattern lining small vessels and producing rosettes or pseudorosettes is characteristic. Increased mitotic activity and vascular proliferation are seen in the more aggressive ependymomas. Because they are commonly located outside the ventricles, subarachnoid seeding is not usual. The term "ependymoblastoma" refers to an undifferentiated primitive ependymoma that belongs to the primitive neuroectodermal tumor group (PNET).

IMAGING FEATURES

Oligodendrogliomas may occur in any lobe, are usually situated in the superficial white matter, and involve the cortex. The inner table of the skull may be scalloped and the meninges invaded. Calcifications are present in 50% of tumors by computed tomography (CT). Oligodendrogliomas tend to be well demarcated, solid, and show variable degrees of contrast enhancement (Fig. 6.06-1A). Cysts, areas of necrosis, and spontaneous hemorrhage are seen (Fig. 6.06-1B). Little or no edema is typical. Pure oligodendrogliomas appear hypodense on CT and hypointense on magnetic resonance (MR) T1-weighted images (Fig. 6.06-1C–E). They tend to have lesser amounts of calcifications and show less enhancement than mixed oligodendrogliomas. The latter usually are indistinguishable from more common astrocytomas.

Ependymomas occur anywhere in the brain, but preferentially in the frontal and parietal regions (Fig. 6.06-2A). They tend to be periventricular in location. Less commonly, they occur within the ventricles, most likely the lateral ones (Fig. 6.06-2B–D). Cysts are common and calcifications are seen in up to

44% of supratentorial ependymomas. Little or no edema is typical; however, if significant edema is present, malignant transformation should be considered. By MR imaging, heterogenicity is typical of ependymomas. Some supratentorial ependymomas are homogenous, however, and indistinguishable from low-grade astrocytomas. Enhancement is variable.

FIGURE 6.06-1.

Oligodendroglioma. **A.** Axial postcontrast magnetic resonance (MR) T1-weighted image shows nonenhancing low-intensity tumor *(arrowheads)* in the left frontotemporal region. There is compression of the foramina of Monroe, resulting in hydrocephalus. **B.** Axial noncontrast computed tomography (CT) shows right temporal acute bleed with intraventricular extension, midline shift to the left, and blood in the ventricles. Angiography was negative in this teenager, and at surgery an oligodendroglioma was found. **C.** Coronal CT in a 6-year-old with chronic seizures shows a small, subcortical, hypodense mass *(arrow)* expanding the overlying gyrus. **D.** Axial postcontrast MR T1-weighted image in the same patient shows nonenhancing hypointense mass *(arrow)*. Mass is anterior to the right central sulcus. **E.** Sagittal view from intraoperative sonogram shows oligodendroglioma *(large arrow)* anterior to the marginal ramus *(small arrow)* of the cingulate sulcus and anterior to the premotor gyrus (P).

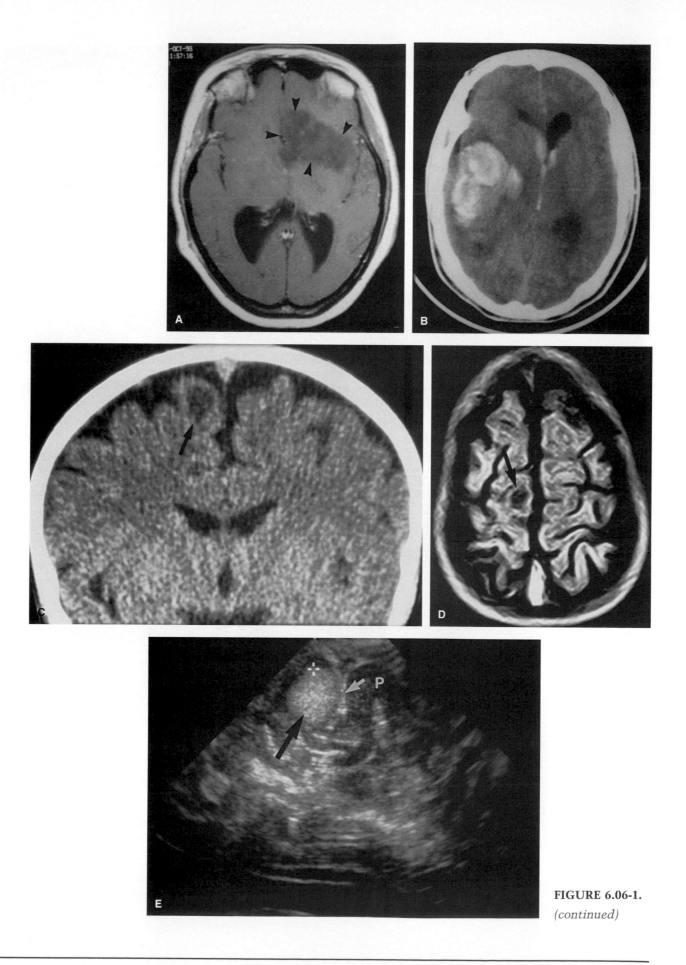

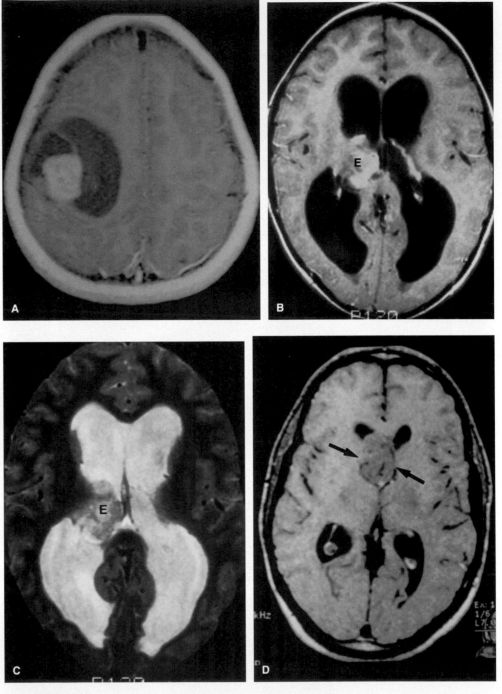

FIGURE 6.06-2.

Ependymoma. **A.** Axial postcontrast MR T1-weighted image in a patient with an anaplastic ependymoma shows mostly cystic-appearing mass with enhancing nodule. The appearance is similar to that of pleomorphic xanthoastrocytoma. (Case courtesy R. Tien, M.D., Duke University Medical Center, Durham, NC.) **B.** Axial postcontrast MR T1-weighted image shows heterogenously enhancing mass (E) in the body of the right lateral ventricle. Hydrocephalus is present. (With permission from Castillo M. Neuroradiology Companion. Philadelphia: JB Lippincott, 1995.) **C.** Corresponding MR T2-weighted image shows the ependymoma (E) to be of low signal intensity. **D.** Axial postcontrast MR T1-weighted image in a different patient shows no enhancement in an inhomogeneous ependymoma *(arrows)* that contains some areas of flow void (vessels?).

SUGGESTED READINGS

1. Edwards-Brown MK. Supratentorial tumors. Neuroimaging Clinics of North America 1994;4:437.
2. Castillo M. Contrast enhancement in primary tumors of the brain and spinal cord. Neuroimaging Clinics of North America 1994;4:63.
3. Tice H, Barnes PD, Goumnerova L, Scott RM, Tarbell NJ. Pediatric and adolescent oligodendrogliomas. AJNR 1993;14:1293.

6.07   Supratentorial: Choroid Plexus Tumors

EPIDEMIOLOGY

Choroid plexus papillomas comprise less than 1% of all childhood intracranial tumors and 5% of supratentorial tumors. Approximately 85% are found during the first 5 years of life. Choroid plexus carcinomas comprise 30% to 40% of choroid plexus tumors in pediatric patients, and tend to occur in older children. Boys are affected more often than girls (both types of tumors). Choroid plexus papillomas are known to occur in utero.

CLINICAL FEATURES

Presentation usually consists of signs of increased intracranial pressure, vomiting, clumsiness, headache, and seizures. Hydrocephalus (80% of patients) is probably the result of overproduction of cerebrospinal fluid (CSF), tumor bleeding, tumor CSF seeding, and mechanical obstruction.

Pathologically, these tumors are reddish, meaty, cauliflower-like masses. They are composed of delicate papillary fronds resembling normal choroid plexus. The cells are cuboidal to columnar and are arranged in an orderly fashion. Mitoses and mucin are absent. Calcifications are common. Surgical resection is the treatment of choice. CSF seeding may occur after surgery. Subtotal resection often leads to recurrence. Malignant degeneration is uncommon. Irradiation and chemotherapy are reserved for recurrences or carcinomas.

Although choroid plexus carcinomas are histologically similar to papillomas, their cells are less organized. With carcinomas there is a tendency toward invasion of the adjacent brain parenchyma. Systemic metastases may occur.

IMAGING FEATURES

Choroid plexus papillomas are found in the lateral ventricles (50%), fourth ventricle (10%), third ventricle, and cerebellopontine angle cisterns. In children, the lateral ventricles are the most common site (Fig. 6.07-1A, B). Inexplicably, the left lateral ventricle is more often involved (the same phenomenon is seen with intraventricular meningiomas). In 3% to 4% of cases they are bilateral. By imaging, they are lobulated, well-marginated masses in the atrium of the lateral ventricle. There is generalized hydrocephalus, but a portion of a ventricle may dilate out of proportion to others secondary to its entrapment. Computed tomography best defines the punctate calcifications present in 25% of tumors. The tumors are of low signal intensity on precontrast magnetic resonance (MR) T1-weighted images and may be of low signal intensity on T2-weighted images (probably reflecting their hypercellularity; Fig. 6.07-1C, D). After contrast administration, these tumors enhance markedly (Fig. 6.07-1E). On MR imaging, multiple areas of signal void may be noted. These are probably related to calcifications and hypertrophied vessels. Cyst formation is relatively common. Spontaneous hemorrhage is uncommon. Contrast-enhanced MR imaging is ideal for identifying seeding of the subarachnoid spaces. Edema is uncommon, but if present is mild with papillomas. Edema is a prominent feature of carcinomas (Fig. 6.07-2). Invasion of the brain parenchyma and subarachnoid tumor seeding are also typical of carcinomas. Carcinomas are very heterogenous by MR imaging, whereas papillomas tend to be homogenous in appearance. Carcinomas may have an identical appearance to primitive neuroectodermal tumors.

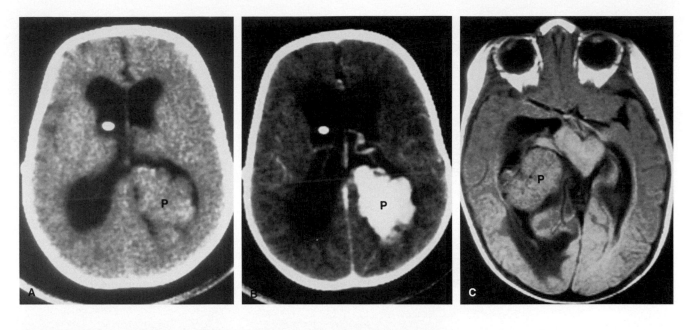

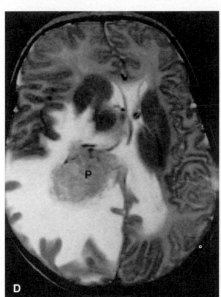
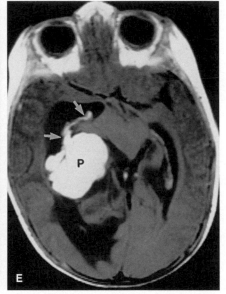

FIGURE 6.07-1.

Choroid plexus papilloma. **A.** Axial noncontrast computed tomography (CT) shows a bulky and slightly hyperdense tumor (P) in the atrium of the left lateral ventricle. There is hydrocephalus and a shunt in the frontal horn of the right lateral ventricle. **B.** Corresponding postcontrast CT image shows significant enhancement of the choroid plexus papilloma (P). **C.** Axial noncontrast magnetic resonance (MR) T1-weighted image shows tumor (P) in the atrium of the right lateral ventricle. Tumor is isointense to brain. There is hydrocephalus and edema adjacent to tumor and significant mass effect on the brain stem. **D.** Axial MR T2-weighted image in the same patient (cephalad to [C]) shows tumor (P) to be of low signal intensity and surrounded by large areas of edema. Multiple areas of flow void (vessels) are seen in the tumor. **E.** Axial postcontrast MR T1-weighted image shows the tumor (P) to enhance markedly. Note that tumor is continuous with the choroid plexus in the temporal horn of the right lateral ventricle. Extensive edema is again noted.

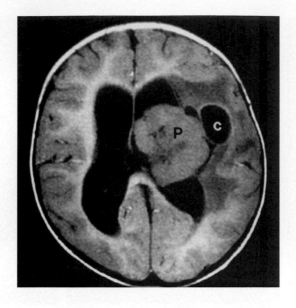

FIGURE 6.07-2.

Choroid plexus carcinoma. Axial noncontrast magnetic resonance T1-weighted image shows mass (P) in the left lateral ventricle and hydrocephalus. The mass has extended outside the ventricle, and there is cyst (c) formation and edema.

SUGGESTED
READING

1. Osborn AG. Astrocytomas and other glial neoplasms. In: Diagnostic Neuroradiology. St. Louis: CV Mosby, 1994:572.

6.08 Supratentorial: Neuronal Origin Tumors

EPIDEMIOLOGY

This group of tumors includes ganglioglioma, ganglioneuroma, gangliocytoma, desmoplastic infantile ganglioglioma, and dysembryonoplastic neuroepithelial tumor. Dysplastic cerebellar gangliocytoma (Lhermitte-Duclos disease) is not discussed here. Tumors of neuronal origin probably comprise less than 1% of all brain tumors, but up to 5% to 6% of childhood brain neoplasms. There is no gender predilection.

CLINICAL FEATURES

These tumors are characterized by intractable seizures. Most patients become symptomatic during the second decade of life. The treatment of choice is surgical resection. Leptomeningeal dissemination of ganglioglioma has been described. Histologically these tumors are divided as follows:

a. Ganglioglioma: composed of well differentiated neoplastic ganglion cells mixed with glial stroma that contains astrocytes and oligodendrocytes.
b. Ganglioneuroma: the dominant component in these tumors is mature neurons. They are usually grouped together with the gangliogliomas because they are often indistinguishable from each other.
c. Gangliocytoma: tumors consisting entirely of ganglion cells with minimal glial stroma.
d. Desmoplastic infantile ganglioglioma: mostly ganglionic elements and glial stroma but with a strong desmoplastic reaction.
e. Dysembryonoplastic neuroepithelial tumor: cellular heterogeneity is typical, and they contain neurons, oligodendrocytes, and astrocytes. They are usually associated with an area of cortical dysplasia.

IMAGING FEATURES

Gangliogliomas tend to occur mainly in the temporal lobes, followed by the parietal lobes and the cerebellum (Fig. 6.08-1). Other parts of the brain and the spinal cord may also be involved. There is no typical appearance by imaging but they tend to be of low signal intensity on magnetic resonance (MR) T1-weighted images and hyperintense on T2-weighted images. However, up to half of the tumors may be cystic and contain mural nodules that enhance. However, hypodense or hypointense areas within neuronal cell tumors are not necessarily cystic. These tumors may be completely solid. At times, total lack of enhancement is seen, and the tumors may be difficult to distinguish from surrounding normal brain. Gangliogliomas contain calcifications in 35% of cases. They may be situated in the periphery of the brain and produce pressure erosion of the inner table of the skull. Rarely, gangliogliomas may extend through the subarachnoid space. In this situation, multiple microcysts (simulating infectious origin) may be seen on computed tomography or MR T2-weighted images. Giant gangliogliomas tend to be of the desmoplastic type histologically, and some of them are actually more akin to hamartomas than to true tumors. Gangliocytomas may be identical to gangliogliomas by imaging (Fig. 6.08-2).

Desmoplastic infantile ganglioglioma is a massive cystic lesion occurring more often in the frontal and parietal lobes. It is attached to the dura and may erode the skull.

Dysembryonoplastic neuroepithelial tumors occur more often in the temporal lobes (60%), followed by the frontal lobes (30%). They predominantly involve the cortex (Fig. 6.08-3). Their imaging features are nonspecific, and they may appear as an area of gray matter thickening. They are hypointense on MR T1-weighted images, hyperintense on T2-weighted images, and may also contain areas of signal void related to calcifications. These lesions may be completely cystic or contain small cysts. Enhancement is variable. They may also produce scalloping of the inner table of the skull due to pressure erosion. As in most tumors of neuronal origin, edema is often lacking and the mass effect produced is mild.

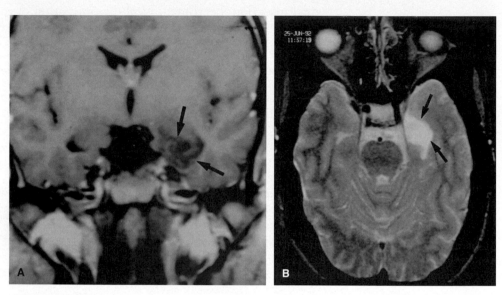

FIGURE 6.08-1.

Ganglioglioma. **A.** Coronal postcontrast magnetic resonance (MR) T1-weighted image shows nonenhancing tumor *(arrows)* in mesial left temporal lobe. The tumor is mostly hypointense in relation to normal brain. **B.** Axial MR T2-weighted image shows the tumor *(arrows)* to be of high signal intensity.

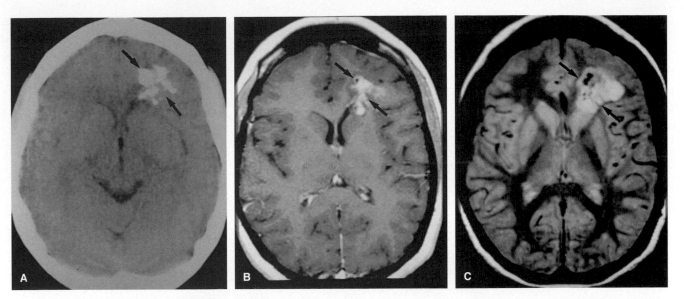

FIGURE 6.08-2.

Gangliocytoma. **A.** Axial noncontrast computed tomography shows a mass *(arrows)* containing multiple calcifications in the left frontal lobe. **B.** Postcontrast magnetic resonance (MR) T1-weighted image shows the mass *(arrows)* to enhance. Note absence of significant mass effect. **C.** Corresponding MR T2-weighted image shows the mass *(arrows)* to be of increased signal intensity and to contain areas of signal void corresponding to calcifications. Note absence of edema.

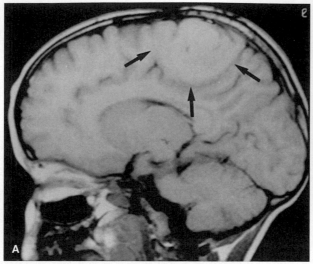

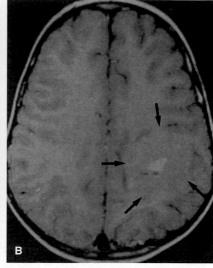

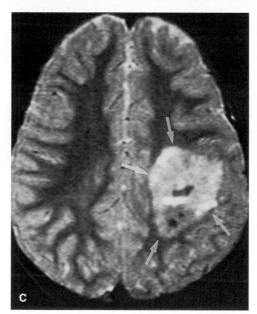

FIGURE 6.08-3.

Dysembryonoplastic neuroepithelial tumor.
A. Parasagittal noncontrast magnetic resonance (MR) T1-weighted image shows tumor *(arrows)* arising in cortex. Note that tumor is isointense with brain. The appearance is similar to that of a meningioma. Note absence of significant mass effect. **B.** Axial postcontrast MR T1-weighted image shows no significant enhancement in the tumor *(arrows)*. **C.** Axial MR T2-weighted image shows that the tumor *(arrows)* is inhomogeneous but relatively hypointense. There is no edema.

SUGGESTED READINGS

1. Castillo M, Davis PC, Takei Y, Hoffman JC. Intracranial ganglioglioma: MR, CT, and clinical findings in 18 patients. AJNR 1990;11:109.
2. Altman NR. MR and CT characteristics of gangliocytoma: a rare cause of epilepsy in children. AJNR 1988;9:917.
3. Koeller KK, Dillon WP. Dysembryonoplastic neuroepithelial tumors: MR appearance. AJNR 1992;13:1319.

6.09 Supratentorial: Neuroblastoma and Other Primitive Neuroectodermal Tumors

EPIDEMIOLOGY

Medulloblastoma and retinoblastoma are probably the most common primitive neuroectodermal tumors (PNETs), and are not addressed here. Neuroblastoma accounts for less than 1% of childhood brain tumors. Approximately 20% of all supratentorial neuroblastomas are found during the first 2 months of life, and most are found before 5 years of age. There is no gender predilection.

CLINICAL FEATURES

The World Health Organization now accepts the following types of PNETs:

> a. Embryonal tumors: medulloepithelioma, neuroblastoma, ependymoblastoma, retinoblastoma, PNETs with multipotential differentiation, medulloblastoma.
> b. Pineal tumors: pineocytoma, pineoblastoma, mixed pineocytoma/pineoblastoma.

Most patients present with headaches, seizures, nausea and vomiting, and hydrocephalus. In younger patients, macrocrania may be present. The treatment of choice is surgical resection. Because these tumors are very large at diagnosis, only debulking is possible in many patients. Because cerebrospinal fluid dissemination is common, prophylactic spinal axis irradiation is recommended. The role of chemotherapy is not established, but because this treatment is effective in many medulloblastomas, it is commonly given for other PNETs. Prognosis is poor, with a 5-year survival rate of less than 30%. Prognosis is slightly better for older children. Metastases to lung, lymph nodes, pericardium, diaphragm, and liver have been described.

Histologically, PNETs are hypercellular. More than 90% of cells are undifferentiated, have abundant mitoses, and scant cytoplasm. Vascular endothelial hyperplasia and necrosis are present. The cells cluster around a fibrinoid matrix, resulting in Homer-Wright rosettes.

IMAGING FEATURES

Most neuroblastomas are large masses with zones of necrosis and cysts. Therefore, by magnetic resonance (MR) imaging, they commonly have multiple zones of mixed signal intensity on both the T1- and T2-weighted images. Intratumoral hemorrhage is not uncommon. Prominent vessels may be present within the tumor. The tumors may be found in any part of the brain, but the frontal and parietal periventricular white matter is more commonly affected. Their most important imaging features are heterogeneity and large size. Some contrast enhancement is always present, particularly within solid tumor portions and along the margins of the cystic components (Fig. 6.09-1A). MR imaging with contrast is preferred over computed tomography because it can also detect subarachnoid tumor seeding. In the spine, both subarachnoid and intramedullary metastases may occur. By MR imaging, many of the solid portions of a neuroblastoma are dark on T2-weighted images (Fig. 6.09-1B, C). This characteristic probably reflects a high nuclei-to-cytoplasm ratio. Neuroblastomas may also be found inside the ventricles and in the basilar cisterns (especially the prepontine and suprasellar cisterns; Fig. 6.09-1D–H).

Secondary neuroblastoma is usually caused by metastases from primary tumors in the abdomen, chest, or pelvis. It presents with cranial neuropathy secondary to metastases to the base of the skull, proptosis due to metastases to the bony orbit, or splitting of the sutures due to calvarial tumor deposits (Fig. 6.09-2). These metastases are commonly of intermediate signal intensity on T1- and T2-weighted images and enhance after contrast administration.

FIGURE 6.09-1.

Primitive neuroectodermal tumors (PNETs). **A.** Axial postcontrast magnetic resonance (MR) T1-weighted image shows complex mass in the left temporal lobe. The laterally located solid components enhance and there is questionable enhancement along the anterior margin of the large cyst. There is midline shift and dilation of the temporal horn of the right lateral ventricle. (With permission from Castillo M. Neuroradiology Companion. Philadelphia: JB Lippincott, 1995.) **B.** Corresponding axial MR T2-weighted image shows the solid portions of the tumor to be hypointense, related to high cellularity. The cysts are hyperintense. **C.** Frontal view from MR time-of-flight three-dimensional angiogram shows upward and medial displacement of the left middle cerebral artery *(arrows)*, indicating that this tumor arises outside the ventricular system. **D.** Axial postcontrast MR T1-weighted image in a different patient shows a mostly hypointense, nonenhancing mass in the body of the left lateral ventricle, and hydrocephalus. There is periventricular edema. **E.** Coronal postcontrast MR T1-weighted image in the same patient shows minimal central enhancement (also present on axial image) of the mass. Note tumor *(arrow)* extending into the third ventricle. **F.** Axial MR T2-weighted image shows the same tumor to be relatively hypointense, probably related to its high cellularity. Periventricular edema from hydrocephalus is well visualized. **G.** Precontrast midsagittal MR T1-weighted image in a different patient shows an inhomogeneous mass (M) in the suprasellar region. Note irregular massa intermedia, pineal gland region, and nodule in floor of fourth ventricle, all of which were metastases from the suprasellar PNET. **H.** Axial MR T2-weighted image in same patient shows the suprasellar tumor *(arrows)* to be of low signal intensity.

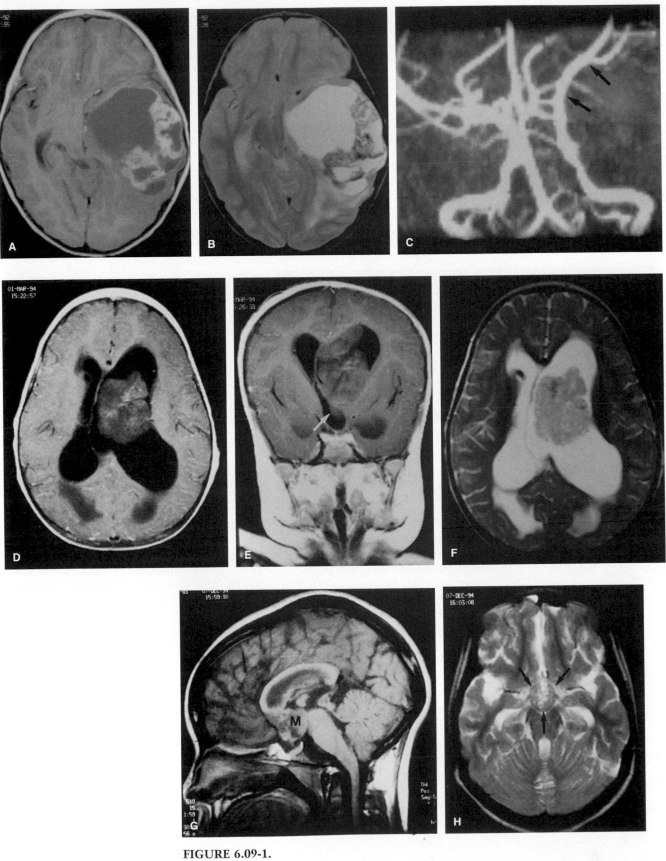

FIGURE 6.09-1.

(continued)

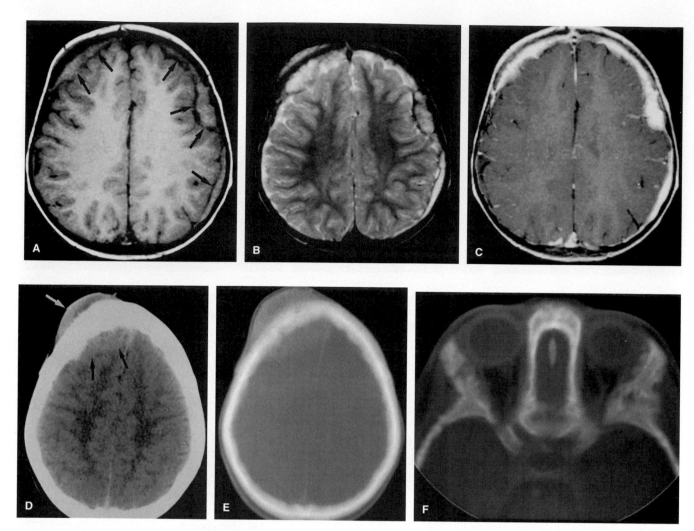

FIGURE 6.09-2.

Metastatic neuroblastoma. **A.** Axial precontrast magnetic resonance (MR) T1-weighted image in a child with metastatic abdominal neuroblastoma to the skull shows lobulated masses *(arrows)* located in the inner table/dura. The lesions are of intermediate signal intensity. **B.** Corresponding MR T2-weighted image shows that some tumor deposits are hyperintense whereas others are of intermediate signal intensity. **C.** Axial postcontrast MR T1-weighted image shows tumor deposits to enhance markedly. **D.** Postcontrast axial computed tomography (CT) shows mass *(arrows)* in right frontal region involving scalp and extraaxial intracranial compartment secondary to solitary metastasis from neuroblastoma. **E.** Corresponding bone window setting shows permeative pattern of involved calvarium, which is also slightly expanded. **F.** Axial CT shows involvement of bony orbits by metastatic neuroblastoma.

SUGGESTED READINGS

1. Davis PC, Wichman RD, Taei Y, Hoffman JC. Primary cerebral neuroblastoma: CT and MR findings in 12 cases. AJNR 1990;11:115.
2. Rorke LB. Primitive neuroectodermal tumors. In: Nelson JS, Parisi JE, Schochet SS, eds. Principles and Practice of Neuropathology. St. Louis: CV Mosby, 1993:185.

6.10 Supratentorial: Pineal Gland Tumors

EPIDEMIOLOGY

Most pineal tumors derive from the germ cell line. In the Western hemisphere, they comprise less than 1% of intracranial tumors, but in the Orient they represent up to 6% of intracranial tumors. Germinomas occur most often between 15 to 20 years of age, and almost exclusively in male patients. Teratomas are the most common congenital tumor, and there is a second peak between 10 to 20 years of age. They are also more common in boys. Primitive neuroectodermal tumors (PNETs; pineocytoma and pineoblastoma) account for 20% of pineal masses. Pineoblastomas tend to occur in young boys, whereas pineocytomas are tumors of adults. Other, less common pineal region tumors include gliomas, embryonal carcinomas, endodermal sinus tumors (yolk sac tumors), and choriocarcinomas.

CLINICAL FEATURES

Clinical signs are usually related to hydrocephalus and compression of the dorsal midbrain. Parinaud syndrome is typical and is characterized by lack of convergence, restricted upward gaze, and abnormal accommodation. Other symptoms include loss of vision, diabetes insipidus, and precocious puberty. Germinomas represent over 50% of masses in the region of the pineal gland. Approximately 35% of germinomas occur in the suprasellar region. In these cases, both genders are equally affected. The triad of visual loss, hypopituitarism, and diabetes insipidus suggests a suprasellar location. Less than 10% of germinomas arise primarily within the brain, mainly in the thalami or basal ganglia. Intraparenchymal germinomas are also more common in boys. Germ cell tumor markers are given in Table 6.10-1.

TABLE 6.10-1. Germ Cell Tumor Markers

Type of Tumor	α-Fetoprotein	Human Chorionic Gonadotropin	Carcinoembryonic Antigen
Germinoma*	−	+	−
Embryonal carcinoma	+ + +	+ + +	−
Endodermal sinus tumor	+ + +	−	−
Choriocarcinoma	−	+ + +	−
Teratoma	−	−	+

* Germinomas may also secrete placental alkaline phosphatase (PLAP).

Biopsy is required for diagnosis, but because some of these tumors may contain different cell populations, open biopsy is recommended rather than needle aspiration. Management depends on histologic type. Germinomas are treated with irradiation and chemotherapy. This treatment provides a 50% to 80% 5-year survival rate. Surgery is the treatment of choice in teratomas and gliomas. Radiation therapy is used for pineoblastomas. Prophylactic irradiation of the spinal axis is also commonly used for pineal PNETs.

IMAGING FEATURES

Germinomas are well defined masses that enhance uniformly by computed tomography or magnetic resonance (MR) imaging (Fig. 6.10-1A). Although most germinomas are bright on MR T2-weighted images, some are hypointense. This is believed to be the result of a high nuclei-to-cytoplasm ratio and decreased free water. Germinomas tend to seed the cerebrospinal fluid spaces and invade the adjacent brain (Fig. 6.10-1B). Teratomas in the pineal gland are often malignant. Heterogeneity is their hallmark; they contain solid enhancing regions, cysts, fat, and calcifications. However, teratomas may also be homogenous and indistinguishable from the more common germinomas. Teratomas are aggressive and may invade the brain. Embryonal carcinoma and endodermal sinus tumors have no specific imaging features. Choriocarcinomas tend to be hemorrhagic. Pineocytomas tend to be well marginated, noninvasive, and slow growing. They may have cysts and calcifications. Although the MR imaging of pineocytomas is nonspecific occasionally they may be cyst-like and indistinguishable from primary pineal cysts. Cystic pineocytomas may contain soft tissue trabeculations and may show enhancement after contrast administration. Cystic pineal masses need to be imaged immediately after the administration of MR contrast material because some benign cysts may show enhancement in delayed images, giving the appearance of neoplasia. Unlike pineocytomas, pineoblastomas are heterogenous, larger, invasive, and tend to occur in younger patients. The solid portions of pineoblastomas always enhance, whereas cysts and zones of necrosis do not (Fig. 6.10-2).

Idiopathic pineal cysts are seen in up to 5% of all MR imaging studies. They usually measure less than 1.5 cm in their greatest dimension. Their rim normally enhances after contrast administration, but, as mentioned earlier, they may show homogenous enhancement on delay postcontrast MR images. They are typically devoid of any internal architecture.

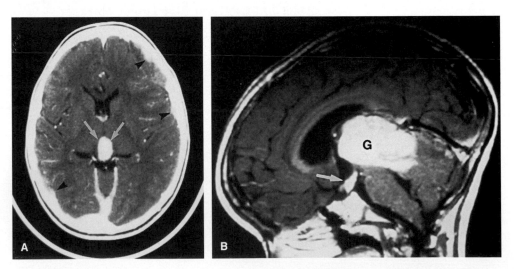

FIGURE 6.10-1.

Germinona. **A.** Axial postcontrast computed tomography shows a densely enhancing and homogenous mass *(arrows)* in the pineal gland in a male adolescent. There are subtle but definite enhancing masses *(arrowheads)* in the subarachnoid spaces related to tumor seeding. **B.** Midsagittal postcontrast magnetic resonance T1-weighted image shows large enhancing mass (G) in the pineal region. There is tumor *(arrow)* seeding of the inferior third ventricle. The ventral surface of the pons shows questionable enhancement, which also could be related to tumor seeding. There is hydrocephalus.

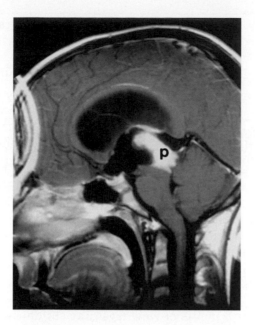

FIGURE 6.10-2.

Pineoblastoma. Postcontrast midsagittal magnetic resonance T1-weighted image shows nonspecific-appearing and enhancing mass (p) in the pineal gland region. There is compression of the aqueduct, resulting in hydrocephalus. (With permission from Castillo M. Neuroradiology Companion. Philadelphia: JB Lippincott, 1995.)

SUGGESTED READINGS

1. Fujimakati T, Matsutani M, Funada N, et al. CT and MRI features of intracranial germ cell tumors. J Neurooncol 1994;19:217.
2. Higano S, Takahashi S, Ishii K, Matsumoto K, Ikeda H, Sakamoto K. Germinoma originating in the basal ganglia and thalamus: MR and CT evaluation. AJNR 1994; 15:1435.

6.11 Supratentorial: Meningioma

EPIDEMIOLOGY

Meningiomas constitute 1.4% to 4% of all childhood intracranial tumors. Most are found between 10 to 20 years of age. They occur in association with neurofibromatosis type II (NF-2) and in patients who have received prior radiation therapy to the head. Contrary to adults, boys are affected more often than girls. Other meningeal tumors in children include fibromas, sarcomas, and melanomas.

CLINICAL FEATURES

Symptoms are related to the tumor's site of origin. Overall, signs of increased intracranial pressure, focal neurologic deficits, and seizures are the most common clinical presentations. Hydrocephalus is common with intraventricular meningiomas. Cranial nerve deficits may also be seen. Up to 20% of children with meningiomas have NF-2. Meningiomas are multiple in 2.5% of children. Multiplicity is also more common in children with NF-2. Radiation-induced meningiomas usually occur anywhere from 7 to 20 years after completion of treatment.

There are two points of view regarding childhood meningiomas. The first (and traditional) one states that these tumors behave clinically and appear by imaging different from those found in adults. For example, it is said that 10% to 50% of childhood meningiomas show malignant degeneration (especially sarcomatous), and that these tumors tend to arise in atypical locations (intraventricular [16%–20%], lack of dural attachments [30%], and optic chiasm). Imaging may differ from adult meningiomas in that those found in pediatric patients tend to have more cysts or may be totally cystic. The second point of view is that pediatric tumors are no different from those seen in adults, with the exception of being somewhat larger at the time of diagnosis.

Surgical resection is the treatment of choice. Incomplete resection or malignant changes may be indications for irradiation. With incomplete removal, the recurrence rate is high.

IMAGING FEATURES

We prefer magnetic resonance imaging for the diagnosis of suspected meningioma. Calcifications and hyperostosis are the only two imaging features that are better seen with computed tomography. Pediatric meningiomas tend to be very large at time of diagnosis, usually measuring more than 5 cm in diameter. They commonly arise from the dura, brain, ventricular lining and choroid plexuses, and in the region of the Sylvian fissure (Fig. 6.11-1A). On T1-weighted images, meningiomas are isointense to gray matter and are surrounded by a thin, hypointense rim. This rim represents either a cerebrospinal fluid cleft between brain and tumor, or a fibrous capsule (or a combination of both). Intratumoral areas of signal void are related to calcifications or vessels. Cysts may be present (Fig. 6.11-1B,C). On T2-weighted images, meningiomas are commonly somewhat hypointense, probably reflecting their cellular compactness or the presence of fibrous components. Hyperintensity on T2-weighted images correlates with atypical histologic features. Meningiomas usually enhance densely after contrast administration. Tumor cysts and areas of necrosis are more common than in adults and do not enhance, but their margins may show contrast enhancement. Peritumoral edema is variable but is often encountered with intraventricular tumors, producing hydrocephalus. In children, dural sarcomas may have an identical imaging appearance to meningiomas, and histologic study is needed for the correct diagnosis (Fig. 6.11-2). Meningiomas may also occur secondary to prior irradiation (Fig. 6.11-3). This is especially seen in children who in the past have received radiation therapy for optic chiasm astrocytoma.

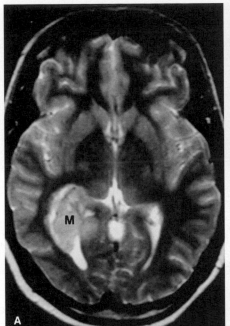

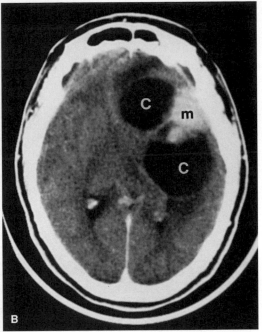

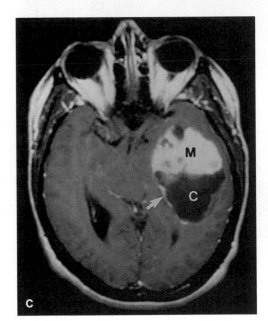

FIGURE 6.11-1.

Meningioma. **A.** Axial magnetic resonance (MR) T2-weighted image shows meningioma (M) in the atrium of the right lateral ventricle. **B.** Axial postcontrast computed tomography shows a laterally located, solid, and enhancing meningioma (m) with two large cystic (C) components and surrounding edema. **C.** Axial postcontrast MR T1-weighted image shows enhancing meningioma (M) in the left temporal lobe with a large cyst (C) posteriorly. Note enhancement (*arrow*) in medial cyst wall. The lesion was atypical meningioma.

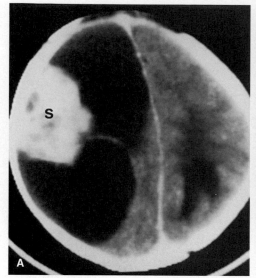

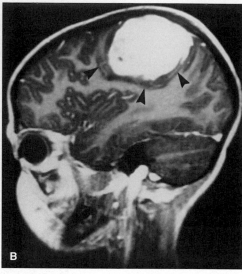

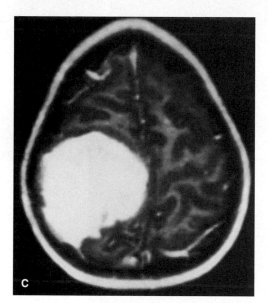

FIGURE 6.11-2.

Dural-based sarcoma. **A.** Axial postcontrast computed tomography shows deeply enhancing dural-based nodule (S) in the right parietal convexity with large cystic components medially. The imaging features of the mass are highly suggestive of meningioma in this newborn, but it proved to be a malignant fibrous hystiocytoma. **B.** Parasagittal postcontrast magnetic resonance T1-weighted image in a different patient shows dural-based (note inward buckling of cortex; *arrowheads*), large, and enhancing fibrosarcoma. **C.** Axial image in same patient shows mass, which proved to be fibrosarcoma.

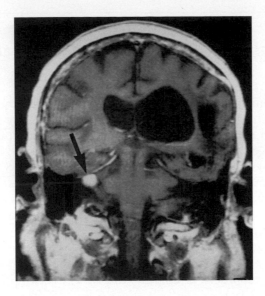

FIGURE 6.11-3.

Radiation-induced meningioma. Coronal postcontrast magnetic resonance T1-weighted image in a patient who received irradiation as a child for a left temporal astrocytoma. At 26 years of age, a right tentorial meningioma *(arrow)* has developed. This meningioma is presumed to be radiation induced.

SUGGESTED
READING

1. Darling CF, Byrd SE, Reyes-Mugica M, et al. MR of pediatric intracranial meningiomas. AJNR 1994;15:435.

6.12 Supratentorial: Lymphoma, Leukemia, and Langerhans Cell Histiocytosis

EPIDEMIOLOGY

Involvement of the central nervous system (CNS) by lymphoma is the result almost exclusively of the non-Hodgkin variety. Five percent to 11% of patients with this disease have CNS involvement. Leptomeningeal involvement is seen in 4% to 9% of patients with non-Hodgkin lymphoma. Brain lymphoma is seen in immunosuppressed patients (AIDS or transplant). CNS complications from leukemia (mainly acute lymphoblastic leukemia) occur in 5% to 10% of patients. Because many of these patients receive craniospinal irradiation and chemotherapy, complications related to treatment (leukoencephalopathies) are not uncommon.

Langerhans cell histiocytosis (histiocytosis X) is the very rare. It commonly involves the skull, meninges, and hypothalamus. There is a 42% cumulative risk for development of diabetes insipidus over the first 4 years after diagnosis of histiocytosis X.

CLINICAL FEATURES

In the past, the main complication of non-Hodgkin lymphoma was spinal cord compression from epidural disease; however, at present, most cases of cord compression are secondary to leptomeningeal metastases. This occurs because the CNS represents a sanctuary for tumor cells. Common sites of involvement include the meninges (46%), spinal cord (38%), and the cerebellum (16%). Most patients present with focal motor or sensory deficits, cranial palsies (often multiple), headaches, nausea, vomiting, and radiculopathies. Treatment include either irradiation or chemotherapy, but there is a role for surgical laminectomy in cases of acute spinal cord compression.

Infiltration of the subarachnoid space is the initial sign of meningeal leukemia. Leukemia may enter the brain via the Virchow-Robin spaces. Signs and symptoms are related to increased intracranial pressure, but fever may be present, making leukemia hard to distinguish from infectious meningitis. Infiltration of the cranial nerves (particularly II, VI, VII, and VIII) is not rare. Optic nerve involvement occurs in almost 9% of patients. Sinus thrombosis and cerebrovascular accidents are secondary to the leukemia or to chemotherapy (particularly with L-asparaginase). Infiltration of the hypothalamus is rare in patients receiving combination chemotherapy and radiation. Seizures in leukemic patients are idiopathic in over two thirds of cases. Spinal cord compression is unusual and occurs in less than 1% of leukemic patients. Bacterial meningitis is surprisingly uncommon in children with leukemia. Granulocytic sarcoma (chloroma) is a solid mass composed of immature granulocytes that occurs in patients with myelogenous or myelomonocytic leukemias. They rarely involve the CNS, but may arise in the orbits or the paranasal sinuses.

With the exception of diabetes insipidus, there are no specific clinical manifestations associated with Langerhans cell histiocytosis. More than 80% of the paraventricular–supraoptic neurons need to be destroyed before diabetes insipidus ensues.

IMAGING FEATURES

Both lymphoma and leukemia may present similar magnetic resonance imaging features. A common imaging finding is enlargement of the ventricles and prominence of the cortical sulci. This probably reflects atrophy secondary to systemic tumor, but may be related to communicating hydrocephalus secondary to meningeal infiltration. Both may cause thick and nodular dural and pial masses that enhance after contrast administration. In the brain, mass lesions from lymphoma are somewhat dark on both T1- and T2-weighted images, probably reflecting hypercellularity and compactness. The masses show marked enhancement after contrast administration (Fig. 6.12-1A–C). Extension of tumor along the Virchow-Robin spaces may account for many intraaxial masses, particularly those in the basal ganglia. In immunocompetent patients, they produce little mass effect and edema, and are located in the deep gray nuclei or white matter (particularly the commissural fibers). In immunocompromised patients, primary brain lymphoma has no specific features, but often appears as ring-enhancing lesions surrounded by edema that are indistinguishable from infectious processes. Both lymphoma and leukemia may involve the calvarium, producing destructive lesions. The cavernous sinuses may also be involved (Fig. 6.12-1D). Leukemic masses (chloromas) may be dural based and indistinguishable from lymphoma. They do, however, occur in patients with known disease. Patients with systemic lymphoma and leukemia are commonly immunosuppressed, and opportunistic infections of the brain are common.

Langerhans cell histiocytosis produces either a solitary lytic skull lesion (eosinophilic granuloma) or multiple skull lesions (Hand-Schüller-Christian disease). Single lesions tend preferentially to involve the outer table (Fig. 6.12-2A). The orbits, paranasal sinuses, and hypothalamus may also be involved (Fig. 6.12-2B). The lesions have a nonspecific appearance and tend to enhance after contrast administration. In the hypothalamus, thickening of the pituitary stalk and absence of high signal intensity from the posterior lobe are typical. Intraaxial ring-enhancing lesions are known to occur. Hand-Schüller-Christian disease presents with multiple, well defined lytic lesions involving bones (Fig. 6.12-3).

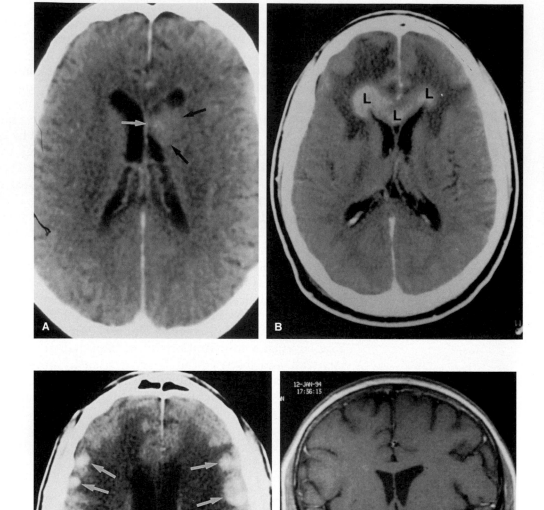

FIGURE 6.12-1.

Lymphoma. **A.** Axial postcontrast computed tomography (CT) shows mildly enhancing mass *(arrows)* in the head of the left caudate nucleus in this adolescent with AIDS. **B.** Axial postcontrast CT in a different adolescent with AIDS shows densely enhancing lymphoma (L) involving the genu of the corpus callosum with surrounding edema and slight mass effect on the ventricle. (With permission from Castillo M. Neuroradiology Companion. Philadelphia: JB Lippincott, 1995.) **C.** Axial postcontrast CT in different adolescent with AIDS shows multiple enhancing cortical nodules *(arrows)* and mild hydrocephalus. **D.** Coronal postcontrast CT shows mass *(arrow)* in right cavernous sinus that proved to be a metastasis from the patient's abdominal Burkitt lymphoma.

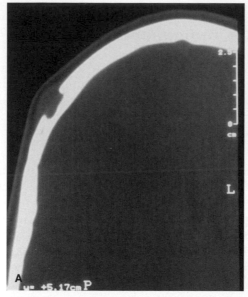 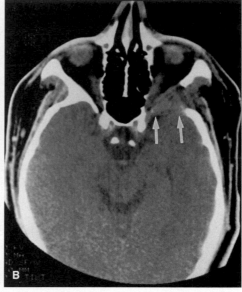

FIGURE 6.12-2.

Eosinophilic granuloma. **A.** Axial computed tomography (CT; bone windows) shows lytic lesion involving mostly the outer table and diploic space. The inner table of the skull is preserved. There is an extension of the process into the subcutaneous tissues. **B.** Axial CT shows destructive lesion *(arrows)* involving the left lateral orbital wall and greater sphenoidal wing.

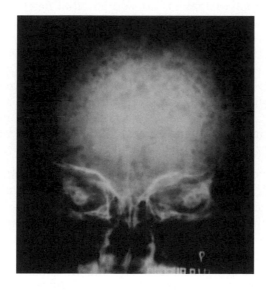

FIGURE 6.12-3.

Hand-Schüller-Christian disease. Frontal radiograph shows multiple lytic skull lesions.

SUGGESTED READINGS

1. Maghnie M, Arico M, Villa A, Genovese E, Beluffi G, Severi F. MR of the hypothalamic–pituitary axis in Langerhans cell histiocytosis. AJNR 1992;13:1365.
2. Ginsberg LE, Leeds NE. Neuroradiology of leukemia. AJR 1995;165:525.

6.13 *Malformative Tumors: Craniopharyngioma and Rathke Cleft Cyst*

EPIDEMIOLOGY

Craniopharyngiomas comprise 5% to 13% of all childhood intracranial tumors. They account for over 50% of suprasellar tumors in childhood. They are more commonly found between 6 to 13 years of age. Boys are affected more often than girls. Rathke cleft cysts represent less than 1% of intracranial tumors, and occur mainly in adults; they are rare in children.

CLINICAL FEATURES

Most patients with craniopharyngiomas present with growth failure, visual difficulties, and hydrocephalus. In children, headaches, vomiting, visual deficits, papilledema, and endocrine dysfunction are prominent. Because the tumor compresses the medial aspect of the optic chiasm, bitemporal hemianopsia is the most common visual defect. Growth hormone deficiency is the most common (> 50%) endocrine abnormality. Less common endocrinopathies include precocious puberty, obesity, and hyperphagia. Diabetes insipidus may occur after surgery. When craniopharyngiomas are completely intrasellar (5%–10%), visual and endocrine problems are more common. Over one half of patients with Rathke cleft cysts have pituitary hormone deficiencies (mainly growth hormone and prolactin). Visual abnormalities are present in 50% of patients, and headaches in one third.

Histologically, the adamantinomatous type of craniopharyngioma is more common in children. These tumors are solid, firm, and nodular and contain one or more cysts filled with an oil-like material. This material may leak out and produce a leptomeningitis. Almost all craniopharyngiomas have calcifications. Craniopharyngiomas are composed of nests of epithelial cells separated by a myxoid stroma. Keratin is present. These tumors are histologically benign. Papillary craniopharyngiomas are less common in children (they are found mostly in adults). They are composed mainly of well differentiated squamous cell epithelium. Rathke cleft cysts have a thin wall composed of goblet or ciliary cells and are filled with a watery to mucinous fluid.

Craniopharyngiomas grow very slowly. Surgical resection is the treatment of choice. Complete resection is achieved in only one third of patients. Most patients with incompletely resected tumor receive radiation therapy.

IMAGING FEATURES

The "rule of the 90s" characterizes craniopharyngiomas: 90% are cystic, 90% have calcifications, 90% enhance, and over 90% are suprasellar in location. The cysts are low density on computed tomography, but may be of either low (high keratin content) or high (high cholesterol content) signal intensity on magnetic resonance (MR) T1-weighted images (Fig. 6.13-1A–E). On T2-weighted images, cysts are hyperintense (Fig. 6.13-1C). Ten percent of craniopharyngiomas are completely solid and are indistinguishable from other suprasellar masses. Many tumors are mixed solid and cystic (Fig. 6.13-1F, G). In 25% of patients, the tumors extend into the middle, anterior, or posterior cranial fossae. Uncommon sites of origin for craniopharyngiomas include the cerebellopontine angle, optic chiasm, third ventricle, pineal gland, nasopharynx, and paranasal sinuses.

Rathke cleft cysts are intrasellar masses that are bright (> 75%) on MR T1-weighted images (Fig. 6.13-2). Their appearance on T2-weighted images is extremely variable. They do not enhance after contrast administration. Most measure between 1 and 2 cm at diagnosis. A significant number of these cysts have suprasellar extension. Distinguishing them from the rare intrasellar craniopharyngioma is not imperative because both are resected through a transphenoidal approach.

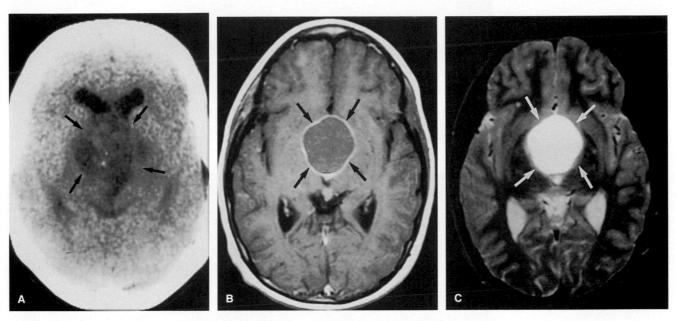

FIGURE 6.13-1.

Craniopharyngioma. **A.** Axial noncontrast computed tomography shows a large, mostly hypodense mass *(arrows)* in the region of the third ventricle. The mass contains some punctate calcifications. There is hydrocephalus. **B.** Axial postcontrast magnetic resonance (MR) T1-weighted image in a different patient shows cystic craniopharyngioma with rim enhancement *(arrows).* Note that although cystic, its signal intensity differs from that of cerebrospinal fluid. **C.** Corresponding MR T2-weighted image shows that the tumor *(arrows)* is bright. **D.** Coronal precontrast MR T1-weighted image in a different patient shows solid but inhomogeneous suprasellar craniopharyngioma. The imaging features in this mass are probably related to high keratin content in the lesion. **E.** Midsagittal precontrast MR T1-weighted image in a different patient shows a bright craniopharyngioma *(arrows).* These imaging features are probably related to high cholesterol content in the lesion. **F.** Coronal postcontrast MR T1-weighted image shows a different craniopharyngioma containing a solid (S) and enhancing component in its right lower aspect. The rim *(arrows)* of the cyst (C) also enhances. (With permission from Castillo M. Neuroradiology Companion. Philadelphia: JB Lippincott, 1995.) **G.** Midsagittal postcontrast MR T1-weighted image shows a different craniopharyngioma with a solid (S) and enhancing component anteriorly and a cystic component (C) posteriorly. The cystic component shows rim enhancement. There is hydrocephalus.

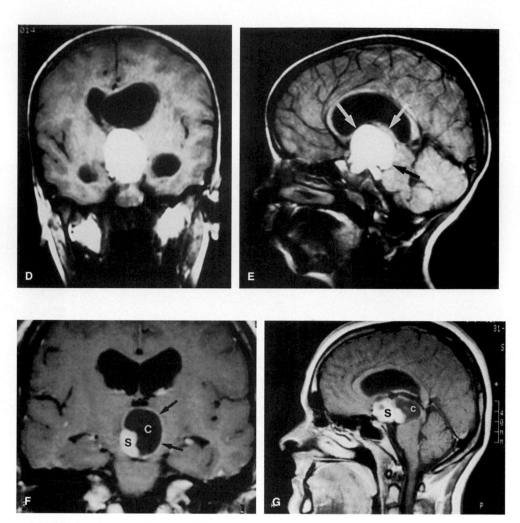

FIGURE 6.13-1.

(continued)

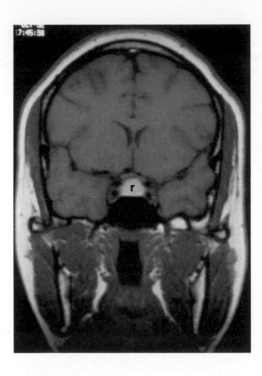

FIGURE 6.13-2.

Rathke cleft cyst. Coronal noncontrast magnetic resonance T1-weighted image shows hyperintense mass (r) in pituitary gland. There is slight upward bowing of the optic chiasm.

SUGGESTED READINGS

1. Voelker JL, Campbell RL, Muller J. Clinical, radiographic and pathological features of Rathke's cleft cysts. J Neurosurg 1991;74:535.
2. Ahmadi J, Destian S, Apuzzo MLJ, et al. Cystic fluid in craniopharyngiomas: MR imaging and quantitative analysis. Radiology 1992;182:783.

6.14 *Malformative Tumors: Teratomas*

EPIDEMIOLOGY

Teratomas account for 0.3% to 1.5% of all childhood intracranial tumors. They are more commonly seen in patients younger than 2 years of age, and perhaps are the most common brain tumor to be discovered in utero and during early neonatal life. They tend to be more common in boys.

CLINICAL FEATURES

Teratomas are more common in the sacrococcygeal area and relatively rare in the spinal cord (almost always associated with spina bifida) and brain. Intracranially, most occur in the pineal gland region. Other sites include the sella turcica, suprasellar region, and the fourth ventricle. Suprasellar teratomas are also more common in boys. Because most arise in the pineal region, the most common clinical presentation is that of hydrocephalus. Teratomas are the second most common pineal germ cell tumor (after germinomas), and account for 15% of all pineal region masses. Some teratomas secrete carcinoembryonic antigen.

Histologically, these tumors may be mature, immature, or malignant. Mature tumors are composed of well differentiated tissues deriving from all three germinal layers. Ectoderm includes skin and neural elements; mesoderm includes cartilage, bone, fat, fibrous tissues, and muscle; and endoderm includes respiratory and gastrointestinal epithelium, liver, pancreas, and salivary glands. Immature teratomas contain embryonic tissues and occur more often in the fourth ventricle. Immature teratomas with abundant embryonic undifferentiated tissues have a potential for rapid growth and metastases, and may be considered malignant. Also, immature malignant teratomas often contain primitive neuroectodermal elements. Malignant teratomas that contain regions of carcinoma, sarcoma, and other germ cell tumors are known as teratocarcinomas. Surgical resection is the treatment of choice for all teratomas. If they are benign, there is no need for chemotherapy or radiation therapy.

IMAGING FEATURES

The typical imaging findings are those of a heterogenous midline mass (Fig. 6.14-1). Computed tomography (CT) readily shows fat and calcium, which are typical. When a midline heterogenous tumor is initially found by magnetic resonance imaging, we then perform CT in an attempt to identify fat and calcifications. The solid components of these tumors show variable degrees of enhancement. Occasionally, teratomas are solid and homogenous. This finding implies less differentiation, and therefore these teratomas tend to be of the immature or malignant types. Epidermoid and dermoid cysts may be associated with teratomas. When epidermoids and dermoids are found in the pineal gland, teratoma should be suspected. Subarachnoid tumor seeding may occur. In one case, proton magnetic resonance spectroscopy showed only a large peak at 1.4 ppm, probably reflecting a high lipid concentration in the tumor.

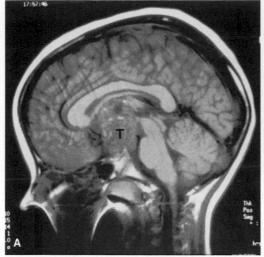
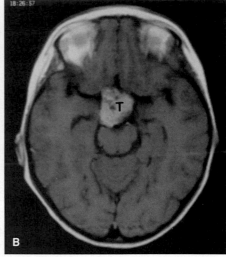
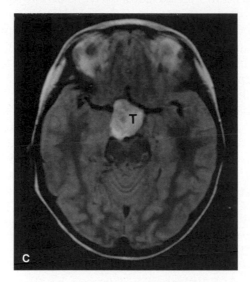

FIGURE 6.14-1.

Teratoma. **A.** Midsagittal noncontrast magnetic resonance (MR) T1-weighted image shows large suprasellar mass (T) with ill-defined borders. Note tumor inhomogeneity. **B.** After contrast administration, coronal MR T1-weighted image shows that most of the tumor (T) enhances. There are central punctate hypointensities. **C.** Axial MR proton density image shows the tumor (T) to be of high signal intensity.

SUGGESTED READINGS

1. Smirniotopoulos JG, Rushing EJ, Mena H. Pineal region masses: differential diagnosis. RadioGraphics 1992;12:577.
2. Tien RD, Barkovich AJ, Edwards MSB. MR imaging of pineal tumors. AJNR 1990; 11:557.
3. Raaijmakers C, Wilms G, Demaerel P, Baert AL. Pineal teratocarcinoma with drop metastases: MR features. Neuroradiology 1992;34:227.

6.15 *Malformative Tumors: Epidermoid and Dermoid*

EPIDEMIOLOGY

Together, these two tumors account for approximately 1.5% of all intracranial tumors. They occur most often in adults. There is no gender predilection for epidermoids, but dermoids are slightly more common in men. Most of these tumors occur in the posterior fossa; dermoids are also common in the spinal canal.

CLINICAL FEATURES

Most epidermoids are found in the cerebellopontine angle cistern. In that location, cranial nerve abnormalities tend to be the initial clinical presentation. Ten percent to 20% occur supratentorially (especially in the midline and the middle cranial fossae). In these cases, hydrocephalus may occur. A small percentage of epidermoids occur in the skull, particularly at sutures, but may be found elsewhere. Epidermoids arising in the brain stem and thalami have been described. All epidermoids are thought to originate from incomplete disjunction of the neuroectoderm from the cutaneous ectoderm at the time of neural tube closure. Histologically, these tumors are composed of a layer of stratified squamous epithelium and are filled with a white, flaky, and keratinous debris. Spillage of this material into the subarachnoid space produces a chemical meningitis.

Dermoids are always located in the midline. They are more often found in the pineal, parasellar, and frontobasal regions. Infratentorially, the fourth ventricle and vermis may be involved. Approximately 20% of all scalp lesions in children are dermoids. Scalp dermoids typically are located over the anterior fontanelle. Histologically, dermoids contain pilosebaceous units with hair shafts and sebaceous glands in addition to the elements found in epidermoids. They are filled with a cheesy, granular material. They spill into the cerebrospinal fluid spaces more commonly than do epidermoids, and produce a meningitis. Malignant degeneration of both types of tumors is known to occur, but is extremely rare. Surgical resection is the treatment of choice.

IMAGING FEATURES

Epidermoids have an appearance that is similar to cerebrospinal fluid (CSF) on both magnetic resonance (MR) imaging and computed tomography (CT) studies (Fig. 6.15-1A–C). They may simulate arachnoid cysts (especially in the cerebellopontine angle cistern). They do not enhance, and occasionally contain calcifications. At times, their surface may be "frond-like." Although they are of similar signal intensity to CSF by MR imaging, in our experience one can always identify intratumoral inhomogeneities (particularly on the T1 and proton density images) that suggest the diagnosis. Occasionally, epidermoids are bright on T1-weighted images and therefore indistinguishable from dermoids. Meningeal enhancement suggests rupture of the tumor. Skull epidermoids are expansile intradiploic masses with well margined and sclerotic borders. They are most commonly seen at sutures. They are commonly of high signal intensity on both T1- and T2-weighted images (Fig. 6.15-1D).

Dermoids have an identical appearance to fat by both CT and MR imaging (Fig. 6.15-2A). They occur in the midline. Fatty droplets or fat/CSF levels in the ventricles may be seen when tumors rupture (Fig. 6.15-2B). Meningeal enhancement also occurs if the dermoid ruptures. The frontal, nasal, and occipital regions should be clinically examined to exclude the presence of a dermal sinus. If a dermal sinus exists, these tumors may become infected. Enhancement is not present unless the dermoid has become infected. Scalp dermoids may occur anywhere but are typical over the anterior fontanelle (Fig. 6.15-2C, D). The may cause scalloping of the underlying outer table. They are solid masses filled with keratin, and are isointense or slightly hypointense on T1-weighted and hyperintense on T2-weighted images.

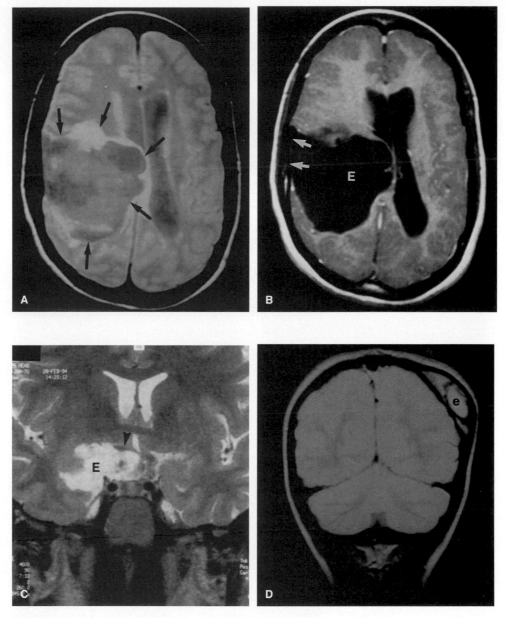

FIGURE 6.15-1.

Epidermoid. **A.** Axial proton density magnetic resonance (MR) image shows large epidermoid *(arrows)* in right temporoparietal region. Note that although the tumor is mainly of low signal intensity (similar to cerebrospinal fluid [CSF]), it contains areas of higher signal, suggesting that it is not a cyst. There is relatively little mass effect for the size of the lesion. **B.** Axial postcontrast MR T1-weighted image in the same patient shows that the epidermoid (E) does not enhance. Note that signal intensity of tumor is similar to that of CSF. The tumor has eroded *(arrows)* the skull. **C.** Coronal MR T2-weighted image in a different patient with partial complex seizures shows epidermoid (E) in the right medial temporal region extending into the suprasellar cistern and displacing the optic chiasm *(arrowhead)* upward. The tumor has the same signal intensity as CSF, but is inhomogeneous. **D.** Coronal proton density MR image shows epidermoid (e) in the left diploic space.

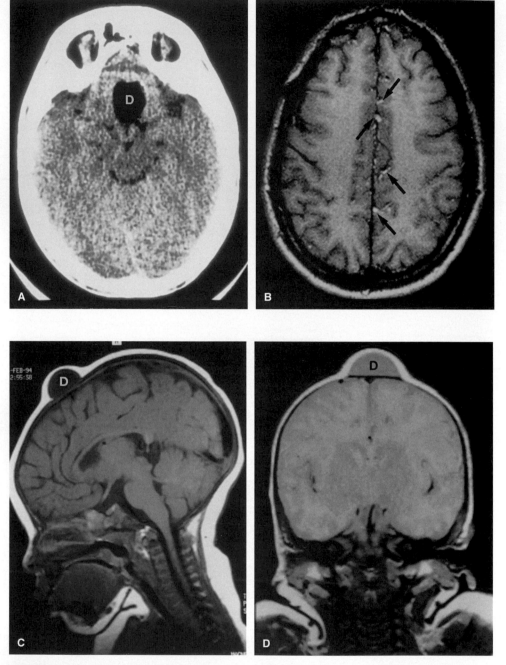

FIGURE 6.15-2.

Dermoid. **A.** Axial precontrast computed tomography (CT) shows midline frontobasal dermoid (D). Its density is that of fat. **B.** Axial precontrast MR T1-weighted image in the same patient shows deposits of fat *(arrows)* in several medial cortical sulci, indicating rupture of the tumor with spilling of its contents into the subarachnoid space. This patient had a history of meningitis. **C.** Midsagittal magnetic resonance (MR) T1-weighted image shows a hypointense dermoid (D) in the region of the bregma. The reason for the low signal intensity of this tumor is probably related to solid keratin content rather than liquid cholesterol, as found in other dermoids. **D.** Coronal MR proton density image in the same patient shows that the dermoid (D) is located under the subcutaneous fat and is of moderately high signal intensity.

SUGGESTED READINGS

1. Tampieri D, Melanson D, Ethier R. MR imaging of epidermoid cysts. AJNR 1989; 10:351.
2. Tatler GLV, Kendall BE. The radiological diagnosis of epidermoid tumors. Neuroradiology 1991;33(Suppl):324.
3. Smith AS. Myth of the mesoderm: ectodermal origin of dermoids. AJNR 1989;10: 449.
4. Smith AS, Benson JE, Blaser SI. Diagnosis of ruptured intracranial dermoid cyst: value of MR over CT. AJNR 1991;12:175.

6.16 Colloid Cyst and Tuber Cinereum Hamartoma

EPIDEMIOLOGY

These hamartomas occur in the portion (tuber cinereum) of the hypothalamus located between the mammillary bodies and the infundibulum. They are rare. Boys are affected more often than girls. The diagnosis is commonly made during the first 4 years of life.

Colloid cysts represent less than 1% of all intracranial tumors. These tumors are mostly found in adults. There is no gender predilection.

CLINICAL FEATURES

Commonly, tuber cinereum hamartomas produce isosexual precocious puberty. The onset of symptoms usually occurs during the first 2 years of life. Diagnosis is made shortly thereafter. The second most common presentation is that of gelastic (laughing) seizures, which are a type of partial complex seizures. Other, less common symptoms are developmental delay, intellectual impairment, psychiatric disorders, and hyperactivity. These masses are composed of heterotopic and hyperplastic tissues containing large and small neurons, astrocytes, and oligodendrocytes. The cause of precocious puberty is uncertain, but it may be related to compression of the hypothalamus with premature activation of its pathways, or to independent secretion of gonadotropin-releasing hormone by the mass. The treatment of choice is pharmacologic manipulation. Long-term infusion of gonadotropin-releasing hormone may inhibit gonadotropic secretion. Antigonadotropic and antiandrogenic agents are of questionable effectiveness. In some cases of pedunculated tumors, surgery may be effective. However, precocious puberty and excessive growth may continue after tumor removal. If hydrocephalus is present, shunting is indicated.

Colloid cysts occur almost exclusively in the roof of the third ventricle between the forniceal columns. However, they have been reported to occur in the posterior fossa and intrasellar space. They obstruct the foramina of Monroe, producing acute hydrocephalus. The obstruction may be episodic, and some patients complain of headaches on wakening up that resolve with standing up. Acute ventricular obstruction may lead to herniation and death. Pathologically, they are often attached to the choroid plexus, and their capsule is composed of a single layer of pseudostratified columnar cells that may be ciliated. Mucin fills these cysts and, if spilled, it may induce a chemical ventriculitis. Although surgical resection results in complete cure, often these patients show some memory deficits. Stereotactic drainage may be attempted but may not be possible in some cysts because of the tenacious nature of their fluid. The cysts may also recur after drainage. A third option is that of shunting both lateral ventricles.

IMAGING FEATURES

The typical appearance of tuber cinereum hamartomas is easily seen on magnetic resonance (MR) sagittal images. The mass hangs from a stalk (Fig. 6.16-1A). It is rounded and isointense with brain on T1-weighted images, and at times it may be large (Fig. 6.16-1B). They may be slightly hyperintense on T2-weighted images (Fig. 6.16-1C). These hamartomas do not enhance after contrast administration and do not contain calcifications (Fig. 6.16-1D). Occasionally, tuber cinereum hamartomas have cystic components, which may be prominent. The differential diagnosis includes low-grade astrocytoma or a tumor of neuronal origin. In our experience, MR spectroscopy shows a pattern remarkably similar to that seen in normal brain.

Colloid cysts have a typical imaging appearance. On computed tomography, most are hyperdense, well margined masses that may occasionally show peripheral enhancement (Fig. 6.16-2A). However, they may also be hypodense. By MR imaging, most are hyperintense to brain on T1-weighted images and of low signal intensity on T2-weighted images (Fig. 6.16-2B, C). This appearance may be caused by proteins and less likely by the presence of paramagnetic ions within the cyst.

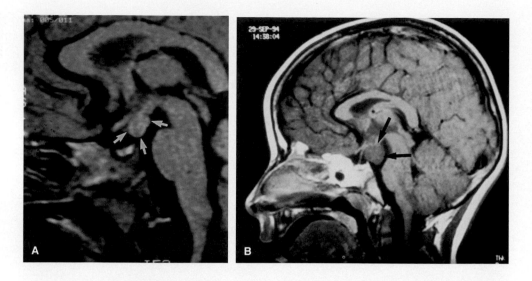

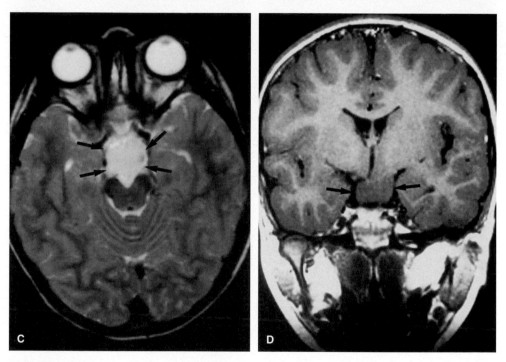

FIGURE 6.16-1.

Tuber cinereum hamartoma. **A.** Midsagittal noncontrast magnetic resonance (MR) T1-weighted image shows pedunculated tuber cinereum hamartoma *(arrows)* of similar signal intensity to gray matter. **B.** Midsagittal noncontrast MR T1-weighted image in an 8-year-old boy with precocious puberty shows a rounded, somewhat pedunculated mass *(arrows)* located anterior to the mamillary bodies and posterior to the infundibulum (region of the tuber cinereum). The mass is slightly hypointense to brain. **C.** Axial MR T2-weighted image in the same patient shows the suprasellar mass *(arrows)* to be hyperintense. **D.** Coronal postcontrast MR T1-weighted image in the same patient shows no enhancement in the mass *(arrows)*. Proton MR spectroscopy of the lesion (not shown) demonstrated minimally decreased *N*-acetyl aspartate and normal choline and creatinine.

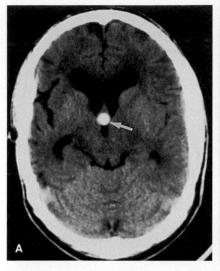

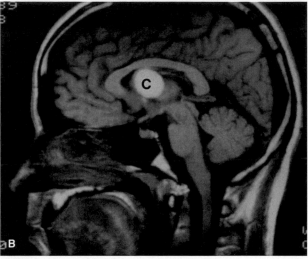

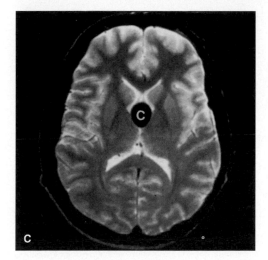

FIGURE 6.16-2.

Colloid cyst. **A.** Axial noncontrast computed tomography shows a well defined, rounded, hyperdense mass *(arrow)* in the anterosuperior third ventricle, producing dilation of the lateral ventricles. **B.** Midsagittal noncontrast magnetic resonance (MR) T1-weighted image shows a bright colloid cyst (C) in a different patient. (With permission from Castillo M. Neuroradiology Companion. Philadelphia: JB Lippincott, 1995.) **C.** Axial MR T2-weighted image in a different patient shows a colloid cyst (C) appearing as an area of signal void.

SUGGESTED READINGS

1. Boyko OB, Curnes JT, Oakes WJ, et al. Hamartomas of the tuber cinereum: CT, MR, and pathologic findings. AJNR 1991;12:309.
2. Wilms G, Marchal G, Van Hecke P, et al. Colloid cysts of the third ventricle: MR findings. J Comput Assist Tomogr 1990;14:527.

Imaging of the Pediatric Head, Neck, and Spine
by Mauricio Castillo and Suresh K. Mukherji,
Lippincott-Raven Publishing, Philadelphia © 1996.

7

Trauma

7.0 Extracerebral: Cephalhematoma, Subgaleal Hematoma, and Caput Succedaneum

EPIDEMIOLOGY

Cephalhematomas are collections of blood under the periosteum of the skull. They occur during birth (seen in 1% of all births) or secondary to other head trauma. An underlying fracture is present in 5% to 20% of cases. In our experience, brain injury is not uncommon in this group of infants. Blood collections under the galea aponeurotica are called subgaleal hematomas. Caput succedaneum refers to a mixture of edema and blood in the subcutaneous tissues. It is commonly seen after uncomplicated vaginal delivery or vacuum extraction.

CLINICAL FEATURES

Cephalhematomas are tense, focal, collections that do not cross sutures because they are delimited by their insertions. Transillumination of the skull is decreased. No treatment is required.

Contrary to cephalhematomas, subgaleal hematomas are diffuse and freely movable. Transillumination of the skull is decreased. Both of these types of hematoma may cause a mild hyperbilirubinemia as they break down. Chronically, they may calcify and result in minor cosmetic defects. Both cephalhematomas and subgaleal hematomas may increase slightly in size during the first few days of life.

Caput succedanea are diffuse, soft, mobile areas of scalp swelling that cross suture lines. Transillumination of the skull is increased. They resolve completely.

We have observed a fourth type of hematoma associated with vacuum extraction or forceps delivery. Its clinical appearance is identical to that of a cephalhematoma. During surgery, however, a well organized hematoma is found in the diploic space. We believe that some of the clinically diagnosed "calcified cephalhematomas" may actually belong to this latter group, which we call "intradiploic" hematomas.

IMAGING FEATURES

In general, there is no indication for imaging patients with these superficial hematomas. Exceptions in the acute period include those patients with suspected brain injury (neurologically symptomatic) or skull fractures (Fig. 7.0-1). In the case of fractures, plain films of the skull usually suffice. When brain injury is suspected, we prefer magnetic resonance imaging. Diffuse and extensive scalp hematomas may occur in the presence of systemic coagulopathies (Fig. 7.0-2). These hematomas often involve many compartments.

Another indication for imaging is a chronically calcified hematoma that results in a cosmetic defect for which the parents/guardians desire correction. In these cases, computed tomography is the imaging method of choice. Calcified cephalhematomas appear as elliptical areas of high density that are separable from or adherent to the outer table. They may produce scalloping of the outer table. Intradiploic hematomas appear as soft tissue masses separating the outer table from the inner table (Fig. 7.0-3). No bone erosion is present.

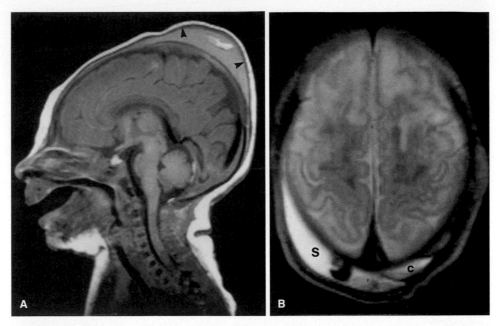

FIGURE 7.0-1.

Subgaleal hematoma. **A.** Midsagittal magnetic resonance (MR) T1-weighted image in a 2-day-old infant with decreased spontaneous movements. Patient was born with vacuum extraction. There is a fluid collection under the galea aponeurotica *(arrowheads)* and superficial to the outer table of the skull. This subgaleal hematoma is mostly hyperintense and contains a well defined hyperintense clot. Note large extension of abnormality crossing sutures. A small subacute clot is also present in the posterior fossa dorsal to the cerebellar vermis. The pituitary is bright, a normal finding in newborns. **B.** Axial MR T2-weighted image in a child with apnea after vacuum delivery shows a subgaleal hematoma(s) in the right parietal region crossing the midline posteriorly. There is also a small cephalhematoma (c) in the posterior left parietal region limited to the posterior midline by the periosteum anchoring in the sagittal suture. Edema in the white matter of both frontal lobes is present.

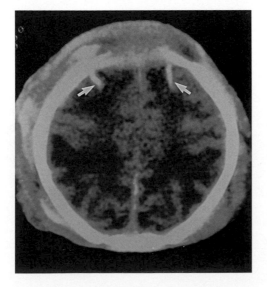

FIGURE 7.0-2.

Diffuse scalp hematomas. Axial computed tomography in a patient born with an idiopathic isoimmune thrombocytopenia shows diffuse hemorrhages probably involving all subcutaneous compartments of the scalp. The two linear hyperdensities *(arrows)* in the frontal lobes may represent shears or thrombosed veins.

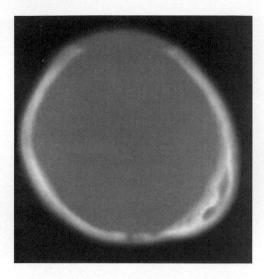

FIGURE 7.0-3.

Calcified hematoma versus intradiploic hematoma. Axial computed tomography, bone windows, shows thickening of skull in the left parietal region, which contains a central lucency. At surgery, a clot was found between the outer and inner tables of the skull (intradiploic hematoma).

SUGGESTED READING

1. Castillo M, Smith JK. Imaging features of acute head and spine injuries secondary to difficult deliveries. Emergency Radiology 1995;2:7.

7.01 *Extracerebral: Skull Fractures*

EPIDEMIOLOGY
Skull fractures are common in children and occur in 2% to 26% of head trauma cases. They occur more commonly before 2 years of age. Over 75% of skull fractures in children are of the linear type. Other types of fractures involving the calvarium include depressed and compound (open) fractures. Diastatic fractures are traumatic separations of sutures seen in the first 4 years of life. Base-of-skull fractures are very rare in children and are of two types, petrous and frontobasal.

CLINICAL FEATURES
Although most fractures are accidental, child abuse should not be overlooked. Many fractures are isolated and, as such, no treatment is needed. Depressed fractures are characterized by inward displacement of bone of 5 mm or more. Brain injury is not uncommonly associated, and these fractures need surgical elevation. Surgery, however, does not decrease the rate of posttraumatic seizures. Compound fractures are accompanied by scalp lacerations. A fully immunized child with a clean laceration, who has had a tetanus booster within the past 10 years, needs no tetanus toxoid or human tetanus immune globulin.

Diastatic fractures usually involve the lambdoid suture. In children younger than 3 years of age, they may become so-called "growing" fractures. Growing fractures are uncommon complications of linear or diastatic fractures seen in 0.6% of all skull fractures. The fracture grows because of herniation of the brain (posttraumatic cephalocele), porencephalic cyst, or a leptomeningeal cyst. Surgical repair of these fractures is indicated.

Base-of-skull fractures produce hemorrhage in the nose, nasopharynx, middle ears, mastoids (Battle sign), and eyes ("raccoon" sign). Cranial nerve deficits may be present. Cerebrospinal fluid (CSF) rhinorrhea or otorrhea may occur. There is an increased risk of meningitis, which is usually caused by *Streptococcus pneumoniae*.

IMAGING FEATURES
Skull fractures themselves are not an indication for imaging except when neurologic symptoms are present (suspicion of brain injury), cosmetic defects are present, or child abuse is suspected and their presence needs to be documented for legal purposes. In the latter situation, plain films are needed because computed tomography (CT) may miss occasional fractures oriented parallel to the plane of imaging that may be partially averaged, making their visualization impossible. We believe that if an unsuspected fracture is found on plain films, then CT is indicated to evaluate the brain parenchyma. Depressed and compound fractures are easily seen on CT, and on plain films appear as overlapping densities (Fig. 7.01-1A). Fractures should not be confused with sutures (Fig. 7.01-1B). Fractures have sharp, nonsclerotic borders and do not follow the expected course of the sutures (in some cases they cross them, and this readily establishes the correct diagnosis). Patent parietal foramina may vary in size and also should not be confused with depressed fractures or lytic lesions (Fig. 7.01-2). Base-of-skull fractures usually are oriented toward the foramen magnum. If such a type of fracture is clinically suspected, thin-section (1–1.5 mm), high-resolution CT imaging should be obtained. The evaluation of CSF leakage may require introduction of iodinated contrast into the subarachnoid space.

In the past, all children with linear or diastatic fractures had a follow-up radiograph of the skull to exclude the possibility of a "growing" fracture. This complication is so uncommon that obtaining follow-up radiographs in these children is no longer justified unless there is a strong clinical suspicion. If a leptomeningeal cyst is suspected, we usually recommend CT (Fig. 7.01-3A). Leptomeningeal cysts may also be seen by magnetic resonance (MR) imaging (Fig. 7.01-3B).

Skull fractures heal by fibrous union and therefore may remain lucent on radiographs for many months. The presence of stellate or multiple skull fractures is always suspicious for child abuse.

Uncommon acute complications of fractures include extrusion of brain through the fracture site (posttraumatic encephalocele) and injury to the superficial venous sinuses (Figs. 7.01-4 and 7.01-5). In both instances, we prefer MR imaging to CT. In the former, the macerated and extruded brain necessitates resection, and MR imaging allows for detailed evaluation of the intracranial structures. In the latter situation, MR imaging and MR venography may help establish patency of a venous sinus. Tears in a sinus may be present, and are almost always accompanied by thrombosis (Fig. 7.01-6).

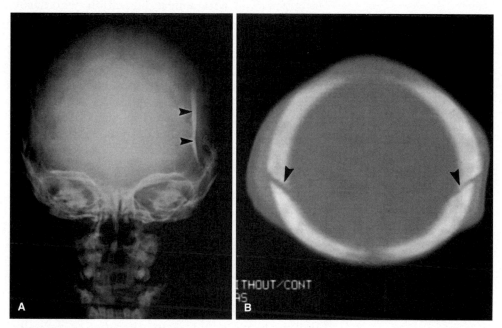

FIGURE 7.01-1.

Skull fractures. **A.** Frontal radiograph shows a left temporal depressed fracture *(arrowheads).* **B.** Axial computed tomography, bone windows, shows bilateral parietal symmetric fractures *(arrowheads)* that are slightly displaced. These fractures should not be confused with normal sutures. Note sharply defined margins and lack of sclerosis, which is commonly present in sutures.

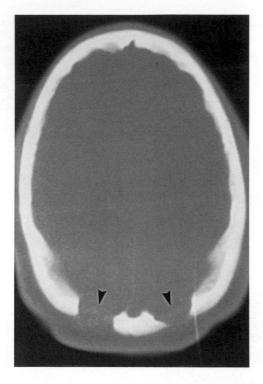

FIGURE 7.01-2.

Patent parietal foramina. Axial computed tomography, bone windows, shows bilateral lucent defects *(arrowheads)*. These should not be confused with depressed fractures or destructive lesions. A clue for the correct diagnosis is their paramedian parietal location.

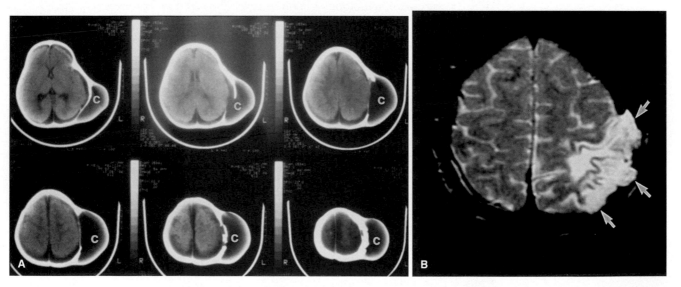

FIGURE 7.01-3.

Postfracture leptomeningeal cysts. **A.** Axial computed tomography sequence in a patient with a cerebrospinal fluid cyst (c) herniating through a gapping fracture in the left posterior parietal region. **B.** Axial magnetic resonance T2-weighted image in a different patient with postfracture leptomeningeal cysts *(arrows)*. There is malacia in the brain underlying the fracture site.

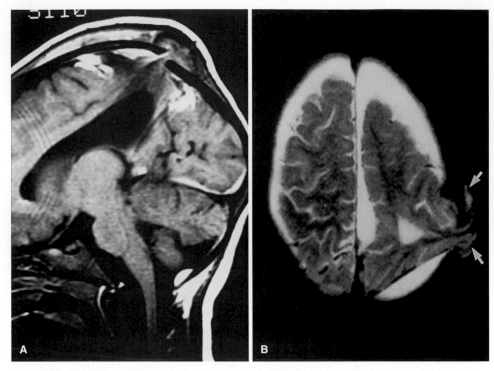

FIGURE 7.01-4.

Skull fractures and posttraumatic encephalocele. **A.** Parasagittal magnetic resonance (MR) T1-weighted image shows parietal skull fracture with hemorrhagic brain extruding through it. **B.** Axial MR T2-weighted image in a different case of displaced left parietal fracture with herniation of brain *(arrows)* through the fracture.

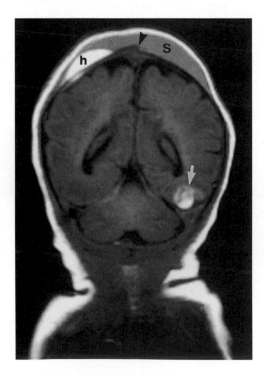

FIGURE 7.01-5.

Fracture with thrombosis of the superior sagittal sinus. Coronal magnetic resonance T1-weighted image in a different case shows a displaced fracture *(arrowhead)* in the convexity, with absent flow void (indicating thrombosis) in the superior sagittal sinus. There is a subgaleal hematoma (s) and a small right parietal subperiosteal hematoma (h). A hemorrhagic contusion *(arrow)* is present in the left temporooccipital region.

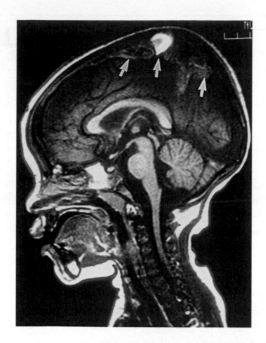

FIGURE 7.01-6.

Fracture with tearing of the superior sagittal sinus. Midsagittal magnetic resonance T1-weighted image in a case of displaced fracture through the parietal convexity that has torn the superior sagittal sinus, which subsequently thrombosed. Note that it is filled with bright clot *(arrows)*.

SUGGESTED READING

1. Harwood-Nash DC. Abuse to the pediatric central nervous system. AJNR 1992;13: 569.

7.02 *Extracerebral: Subdural, Epidural, and Intradural Hematomas*

EPIDEMIOLOGY

The incidence of subdural and epidural hematomas in accidental childhood trauma is unknown. It is known, however, that subdural hematomas are 5 to 10 times more common than epidural hematomas. Subdural hematomas are seen in up to 65% of abused children. Intradural hematomas are unusual, and seen after birth assisted with vacuum extraction or forceps.

CLINICAL FEATURES

Subdural hematomas are collections of blood between the arachnoid and the dura. Subdural hematomas are usually seen in children younger than 2 years of age. Underlying fractures are detected in 30% of patients. They originate from rupture of the veins bridging the subdural space. They are commonly located in the frontoparietal region but may occur anywhere, including the posterior fossa. Subdural hematomas in children are bilateral in up to 75% of patients. Bilateral hematomas, hematomas along the falx cerebri, and hematomas in different stages of evolution are commonly seen in child abuse. Approximately 75% of patients experience postinjury seizures because the incidence of trauma to the brain parenchyma is higher than with epidural hematomas. Also, morbidity and mortality are higher with subdural than with epidural hematomas. Surgical evacuation is the treatment of choice, unless the lesion is small in size, in which case it may be observed with the hope of spontaneous resolution.

Epidural hematomas occur less commonly than subdural hematomas in the supratentorial compartment. However, in the posterior fossa, they are two to three times more common than subdural collections. Epidural hematomas are usually seen in children older than 2 years of age. Fractures are identified in 70% to 90% of cases (less than in adults). The origin of these hematomas is commonly a ruptured venous sinus and not laceration of the middle meningeal artery, as it tends to be in adults. They are commonly unilateral and are located in the temporoparietal regions. Surgical evacuation is the treatment of choice.

Intradural hematomas occur when the leaves of the tentorium are sheared apart from each other as a result of excessive vertical forces, such as produced by vacuum extraction or forceps deliveries. Although they tend to produce mass effect, this is relatively minor, and in our experience most cases do not require surgical decompression.

IMAGING FEATURES

As in adults, computed tomography (CT) is the ideal method for the evaluation of patients suspected of having extraaxial blood collections. Indeed, CT is the imaging method of choice when an acute extraaxial hematoma is suspected. Magnetic resonance (MR) imaging is useful in dating these hemorrhages and in detecting smaller ones not visible by CT (Fig. 7.02-1A). MR imaging is especially helpful in dating these hematomas in cases of child abuse (Fig. 7.02-1B). Subdural hematomas are curvilinear or crescentic in shape and of high density acutely by CT (Fig. 7.02-1C,D). Up to 40% of acute subdural hematomas contain areas of both high and low density. At approximately 2 weeks of age, subdural hematomas become isodense with the brain. Secondary signs, which include mass effect and inward buckling of the gray–white junction, are present. Contrast enhancement may be useful to outline the membrane delimiting the inner surface of these collections. Chronic subdural hematomas have a density equal to cerebrospinal fluid and therefore are indistinguishable by CT from widened subarachnoid spaces. In these cases, MR imaging helps differentiate them from each other.

In epidural hematomas, CT is the imaging modality of choice. These biconvex or lenticular collections have a typical appearance (Fig. 7.02-2). Epidural hematomas with components on either side of the tentorium should suggest laceration of the transverse sinuses.

Intradural hematomas occur simultaneously with other birth-related central nervous system injuries. We prefer to evaluate neurologically symptomatic newborns with MR imaging because it permits identification of extraaxial blood collections, parenchymal injuries, and venous thromboses. Intradural hematomas are typically seen splaying the tentorium (Fig. 7.02-3). They have a biconvex shape in sagittal and coronal images.

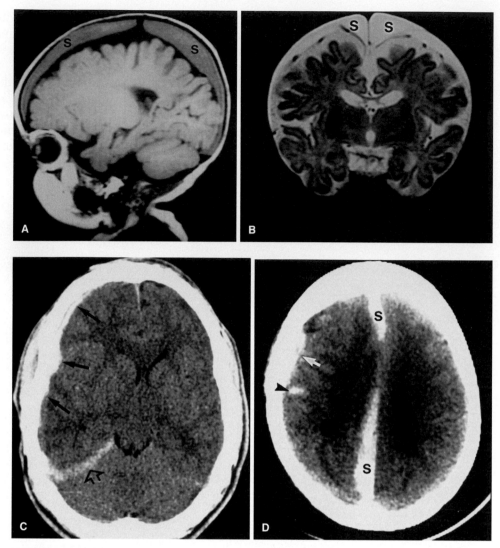

FIGURE 7.02-1.

Subdural hematoma. **A.** Parasagittal magnetic resonance (MR) T1-weighted image in an abused child shows a subacute and slightly hyperintense subdural hematoma (S). Note low signal intensity from normal cerebrospinal fluid (CSF) in subarachnoid space between subdural hematoma and surface of brain. **B.** Coronal MR T2-weighted image shows bilateral hemispheric chronic subdural hematomas (S) in this abused child. There is underlying thickening of the dura and cerebral atrophy with widening of the CSF spaces. **C.** Axial noncontrast computed tomography (CT) in an adolescent after a motor vehicle accident shows a right hemispheric acute subdural hematoma *(arrows)* with midline shift to the left. There is blood *(open arrow)* layering on the right tentorium. This blood could be subarachnoid or subdural in location. **D.** Axial CT shows a right parafalcine subdural hematoma (S), a small right frontal extraaxial hematoma *(arrow)*, and a hemorrhagic shearing injury *(arrowhead)* in the right frontal region.

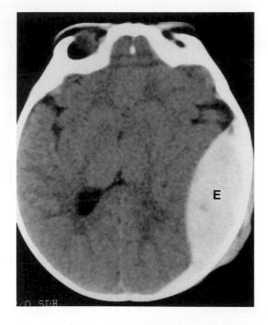

FIGURE 7.02-2.

Epidural hematoma. Axial computed tomography shows acute left temporooccipital epidural hematoma (E) with compression of the atrium of the left lateral ventricle.

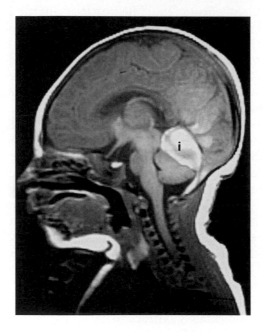

FIGURE 7.02-3.

Intradural hematoma. Midsagittal magnetic resonance T1-weighted image in a patient delivered by vacuum extraction 2 days previously. There is a subacute bright (methemoglobin) hematoma (i) confined by the leaves of the tentorium. There is a mass effect on the superior vermis and mild compression of the fourth ventricle, but no hydrocephalus. A small posterior fossa subdural hematoma is present. The hyperintensity in the occipital region was caused by a posterior falcine subdural hematoma. The bright pituitary gland is a normal finding in newborns.

SUGGESTED
READINGS

1. Zimmerman RA, Bilaniuk LT. Pediatric head trauma. Neuroimaging Clinics of North America 1994;4:349.
2. Castillo M, Fordham LA. MR of neurologically symptomatic newborns after vacuum extraction delivery. AJNR 1995;16:816.

7.03 *Extracerebral: Subarachnoid Hemorrhage and Superficial Siderosis*

EPIDEMIOLOGY

Subarachnoid hemorrhage is usually posttraumatic in children. Subarachnoid hemorrhage secondary to ruptured aneurysms or arteriovenous malformations is uncommon in pediatric patients. Between 25% to 75% of abused children have subarachnoid hemorrhage.

CLINICAL FEATURES

As noted, subarachnoid hemorrhage secondary to ruptured aneurysms is uncommon. When it occurs, it has a sudden onset with acute headaches, meningismus, altered consciousness, and coma. Aneurysms are rare in children younger than 10 years of age. Before 2 years of age, aneurysms are usually larger than 1 cm in diameter and are commonly located in the anterior communicating or internal carotid arteries (see section 5.09).

Subarachnoid hemorrhage associated with trauma is usually accompanied by intraparenchymal lesions. Subarachnoid hemorrhage secondary to trauma rarely induces vasospasm. Communicating hydrocephalus is a chronic sequela of this type of bleed.

IMAGING FEATURES

The diagnosis of subarachnoid hemorrhage should be made based on cerebrospinal fluid analysis. However, computed tomography (CT) is usually obtained in these children before lumbar puncture to exclude other causes of increased intracranial pressure. The reason for this is that funduscopic abnormalities (blurring of the optic disc margins) require some time to develop and may not be present acutely. CT detects more than 90% of all subarachnoid hemorrhages during the initial 24 hours. After 3 days, less than 50% of subarachnoid hemorrhages are visible on CT. On CT images, acute subarachnoid blood appears as high density in the basilar cisterns, along the surface of the tentorium and falx, and outlining the posterior aspects of the superior sagittal sinus (Fig. 7.03-1). Reflux into the ventricles is not unusual. Focal subarachnoid hematomas in the cisterns may suggest the site of an aneurysm. For example, hematomas along the anterior interhemispheric fissure, septum pellucidum, and frontal horns of the lateral ventricles suggest a ruptured aneurysm in the anterior communicating artery region. Hematoma in the Sylvian fissure suggests a ruptured aneurysm in the bifurcation of the middle cerebral artery. High density along the falx cerebri may be the only sign of subarachnoid hemorrhage. Acute subarachnoid hemorrhage is difficult to visualize by magnetic resonance (MR) imaging, and therefore the use of this modality is not indicated. Contrary to this view, some authors have reported a greater sensitivity of MR imaging in the detection of subarachnoid hemorrhage compared to CT. We do not subscribe to this point of view, and believe that CT is a better method. However, we have seen a patient in whom acute and fairly massive subarachnoid hemorrhage developed during imaging in the MR unit. In this patient, the blood was fairly obvious and bright on T1-weighted images. MR imaging using fluid attenuation inversion recovery sequences may be helpful to detect subarachnoid blood. MR imaging, however, is the only technique that detects so-called "superficial siderosis." This term refers to the deposition of hemosiderin on the pia secondary to repeated subarachnoid hemorrhages. It is seen as very low signal intensity along the surface of the brain, especially on T2-weighted images (Fig. 7.03-2). We have seen superficial siderosis in cases of child abuse presumably secondary to repeated shaking, resulting in subarachnoid hemorrhages. Superficial siderosis may also be secondary to "sentinel" bleeds from aneurysms, occult vascular malformations, and unknown tumor (particularly ependymomas of the spinal cord). A single episode of subarachnoid hemorrhage does not result in superficial siderosis. If no cause is found by clinical history or MR imaging of the brain, patients with superficial siderosis may require MR imaging of the entire spine.

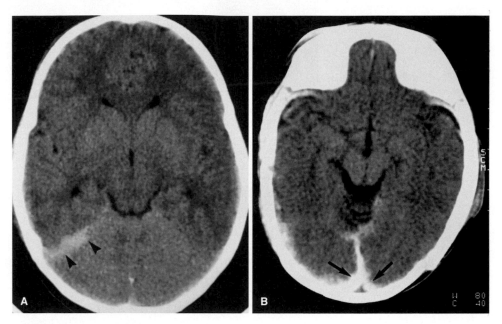

FIGURE 7.03-1.

Subarachnoid hemorrhage. **A.** Axial noncontrast computed tomography (CT) shows asymmetric hyperdensity *(arrowheads)* in the region of the right tentorium. The finding in this case is related to subarachnoid hemorrhage after nonintentional trauma. **B.** Axial noncontrast CT after trauma shows hyperdense blood *(arrows)* layering along margins of the posterior aspect of the superior sagittal sinus and along the posterior falx cerebri (pseudodelta sign).

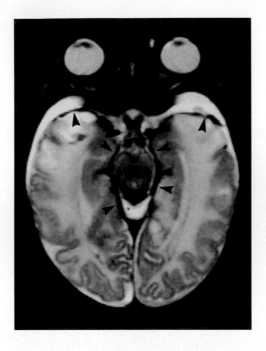

FIGURE 7.03-2.

Pial siderosis. Axial magnetic resonance T2-weighted image in a child with a history of chronic abuse shows very dark signal intensity *(arrowheads)* in the surface of the anterior and medial temporal lobes, pons, and in the occipital lobes. The finding is related to superficial (pial) siderosis occurring as a result of repeated subarachnoid bleeds. The white matter is abnormally hyperintense.

SUGGESTED READING

1. Sato Y, Smith WL. Head injury in child abuse. Neuroimaging Clinics of North America 1991;1:475.

7.04 Intracerebral: Shears, Contusions, and Edema

EPIDEMIOLOGY

Shearing injuries are axonal tears secondary to excessive acceleration–deceleration and rotational forces. They are more common than contusions, in which the brain is directly (coup) or indirectly (contrecoup) injured by compression by adjacent bone. Contusions in patients younger than 5 years of age are large white matter injuries accompanied by microscopic tears in the cortex. Diffuse brain edema usually accompanies child abuse and may also be related to strangulation and suffocation.

CLINICAL FEATURES

The clinical presentation of brain shears is that of diffuse axonal injury syndrome. The patients are devastated, often in a vegetative state despite relative absence of abnormalities in computed tomography (CT) scans. Lumbar puncture demonstrates blood, but usually is not indicated in the management of head injury except in those patients with secondary meningitis. Posttraumatic seizures are more common with shears than with contusions. Approximately 5% of patients with head injuries show seizures within 1 week of the accident. Posttraumatic seizures are more common in the youngest patients. Approximately 60% to 70% of these patients will have more than one seizure, and 20% to 30% will experience permanent seizures. Late posttraumatic epilepsy is characterized by the development of seizures within 1 year of the injury. It occurs in up to 5% of all children who suffer head trauma. The clinical presentation of contusions is less severe because they tend to involve regions of the brain that are relatively "silent," such as the basal portion of the frontal lobes. Complications are similar to those described for shearing injuries.

Diffuse brain edema in child abuse is secondary to contusions, white matter shears, interruption of venous drainage, or interruption of arterial supply with hypoxia. Loss of consciousness with seizures and respiratory arrest may occur.

IMAGING FEATURES

Most shearing injuries are nonhemorrhagic and therefore not clearly seen by CT. Shearing lesions containing only edema are better seen on magnetic resonance T2-weighted images. Shears tend to involve the gray–white matter interfaces. The lesions are usually ovoid or rounded. They are seen in the splenium of the corpus callosum, the peripheral gray–white junctions, the dorsolateral aspect of the midbrain, and the basal ganglia (Fig. 7.04-1). Intraventricular hemorrhage may be present secondary to shearing of the subependymal veins or the choroid plexus. Contusions tend to be hemorrhagic and are commonly located in the inferior surface of the frontal lobes and the anterior portion of the temporal lobes. On early follow-up studies, both types of injuries appear slightly larger than they initially did. Both types of injuries may be seen with child abuse; however, large linear white matter shears should raise high suspicion for nonaccidental trauma (Fig. 7.04-2). Severe brain atrophy may be present on long-term follow-up studies.

Brain swelling is well seen by CT. CT findings may, however, take 24 to 48 hours to develop. The edematous brain is of low density and there is effacement of the gray–white interfaces. The deep gray matter may be hypodense or occasionally hyperdense. The cortical sulci and basilar cisterns may be obliterated.

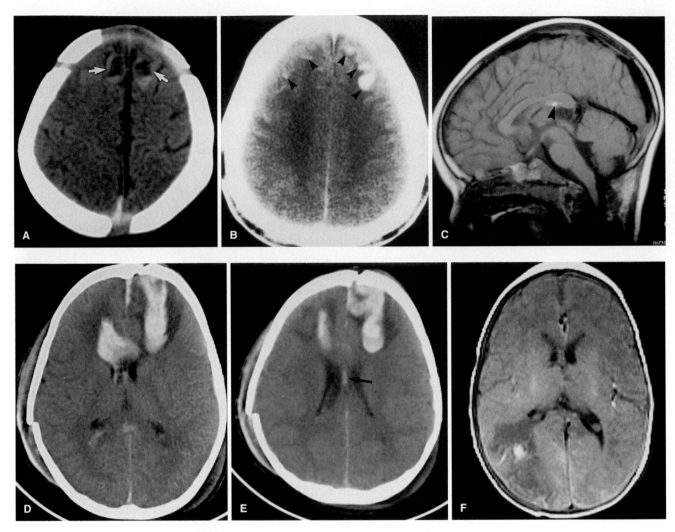

FIGURE 7.04-1.

Shearing injuries.   **A.** Axial computed tomography (CT) shows left frontal hemorrhagic shears *(arrows)* and small extraaxial hematoma in this abused child. Note blood levels within the lesions. **B.** Axial CT shows multiple bilateral hemorrhagic shearing injuries *(arrowheads)* at the gray–white junctions. **C.** Midsagittal magnetic resonance (MR) T1-weighted image after motor vehicle accident shows enlargement (edema) of the splenium of the corpus callosum and small hemorrhage due to shearing injury *(arrowhead)*. Incidental pineal cyst is present. **D.** Axial CT shows large hemorrhagic contusion in the left frontal lobe and genu of the corpus callosum. There is questionable hemorrhage in the splenium of the corpus callosum and atrium of the right lateral ventricle. Note left frontal and right temporal skull fractures. **E.** Axial CT in same patient shows hemorrhage *(arrow)* in body of corpus callosum. **F.** Axial MR T1-weighted image shows hemorrhagic lesion (shear?) in right occipital region with surrounding hyperintensity related to edema in this case of child abuse. Note mass effect on the atrium of the right lateral ventricle.

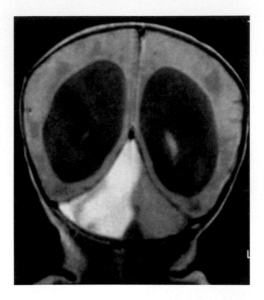

FIGURE 7.04-2.

Shearing injury versus hemorrhagic infarction. Coronal magnetic resonance T1-weighted image shows subacute hemorrhage involving the right cerebellar hemisphere in an infant born with vacuum extraction assistance. The hemorrhage may be related to shearing of the draining veins with subsequent intraparenchymal hemorrhage. Also seen is a small, right-sided subdural hematoma. The aqueduct of Sylvius was compressed, resulting in massive hydrocephalus.

SUGGESTED READING

1. Bird CR, McMahan JR, Gilles FH, et al. Strangulation in child abuse: CT diagnosis. Radiology 1987;163:373.

8

Inflammation and Infection

Imaging of the Pediatric Head, Neck, and Spine
by Mauricio Castillo and Suresh K. Mukherji,
Lippincott-Raven Publishing, Philadelphia © 1996.

8.0 *Multiple Sclerosis and Its Variants*

EPIDEMIOLOGY

Only 2% of patients with multiple sclerosis present during childhood, more often between 10 to 15 years of age. Multiple sclerosis before 5 years of age is very rare. Although there is no clear genetic factor implicated, multiple sclerosis is more common among family members, especially siblings. Its incidence is high in monozygotic twins.

CLINICAL FEATURES

Multiple sclerosis is clinically characterized by remissions and exacerbations. Over 50% of patients have this type of history at presentation. Occasionally, the patients present with an atypical course characterized by continued progression of symptoms, most commonly paraplegia. In some cases, death occurs within months of presentation. Weakness and coordination problems are common initial symptoms. The second most common presentation is that of visual problems, which include blurred vision, partial blindness, and diplopia. Approximately 20% of children with multiple sclerosis complain of headaches. The combination of optic neuritis and transverse myelitis is termed "Devic disease." This term is based on the clinical presentation rather than imaging features. Schilder disease is characterized by a monophasic, continuous presentation. In this disorder, there is demyelination with axonal damage; it may be confused with adrenoleukodystrophy. Balo concentric sclerosis is a rare acute variant of multiple sclerosis occurring in children and young adults. It is characterized by concentric areas of demyelination alternating with lamellae of preserved white matter. There is little associated inflammation. This disease has a rapid course and is fatal.

In multiple sclerosis pathologically there is demyelination with axonal sparing and a mononuclear infiltrate. Cerebrospinal fluid analysis shows increased immunoglobulin G, increased protein, or mild mononuclear pleocytosis.

There is no definite treatment. Corticosteroids diminish the severity of the acute episodes but do not alter the outcome. Azathioprine and other immunosuppressants may alter the duration of acute episodes and halt the clinical progression of the disease. Children may have an especially fast course, with death being the result of pulmonary complications (ie, pneumonia).

IMAGING FEATURES

Magnetic resonance is the imaging modality of choice (Fig. 8.0-1). On T2-weighted images, all lesions are bright. On T1-weighted images, the lesions are slightly hypointense and may have a rim of slight hyperintensity. Lesions that are active enhance after contrast administration. Periventricular lesions have an ovoid configuration, with their long axis perpendicular to the axis of the lateral ventricles (so-called "Dawson fingers"). This is caused by inflammation and demyelination along the deep venules. Children often have lesions in the brain stem and posterior fossa (particularly middle cerebellar peduncles). Identical findings may be present with Lyme disease. Enhancement of one or more cranial nerves (predominantly sensory ones) is also typical of Lyme disease. Rarely, multiple sclerosis presents as a solitary mass with rim enhancement surrounded by edema. Obviously, such appearance is indistinguishable from a tumor. In Devic disease, focal hyperintense lesions are present in the spinal cord, particularly in the cervical region (Fig. 8.0-2). Identification of lesions in the optic nerves is better done with fat-suppression techniques. However, the entire spinal cord may be involved. In Schilder disease, multiple cannonball-like lesions are seen on T2-weighted images. These lesions have an appearance reminiscent of acute disseminated encephalomyelitis. In Balo concentric sclerosis, the lesions are round and large and contain alternating rings of high and low signal intensity similar to those seen in the cross-section of a tree trunk.

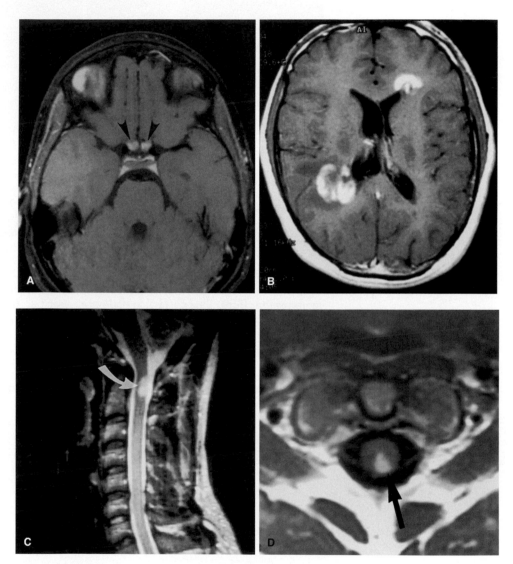

FIGURE 8.0-1.

Multiple sclerosis. **A.** Axial postcontrast fat-suppressed magnetic resonance (MR) T1-weighted image shows intense enhancement of the prechiasmatic optic nerves *(arrowheads)* in this child with proven multiple sclerosis. **B.** Axial postcontrast MR T1-weighted image shows two enhancing mass-like lesions. The right-sided one has surrounding edema. **C.** Midsagittal MR T2-weighted image in the same patient shows hyperintense lesion *(arrow)* in posterior upper cervical spinal cord. **D.** Axial postcontrast MR T1-weighted image in the same patient shows lesion *(arrow)* to enhance and have the configuration of dorsal white matter columns. This appearance is typical of multiple sclerosis. Biopsy of the brain lesion showed demyelination. (**B–D** with permission from Castillo M. Neuroradiology Companion. Philadelphia: JB Lippincott, 1995.)

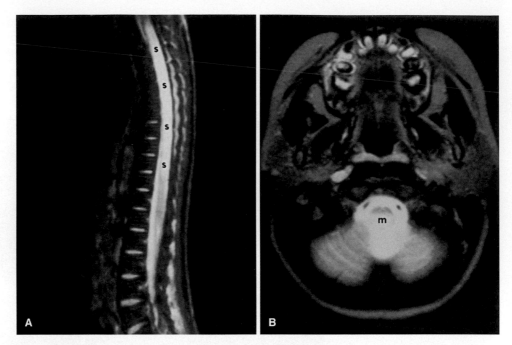

FIGURE 8.0-2.

Devic disease. **A.** Midsagittal magnetic resonance (MR) T2-weighted image in a different patient shows that the entire spinal cord (s) is hyperintense and inseparable from cerebrospinal fluid. This child also had optic neuritis. **B.** Axial MR T2-weighted image in the same patient shows abnormal hyperintensity (m) extending into the medulla. The clinical diagnosis was Devic disease.

SUGGESTED READING

1. Osborn AG, Harnsberger HR, Smoker WRK, et al. Multiple sclerosis in adolescents: CT and MR findings. AJNR 1990;11:489.

8.01 Bacterial Meningitis, Uncomplicated

EPIDEMIOLOGY Bacterial meningitis is a common cause of neurologic disease in the pediatric population. It is almost always fatal without appropriate antibiotic treatment. Before 5 years of age, the incidence is 87:100,000, whereas after 5 years of age, the incidence decreases to 2:100,000. During the first month of life, enterobacteria, particularly *Escherichia coli* and the *Citrobacter* strains, beta streptococci *(Streptococcus agalactiae),* and *Listeria monocytogenes* are responsible for this disease. In older children, the most common causative organisms are *Hemophilus influenzae, Neisseria meningitidis,* and *Streptococcus pneumoniae.* In adolescents, *S pneumoniae* and *N meningitidis* are common. Meningitis is more common during winter, except that caused by *H influenzae,* which tends to occur predominantly during spring and fall. In industrialized countries, the incidence of meningitis due to *H influenzae* is decreasing, a fact probably related to immunization, better living standards, and widespread use of third-generation cephalosporins (which are effective against this microorganism) for routine treatment of upper respiratory tract infections.

CLINICAL FEATURES Onset of symptoms is usually abrupt and relates to meningeal inflammation and increased intracranial pressure. Fever, alteration of consciousness, and full and tense fontanelles are typical in young patients. Older patients also present with irritability, stiff neck, and headache. Seizure and focal neurologic deficits are uncommon in uncomplicated bacterial meningitis. Grounds for clinical suspicion are not always clear. Meningitis is correctly diagnosed in only 50% of cases during the initial clinical visit. Electroencephalography may be normal, slow, or epileptiform. Accurate evaluation of the optic fundi is not often possible, and computed tomography (CT) is (at some institutions) ordered before the lumbar puncture. The reasoning behind this is the fact that the blurring of the optic disc may not occur until later, and therefore does not reflect acute increases in the intracranial pressure. Cerebrospinal fluid (CSF) (3 mL usually is needed) shows pleocytosis (300–10,000 cells/mm^3, predominantly polymorphonuclear cells), low glucose level (<20 mg/dL), and elevated protein. Bacterial cultures are imperative. Two to 3 days after antibiotic treatment, CSF analysis usually returns to normal.

IMAGING FEATURES Initially, a noncontrast CT may be obtained to rule out hydrocephalus. However, plain CT in the setting of acute meningitis is often negative. If iodinated contrast is given, meningeal enhancement along the convexities or tentorium may be visible (Fig. 8.01-1). Contrast-enhanced magnetic resonance imaging shows meningeal enhancement to a better advantage. However, imaging of uncomplicated meningitis usually is not indicated. Imaging should be reserved for patients with suspected complications. It is to be remembered that with the use of magnetization transfer in the postcontrast MR images, enhancement of the dura and the ventricular ependyma may be normally seen.

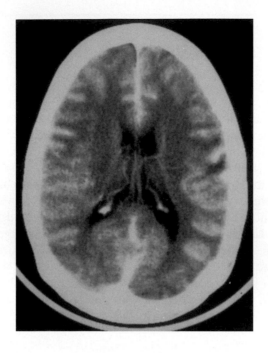

FIGURE 8.01-1.

Meningitis. Axial postcontrast computed tomography shows diffuse enhancement of all subarachnoid spaces in cortical sulci. The ventricles are minimally prominent.

SUGGESTED READINGS

1. Snyder RD. Bacterial and spirochetal infections of the nervous system. In: Swaiman KF, ed. Pediatric Neurology: Principles and Practice, 2nd ed. St. Louis: CV Mosby, 1994:611–620.
2. Harris TM, Edwards MK. Meningitis. Neuroimaging Clinics of North America 1991;1:39–55.

8.02 *Bacterial Meningitis, Complications*

EPIDEMIOLOGY

Persistence of fever for 5 days after initiation of antibiotic treatment is not predictive of complications arising from bacterial meningitis. Twenty to 50% of all children with meningitis will have some complication. These are divided into common and uncommon ones.

CLINICAL FEATURES

Seizure is the most common complication, and is seen in up to 50% of meningitis patients. The etiology is multifactorial, including cortical irritation, vasculitis, fever, and electrolyte imbalance. They may persist after the meningitis has resolved, but are usually self-limited. They may be focal or generalized; chronic seizures are rare.

Increased intracranial pressure is manifested by full fontanelles. The most likely etiology is noncommunicating hydrocephalus. Overhydration may predispose to cerebral edema, which may be complicated by herniation from hydrocephalus.

Electrolyte imbalance in the form of hyponatremia is seen in up to 20% of bacterial meningitis cases. It results from the syndrome of inadequate secretion of antidiuretic hormone.

Extraaxial fluid collections are found in 50% of meningitis patients. Widening of the subarachnoid space is probably related to lack of cerebrospinal fluid (CSF) resorption, although fluid may also accumulate in the subdural compartment. These collections usually are benign and asymptomatic.

Vasculitis is uncommon but may lead to cerebral infarctions. The largest blood vessels are affected as they traverse the inflamed meninges and subarachnoid space at the base of the brain. Cerebral infarctions are associated with a poor prognosis, including hemiparesis and cognitive and speech problems. Inflammation of veins and venous sinuses may lead to thrombosis and result in intracranial hypertension or cerebral infarctions. Venous thrombosis may be secondary to infection of paranasal sinuses or mastoids.

Involvement of the cranial nerves is relatively common. The most likely ones to be affected are VIII, VI, and III. Deafness complicates 5% to 30% of all bacterial meningitis cases. Sensorineural hearing loss is secondary to inflammation of the nerve or cochlea. Conductive deafness may be secondary to otitis media. Most cases of deafness resolve spontaneously, but some are permanent.

Other, less common complications of bacterial meningitis include brain abscess (rare before 2 years of age, and most secondary to anaerobes), disseminated intravascular coagulation, systemic shock, and recurrent bouts of meningitis.

IMAGING FEATURES

Dilation of the lateral ventricles accompanied by diffuse enhancement of the subarachnoid spaces is diagnostic of hydrocephalus (Fig. 8.02-1). Hydrocephalus secondary to meningitis is usually of the communicating type. However, increased signal intensity in periventricular regions on magnetic resonance (MR) T2-weighted images indicates transependymal edema due to noncommunicating hydrocephalus. The ependymal surfaces of the ventricles may also enhance, indicating ventriculitis (Fig. 8.02-2). Ventriculitis occurs more commonly in neonates. Overgrowth of the ependyma may lead to entrapment of a portion of a ventricle with subsequent dilation.

Subdural effusions usually are large, and involve the frontoparietal regions predominantly (Fig. 8.02-3). Most contain sterile fluid. Their walls may show contrast enhancement, and hence this finding may not be used to differentiate them from empyemas (Fig. 8.02-4). However, on MR imaging, the signal intensity of sterile subdural collections tends to closely follow that of CSF on all sequences. Empyemas show slightly increased MR signal intensity with respect to CSF on T1-weighted images.

Vasculitis may be shown by MR angiography, but is better evaluated by conventional angiography. Venous thrombosis is easily diagnosed on MR T1-weighted images, which show replacement of flow void phenomena with bright clot. Absence of blood flow in venous sinuses is well demonstrated on two-dimensional MR venograms. It is important to evaluate the paranasal sinuses and mastoids because infection of these may be the cause of venous thrombosis. High signal intensity on MR T2-weighted images in the paranasal sinuses indicates retained secretions. Venous infarctions do not conform to arterial distributions, are often multifocal and bilateral, and are hemorrhagic in up to 25% of instances (Figs. 8.02-5 and 8.02-6).

Children with recurrent bouts of meningitis should be evaluated for anatomic defects such as occult cephaloceles, dermal sinus tracts, nasal dermoids and epidermoids, and defects secondary to fractures involving the base of the skull. In these cases computed tomography is the imaging method of choice; otherwise, MR imaging is recommended as the first study when complications from meningitis are considered.

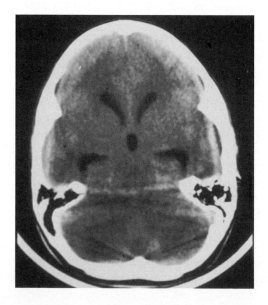

FIGURE 8.02-1.

Hydrocephalus. Axial noncontrast computed tomography shows nonvisualization of basilar cisterns secondary to increased density due to pus. There is mild hydrocephalus.

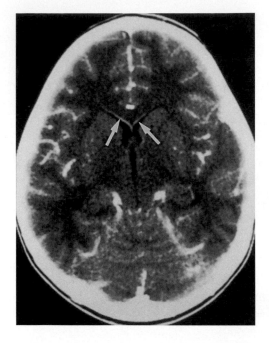

FIGURE 8.02-2.

Ventriculitis. Axial postcontrast computed tomography shows diffuse enhancement of the subarachnoid spaces in cortical sulci and of the ependyma *(arrows)* in the frontal horns of the lateral ventricles. (With permission from Castillo M. Neuroradiology Companion. Philadelphia: JB Lippincott, 1995.)

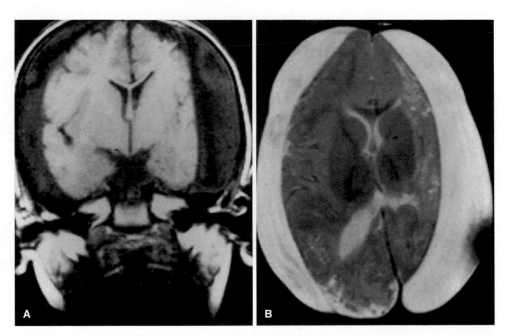

FIGURE 8.02-3.

Subdural effusions. **A.** Coronal magnetic resonance (MR) T1-weighted image in patient with meningitis due to *H influenzae* shows bilateral large subdural fluid collections. Note that collections are of slightly higher signal intensity than cerebrospinal fluid, and therefore may contain an increased amount of proteins or be infected.
B. Axial MR T1-weighted image in the same patient shows the collections to have increased signal intensity. Note slight hyperintensities from the left temporal and right occipital region, suggesting compressive infarctions.

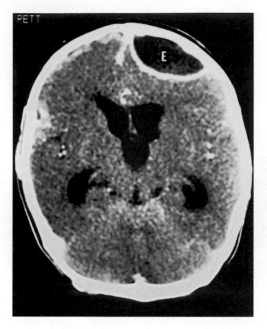

FIGURE 8.02-4.

Empyema. Axial postcontrast computed tomography in a patient with partially treated meningitis shows left frontal subdural empyema (E; surgically proven) with enhancing rim and compression of the frontal horn of the left lateral ventricle. There is hydrocephalus. (With permission from Castillo M. Neuroradiology Companion. Philadelphia: JB Lippincott, 1995.)

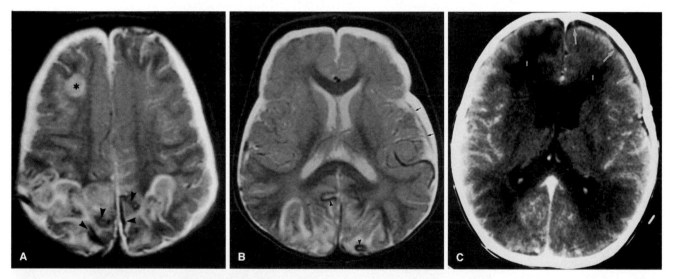

FIGURE 8.02-5.

Venous infarctions. **A.** Axial magnetic resonance (MR) T2-weighted image in a patient with meningitis. There are bilateral, fairly symmetric posterior parietal infarctions that contain edema and hemorrhage *(arrowheads)*. There is also an area of abnormal hyperintensity (*) in the right frontal region. The findings suggest venous infarctions. Small bilateral extraaxial fluid collections are present. **B.** Axial MR T2-weighted image in the same patient shows bilateral extraaxial fluid collections and thickened meninges *(small arrows)* in left temporal region. Note extension of the infarction into the occipital lobes. Note areas of hypointensity *(arrowheads)*, suggesting cortical hemorrhages. **C.** Axial postcontrast computed tomography in a different patient shows hydrocephalus, meningeal enhancement, a small left frontotemporal extraaxial fluid collection *(arrows)*, and bifrontal white matter infarctions (l).

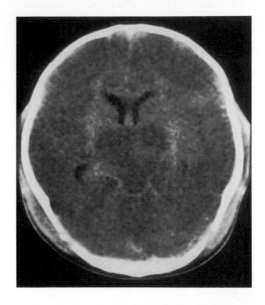

FIGURE 8.02-6.

Infarctions. Axial noncontrast computed tomography shows diffuse hypodensity in the brain with obliteration of cortical sulci in this patient with hemispheric infarctions secondary to meningitis.

SUGGESTED READINGS

1. Castillo M. Magnetic resonance imaging of meningitis and its complications. Topics in Magnetic Resonance Imaging 1994;6:53.
2. Weingarten K, Zimmerman RD, Becker RD, et al. Subdural and epidural empyema: MR imaging. Am J Neuroradiol 1989;10:81.
3. Snyder RD. Bacterial and spirochetal infections of the nervous system. In: Swaiman KF, ed. Pediatric Neurology, 2nd Ed. St. Louis: CV Mosby, 1994:611.

8.03   *Cerebritis and Abscesses*

EPIDEMIOLOGY

Nonfocal, early inflammations of the brain are known as cerebritis. Brain abscesses are very rare, occurring in 1:100,000 people. Approximately 25% of these are found in children younger than 15 years of age. Predisposing conditions include congenital heart disease, cystic fibrosis (and other chronic lung disorders), paranasal sinus or mastoid infections, trauma (including surgery), sepsis, endocarditis, pulmonary arteriovenous malformations, and immunosuppression.

CLINICAL FEATURES

Most abscesses are the result of hematogenous spread. Examples of direct inoculation include trauma (particularly compound fractures) and surgery. Extension from nearby foci of infection (middle ear and paranasal sinuses) may involve the brain directly or be the result of septic thrombophlebitis of the bridging veins. The most common symptoms are fever, headaches, confusion, altered consciousness, seizures, nuchal rigidity, papilledema, hemiparesis, and dysphasia. Infecting agents vary according to the child's age. In prematures, *Citrobacter* is common. In older children, *Streptococcus* and *Staphylococcus* species are often responsible. *Bacteroides fragilis* and *Proteus* species are not uncommon. In over 70% of intracranial abscesses, anaerobic bacteria are found. *Listeria monocytogenes* infection produces inflammatory changes in the brain stem and thalami (rhombencephalitis), and should be suspected if there is history of ingestion of unpasteurized milk products. Clinical suspicion of an intracranial abscess requires confirmation by imaging. Lumbar puncture may result in herniation and is therefore not performed. In cases of early cerebritis, however, the cerebrospinal fluid (CSF) may show mild polymorphonuclear or lymphocytic pleocytosis, elevated proteins, and a normal glucose level. Gram stain is negative unless the abscess has ruptured into the CSF spaces. Appropriate antibiotic administration with or without surgical drainage is the treatment of choice. Chronic seizure disorder is common after abscesses.

Pathologically, the first stage of the disease is characterized by early cerebritis, in which there is diffuse inflammation and early central necrosis without a capsule. This is seen during the initial 5 days. In the second stage, late cerebritis, there is a well defined necrotic center with granulation along its margins, but no true abscess capsule. In the third stage, early capsule formation, there is deposition of reticulin fibers along the periphery of the necrotic center, indicating the start of true capsule formation. This is seen between 5 to 10 days. In the last stage (chronic capsule formation), there is a well defined, thick capsule composed of collagenous tissue and a reduction of the inflammatory process. This occurs between 10 to 14 days after initial inoculation. Edema is present throughout all these stages but tends to decrease with true capsule formation.

IMAGING FEATURES

We consider magnetic resonance (MR) the imaging modality of choice when brain infections are suspected. In the early cerebritis stage, MR imaging shows edema on T2-weighted images and subtle, diffuse, and mild enhancement on postcontrast T1-weighted images (Fig. 8.03-1). In the late cerebritis stage, the forming neocapsule is slightly hyperintense on T1-weighted images and slightly hypointense on T2-weighted images. The center of the abscess is of heterogenous signal intensity on all imaging sequences. The margins of the abscess may show enhancement, and on delayed images, the center of the abscess may enhance. In the subacute abscess stage (early capsule formation), edema is again seen, but there is a well defined necrotic center. At this stage there is a peripheral thin ring of enhancement and better defined peripheral hypointensity on T2-weighted images. Because a true and complete capsule is not present at this time, this ring enhancement is probably related to the presence of granulation tissue in the periphery of the abscess. In the chronic abscess stage (late capsule formation), the capsule enhances and is seen as a ring of low signal intensity on T2-weighted images. The reason for this is not clear, but some paramagnetic substance found in macrophages is probably responsible. The abscess capsule tends to be thin, uniform, and slightly thicker in areas where it abuts gray matter (Fig. 8.03-2). This occurs because of the increased vascularity of gray matter. In this last stage, the degree of edema and mass effect begins to subside. After successful treatment, the abscess capsule changes from hypointense to isointense. This occurs approximately 4 months after treatment. On MR imaging abscess may be seen up to 8 months after treatment, and should not be regarded as a failure of treatment.

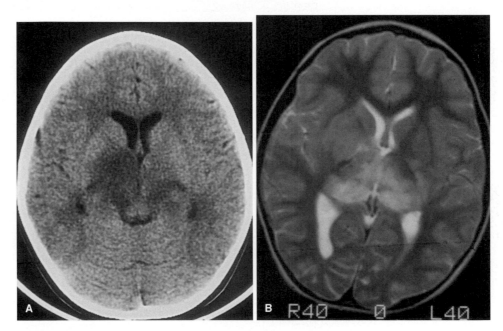

FIGURE 8.03-1.

Cerebritis. **A.** Axial noncontrast computed tomography in a patient with cerebritis secondary to *Listeria monocytogenes* infection shows low density in the thalami and extending into the right internal capsule/lentiform nucleus. **B.** Axial magnetic resonance T2-weighted image in the same patient shows abnormal hyperintensities in the thalami, posterior limbs of both internal capsules, and right lentiform nucleus. After contrast administration (not shown), there was minimal enhancement of the thalamic lesions.

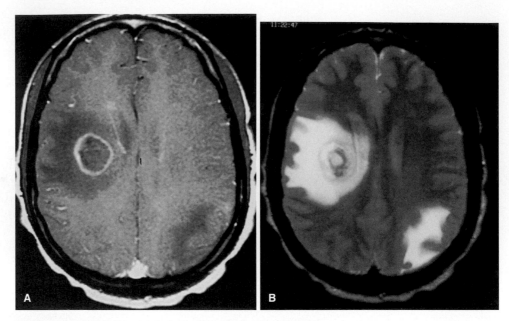

FIGURE 8.03-2.

Abscesses. **A.** Axial postcontrast magnetic resonance (MR) T1-weighted image shows an abscess in the right centrum semiovale. Note that rim of enhancement is thicker in its lateral aspect because of proximity to the cortex, which receives more blood supply than white matter. There is a zone of edema in the left posterior parietal region with enhancement, suggesting cerebritis. **B.** Axial MR T2-weighted image in same patient shows mild hypointensity from capsule of right-sided abscess. This is typical of a true abscess capsule. Note edema in both lesions.

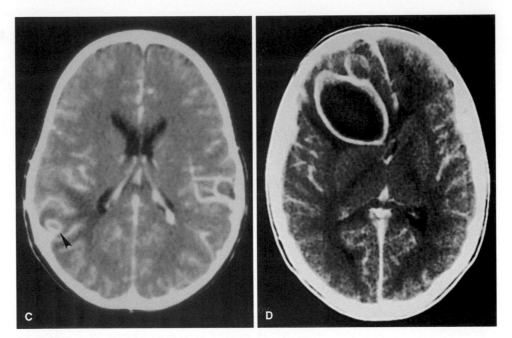

FIGURE 8.03-2. *Continued*

C. Axial postcontrast computed tomography (CT) in a patient with a cervical spine fracture in whom the right posterior pin for the traction halo penetrated the skull, resulting in meningitis (note diffuse enhancement of the subarachnoid space) and a small right temporoparietal abscess *(arrowhead)* with surrounding edema. **D.** Axial postcontrast CT in a young man with endocarditis shows large right frontal abscess and probable daughter abscess anteriorly. Note that rim of enhancement is thicker laterally where it is in the vicinity of cortex. In all abscesses, the rim of enhancement is smooth, whereas in tumors it tends to be nodular. (With permission from Castillo M. Neuroradiology Companion. Philadelphia: JB Lippincott, 1995.)

SUGGESTED READING

1. Buff BL, Mathews VP, Elster AD. Bacterial and viral parenchymal infections of the brain. Topics in Magnetic Resonance Imaging 1994;6:11.

8.04 *Acute Disseminated Encephalomyelitis*

EPIDEMIOLOGY

This rare disorder usually occurs 2 to 3 weeks after a viral illness such as measles, varicella, smallpox, infectious mononucleosis, herpes zoster, mumps, or influenza, or after vaccine immunizations. Rabies may also rarely precede this disease. Acute disseminated encephalomyelitis (ADEM) may also occur spontaneously, possibly secondary to prior subclinical viral infections. Children between 6 to 10 years of age are commonly affected, but younger (2 years of age or less) or older individuals may also contract this disease. ADEM is probably related to allergic encephalomyelitis, multiple sclerosis and variants, Schneider encephalitis periaxialis diffusa, and subacute sclerosing panencephalitis.

CLINICAL FEATURES

Symptoms may have an insidious or abrupt onset. Most common symptoms include motor abnormalities, seizures, altered consciousness, and stiff neck. If spinal cord involvement is present, a transverse myelitis-like picture occurs (flaccid paraplegia, incontinence, and absent plantar and deep tendon reflexes). The course of ADEM is usually monophasic, extending from 2 to 4 weeks, after which there is complete recovery in 60% to 75% of cases. Death occurs in 15% to 20% of patients. Permanent neurologic damage occurs in 10% to 20% of patients and includes mainly optic atrophy, mild mental impairment, cranial nerve deficits, and pyramidal dysfunction. Recurrence of the disease is rare. A form of ADEM isolated to the spinal cord is known to exist. Cerebrospinal fluid analysis reveals mild pleocytosis (mainly lymphocytic), mildly elevated total proteins, and oligoclonal immunoglobulin G bands. Histologically, there is perivenular demyelination and infiltration by lymphocytes, plasma cells, and monocytes. There is sparing of the axons, and microglial proliferation. Although the disease tends to be supratentorial, involvement of the cerebellum is not unusual. The etiology of ADEM is not certain, but it is presumed to be related to an immune-mediated reaction to similar proteins located on the surfaces of a virus and cells of the central nervous system. The agent responsible for this disease has not been isolated. The treatment is usually supportive, but corticosteroids may be used in an attempt to shorten the course of the disease and prevent sequelae.

IMAGING FEATURES

The hallmark of acute demyelination is increased concentration of water. Therefore, magnetic resonance (MR) T2-weighted images readily demonstrate the abnormalities seen in ADEM (Fig. 8.04-1). Most lesions are located in the subcortical white matter, centra semiovale, corona radiata, and periventricular white matter. The lesions are hyperintense, sharply marginated, have mild to moderate mass effect, and have no surrounding edema. Approximately 60% of patients have lesions in gray matter structures such as the thalami, head of caudate nuclei, globi pallidi, and putamina. The cerebellum, brain stem, and spinal cord may also be involved (Fig. 8.04-2). Deep gray matter involvement tends to be bilateral but not symmetric. Because involvement of the deep gray matter nuclei is rare in multiple sclerosis, this feature may help to differentiate both entities. Involvement of the white matter is always seen when gray matter involvement has occurred. On precontrast MR T1-weighted images, the lesions are mildly hypointense with respect to normal white matter. After contrast administration, enhancement is not uncommon. Computed tomography (CT) is less sensitive, but may show hypodense lesions with little mass effect. By CT, the lesions only rarely show enhancement. Occasionally, both MR imaging and CT may be normal. Rarely, the lesions may be hemorrhagic.

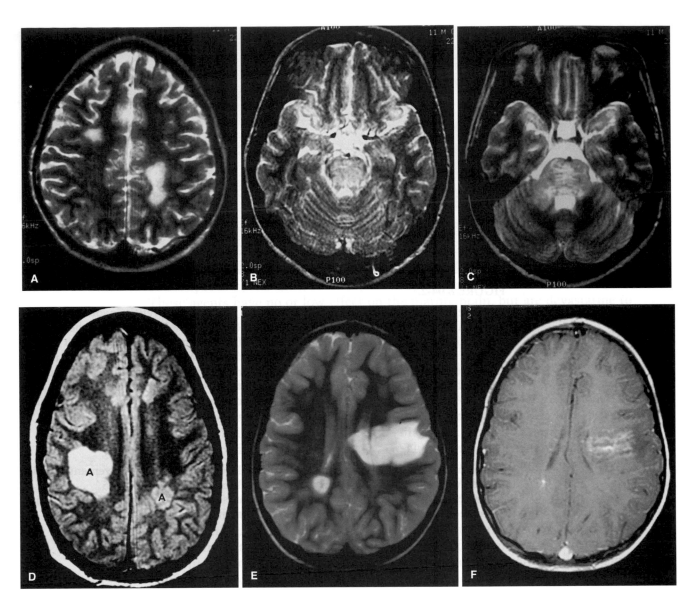

FIGURE 8.04-1.

Acute disseminated encephalomyelitis. **A.** Axial magnetic resonance (MR) T2-weighted image shows hyperintense lesions (A) in the centra semiovale of both hemispheres. **B.** Axial MR T2-weighted image (same patient) shows diffuse hyperintensity in pons. **C.** Axial MR T2-weighted image again shows hyperintensity in pons, extending into both middle cerebellar peduncles (right > left). This child presented with a "locked-in" syndrome and was discharged basically asymptomatic 10 days later. (Case courtesy of N. Nieves, M.D., Brooke Army Medical Center, San Antonio, TX.) **D.** Axial MR proton density image in a different patient shows well marginated hyperintense lesions (A) in both centra semiovale. Note absence of edema and very little mass effect. **E.** In a different patient, MR T2-weighted image shows hyperintense lesions in the centra semiovale bilaterally. Note left-sided lesion extends medially into the corpus callosum. **F.** Corresponding postcontrast MR T1-weighted image shows enhancement in both lesions.

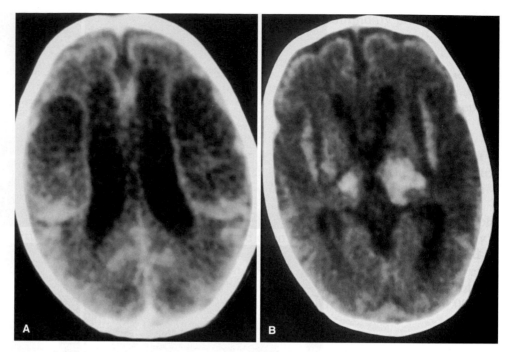

FIGURE 8.05-2.

Herpes encephalitis. **A.** Axial noncontrast computed tomography (CT) in a newborn shows multiple areas of cystic malacia, parenchymal densities (blood vs. early calcifications?), and ventricular prominence. **B.** Axial noncontrast CT in the same patient shows hyperdensity (presumed early calcification) in the insular cortices, right lentiform nucleus, and thalami.

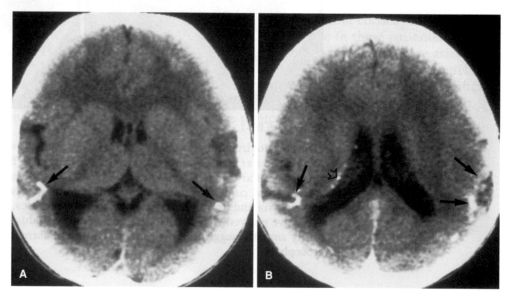

FIGURE 8.05-3.

Toxoplasmosis. **A.** Noncontrast computed tomography (CT) shows cortical calcifications *(arrows)* **B.** Axial CT in same patient shows cortical calcifications *(arrows)* as well as right periventricular calcifications *(open arrow).* (Case courtesy of R. Jinkins, University of Texas, San Antonio, TX.)

SUGGESTED READING

1. Fitz CR. Inflammatory diseases of the brain in childhood. AJNR 1992;13:551.

8.06 Viral Infections in Older Children

EPIDEMIOLOGY

The most common sporadic viral encephalitides occurring in the United States are caused by herpes simplex viruses, and over 30% are found in children less than 20 months of age. Type 2 herpes virus usually affects neonates, whereas type 1 infection occurs in older children and adults. Epidemic viral encephalitides are caused by arbotogaviruses and bunyaviruses. Most of these infections are seasonal (particularly summer and fall) and arthropod borne.

CLINICAL FEATURES

Viral central nervous system infections manifest as aseptic meningitis, encephalitis, and meningomyeloradiculitis. In aseptic meningitis, symptoms begin abruptly, including fever, headaches, vomiting, and stiffness of the neck. These symptoms occur in over 60% of patients. Mild mental alterations may be present. Aseptic meningitides frequently accompany other viral illnesses such as mumps, parotiditis, measles, and pharyngitis. Symptoms of prior upper respiratory tract infection were present in 30% of patients with viral meningitis. Symptoms resolve slowly, in approximately 2 weeks. There may be recurrent episodes. Cerebrospinal fluid (CSF) may show mild elevation of proteins, and the electroencephalogram (EEG) shows diffuse slowing. Treatment consists of supportive measures only. Histologically, there is neuronal degeneration and inflammation in all viral encephalitides.

Encephalitis is clinically characterized by alterations in consciousness, abnormal behavior, seizures, and signs of increased intracranial pressure. Spinal cord involvement is rare. CSF shows mild elevation of cells and protein, and a mild reduction in the glucose level. EEG is always abnormal. If herpes encephalitis is suspected, early treatment with acyclovir decreases mortality from 70% (without treatment) to 8%.

Subacute sclerosing panencephalitis is a disorder mostly of children, usually encountered between 5 to 15 years of age. Clinically it is characterized by mental status changes, ataxia, myoclonus, and seizures. It is probably secondary to reactivation of prior measles infection. Imaging features are nonspecific.

Meningomyelitis is typified by poliomyelitis and transverse myelitis. Polio leads to involvement of the anterior gray matter horns. In this era of postpoliovirus immunization, this disease is usually related to polio-like syndromes, or seen very rarely after vaccination. Transverse myelitis is characterized by weakness and tingling of the extremities, with back pain and a sensory level. Bladder dysfunction and paralysis may occur. Polyradiculitis is seen after infectious mononucleosis, varicella, measles, mumps, and parainfluenza virus infections.

Rassmussen encephalitis is a syndrome of presumed viral etiology (Fig. 8.06-1). Clinically it is characterized by seizures (particularly epilepsia partialis continua), mental deterioration, and progressive loss of motor function, which may lead to hemiparesis. CSF may demonstrate lymphocytosis. Pathologically, the abnormalities usually are confined to one hemisphere and include perivascular lymphocytic infiltration, glial nodules, loss of cortical neurons, gliosis, and atrophy. Hemispherectomy may help in controlling the seizures. If untreated, the disease is progressive and leads to death.

IMAGING FEATURES

Magnetic resonance (MR) is the imaging modality of choice in these disorders. Most viral encephalitides show patchy areas of increased intensity on T2-weighted images. These abnormalities involve both the white and gray matter. Herpes virus type 1 tends to reside in the trigeminal or geniculate ganglia. Active infection of the brain is caused by reactivation of the virus, and commonly involves the medial temporal lobe and the brain stem (Fig. 8.06-2A). A second pathway is that of extension of the virus from the trigeminal nerves to the nasal mucosa, then into the brain via the olfactory nerves, therefore affecting preferentially the frontal lobes. In most cases, MR imaging shows edema of the medial temporal lobe and the subinsular cortex. The basal ganglia usually are spared. These areas show enhancement. Hemorrhage (particularly petechial) may occur during the first week. Necrosis and cystic malacia occur chronically. Symmetric bilateral abnormalities are typical, but occur less often than unilateral abnormalities. When the frontal lobes are involved, the process tends to initiate at the cingulate gyri. Herpes type 1 infection produces generalized white matter abnormalities with minimal enhancement (Fig. 8.06-2B). Atrophy, malacia, and deep and superficial calcifications appear rapidly after the infection. Other viral encephalitis may also be hemorrhagic (Fig. 8.06-3).

In our experience, most MR imaging studies performed for transverse myelitis are negative. Occasionally, one may see areas of increased T2 signal that may or may not enhance. In postvaccination poliomyelitis, we have seen enhancement of the anterior horns. In Guillain-Barré syndrome, the ventral nerve roots from the cauda equina enhance. In cases of polyradiculitis, the nerve roots are enlarged and enhance.

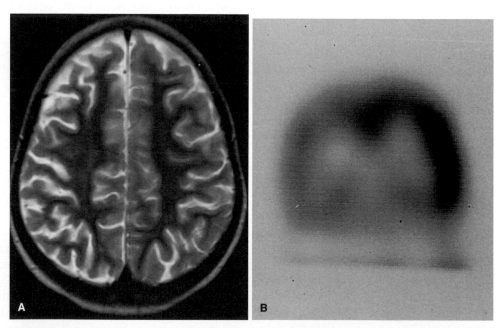

FIGURE 8.06-1.

Rasmussen encephalitis. **A.** Axial magnetic resonance T2-weighted image in a patient with chronic seizures and atrophy of the right cerebral hemisphere. Biopsy was compatible with chronic encephalitis of the Rasmussen type. **B.** Coronal view from Tc 99m HMPAO single photon emission computed tomography study shows decreased activity in the corresponding hemisphere.

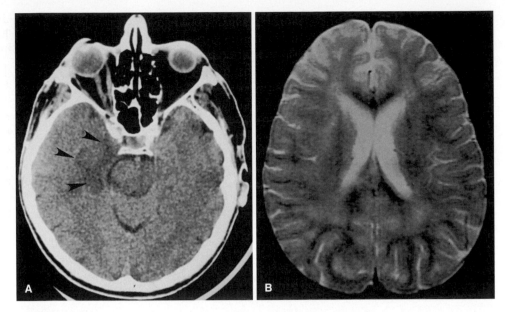

FIGURE 8.06-2.

Herpes encephalitis. **A.** Axial noncontrast computed tomography in an adolescent shows low density *(arrowheads)* in the medial right temporal lobe (herpes simplex type 1). **B.** Axial magnetic resonance T2-weighted image in a different patient shows multiple, diffuse, patchy hyperintense areas throughout the white matter of both cerebral hemispheres (herpes simplex type 2). (With permission from Castillo M. Neuroradiology Companion. Philadelphia: JB Lippincott, 1995.)

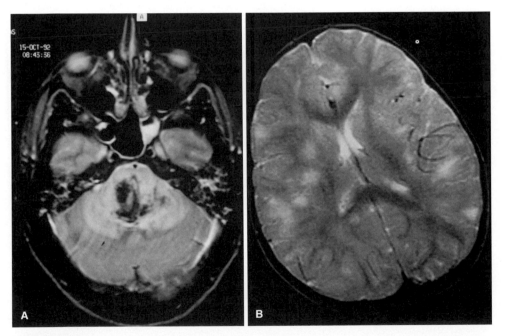

FIGURE 8.06-3.

Hemorrhagic leukoencephalitis. **A.** Axial magnetic resonance (MR) T2-weighted image in a patient with prior viral illness with autopsy-proven acute hemorrhagic leukoencephalitis shows acute hemorrhage in pons with surrounding edema. The initial differential diagnosis was basilar artery thrombosis, but note that this artery is patent (angiographically confirmed). **B.** Axial MR T2-weighted image in the same patient shows multiple, patchy, hyperintense areas throughout both cerebral hemispheres.

SUGGESTED
READINGS

1. Shaw DWW, Cohen WA. Viral infections of the CNS in children: imaging features. AJR 1993;160:125.
2. Tien RD, Felsberg GJ, Osumi AK. Herpesvirus infections of the CNS: MR findings. AJR 1993;161:167.
3. Noorbehescht B, Enzmann DR, Sullender W, Bradley JS, Arvin AM. Neonatal herpes simplex encephalitis: correlation of clinical and CT findings. Radiology 1987;162:813.

8.07 Parasitic Infections: Toxoplasmosis

EPIDEMIOLOGY

Infection with the protozoon, *Toxoplasma gondii*, may occur on a congenital basis or later in life, when it is usually seen in immunosuppressed patients. Toxoplasmosis affects 0.1% or less of all pregnancies in the United States. Infection most commonly occurs during the third trimester of pregnancy, but earlier infection produces more severe damage. Toxoplasmosis also occurs in immunosuppressed children (transplants and AIDS), but it is much less common than in immunosuppressed adults.

CLINICAL FEATURES

During pregnancy, the infection is asymptomatic in the mother but produces damage to the spleen, liver, eyes, and brain in the fetus. The most common manifestations include microcephaly (20%), hydrocephalus (25%), microphthalmia (35%), and chorioretinitis (95%). Mental retardation is seen in over 80% of survivors. Other manifestations include seizures and hydranencephaly. The diagnosis is made by positive indirect fluorescent antibody test or hemagglutination test. Treatment is controversial, but early administration of sulfadiazine, pyrimethamine, and folinic acid may be beneficial. Of infectious disorders, toxoplasmosis is second in prevalence to cytomegalovirus infection in neonates (see section 8.05).

In immunosuppressed patients, disseminated toxoplasmosis may occur, and presents with signs and symptoms of meningoencephalitis. Treatment with the above-mentioned drug regimen is highly effective.

IMAGING FEATURES

Cerebral calcifications are detected by computed tomography (CT) in over 60% of patients and are the most common radiologic manifestation. Calcifications may also be seen in the basal ganglia, white matter, and the cortex. Hydrocephalus is commonly present and is related to stenosis of the aqueduct of Sylvius. Microcephaly is also common. Areas of malacia are rare, and hydranencephaly has been described. Because calcifications are so common in this disease, CT is the imaging method of choice.

In immunosuppressed patients with suspected toxoplasmosis, magnetic resonance is the imaging modality of choice. The findings are nonspecific and consist of single or multiple ring-enhancing lesions located mainly at the gray–white junctions (Fig. 8.07-1). Surrounding edema is usually present. Pial enhancement is also seen.

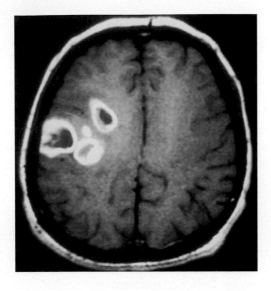

FIGURE 8.07-1.

Toxoplasmosis. Axial postcontrast magnetic resonance T1-weighted image in a patient with AIDS shows four ring-enhancing lesions (three of them necrotic) in the right frontoparietal region.

SUGGESTED READING

1. Becker LE. Infections of the developing brain. AJNR 1992;13:537.

8.08 *Parasitic Infections: Cysticercosis*

EPIDEMIOLOGY

Almost 100% of patients with cysticercosis have involvement of the central nervous system. Approximately 90% of patients are immigrants, particularly from Latin America. In endemic countries, the rate of infection may be as high as 3% of the general population.

CLINICAL FEATURES

Over 90% of patients are infected by ingesting ova-containing food and water. In 10% of patients, the fecal–oral route is responsible for the infection. The latter is typically responsible for cysticercosis in children. The ova release oncospheres, which penetrate the gastrointestinal mucosa and then invade the bloodstream. The parasites lodge in the distal arterioles and penetrate through them into the brain, ventricles, and subarachnoid spaces. The parasites form a cyst (bladder) containing a scolex. In the brain, these cysts are surrounded by a thin layer of granulation tissue. Eventually, the parasites die and the cysts release their fluid, which produces an inflammatory reaction. At this time, immunoglobulins M (IgM) and G (IgG) are detectable in cerebrospinal fluid (CSF) and serum. When the inflammation subsides, the dead parasites calcify. In the CSF spaces, the cysts form but there should be no scolex (this is not always true; we have seen cases in which the scolex is identifiable by magnetic resonance [MR] imaging in intraventricular parasites). These parasites produce an intense inflammatory reaction of the leptomeninges.

Clinically, over 60% of patients present with seizures. Headaches occur in 15% of patients. Other findings include papilledema, altered mental status, focal neurologic findings, chronic meningitis, ataxia, positional headache, nausea, and vomiting. Electroencephalographic abnormalities (mainly generalized) are detected in half of the patients. Inflammation of the subarachnoid spaces leads to vasculitis in 10% of cases. The most common manifestation of this vasculitis is lacunar infarctions in the basal ganglia. One third of patients with neurocysticercosis remain asymptomatic. The diagnosis is made by enzyme-linked immunosorbent assay to detect specific IgM and IgG antibodies. Most patients require treatment with anticonvulsants, and administration of praziquantel is controversial in children. Surgery may be needed for the removal of intraventricular and spinal cysts. Albendazole is a drug that has been recently used; it is effective for parenchymal and subarachnoid cysts.

IMAGING FEATURES

We prefer MR imaging in suspected cases of cysticercosis. MR imaging allows for identification of intraventricular and subarachnoid cysts, which are difficult to visualize by computed tomography. The lesions appear as well defined, low signal intensity cysts on T1-weighted images (Fig. 8.08-1). Most parenchymal cysts are located at the gray–white junctions. These cysts usually measure 1 to 2 cm and are devoid of surrounding edema on T2-weighted images. With death, pericyst edema develops and there is intense enhancement of a capsule, which may be thin or thick but is always smooth. Death of multiple cysts produces an encephalitis-like picture. Miliary encephalitic cysticercosis is typically encountered in young children (Fig. 8.08-2). Dead parasites calcify (Fig. 8.08-3). Intraventricular and subarachnoid cysts have a wall of slight hyperintensity on T1-weighted images, and their fluid is slightly brighter than CSF (Figs. 8.08-4 and 8.08-5). Diffuse meningeal enhancement may be present (Fig. 8.08-6). The fourth and third ventricles and the atria of the lateral ventricles are favorites sites. In the subarachnoid spaces, the suprasellar cistern and cisterns around the brain stem are commonly affected. Cysticercosis may be found in unusual locations, such as spinal cord and the eyes (Figs. 8.08-7 and 8.08-8)

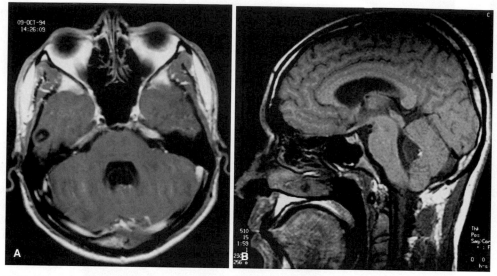

FIGURE 8.08-4.

Cysticercosis, intraventricular. **A.** Axial postcontrast magnetic resonance (MR) T1-weighted image shows parasitic cyst inside the fourth ventricle. Note absence of scolex, which is typical of cysticerci in the cerebrospinal fluid (CSF) spaces. There is another cystic lesion with a central scolex in the right temporal region. **B.** Midsagittal precontrast MR T1-weighted image shows that the fluid of the fourth ventricular cystic lesion is of different signal intensity than CSF.

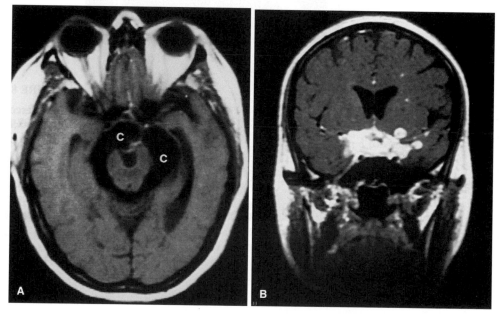

FIGURE 8.08-5.

Cysticercosis, cisternal. **A.** Axial noncontrast magnetic resonance (MR) T1-weighted image shows multiple cysticerci (c) in the perimesencephalic and interpenduncular cistern. **B.** Coronal postcontrast MR T1-weighted image in a different patient shows multiple solid-enhancing cysticerci in the sella, suprasellar region, and brain parenchyma. (**A** and **B** courtesy of R. Rojas, M.D., ABC Hospital, Mexico City, Mexico.)

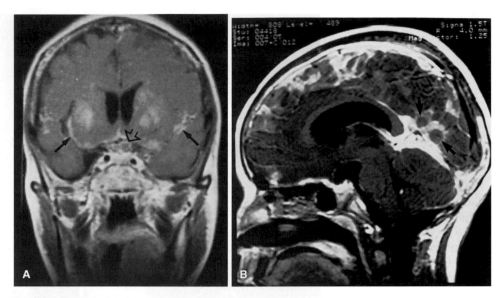

FIGURE 8.08-6.

Cysticercosis, meningitis. A. Coronal postcontrast magnetic resonance (MR) T1-weighted image shows enhancement of Sylvian fissures *(arrows)*, cysticerci *(open arrow)* in the suprasellar cistern, and hydrocephalus. We have seen infarcts develop in similar situations as a result of basilar meningitis and vasculitis. **B.** Midsagittal postcontrast MR T1-weighted image shows significant meningeal enhancement and two cysticerci *(arrows)* in the posterior interhemispheric fissure. (**A** and **B** courtesy of R. Rojas, M.D., ABC Hospital, Mexico City, Mexico.)

8.09 *Fungal Infections*

EPIDEMIOLOGY

Overall, fungal infections involving the central nervous system in children are very rare. Cryptococcosis, coccidioidomycosis, and histoplasmosis are probably the most common ones in hosts with a normal immune response. In immunocompromised patients, *Cryptococcus, Candida, Aspergillus,* and the phycomycoses are common.

CLINICAL FEATURES

Cryptococcus is globally distributed, with most coming from bird feces. It is acquired by inhalation–ingestion. Patients usually present with nausea, vomiting, headaches, and fever. Immunocompromised patients may be asymptomatic. In patients with AIDS, meningismus, photophobia, and altered mental status are the most common symptoms. The organism is found in the cerebrospinal fluid (CSF) in 75% of cases, and latex agglutination test of the CSF is 90% reliable. Amphotericin B, flucytosine, or fluconazole are the drugs of choice.

Coccidioidomycosis is endemic in the southwestern United States, Mexico, and Central America. It is acquired by inhalation or transcutaneously through abrasions. Patients present with a nonspecific meningitis preceded 3 weeks earlier by pulmonary infection. Complement fixation and precipitin tests provide the diagnosis in 99% of cases. Amphotericin B, fluconazole, and intraconazole are effective drugs.

Histoplasmosis is endemic in the Mississippi River region, Mexico, and Central and South America. Up to 80% of children younger than 5 years of age have a positive skin test. The infection is acquired by inhalation and produces a tuberculosis-like picture in the lungs and brain. Diagnosis requires isolation of the organism from bone marrow, liver, nodes, blood, or CSF. Amphotericin B is the drug of choice.

Candidiasis, nocardiosis, and aspergillosis are exceedingly rare in children and usually occur in the setting of immunosuppression or chronic pulmonary disorders. All may produce a meningitis, meningoencephalitis, single or multiple brain abscesses, hemorrhagic necrosis, or solitary granulomas. Aspergillosis tends to involve the posterior circulation.

The phycomycoses usually occur in the setting of poorly controlled diabetes mellitus. They extend into the brain from the nose, nasopharynx, and nasolacrimal ducts.

IMAGING FEATURES

Cryptococcoses lead to hydrocephalus in 20% to 60% of patients. Computed tomography scans tend to be negative, but meningeal enhancement may be seen. By magnetic resonance imaging, the basal ganglia may demonstrate cryptococcomas. These are usually less than 3 mm in size, and may enhance. They are believed to represent extension into the Virchow-Robin spaces from the basilar cisterns. Larger cryptococcomas may be of low signal intensity on T1-weighted images and hyperintense on T2-weighted images (Fig. 8.09-1A, B). They rarely enhance, and are called "gelatinous pseudocysts." Cryptococcal abscesses appear as nonspecific ring-enhancing lesions (Fig. 8.09-1C).

Coccidioidomycosis produces basilar cistern enhancement and may lead to occlusion of vessels. Histoplasmosis is indistinguishable from the more common pyogenic abscesses. Candidal infection produces multiple, small, abscess-like lesions at the gray–white junctions (Fig. 8.09-2). Nocardial infection results in similar findings to those of candidiasis (Fig. 8.09-3). Phycomycosis and aspergillosis present as masses in the paranasal sinuses and nasal cavity, which may extend to the brain and are of low signal intensity on both T1- and T2-weighted images (Fig. 8.09-4). They enhance and may invade the brain and cavernous sinuses. They may cause vascular occlusions with cerebral infarctions.

SUG(
REAI

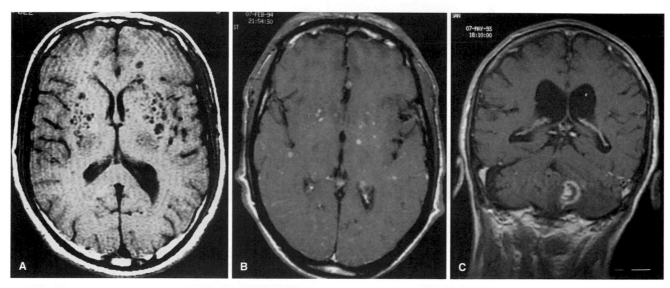

FIGURE 8.09-1.

Cryptococcus. **A.** Axial noncontrast magnetic resonance (MR) T1-weighted image shows multiple cysts ("gelatinous pseudocysts") in the region of the perforating vessels of the basal ganglia in this patient with AIDS and cryptococcosis. (With permission from Castillo M. Neuroradiology Companion. Philadelphia: JB Lippincott, 1995.) **B.** Axial postcontrast MR T1-weighted image in a different patient with AIDS and cryptococcosis shows punctate-enhancing lesions in the basal ganglia. **C.** Coronal postcontrast MR T1-weighted image in a different patient with AIDS shows cryptococcal abscess in left cerebellum. Note thicker rim facing gray matter (dentate nucleus). There are no specific features in this lesion to suggest the diagnosis. The ventricles are prominent.

8.10 Granulomatous Diseases

EPIDEMIOLOGY

Tuberculosis involving the central nervous system (CNS) is not as common as the pulmonary type. It is rare before 3 months of age but not uncommon during the first 5 years of life. The number of new cases of tuberculosis in the United States has increased at a rate of 16% per year since 1985.

Neurologic complications from sarcoidosis occur in 5% of all patients. Approximately 6% of all cases of neurosarcoidosis occur in children. Most affected children are between 10 to 15 years of age.

CLINICAL FEATURES

Central nervous system tuberculosis presents as a chronic meningitis in 50% of children and has an acute onset in the other 50%. Tuberculous meningitis almost always occurs in the setting of disseminated miliary tuberculosis. Symptoms include alteration of consciousness, irritability, headaches (20%), nuchal rigidity (50%), apathy, seizures, low-grade fever (50%), nausea, vomiting, and cranial nerve deficits (particularly cranial nerve VI). Electroencephalography shows slowing, and there may be epileptiform activity. Involvement of the brain and spinal cord is the result of hematogenous spread. Spread to the subarachnoid space is probably secondary to rupture of superficial or choroid plexus tuberculomas. Tuberculosis induces an inflammation of the basal meninges that may result in a vasculitis (with secondary infarctions) or venous thrombosis. Isoniazid, rifampin, and pyrazinamide are the drugs of choice. The use of steroids is controversial. Mortality varies between 10% to 20% for tuberculous meningitis. If untreated, death may occur as soon as 3 weeks after the onset of the disease.

Clinical findings in patients with neurosarcoidosis include headaches, cranial nerve deficits (particularly cranial nerves II, V, VII, and VIII), seizures, hydrocephalus, pituitary and hypothalamic dysfunction, peripheral neuropathy, myelopathy, and vasculitis. The most common form of the disease is basilar meningitis. In these patients, cerebrospinal fluid (CSF) shows elevated protein, decreased glucose, elevated immunoglobulin G, and positive angiotensin-converting enzyme. Peripheral neuropathy and myopathy may also be present. Treatment with steroids is beneficial.

IMAGING FEATURES

We prefer magnetic resonance (MR) to image patients with suspected CNS tuberculosis (Fig. 8.10-1). On noncontrast T1-weighted images, the CSF in the basilar cisterns may appear slightly hyperintense (similar to muscle signal intensity), and hydrocephalus is present in 50% to 75% of patients. After contrast is given, there is intense enhancement in the basilar cisterns. On T2-weighted images, the exudate in the subarachnoid spaces is of high signal intensity and inseparable from normal CSF. The perivascular spaces, particularly those of the lenticulostriate vessels, may also enhance. The presence of infarctions suggests vasculitis. Cortical infarctions may also occur. Because this vasculitis involves large vessels in the base of the brain, MR angiography may be positive. Identical findings may be seen with meningovascular syphilis. Tuberculomas are seen as small (usually less than 2 cm in diameter), ring-enhancing lesions at the gray–white junctions. Central necrosis or calcifications may be found in tuberculomas. As with pyogenic abscesses, the capsule of the tuberculomas is of low signal intensity on T1- and T2-weighted images. Tuberculomas usually have surrounding edema.

In patients with suspected sarcoidosis, MR is also the imaging modality of choice (Fig. 8.10-2). The findings include meningeal thickening and enhancement, enhancement along the perivascular spaces (especially those in the basal ganglia), enhancing cerebral lesions, hydrocephalus, and enhancing cranial nerves. The lesions may also have an appearance indistinguishable from demyelinating disease or Lyme disease. Intraparenchymal foci have no surrounding edema. Mass-like lesions may be present in the pituitary gland or the hypothalamus. Dural-based granulomas may be confused with meningiomas.

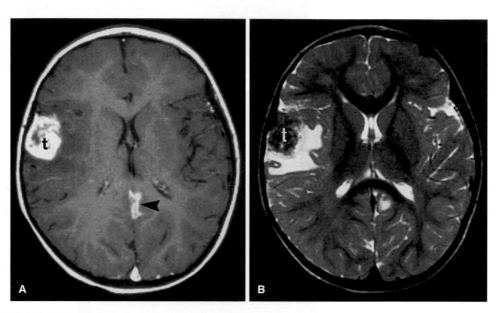

FIGURE 8.10-1.

Tuberculosis. **A.** Axial postcontrast magnetic resonance (MR) T1-weighted image shows solid but inhomogenous enhancing lesion (t) in right temporal region. It is difficult to determine if the lesion is extraaxial or intraaxial. There is surrounding hypointensity, suggesting edema. A second lesion *(arrowhead)* is seen posteriorly along the falx. **B.** Axial MR T2-weighted image shows that the lesion in the right temporal region (t) is mostly hypointense, with surrounding bright edema. The posterior lesion is only partly seen. Biopsy revealed tuberculosis. (Both figures with permission from Castillo M. Neuroradiology Companion. Philadelphia: JB Lippincott, 1995.)

9.0 *Aqueductal Stenosis*

EPIDEMIOLOGY

This anomaly occurs in approximately 0.1% of the population and accounts for 20% of hydrocephalus cases. It is four times more common in the siblings of affected patients. Aqueductal stenosis may be slightly more common in boys. Most cases are sporadic, but the hereditary type is transmitted as a gender-linked recessive trait.

CLINICAL FEATURES

The etiology for aqueductal stenosis usually is not found, but it may be associated with intrauterine viral infections, neurofibromatosis type 1, and Chiari malformations. Conversely, it may also be acquired postnatally because of intraventricular hemorrhage or meningitis, which results in aqueductal gliosis. Also, direct compression of the aqueduct by vascular malformations or tumors of the tectum may produce similar findings. Some patients have hydrocephalus at birth, but it may develop at any age. The onset of symptoms is usually insidious and the disorder may not manifest itself until late in life. The clinical manifestations are those of chronic intracranial hypertension. The symptoms include an enlarged head, decreased visual acuity, headaches, seizures, gait disturbances, dementia, and, rarely, cerebrospinal fluid rhinorrhea. Dilation of the third ventricle may lead to compression of the hypothalamus, resulting in delayed or precocious puberty, impotence, short stature, obesity, hypothyroidism, temperature instability, and multiple hormonal deficiencies. After shunting, these endocrinopathies resolve or improve markedly.

IMAGING FEATURES

Magnetic resonance is the imaging modality of choice (Fig. 9.0-1). Sagittal, thin-section T1-weighted images show dilation of the third and lateral ventricles. The aqueduct may show a narrowing that is commonly located at the level of the superior colliculi or the intercollicular sulcus. The tectum may be deformed and the colliculi fused. The aqueduct may be divided into several channels shortly after its origin (so-called "aqueductal forking"). Forking is commonly associated with spina bifida. In other cases, the patent segment of the aqueduct may be dilated and a web may be present within its lumen. This web may be a stretched area of stenosis or represent a true membrane. A true membrane is very rare and may be the consequence of prior infection or glial overgrowth. Axial T2-weighted images may show increased signal intensity in the periaqueductal region. This finding may be related to gliosis, but a tumor needs to be excluded. Contrast administration is needed. If the abnormality enhances, then tumor is a strong consideration. If no enhancement is seen, we believe that a low-grade astrocytoma continues to be a consideration, and that these patients should be followed carefully. In patients with neurofibromatosis, masses in the tectum may be caused by low-grade tumors or hamartomas. Although the distortion of the tectum may be the cause of the obstruction, it may also be secondary to compression by the dilated ventricles. In these cases, the tectum may return to normal after adequate shunting.

320   *Chapter 9. Hydrocephalus*

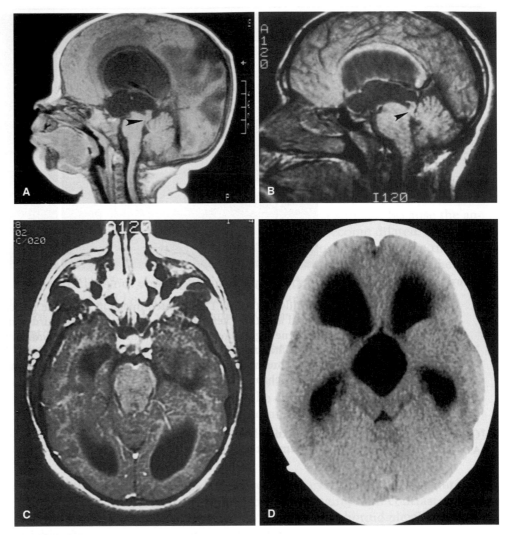

FIGURE 9.0-1.

Aqueductal stenosis. **A.** Midsagittal magnetic resonance (MR) T1-weighted image shows markedly dilated lateral and third ventricles. Note thick area of stenosis *(arrowhead)* in mid- to distal aqueduct. The fourth ventricle is of normal size. The chiasmatic and infundibular recesses of the third ventricle are herniating inferiorly. **B.** Midsagittal MR T1-weighted image in an adolescent with atresia *(arrowhead)* of the distal aqueduct resulting in hydrocephalus. The tectum is distorted but showed no abnormal signal intensity or enhancement. The third ventricle herniates into the pineal gland and suprasellar regions. **C.** Axial T1-weighted flow-sensitive (single-slice) gradient echo image in the same patient shows no flow-related enhancement in the aqueduct. **D.** Axial computed tomography (CT) in a different patient shows marked dilation of the lateral and third ventricles. Aqueduct is not seen.

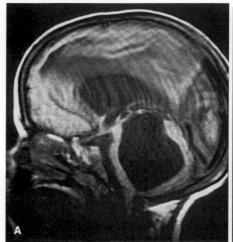

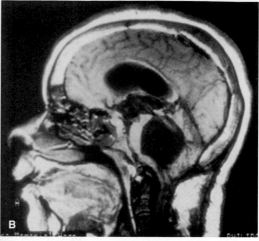

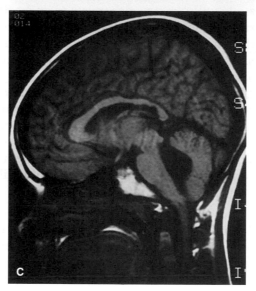

FIGURE 9.01-1.

Trapped fourth ventricle. **A.** Midsagittal magnetic resonance (MR) T1-weighted image shows markedly dilated and entrapped fourth ventricle in a patient with a history of prior meningitis. Also note lateral ventricles. **B.** Midsagittal MR T1-weighted image in a different case shows markedly dilated fourth ventricle of uncertain etiology. **C.** Midsagittal MR T1-weighted image in a different patient with a mildly to moderately dilated and trapped fourth ventricle. The etiology of the disorder in this patient is unknown. The aqueduct of Sylvius is not seen. The lateral ventricles are not distended because the patient has been shunted.

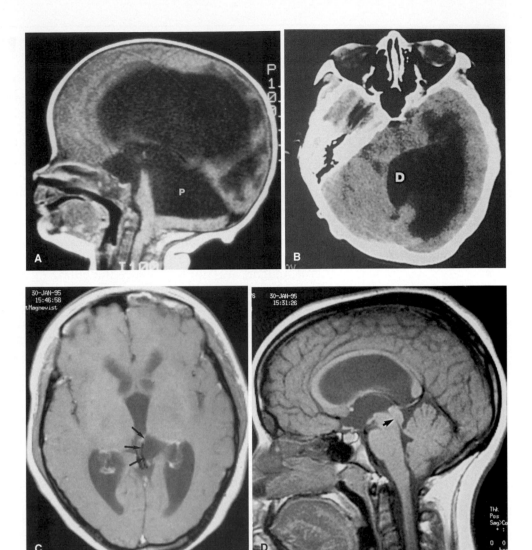

FIGURE 9.01-2.

Ventricular diverticula. A. Midsagittal magnetic resonance (MR) T1-weighted image with presumed aqueductal stenosis and massive dilation of the lateral ventricles and third ventricle. Note pineal recess (P) of third ventricle has herniated under the tentorium and compresses the cerebellum. This abnormality could be confused with a quadrigeminal plate cistern arachnoid cyst. The chiasmatic and infundibular recesses of the third ventricle have also herniated inferiorly. **B.** Axial noncontrast computed tomography (tilted to right) shows large diverticulum (D) arising from the medial border of the atrium of the left lateral ventricle. This patient had aqueductal stenosis. **C.** Axial MR T1-weighted image shows small diverticulum *(arrows)* arising from the medial aspect of the atrium of the left lateral ventricle. **D.** Midsagittal MR T1-weighted image in the same patient shows stenosis of mid-portion *(arrow)* of the aqueduct. Note somewhat bulbous tectum, which did not enhance or show abnormal T2 signal intensity.

SUGGESTED READING

1. Barkovich AJ. Hydrocephalus. In: Pediatric Neuroimaging. New York: Raven Press, 1995:439.

9.02 Complications from Ventricular Shunts

EPIDEMIOLOGY

Shunt malfunction occurs in 25% to 60% of patients. Infections occur in 1% to 5% of patients harboring shunts. Postshunt subdural hematomas are uncommon before 3 years of age and are usually related to the use of low-pressure valves or arise after vigorous drainage of very large ventricles. Slit-like ventricle syndrome is rare and refers to symptoms of increased intracranial pressure in the presence of normal ventricular size. Other, less common complications include perishunt edema and cyst formation.

CLINICAL FEATURES

Follow-up of patients with ventricular shunts is easily accomplished with noncontrast computed tomography (CT). Prior studies are very helpful. The usual symptoms of shunt function failure are headaches, lethargy, altered mental status, bulging anterior fontanelle, and enlarging head circumference. The most common causes for shunt malfunction are growth of choroid plexus or glial tissue into the tube or disconnection of the system.

In shunt infections, the clinical symptoms include intermittent low-grade fevers, anemia, dehydration, and hepatosplenomegaly. There may be signs of inflammation in the skin covering the tract of the shunt. In patients with complications involving the distal shunt segment, signs of peritonitis, intestinal obstruction, visceral perforation, pseudocyst formation, or ascites may be present. Infection of the distal shunt may produce peritonitis. We have seen one case of peritoneal seeding by "normal choroid plexus" in which intractable ascites developed in the patient.

Slit-like ventricle syndrome probably results from low-pressure headaches, intermittent shunt malfunction, or venous hypertension. Patients with this syndrome may have small heads secondary to sutural synostosis.

IMAGING FEATURES

Computed tomography is the ideal method to evaluate suspected shunt malfunction. Progressive enlargement of the ventricles, even when slight, is indicative of shunt failure (Fig. 9.02-1). Enlargement of the ventricles may be subtle because the walls become scarred in these patients. The shunts usually enter the skull through occipitoparietal or frontal burr holes. Regardless of the site of entry, the tip of the shunt ideally should be located anterior to the foramina of Monroe in the frontal horns of the lateral ventricles. At this level, there is no choroid plexus and ingrowth of this structure into the catheter is avoided. At times, several shunts are located in different parts of the ventricles. This is usually seen in patients whose ventricles are segmented by scars. The intracranial shunt portions may be connected to a single or multiple reservoirs. Discontinuity of shunts is better evaluated with plain radiographs, which should include the entire course of the catheters.

Evaluation of suspected shunt infection needs contrast enhanced CT or magnetic resonance (MR) imaging (Fig. 9.02-2). The most common finding is that of enhancement of the ependymal lining of the lateral ventricles, suggesting ventriculitis. Enhancing septations in the ventricles may also be present. The slit-like ventricle syndrome is characterized by small lateral ventricles and a thick calvarium. It probably occurs because of fibrosis of the ventricular walls or intraventricular synechiae. If the tip of a shunt becomes obstructed, cerebrospinal fluid (CSF) may leak around the catheter, producing parenchymal edema or formation of perishunt cysts (Fig. 9.02-3). The evaluation of abdominal complications of shunts requires sonograms or CT of that area. Knowledge of where the distal shunt tip was originally placed is important to avoid mistakes. The tip of the shunt may end in the peritoneal cavity, right heart, and even the gallbladder. Occasionally, patients show a granulomatous reaction where the shunt enters the ventricles. These reactive tissues may grow along the catheter and obstruct it. They appear as enhancing, small, irregular masses along the intraventricular segment of the shunt. Subdural hematomas are secondary to rapid collapse of the ventricles associated with low-pressure systems (Fig. 9.02-4). The use of medium- or high-pressure valves avoids this complication. These subdural collections usually are small, asymptomatic, and do not require drainage. MR imaging is more sensitive for the detection of small subdural hematomas. On CT and noncontrast MR imaging, subdural hematomas may be indistinguishable from meningeal fibrosis. Meningeal fibrosis may develop rapidly after shunting and enhances after contrast administration (Fig. 9.02-5).

We have used single-slice, T1-weighted gradient echo imaging obtained perpendicular to the axis of the shunt to detect CSF flow through it. Active flow appears as a tiny dot of high signal intensity inside the shunt (Fig. 9.02-6). Lack of flow-related enhancement may be caused by intermittent CSF flow or low-velocity flow, and therefore should not be interpreted as a nonfunctioning shunt in the absence of symptoms.

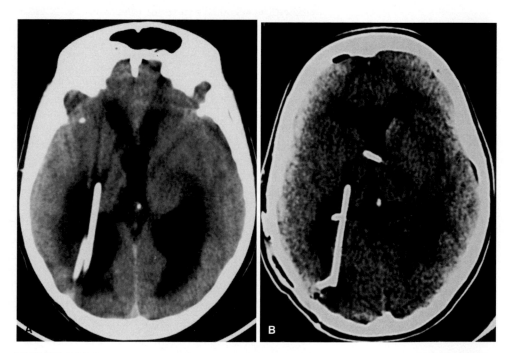

FIGURE 9.02-1.

Shunt malfunction. **A.** Axial computed tomography (CT) in a patient with two ventricular shunts (one with its tip outside the right atrium) shows moderate ventricular dilation with periventricular low densities, suggesting shunt malfunction. **B.** Axial CT in the same patient shortly after insertion of a third shunt via a right frontal approach shows tip of new shunt in region of foramina of Monroe and that the ventricles have returned to a more normal appearance. Posterior shunts could not be removed because they probably were embedded in choroid plexus and fixed in that location.

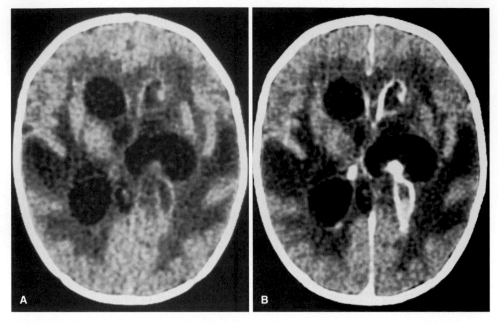

FIGURE 9.02-2.

Ventriculitis secondary to shunt infection. **A.** Noncontrast computed tomography (CT) after removal of infected shunt shows hydrocephalus and multiple ventricular loculations. There is periventricular white matter edema. **B.** Corresponding postcontrast CT image shows marked enhancement of the ependymal surface of the left lateral ventricle, compatible with ventriculitis. Mild ependymal enhancement is present in the atrium and medial-frontal horn of the right lateral ventricle. (Courtesy of S. Birchansky and N. Altman, Miami Children's Hospital, Miami, FL.)

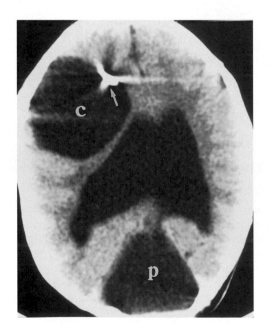

FIGURE 9.02-3.

Perishunt cyst. Axial noncontrast computed tomography in a patient with shunt malfunction shows cyst (c) surrounding the shunt catheter *(arrow)*. The lateral ventricles are dilated and there is a posterior fossa cyst (p) secondary to a Dandy-Walker malformation.

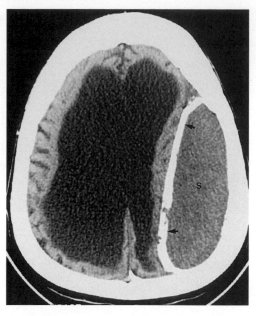

FIGURE 9.02-4.

Chronic subdural hematoma. Axial computed tomography in a patient with shunt malfunction and hydrocephalus shows left chronic subdural hematoma (S) with calcified inner wall *(arrows).*

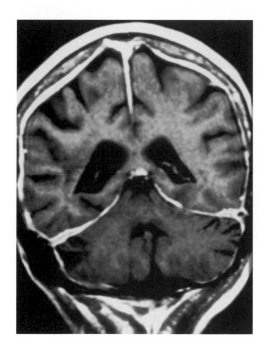

FIGURE 9.02-5.

Meningeal fibrosis. Coronal postcontrast magnetic resonance T1-weighted image 2 weeks after shunting shows marked and diffuse dural enhancement, suggesting fibrosis.

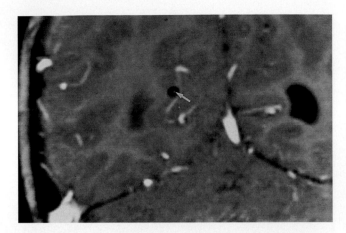

FIGURE 9.02-6.

Flow in shunt. Oblique magnetic resonance T1-weighted, single-slice gradient echo image parallel to course of intracranial segment of ventricular shunt catheter in an asymptomatic patient. There is a dot of high signal intensity *(arrow)* inside the shunt, indicating cerebrospinal fluid flow.

SUGGESTED READING

1. Castillo M, Hudgins PA, Malko JA, Burrow BK, Hoffman JC. Flow-sensitive MR imaging of ventriculoperitoneal shunts: in vitro findings, clinical applications, and pitfalls. AJNR 1991;12:667.

Imaging of the Pediatric Head, Neck, and Spine
by Mauricio Castillo and Suresh K. Mukherji,
Lippincott-Raven Publishing, Philadelphia © 1996.

10

Neurocutaneous Disorders

10.0 *Neurofibromatosis Type I*

EPIDEMIOLOGY

Neurofibromatosis type I (NF-1) affects approximately 1:4000 to 5000 individuals. It has been mapped to band 11.2 of the long arm of chromosome 17. There is a linkage with the nerve growth factor receptor gene. The rate of penetrance for this trait is almost 100%, and the rate of spontaneous mutation is about 50%. There may be a slight male predominance. Approximately 15% of NF-1 patients have central nervous system involvement.

CLINICAL FEATURES

Café-au-lait spots are commonly present at birth. They are commonly located on the trunk, measure more than 1.5 cm in diameter, and number more than six. Because 10% of normal individuals harbor these spots, they are not diagnostic of NF-1. Other cutaneous manifestations include cutaneous tumors (fibroma molluscum) and hypopigmented areas. Melanocytic hamartomas of the iris (Lisch nodules) are present in 10% of children. Optic gliomas are seen in 15% to 20% of NF-1 patients, who present with decreased visual acuity, precocious puberty, or signs of increased intracranial pressure. Tumor extension posteriorly along the optic pathways may lead to diencephalic syndrome. Approximately 75% of patients with optic pathway tumors are asymptomatic, and 65% have negative ophthalmologic examinations. Because less than 10% have progression of symptoms or deterioration of vision, screening NF-1 patients for optic pathway tumors with magnetic resonance (MR) imaging is of questionable utility. The incidence of brain astrocytomas is also increased, particularly in the tectum, where they should be differentiated from periaqueductal gliosis. So-called cerebral hamartomas are found by MR imaging studies in 60% to 80% of patients and are more common in patients who also have an optic astrocytoma. The pathology and significance of these lesions are poorly understood. Their number and location are not related to clinical symptoms. Plexiform neurofibromas involving the cranial nerves are relatively rare in NF-1 patients. Most patients with intracerebral abnormalities and cranial nerve masses probably represent an overlap between NF-1 and NF-2, and these patients may be considered as having NF-3. The main manifestation of mesodermal dysplasia is hypoplasia or absence of the greater wing of the sphenoid bone, leading to pulsatile exophthalmos or cephaloceles. The spinal canal is widened and the posterior surface of the vertebral bodies scalloped. Lateral thoracic meningoceles are common. The eyeball may be enlarged secondary to congenital glaucoma, producing buphthalmos in up to 50% of NF-1 patients. Macrocephaly and short stature are present in 10% to 40% of these patients. The rate of sarcomatous degeneration of neural tumors in NF-1 patients varies between 2% to 7%. Intracranial arterial narrowing and occlusions producing a moyamoya-like appearance may occur in 50% to 60% of NF-1 patients. Histologically, this dysplasia corresponds to intimal proliferation, which results in stenoses or occlusions. Aneurysms may also occur.

IMAGING FEATURES

Magnetic resonance is the imaging modality of choice to evaluate these patients. Optic nerve gliomas are isointense or hypointense on T1-weighted images and hyperintense on T2-weighted images (Fig. 10.0-1). Contrast enhancement is variable, but usually is absent or subtle. Occasionally it may be striking or patchy. Signal intensity abnormalities in the region of the posterior optic pathways may be related to extension from the glioma or to the presence of hamartomas. Contrast enhancement suggests glioma. Hamartomas are seen as areas of increased signal intensity on proton density and T2-weighted images, and may be slightly hyperintense on T1-weighted images

(Fig. 10.0-2A,B). They usually have little or no mass effect and do not enhance. They may show slight growth, but tend to decrease in size after 10 years of age. Hamartomas in the globus pallidi are slightly larger and may have mass effect. Pathologically, hamartomas contain spongiotic and vacuolar white matter changes. Their increased signal intensity on noncontrast MR T1-weighted images may be caused by the presence of perivascular schwannomas, piloid astrocytes, and microcalcifications. Increased T2 signal may result from intermyelinic edema, which may resolve, explaining the improvement of some of these abnormalities over time (data from DiPaolo DP, Zimmerman RA, Rorke LB, Yachnis AT. Radiologic–pathologic correlation of high-signal-intensity foci in type 1 neurofibromatosis. RSNA 1994). We have used hydrogen MR spectroscopy to differentiate them successfully from gliomas (Fig. 10.0-2C). Plexiform neurofibromas follow the course of the cranial nerves and are slightly hyperintense to muscle on T1-weighted images. They are bright on T2-weighted images and may show a central linear hypointensity, probably related to fibrous components. The greater wing of the sphenoid may be partially or completely absent, leading to protrusion of the temporal lobe and exophthalmos (Fig. 10.0-3). Temporal arachnoid cysts may occur in this setting. Moyamoya phenomenon results in stenosis or occlusion of the supraclinoid internal carotid, anterior cerebral, or middle cerebral arteries (Fig. 10.0-4). This complication is better seen on conventional angiograms, but screening may be performed with MR angiography. Calcifications on the surface of the cerebellum have been described (Fig. 10.0-5). Their significance and etiology are uncertain, but they may be related to meningoangiomatosis.

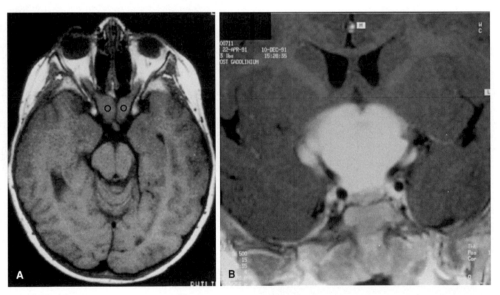

FIGURE 10.0-1

Optic astrocytoma. **A.** Noncontrast axial magnetic resonance (MR) T1-weighted image shows enlargement (O) of both prechiasmatic optic nerves in patients with neurofibromatosis type I. **B.** Postcontrast coronal MR T1-weighted image shows enhancing mass in the optic chiasm.

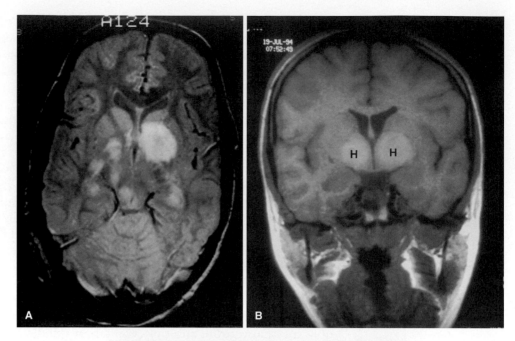

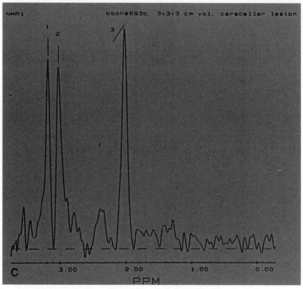

FIGURE 10.0-2

Hamartomas. **A.** Axial magnetic resonance (MR) proton density image shows multiple areas of increased signal intensity with no mass effect. The lesion in the left globus pallidus is larger than the others. Some lesions are located in the region of the posterior optic pathways and the midbrain. None of the lesions enhanced after contrast administration. (With permission from Castillo M. Neuroradiology Companion. Philadelphia: JB Lippincott, 1995.) **B.** Coronal noncontrast MR T1-weighted image shows slightly hyperintense hamartomas (H) in basal ganglia bilaterally. **C.** Proton MR spectra from a presumed hamartoma in a different patient with neurofibromatosis type I shows mild reduction in N-acetyl aspartate in an otherwise unremarkable pattern. The pattern shown is not consistent with astrocytoma. 1, creatinine; 2, choline; 3, N-acetyl aspartate.

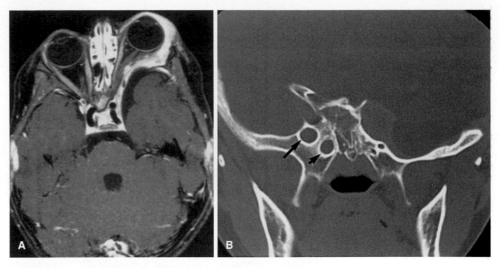

FIGURE 10.0-3.

Neurofibromas and dysplasia of greater sphenoidal wing.   **A.** Axial postcontrast fat-suppressed magnetic resonance T1-weighted image shows absence of the left greater sphenoidal wing with protrusion of the brain and cerebrospinal fluid spaces, resulting in proptosis. There is an enhancing plexiform neurofibroma arising in the left cavernous sinus and following the course of cranial nerve VI. **B.** Coronal computed tomography in a different patient with dysplasia of sphenoid on left side shows marked widening of right foramen rotundum *(longer arrow)* and vidian canal *(shorter arrow)* resulting from plexiform neurofibromata.

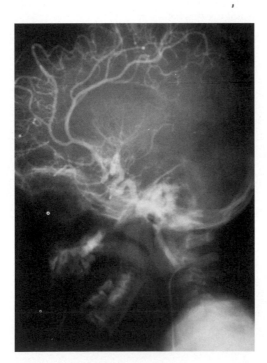

FIGURE 10.0-4.

Vascular dysplasia.   Lateral view from catheter angiogram in a patient with neurofibromatosis type I shows occluded middle cerebral artery and proliferation of perforating arteries (moyamoya phenomenon).

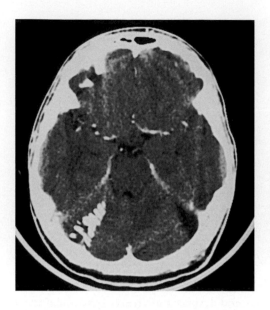

FIGURE 10.0-5.

Possible meningoangiomatosis. Axial postcontrast computed tomography shows calcifications on the superior surface of the right cerebellar hemisphere. Note that these calcifications follow the configuration of the folia. There is a suprasellar mass (optic chiasm astrocytoma).

SUGGESTED READINGS

1. Castillo M, Green C, Kwock L, et al. Proton MR spectroscopy in patients with neurofibromatosis type 1: evaluation of hamartomas and clinical correlation. AJNR 1995;16:141.
2. Braffman B, Naidich TP. The phakomatoses: part 1. Neurofibromatosis and tuberous sclerosis. Neuroimaging Clinics of North America 1994;4:299.
3. Lisernick R, Charrow J, Greenwald M, Mets M. Natural history of optic pathway tumors in children with neurofibromatosis type 1: a longitudinal study. J Pediatr 1994;125:63.
4. DiPaolo DP, Zimmerman RA, Rorke LB, Zackai EH, Bilaniuk LT, Yachmis AT. Neurofibromatosis type I: pathologic substrate of high-signal-intensity foci in the brain. Radiology 1995;195:721.

10.01 *Neurofibromatosis Type II*

EPIDEMIOLOGY

Neurofibromatosis type II (NF-2) is approximately 10 times less common than NF-1, and occurs in 1:50,000 individuals. It has been mapped to the middle of the long arm of chromosome 22. This trait is autosomal dominant. It usually manifests during adulthood and is uncommon in children.

CLINICAL FEATURES

To make the diagnosis of NF-2, one of the following criteria must be met: 1) bilateral vestibular schwannomas on imaging studies, preferably magnetic resonance imaging (Fig. 10.01-1A), and 2) a first-degree relative with NF-2 and either one vestibular schwannoma or two of the following: neurofibroma, meningioma, astrocytoma, schwannoma, and juvenile posterior subcapsular lenticular opacity.

Less than 50% of NF-2 patients have café-au-lait spots, and cutaneous neurofibromas are rare. The most common cranial nerves in which schwannomas develop are VIII, V, and III through IX. Schwannomas do not involve the nerve fibers, but rather occur in the coverings of the nerves. Therefore, some are amenable to surgical resection. Vestibular schwannomas usually become clinically evident in NF-2 patients during the third decade of life. Meningiomas (Fig. 10.01-1B) are also initially detected during the same decade. Meningiomas in NF-2 patients tend to be multiple and may be located in unusual sites. Sixteen percent of them occur inside the lateral ventricles in these patients (Fig. 10.01-2).

There are a number of other types of neurofibromatoses, which are not recognized in the World Health Organization. Type III is an overlap syndrome between types I and II. Type IV is a diverse category with multiple variants. Type V is a segmental disease, usually involving only one extremity. Type VI patients have café-au-lait spots without neurofibromas. Type VII is the same disease as type I, but has its onset late in life. Type VIII refers to variants of the disease that do not fit into any of the previous categories.

IMAGING FEATURES

Magnetic resonance is the imaging method of choice in NF-2 patients. Vestibular schwannomas are hypointense to isointense with brain on precontrast T1-weighted images. On T2-weighted images, these tumors usually are hyperintense. They enhance markedly and homogenously after contrast administration. They are centered on the internal auditory canal and have a tail of tumor extending into the canal. Occasionally, they may be internal areas of necrosis, tumor cysts, surrounding arachnoid cysts, or be completely cystic. Meningiomas are minimally hypointense to gray matter on T1-weighted images and isointense to gray matter on T2-weighted images. They may contain areas of signal void, which are related to vessels or calcifications. They enhance homogenously (but at times patchily) after contrast administration. Meningiomas and schwannomas may be very small and escape detection if contrast is not administered.

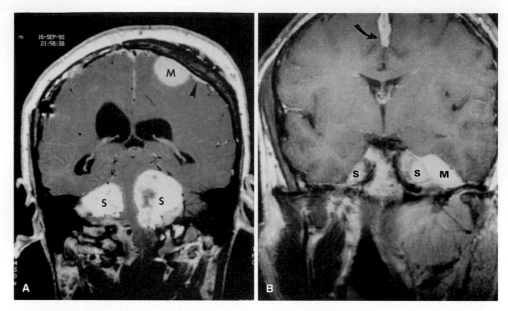

FIGURE 10.01-1.

Schwannomas and meningiomas. **A.** Coronal postcontrast magnetic resonance (MR) T1-weighted image shows large bilateral vestibular schwannomas (S) and a left parasagittal meningioma (M; note dural tail, *arrowhead*). A right-sided craniotomy for prior meningioma resection is present. **B.** Coronal postcontrast MR T1-weighted image in a different patient shows parafalcine *(curved arrow)* and left middle cranial fossa meningioma (M). There are bilateral cavernous sinus schwannomas (S).

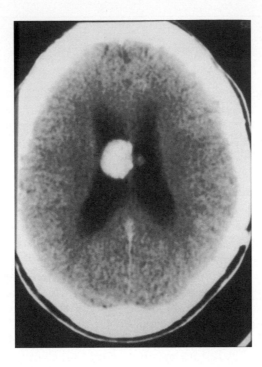

FIGURE 10.01-2.

Intraventricular meningioma. Axial noncontrast computed tomography shows markedly calcified meningioma inside the body of the right lateral ventricle. In this young adult, other meningiomas and a family history of neurofibromatosis type II were present.

SUGGESTED READING

1. Smirniotopoulos JG, Murphy FM. The phakomatoses. AJNR 1992;13:725.

10.02 *Tuberous Sclerosis*

EPIDEMIOLOGY

Tuberous sclerosis occurs in 1:29,000 to 100,000 people. It is inherited as an autosomal dominant trait with variable penetrance, but there is a 60% spontaneous mutation rate. It has been mapped to a deletion on chromosome 9. However, this finding is not always consistent, and abnormalities in chromosome 11 have also been implicated. There is no gender or racial predilection.

CLINICAL FEATURES

Seizures often begin after the first year of life, and are the most common symptom. They commonly are of the infantile spasm or partial types. In more than 25% of patients with infantile spasms, other signs of tuberous sclerosis eventually develop. There are no typical electroencephalographic findings. The degree of mental retardation is variable, and up to one-third of patients are intellectually normal. Recent data indicate that mental retardation may not be as common as previously thought. The outcome of patients with both mental retardation and seizures is poor. Facial angiofibromas (adenoma sebaceum) are first noted between 1 to 4 years of age. The lesions are located in the nose, cheeks, and chin, and enlarge with time. Hypopigmented, ash-leaf–shaped skin lesions are more common than facial angiofibromas and occur predominantly in the trunk. Retinal hamartomas occur in 50% of patients, but are often clinically silent. They tend to involve both eyes and may be multiple. The cerebral hamartomas are composed of large, bizarre, and vacuolated neurons. Also seen are areas of proliferation of fibrillary astrocytes, abnormal cortical organization, and demyelination. The treatment of these patients is geared toward the management of the seizure disorder. Outside the central nervous system, other common manifestations of this disorder include subungual fibromas, renal angiomyolipomas, heart tumors, and interstitial lung disease.

IMAGING FEATURES

Magnetic resonance (MR) is the imaging modality of choice in these patients. The most common lesions are cerebral hamartomas (Figs. 10.02-1–10.02-3). Hamartomas are seen as linear areas of abnormal signal intensity extending in a radial fashion from the periventricular regions to the subcortical regions. Less commonly, these lesions have a wedge-like configuration with their apex pointing toward the ventricles. These lesions also may have a mass-like appearance. The overlying cortex may be normal or appear flat and broad. Hamartomas are almost always hypointense to isointense on T1-weighted images, and hyperintense on T2-weighted images (Fig. 10.02-1A,B). They are more common in the frontal lobes, and may enhance after contrast administration (Fig. 10.02-2). A greater number of hamartomas are found in patients with infantile spasms, early onset of seizures, and mental disabilities. Hamartomas are also found in the cerebellum in 10% of patients. Subependymal nodules are probably the second most common MR imaging finding. Their signal intensity is variable, and they may simulate gray matter heterotopias. On postcontrast MR images, they may enhance intensely, moderately, mildly, or remain unchanged. On computed tomography, they may be calcified (Fig. 10.02-3).

Giant cell astrocytomas occur in 2% to 26% of patients with tuberous sclerosis (Fig. 10.02-1C). They arise from subependymal nodules or from germinal matrix cells that have failed to migrate. They almost always arise at the foramina of Monroe, but are rarely seen in the temporal horns and atria of the lateral ventricles or the cerebral hemipheres. Unilateral hydrocephalus is commonly present, but if the mass is large, both lateral ventricles may be dilated. The tumors are hypointense to isointense on T1-weighted images and hyperintense on T2-weighted images. Some have areas of signal void related to calcification of vessels. All giant cell astrocytomas enhance after contrast administration. Other cerebral tumors known to occur in these patients are pilocytic astrocytomas, fibrillary astrocytomas, and gliomatosis.

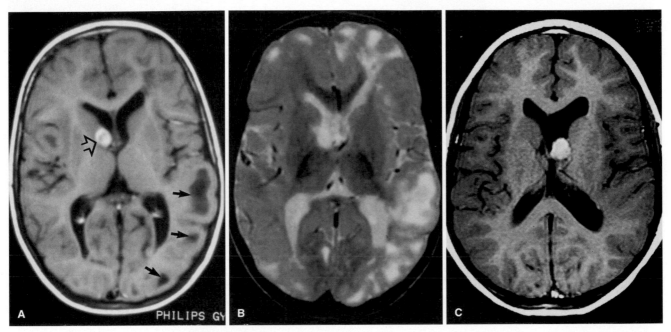

FIGURE 10.02-1.

Giant cell astrocytoma and hamartomas. **A.** Axial postcontrast magnetic resonance (MR) T1-weighted image shows multiple nonenhancing subcortical hamartomas *(solid arrows)*. Note that cortex overlying these lesions is somewhat flattened. There is an enhancing presumed giant cell astrocytoma *(open arrow)* in the region of the right foramen of Monroe. **B.** Corresponding axial MR T2-weighted image shows that all lesions (including the one at the right foramen of Monroe) are hyperintense. This sequence shows to a better advantage the full extent of the hamartomas. **C.** Axial postcontrast MR T1-weighted image shows enhancing giant cell astrocytoma (presumed) at the left foramen on Monroe. There is some dilation of the left lateral ventricle.

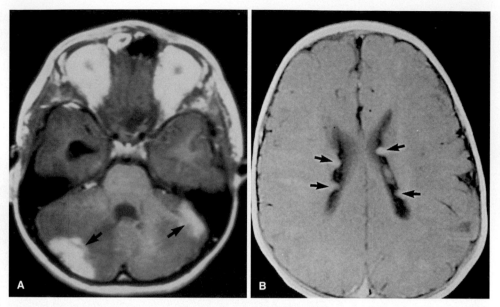

FIGURE 10.02-2.

Enhancing hamartomas.   **A.** Axial postcontrast magnetic resonance (MR) T1-weighted image shows somewhat wedge-shaped enhancing hamartomas *(arrows)* in the cerebellum of a patient with tuberous sclerosis. Note dilated right temporal horn of the lateral ventricle secondary to giant cell astrocytoma at foramen of Monroe. These enhancing abnormalities could be confused with infarctions, which also occur in these patients who have an abnormal cerebral vasculature. **B.** Axial postcontrast MR T1-weighted image shows multiple enhancing hamartomas *(arrows)* along the outer walls of both lateral ventricles.

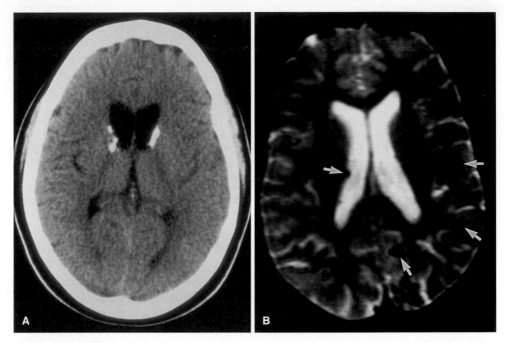

FIGURE 10.02-3.

Calcified hamartomas. **A.** Axial noncontrast computed tomography shows calcified hamartomas in the outer walls of the frontal horns of the lateral ventricles. **B.** Axial gradient echo magnetic resonance T2-weighted image (different patient) shows signal void *(arrows)* from several calcified hamartomas.

SUGGESTED READINGS

1. Braffman BH, Bilaniuk LT, Naidich TP, et al. MR imaging of tuberous sclerosis: pathogenesis of this phakomatosis, use of gadopenetate dimeglumine, and literature review. Radiology 1992;183:227.
2. Shepherd CW, Houser OW, Gomez MR. MR findings in tuberous sclerosis complex and correlation with seizure development and mental impairment. AJNR 1995;16: 149.

10.03 *Sturge-Weber Syndrome*

EPIDEMIOLOGY

The exact incidence of this rare syndrome is not known. The mode of inheritance has been described as both autosomal dominant and recessive. There is no gender predilection.

CLINICAL FEATURES

The most typical sign is that of a facial angioma (nevus flammeus or port wine nevus) involving the territory innervated by the first and second divisions of the trigeminal nerves. The presence of an angioma in the forehead and superior eyelid is highly indicative of Sturge-Weber syndrome. The oral and upper airway mucosas may be involved. The facial angioma is commonly unilateral, but may be bilateral, and usually involves the ipsilateral choroid plexus and occipitoparietal lobes. The temporal lobes may also be involved, and occasionally the abnormality is bilateral. Ocular findings include glaucoma (25%), iris heterochromia, strabismus, optic atrophy, and prominent retinal veins. Prominent symptoms include hemiparesis, homonymous hemianopsia, and seizures, which are primarily partial motor. Seizures occur in over 75% of patients. Electroencephalography shows decreased amplitude and frequency of activity in the affected cerebral hemisphere. Hemiparesis develops in up to 30% of patients. Some patients are mentally retarded.

Pathologically, the vascular malformation is a low-pressure, low-flow angioma of the leptomeninges. There is absence of cortical veins and, as such, the deep medullary veins become hypertrophied and redirect the blood drainage toward the choroid plexus, which also shows angiomatous changes. The underlying brain shows cortical calcifications (layers 2 and 3), atrophy, gliosis, ischemic damage, and demyelination. Treatment is geared toward the management of seizures. Mentally retarded patients with unilateral brain abnormalities and intractable seizures may benefit from hemispherectomy. Patients with bilateral abnormalities have a very poor prognosis.

IMAGING FEATURES

Intracortical calcifications are seen in over 90% of patients by plain radiographs or computed tomography scans, and may be bilateral in 20% of cases (Fig. 10.03-1). By magnetic resonance (MR) imaging, these calcifications are hypointense on all sequences. The involved brain is atrophic. There may be hyperpneumatization of the paranasal sinuses and mastoids as well as elevation of the petrous bone and thickening of the calvarium in an attempt to compensate for the loss of cerebrum. On postcontrast MR imaging, the affected leptomeninges are thick and show prominent enhancement (Fig. 10.03-2). The ipsilateral choroid plexus may appear enlarged (Fig. 10.03-3). The affected choroid plexus may be hyperintense on T2-weighted images. The underlying white matter may show increased signal intensity on T2-weighted images, probably related to gliosis. The underlying white matter also may show punctate or serpiginous areas of signal void related to hypertrophy of the deep draining veins. Occasionally, the myelination of the white matter underlying the pial angioma may be accelerated. Anomalies of neuronal migration such as pachygyria and lissencephaly may occur in patients with Sturge-Weber syndrome. Polymicrogyria may also occur. In the eye, the choroid may be thickened and enhance. Retinal detachments may be present. Congenital glaucoma with secondary buphthalmos may occur. Eye abnormalities are present in up to 30% of patients with Sturge-Weber syndrome

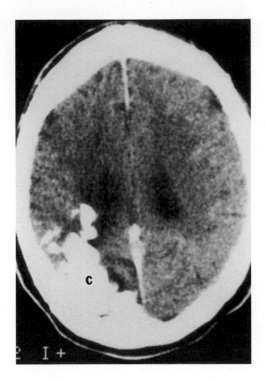

FIGURE 10.03-1.

Calcified cortex. Axial postcontrast computed tomography shows heavily calcified cortex (C) and underlying white matter in the right posterior parietal region in a patient with Sturge-Weber syndrome. The right cerebral hemisphere is smaller than the left one. (With permission from Castillo M. Neuroradiology Companion. Philadelphia: JB Lippincott, 1995.)

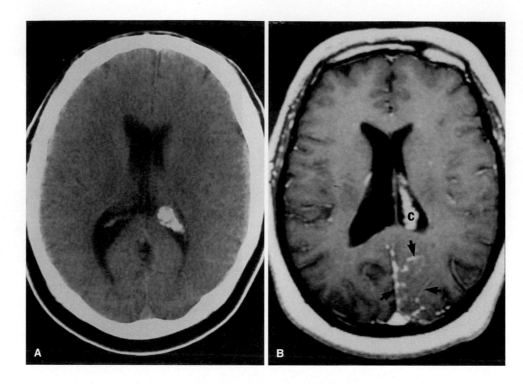

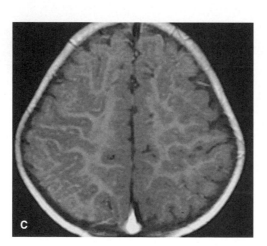

FIGURE 10.03-2.

Noncalcified pial angioma. **A.** Axial noncontrast computed tomography shows large calcification in the left choroid plexus and slight reduction in the size of the ipsilateral cerebral hemisphere. **B.** Axial postcontrast magnetic resonance (MR) T1-weighted image in the same patient shows enhancing and enlarged left choroid plexus (C) and pial enhancement (*arrows;* presumably secondary to angioma) in the left parietooccipital region. **C.** Axial postcontrast MR T1-weighted image shows diffuse pial enhancement throughout right cerebral hemisphere in a boy with an ipsilateral facial nevus. This was the only finding in the brain of this child.

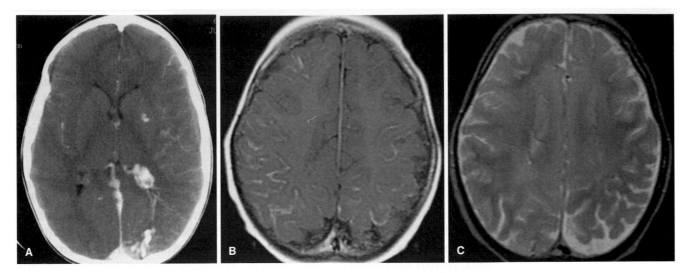

FIGURE 10.03-3.

Combination of calcified and noncalcified angioma. **A.** Postcontrast computed tomography shows calcified left occipital cortex and enlarged left choroid plexus. The pial vessels of the left hemisphere are increased in size and number and are well visualized. There is a small focus of calcification in the left basal ganglia. **B.** Axial postcontrast magnetic resonance (MR) T1-weighted image shows diffuse pial enhancement in both cerebral hemispheres. **C.** Corresponding axial MR T2-weighted image shows atrophy in the left posterior parietal region with reduction in the overall size of the left hemisphere.

SUGGESTED READINGS

1. Elster AD, Chen MYM. MR imaging of Sturge-Weber syndrome: role of gadopentetate dimeglumine and gradient-echo techniques. AJNR 1990;11:685.
2. Stimac GK, Solomon MA, Newton TH, et al. CT and MR of angiomatous malformations of the choroid plexus in patients with Sturge-Weber disease. AJNR 1986;7: 623.

10.05 Uncommon Phakomatoses

Table 10.05-1 lists the epidemiologic, clinical, and imaging features of the less common phakomatoses.

TABLE 10.05-1. *Epidemiologic, Clinical, and Imaging Features of the Uncommon Phakomatoses*

Disorder	Genetics	Clinical Features	Imaging Features
Klippel-Trenaunay-Weber syndrome	Unknown	Skin hemangiomas, varicosities, hypertrophy of limbs	Macrocephaly, findings similar to Sturge-Weber syndrome
Osler-Weber-Rendu disease	Unknown	Pulmonary arteriovenous fistulae, capillary telangiectasias in multiple sites	Skull and dura arteriovenous malformations, cerebral infarcts
Multiple hemangioma syndrome	Unknown	Vascular anomalies of skin, brain (seizures), liver, kidney, retina, optic nerve, and bones	Multiple cerebral cavernous angiomas (Fig. 10.05-1)
Wyburn-Mason syndrome	Unknown	Visual disturbances, seizures, headache, subarachnoid hemorrhage	Vascular malformations in face, retina, and brain
Ataxia–telangiectasia	Autosomal recessive, 1:40,000 live births, abnormality in chromosome 11q22–23	Ataxia, oculomotor abnormalities, telangiectasias in exposed skin, recurrent sinopulmonary infections, elevated α-fetoprotein, lymphoma, leukemia	Cerebellar atrophy, atrophy of vermis and dentate nuclei, abnormal meningeal vessels (Fig. 10.05-2), increased incidence of medulloblastoma
Neurocutaneous melanosis	Unknown but nonfamilial	Abnormally pigmented skin, malignant leptomeningeal melanoma	Areas of high signal intensity in anteromedial temporal lobes and cerebellum
Incontinentia pigmenti	X-linked trait mapped to Xpll.21	Stages of skin lesions: vesicles, verrucae, pigmented, and atrophic scars	Hemorrhagic cerebral infarcts, microcephaly, optic nerve atrophy, hydrocephalus, polymicrogyria, skull deformities
Hypomelanosis of Ito	Autosomal dominant, mostly girls	Linear whorled skin lesions, abnormal skin, hair, teeth, nails, bones, and eyes, optic nerve hypoplasia	CNS findings in 50% of patients, gray matter heterotopias, cortical dysplasias, hemimegalencephaly, porencephaly, gliosis, agenesis of corpus callosum
Epidermal nevus syndrome	Unknown	Yellow-brown hairless plaque in midline of face and scalp, mental retardation, seizures, eye abnormalities	50% of patients have CNS anomalies, most commonly hemimegalencephaly with multiple neuronal migration defects (Fig. 10.05-3)
Cowden disease	Autosomal dominant	Gastrointestinal polyps, breast cancer and fibrocystic disease, thyroid tumors, ovarian cysts, liver hemangiomas and hamartomas, neurofibromas, meningiomas	Lhermitte-Duclos disease of the cerebellum
Hypomelanosis of Ito	Unknown	Decreased size and number of melasomes and melanocytes	Cerebral atrophy, migration anomalies, gliosis, dysgenesis of corpus callosum, porencephaly, cysts, white matter abnormalities, macrocephaly (Fig. 10.05-4)

CNS, central nervous system.

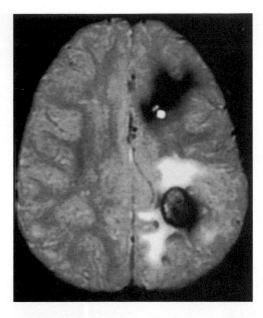

FIGURE 10.05-1.

Multiple cerebral cavernous angiomas.
Axial magnetic resonance T2-weighted
image shows two of many cavernous angiomas in the brain of this child who
had a sibling with similar findings. Note
that the posterior angioma is surrounded
by high signal intensity, which could be
related to gliosis. The outer core of hypointensity probably results from hemosiderin.

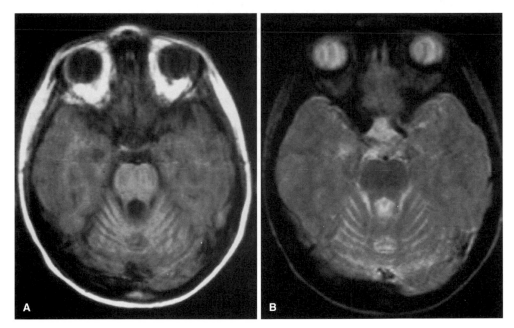

FIGURE 10.05-2.

Ataxia–telangiectasia. **A.** Axial magnetic resonance (MR) T1-weighted image shows
diffuse atrophy of the cerebellum. **B.** Corresponding MR T2-weighted image shows atrophy again and no hemorrhages. (Case courtesy of M. Tennison, M.D., University of
North Carolina, Chapel Hill, NC.)

PART TWO
HEAD AND NECK

Imaging of the Pediatric Head, Neck, and Spine
by Mauricio Castillo and Suresh K. Mukherji,
Lippincott-Raven Publishing, Philadelphia © 1996.

11
Orbit

11.0 *Applied Embryology*

Three different cell layers contribute to the formation of the eye: the forebrain neuroectoderm (retina, iris, optic nerve), the surface ectoderm (lens), and the mesoderm (vascular structures, sclera, choroid).

Step 1. Formation of the Optic Vesicles

The formation of the eye begins during the fourth week of gestation when grooves appear in the neural folds (optic sulci) of the forebrain in the developing embryo (Fig. 11.0-1A). The optic sulci invaginate to form the optic vesicles, which are the precursors of most of the structures that comprise the globe (Fig. 11.0-1B). Progressive growth of the optic vesicles results in flattening of the lateral surfaces and constriction of the connections with the forebrain, forming the optic stalk. The optic stalk is the precursor to the optic nerve. With further development, the optic vesicle invaginates, forming a double-walled structure referred to as the optic cup (Fig. 11.0-1C,D). Linear defects referred to as the optic fissures, which contain vascular mesenchyme, develop along the inferior surface of the optic cups. The margins of the optic fissure eventually fuse, thus trapping the developing hyaloid vessels within the optic stalk. Abnormalities resulting from insults at this stage include colobomas.

Step 2. Formation of Vascular Structures

The vascular mesenchyme gives rise to several important components, including the hyaloid blood vessels, sclera, and choroid. The innermost mesenchyme forms the choroid and is adherent to the underlying retinal pigment epithelium. The outer mesenchyme gives rise to the sclera and is continuous with the dura. The fetal vascular system can be divided into anterior and posterior compartments based, in part, on the expected position of the lens. The anterior component consists of the pupillary membrane, which develops from small vascular buds that grow inward to supply the vascular mesoderm anterior to the lens. The posterior component is located within the vitreous and includes the main hyaloid artery, vasa hyaloidea propria, and the tunica vasculosa lentis. The hyaloid artery develops in the third week of gestation and arises from a branch of the dorsal ophthalmic artery (Fig. 11.0-1E). This artery extends from the posterior aspect of the globe to the lens. The hyaloid artery provides blood supply to the lens (posterior tunica vasculosa lentis), optic nerve, and vitreous (vasa hyaloidea propria). Normally, the hyaloid vascular system involutes by the eighth month of gestation. The vasa hyaloidea is usually the first system to regress, followed by the tunica vasculosa lentis and eventually the main hyaloid artery itself.

Step 3. Formation of the Lens and Vitreous

Induction of the surface ectoderm by the adjacent optic vesicles results in the formation of the lenses. Initially, the surface ectoderm forms the lens placode, which eventually separates from the surrounding ectoderm. The edges of the placode fuse to form the lens vesicle. Progressive growth eventually results in the obliteration of the lens cavity and completes the formation of the lenses.

The vitreous develops in the hollow of the optic vesicle. The primary vitreous arises from the vesicular mesenchyme within the optic cup. The primary vitreous is engulfed by the secondary vitreous. The secondary vitreous is gelatinous, and its origin is unknown.

The retina is derived from the forebrain and from the two walls of the optic cup. The inner wall forms the neural retina, which differentiates into the photoreceptors (rods, cones, and ganglion cells). The outer wall forms the retinal pigment epithelium and becomes firmly attached to the underlying choroid. More anteriorly, the outer layer of the optic cup forms the ciliary body. The ciliary muscles arise from the mesenchyme located at the margin of the optic cup. The iris develops from both layers of the optic cup and is in continuity with the neural retina and the ciliary body. The iris grows centrally and eventually surrounds the lens.

The embryogenesis of the vitreous begins in the first month of gestation. The primary vitreous develops in the space between the retina and the developing lens. It is composed of mesodermally derived tissue, which includes the hyaloid vessels and its various branches and a fibrillar meshwork that is thought by some to be of neuroectodermal origin. The secondary is the adult vitreous, and begins to appear during the second month of gestation. It is composed primarily of water (99%) bound to collagen fibers and hyaluronic acid. The secondary vitreous normally fills the vitreous cavity by the sixth month of gestation. The primary vitreous is confined to a small central canal (Cloquet canal) that extends from the optic disc to the posterior surface of the lens. A tertiary vitreous forms during the fourth month of gestation and is the precursor to the zonules of Zinn, which are the suspensory ligaments of the lens. Failure of the normal regression of the primary vitreous and associated fetal hyaloid vascular system results in persistent hyperplastic primary vitreous.

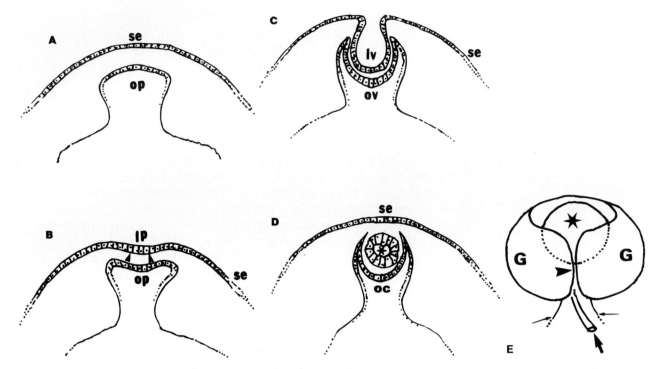

FIGURE 11.0-1.

Diagram illustrating the embryogenesis of the eye. **A.** At approximately 24 days of life, the optic pit (op) evaginates towards the surface ectoderm (se). The neural tube is closed at this stage. **B.** At approximately 28 days of life, the optic pit (op) induces thickening and elongation of the cells in the mid-portion of the surface ectoderm (se). This forms the lenticular plate (lp), which is slightly invaginated into the optic pit (now in the process of becoming the optic vesicle). The lenticular plate will become the lens placode and later the lens vesicle. **C.** During the second month of life, the invagination of the lens vesicle (lv) into the optic vesicle (ov) is well advanced. The neck of the lens vesicle begins to narrow. se, Surface ectoderm. **D.** The lens vesicle (star) is now completely detached from the surface ectoderm (se), which again becomes smooth. The optic cup (oc) is now a bilayered structure. **E.** The globe (G) is now formed and encloses the lens vesicle (star). In its inferionasal aspect, the globe contains the embryonic fissure *(arrowhead)*, which traps the hyaloid artery *(broader arrow)* in the region of the developing optic disc *(thin arrows)*. Failure of embryonic fissure closure results in colobomas anywhere from the iris (anterior) to the optic disc (posterior).

SUGGESTED READINGS

1. Moore KL, ed. The eye and ear in the developing human: clinically oriented embryology, 4th ed. Philadelphia: WB Saunders, 1988:402–420.
2. Mafee MF, Goldberg MF. Persistent hyperplastic primary vitreous (PHPV): role of computed tomography and magnetic resonance. Radiol Clin North Am 1987;25: 683.
3. Sahel JA, Brini A, Albert DM. Pathology of the retina and vitreous. In: Albert DM, Jakoviec FA, eds. Principles and Practice of Ophthalmology. Philadelphia: WB Saunders, 1994:2242.

11.01 *Anophthalmos*

EPIDEMIOLOGY

Anophthalmos is absence of one or both globes. Most cases of anophthalmos are sporadic, although hereditary forms have been recorded, including autosomal recessive, autosomal dominant, and X-linked recessive. Anophthalmos has also been associated with chromosomal anomalies, including Kleinfelter syndrome and trisomy 13. Anophthalmos has been produced in laboratory animals by applying minute trauma at a specific time in development. A number of toxins and drugs have also been used to induce anophthalmos. Deficiencies of vitamin A, galactose, adenine, and leucine have also been associated with anophthalmos.

CLINICAL FEATURES

True anophthalmos is extremely rare, and definitive diagnosis requires histologic evaluation to exclude the presence of normal neuroectodermal structures such as the retina and optic nerve. Intraorbital structures that are not derived from neuroectoderm, including the conjunctiva, lacrimal apparatus, and extraocular muscles, are normally present in microphthalmos. Most cases of anophthalmos are severe forms of microphthalmos, and therefore the term "clinical anophthalmos" is preferred by some.

True anophthalmos is caused by a failure of outgrowth of the optic vesicles from the diencephalon. Anophthalmos is divided into three types. Primary anophthalmos occurs in otherwise normal children and results from an isolated failure of invagination of the optic pit. Secondary anophthalmos results from a generalized suppression of forebrain development. The corpus callosum may be absent in these patients. A third type is a degenerative form caused by regression of initially normal ocular development.

There is no definitive treatment for anophthalmos. Early use of ocular implants is helpful for stimulating growth of the bony orbit and preventing cosmetic deformities.

IMAGING FEATURES

Both computed tomography and magnetic resonance (MR) imaging may be used in patients with anophthalmos; however, we prefer MR imaging (Fig. 11.01-1). Primary anophthalmos is associated with lack of formation of the visual pathways. Besides absence of the globes, this condition is associated with absence of the optic nerves and chiasm. The remainder of the visual pathway, including the optic tracts, lateral geniculate bodies, and calcarine cortex, may be gliotic and atrophic. Ocular soft tissues may be present within the orbit in patients with clinical anophthalmos. Coalescent tissue may be found in the orbits of patients with true anophthalmos. Differentiating this from rudimentary globes due to severe microphthalmos may be difficult by imaging alone. However, the absence of the optic nerves and chiasm is helpful in confirming the diagnosis of true anophthalmos.

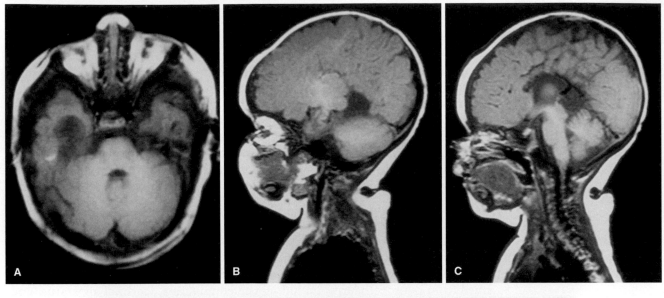

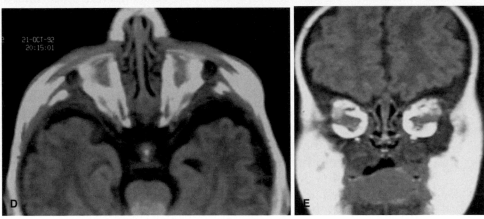

FIGURE 11.01-1.

Anophthalmos. **A.** Axial magnetic resonance (MR) T1-weighted image shows absent globes. **B.** Parasagittal MR T1-weighted image shows absent globe (same patient). **C.** Midsagittal MR T1-weighted image in same patient shows absent corpus callosum. This finding implies an anomaly of forebrain and optic placode formation. **D.** Axial MR T1-weighted image in a different patient shows bilateral anophthalmos. **E.** Coronal MR T1-weighted image (same patient) shows absent globes. The brain was normal, implying primary failure of invagination of the optic pit.

SUGGESTED READINGS

1. Sarraf D, Schwartz JS, Lee DA. Ocular size and shape. In: Isenberg SJ, ed. The Eye in Infancy. St. Louis: CV Mosby, 1994:275.
2. Sobol DF, Salvolini U, Newton TH. Computed tomography: ocular and orbital pathology. In: Newton TH, Bilaniuk LT, eds. Modern Neuroradiology: Radiology of the Eye and Orbit. Kentfield: Clavadel, 1990:9.1.

11.02 Microphthalmos

EPIDEMIOLOGY

Microphthalmos refers to a small globe. Microphthalmos has been reported to occur in 1:2000 live births, and there is no gender predilection. Seventy-five percent of cases are sporadic, although autosomal recessive, autosomal dominant, and X-linked forms have been reported. Microphthalmos has been associated with a variety of other conditions, such as persistent hyperplastic primary vitreous, buphthalmos and congenital glaucoma, congenital rubella syndrome, fetal alcohol syndrome, basal cell nevus syndrome, Hallermann-Streiff syndrome, Treacher Collins syndrome, Sjögren-Larsson syndrome, Lenz microphthalmos syndrome, CHARGE syndrome, epidermal nevus syndrome, Rubinstein-Taybi syndrome, Fanconi syndrome, and Diamond-Blackfan syndrome. Microphthalmos is also associated with a variety of chromosomal anomalies, including trisomies, duplications, and deletions.

CLINICAL FEATURES

The reduced volume of an eye may be the result of either congenital underdevelopment or acquired causes. Over 95% of ocular growth occurs within the first year of life. The transverse diameter of the globe at 1 year of age is 20 to 21 mm. Strict criteria for diagnosing microphthalmos do not exist; however, an adult eye with an axial diameter of less than 20 mm may be considered microphthalmic.

Microphthalmos covers a spectrum of anomalies and is not caused by a specific developmental insult. Rather, interruption of growth of the optic vesicle at almost any time may lead to this condition. The earlier the insult occurs in development, the more severe the microphthalmos. The term "microphthalmos" includes a spectrum of anomalies, ranging from "clinical anophthalmos" to a slightly reduced volume with normal visual acuity. Microphthalmos may be isolated or may occur in association with other ocular or systemic abnormalities. The isolated form is frequently mild and is often associated with normal vision. Nanophthalmos is a form of microphthalmos in which there is a small globe with a small cornea. It is caused by a developmental arrest after closure of the embryonic fissure. In these patients, ophthalmoscopic examination reveals a narrow angle, shallow anterior chamber, and a high lens–volume ratio, which predisposes to the development of acute-angle glaucoma. Microphthalmos with cyst is a severe malformation often seen in association with scleral coloboma. The cyst may be in direct communication with the coloboma. The coloboma results from developmental arrest in the closure of the embryonic fissure, with the cyst representing herniation of the embryonic neuroectoderm. The cyst may vary in size from a small outpouching to a mass large enough to displace the globe. The walls of the cyst are composed of collagenous connective tissue, which is histologically similar to sclera, but is lined by neuroectoderm. Microphthalmos with cyst is usually sporadic and unilateral. Funduscopic examination in mild cases may be unremarkable. Patients with microphthalmos with cyst often have severe refractive amblyopia and a poor visual prognosis.

Occasionally, microphthalmos may result from previous trauma, inflammation, infection, and other processes in which there is destruction of the globe. An acquired small eye is referred to as *phthisis bulbi*.

IMAGING FEATURES

Either computed tomography (CT) or magnetic resonance (MR) imaging may be used initially to evaluate patients suspected of having microphthalmos (Fig. 11.02-1). Most patients may be adequately screened with CT. MR imaging is preferred for evaluating the presence of associated intracranial abnormalities, including dysgenesis of the corpus callosum, lipomas, and the medial cleft syndrome (Fig. 11.02-2). The optic nerves and chiasm may be small.

Imaging studies typically show a small globe(s), which may be associated with a retroocular cyst (Fig. 11.02-3). In long-standing cases, the bony orbit may be hypoplastic. As mentioned, the size of an associated cyst is variable, and it may at times be larger than the globe, causing proptosis or displacement of the small eye. Patients with phthisis bulbi demonstrate a hyperdense, shrunken globe that may contain intraocular calcification or ossification (Fig. 11.02-4).

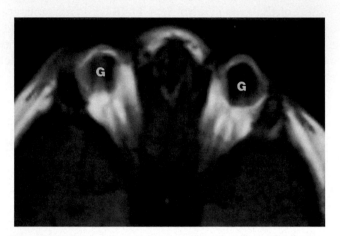

FIGURE 11.02-1.

Primary microphthalmos. Axial magnetic resonance T1-weighted image shows marked bilateral microphthalmos (G).

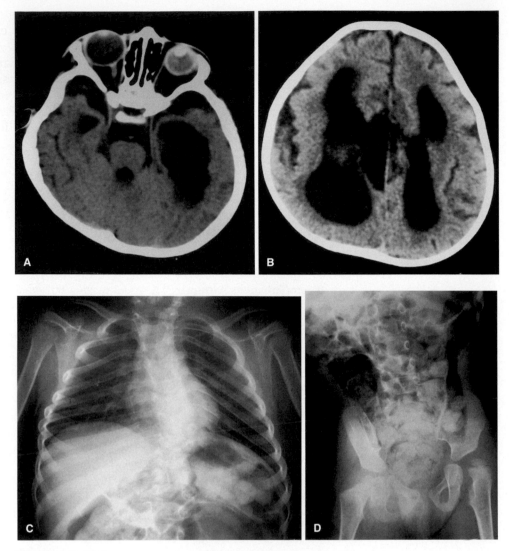

FIGURE 11.02-2.

Microphthalmos in Aicardi syndrome. **A.** Axial computed tomography (CT) shows small left globe, which is hyperdense. Note dilation of temporal tips (left > right) of lateral ventricles. **B.** Axial CT shows parallel lateral ventricles with colpocephaly and interhemispheric cyst compatible with agenesis of corpus callosum. **C.** Frontal chest radiograph shows thoracic levoscoliosis secondary to vertebral segmentation defects. **D.** Frontal radiograph shows dysplastic hips. This syndrome occurs in girls, who present with infantile spasms, mental retardation, cleft palate, and chorioretinal lacunae.

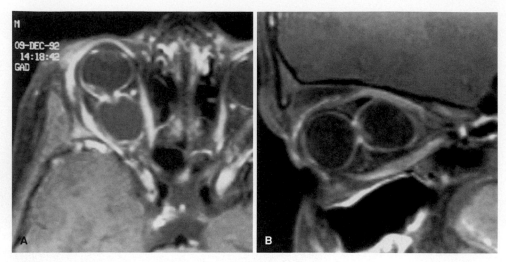

FIGURE 11.02-3.

Microphthalmos with cyst.   A. Axial magnetic resonance (MR) T1-weighted image shows right small eye with large posterior cyst. **B.** Oblique MR T1-weighted image shows cyst arising at optic nerve insertion similar to a coloboma. (Case courtesy of J. Alarcon, Scottish Rite Childrens Hospital, Atlanta, GA.)

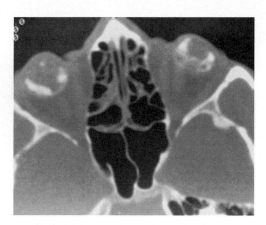

FIGURE 11.02-4.

Acquired microphthalmos.   Axial computed tomography shows small, shrunken, and calcified globes (phthisis bulbi).

SUGGESTED READINGS

1. Sarraf D, Schwartz JS, Lee DA. Ocular size and shape. In: Isenberg SJ, ed. The Eye in Infancy. St. Louis: CV Mosby, 1994:275.
2. Sobol DF, Salvolini U, Newton TH. Computed tomography: ocular and orbital pathology. In: Newton TH, Bilaniuk LT, eds. Modern Neuroradiology: Radiology of the Eye and Orbit. Kentfield: Clavadel, 1990:9.1.

11.03 *Buphthalmos*

EPIDEMIOLOGY

Buphthalmos refers to an enlarged globe resulting from increased intraocular pressure. This disorder occurs mostly in infants and young children. There is no gender predilection.

CLINICAL FEATURES

The term "buphthalmos" is derived from the Greek *bous*, meaning "ox," and *ophthalmos*, meaning "eye." Buphthalmos is believed to be secondary to obstruction of the Schlemm canal by masses or membranes composed of aberrant mesodermal tissues. Increased intraocular pressure leading to glaucoma distends the elastic outer coat of the globe over time. The globe in infants is especially prone to enlargement from increased intraocular pressure because its collagen filaments are not yet rigid and may be easily stretched. Buphthalmos may be an isolated finding or associated with a multisystem disease. Buphthalmia is an unusual autosomal recessive disorder characterized by bilaterally enlarged globes but not associated with glaucoma or increased intraocular pressure. This disorder is associated with Sturge-Weber syndrome, neurofibromatosis type I, Lowe (cerebrohepatorenal) syndrome, ocular mesodermal dysplasia (Axenfeld or Rieger anomaly), homocystinuria, and aniridia.

Clinically, newborns with congenital glaucoma present with hazy corneas, whereas older children present with epiphora (tearing), a large eye, or both. Other findings include proptosis and lid swelling. Once increased intraocular pressure has been identified, immediate treatment is essential. Mild cases may be treated with acetozolamide. More severe cases may require surgical decompression by performing a goniotomy or a trabeculotomy.

IMAGING FEATURES

Either computed tomography (CT) or magnetic resonance (MR) imaging may be used to image patients with buphthalmos. The preferred imaging modality may depend on proper identification of associated anomalies when buphthalmos occurs in combination with a multisystem disorder. Radiographically, the eye is diffusely enlarged (Fig. 11.03-1). The CT attenuation and MR imaging signal characteristics of the vitreous are normal in early stages of the disease. The sclera may be thin, the anterior chamber enlarged, and the ventral surface of the lens flattened. Microphthalmos and phthisis bulbi may occur later in the course of the disease secondary to uncontrolled elevated intraocular pressure.

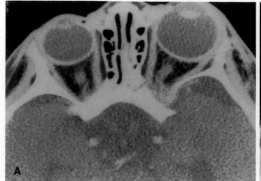

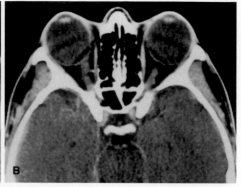

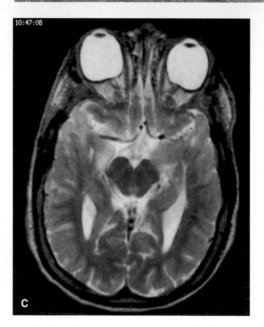

FIGURE 11.03-1.

Buphthalmos. **A.** In a patient with neurofibromatosis type I, axial computed tomography (CT) shows enlarged left globe. Note dysplasia of greater wing of left sphenoid with abnormal enhancing soft tissues (neurofibromas?) in enlarged superior orbital fissure. (With permission from Castillo M, Quencer RM, Glaser J, Altman N. Congenital glaucoma and buphthalmos in a child with neurofibromatosis. J Clin Neuro Ophthalmol 1988; 8:69.) **B.** Axial CT shows bilateral buphthalmos in a patient with glaucoma. **C.** Axial magnetic resonance T2-weighted image shows bilateral buphthalmos with posterior staphylomas in a patient with Cockayne syndrome.

SUGGESTED READINGS

1. Castillo M, Quencer RM, Glaser J, Altman N. Congenital glaucoma and buphthalmos in a child with neurofibromatosis. J Clin Neurol Ophthalmol 1988;8:69.
2. Sarraf D, Schwartz JS, Lee DA. Ocular size and shape. In: Isenberg SJ, ed. The Eye in Infancy. St. Louis: CV Mosby, 1994:275.

11.04 *Colobomas*

EPIDEMIOLOGY

Colobomas are congenital fissures or gaps of the globe that may involve the eyelid, iris, retina, lens, or optic nerve. Colobomas may be acquired or congenital. The exact incidence of this entity in the general population is not known, but it probably occurs in less than 1:1000 individuals. Children of an affected parent have a greater than 40% probability of having a coloboma. The incidence is equal in boys and girls. Most colobomas are inherited as an autosomal dominant trait with variable penetrance. A sporadic variety also exists. Colobomas may be associated with multisystem disorders such as Lenz microphthalmia syndrome, Goltz's focal dermal hypoplasia, Meckel syndrome, Warburg syndrome, Aicardi syndrome, and CHARGE (colobomatous microphthalmos, heart defects, choanal atresia, retarded growth, genital anomalies, ear anomalies) syndrome.

CLINICAL FEATURES

Colobomas may be isolated or associated with other ocular abnormalities, including microphthalmos, optic nerve sheath cyst, tilted disc syndrome (Fuchs coloboma), and congenital optic pit. Colobomas may be unilateral but are more commonly bilateral. They are asymmetric in size when they are bilateral. Colobomas arise from a defect in the closure of the optic fissure. The optic fissure is a groove that extends along the inferonasal aspect of the optic cup and stalk. Normally, this fissure closes 33 to 40 days after conception. Therefore, all structures adjacent to this fissure or those containing primordial vascular mesenchyme are predisposed to the development of colobomas. A defect within the anterior aspect of the embryonic fissure causes a cleft in the iris pigment epithelium, resulting in iris coloboma. Retinochoroidal colobomas are formed when the sensory elements of the retina fail to converge with the retinal pigment layer. Posteriorly, the optic nerve head may be involved in colobomas. The location of the defects is characteristically inferior and slightly medial. Colobomas may also occur in other locations and are caused by an atypical location of the optic fissure.

Findings on funduscopic evaluation range from slightly increased physiologic cupping to large excavations. Retinal colobomas appear as well demarcated, whitish lesions in the inferior fundus and may extend into the optic disc. Optic nerve colobomas may demonstrate incomplete or total excavation of the optic disc. Some patients present with a reduced red reflex; therefore, other etiologies of leukokoria such as retinoblastoma must be excluded.

"Morning glory syndrome" refers to the appearance of a large optic nerve head coloboma with involvement of the adjacent retina. On funduscopy, the optic disc is excavated with a central core of white or tan glial tissue. Recent reports suggest that morning glory syndrome, optic nerve pits, and congenital tilted disc syndrome (Fuchs coloboma) are all derived from the same abnormality that produces the typical coloboma. Morning glory syndrome is commonly unilateral.

Most colobomas are associated with microphthalmos. The degree of visual loss depends on the degree of the ocular malformation and the degree of microphthalmia. Other commonly associated ocular anomalies include cysts and optic nerve atrophy. Intracranial abnormalities in patients with colobomas include basal encephalocele, midline facial clefts, dysgenesis of the corpus callosum, mental retardation, and hearing loss; cardiac anomalies also may be seen.

IMAGING FEATURES

Computed tomography (CT) is preferred for imaging patients suspected of having a coloboma (Fig. 11.04-1). CT may be helpful for detecting the presence of colobomas in uncooperative patients or those patients with intrabulbar opacities that do not permit adequate funduscopic examination. Magnetic resonance (MR) imaging and ultrasound may be used as alternatives. Colobomas appear as focal cystic outpouchings arising from the periphery of the globe. The lesions communicate with the vitreous humor and are enclosed by a deformed and enhancing sclera. Retinal colobomas, also termed retinochoroidal colobomas, arise from the wall of the globe, whereas optic nerve colobomas characteristically involve the insertion of the optic disc. The globe is reduced in size in the vast majority of patients. The anterior chamber is small. Retroocular cysts (colobomatous cysts) may be present. Colobomatous cysts and microphthalmos may be considered a variant of coloboma. Colobomas are bilateral in 60% to 90% of cases. Colobomas may also arise from atypical locations such as the macula, and are probably secondary to postinflammatory retinochoroidal scars or macular dystrophy. Colobomas involving the eyelid and iris are readily apparent on clinical examination, and CT and MR imaging are probably not indicated in the presence of a negative funduscopic examination. The imaging differential diagnosis of colobomas includes staphyloma, retroocular cysts, and orbital dermoids.

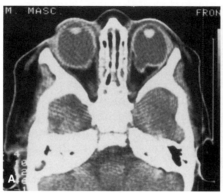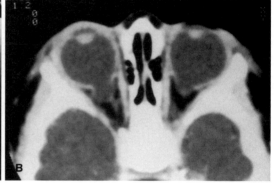

FIGURE 11.04-1.

Colobomas. **A.** Axial computed tomography (CT) shows coloboma in posteromedial left globe, which also is small. The left lens is dysplastic. **B.** Axial CT shows bilateral colobomas (right > left).

SUGGESTED READINGS

1. Robb R. Developmental abnormalities of the eye affecting vision in the pediatric years. In: Albert DM, Jakoview FA, eds. Principles and Practice of Ophthalmology. Philadelphia: WB Saunders, 1994:2793.
2. Murphy BL, Griffen JF. Optic nerve coloboma (morning glory syndrome): CT findings. Radiology 1994;191:59.
3. Mafee MF, Jampol LM, Langer BG, Tso M. Computed tomography of optic nerve colobomas, morning glory anomaly, and colobomatous cyst. Radiol Clin North Am 1987;25:693.

11.05 *Persistent Hyperplastic Primary Vitreous*

EPIDEMIOLOGY

Persistent hyperplastic primary vitreous (PHPV) is an intraocular developmental anomaly caused by failure of involution of the primary vitreous and of the fetal hyaloid vasculature. There is no gender predilection. Sporadic PHPV is usually unilateral. PHPV may occur as part of a multisystem disease such as Norrie disease, primary vitreolental dysplasia, and Warburg disease. Bilateral PHPV is more commonly seen in the presence of a multisystem syndrome.

CLINICAL FEATURES

The lesion results from persistent remnants of the primary vitreous and lenticular branches of the primitive hyaloid artery (tunica vasculosa lentis). These remnants occur along the course of Cloquet's canal. They may be detected on the dorsal surface of the lens (Mittendorf's dot), posteriorly (Bergmeister's papilla at the optic disc), or be extensive (hyaloid vessel). Histologically, a fibrovascular plaque of tissue that is a remnant of the tunica vasculosa lentis is found adherent to the posterior surface of the lens. This retrolental tissue may undergo extensive proliferation and can extend to the ciliary processes. Other tissues, including smooth muscle, cartilage, and fat, may also be present within the lesion.

Patients usually present with leukokoria, microphthalmos, vitreous hemorrhage associated with a retinal detachment, or with an opacified lens. Funduscopic examination reveals a white or pink vascularized membrane behind the lens. The involved globe is often small with a shallow anterior chamber. The lens is clear at birth; however, it eventually becomes swollen and opaque. Swelling of the lens results in narrowing of the anterior chamber. If untreated, the eye develops angle-closure glaucoma, and may eventually become nonfunctional. Spontaneous hemorrhage is another complication. PHPV is the second most common cause of leukokoria (after retinoblastoma) during childhood. Patients may also have seizures, hearing loss, and mental retardation, often as a part of a multisystem disorder.

Surgical extraction of the retrolental membrane is recommended if the eye is not severely microphthalmic. Resection of the vascularized tissues may prevent glaucoma and spontaneous hemorrhage. Successful surgery results in preservation of some peripheral vision in selected cases, with only limited development of central vision.

IMAGING FEATURES

Both computed tomography (CT) and magnetic resonance (MR) imaging may be used to evaluate patients with PHPV. Noncontrast CT should be performed to exclude the presence of a calcified intraocular mass (retinoblastoma) in patients in whom funduscopic examination cannot be adequately performed.

In patients with PHPV, CT demonstrates generalized increased attenuation of the vitreous chamber and a small globe. Calcifications are not present. There may be small, discrete, intravitreal hyperdense masses that likely represent remnants of the embryonic hyaloid vascular system (Fig. 11.05-1A). These masses may enhance after contrast administration. There is a fine linear hyperdensity extending from the retina to the posterior surface of the lens, representing Cloquet's canal. Retinal detachment may be present and accompanied by serosanguinous fluid within the subretinal or subhyaloid space, which is better seen on MR imaging. Congenital retinal detachment is often difficult to differentiate from a hyaloid remnant on CT. MR imaging shows increased signal intensity on both T1- and T2-weighted images within the vitreous cavity, which represents highly proteinaceous fluid (Fig. 11.05-1B). MR imaging is also sensitive for detecting fluid levels, which may result from hemorrhages arising spontaneously or be associated with retinal detachments. Elevation of the retina eccentric to the optic nerve is suggestive of developmental nonattachment of the retina, whereas retinal elevation away from the optic disc suggests the acquired type of retinal detachment.

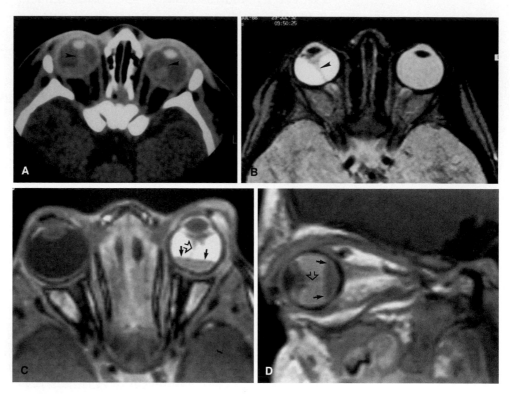

FIGURE 11.05-1.

Persistent hyperplastic primary vitreous.   **A.** Axial computed tomography shows bilateral small eyes with increased density posteriorly (primary vitreous) and Cloquet's canals *(arrowheads)* extending across midline. **B.** In a different patient, magnetic resonance T2-weighted image shows Cloquet's canal *(arrowhead)* in right globe, which is slightly smaller than left globe. **C.** Axial MR T1-weighted image in a different patient shows bright left vitreous with dependent fluid level *(solid arrows)* from hemorrhage. Note Cloquet's canal *(open arrow)* and slight microphthalmia. **D.** Oblique sagittal MR T1-weighted image again shows blood level *(solid arrows)* and Cloquet's canal *(open arrow).* (Case illustrated in parts C and D courtesy of J. Alarcan, Scottish Rite Children's Hospital, Atlanta, GA.)

SUGGESTED READINGS

1. Mafee MF, Goldberg MF. Persistent hyperplastic primary vitreous (PHPV): role of computed tomography and magnetic resonance. Radiol Clin North Am 1987;25: 683.
2. Sahel JA, Brini A, Albert DM. Pathology of the retina and vitreous. In: Albert DM, Jakoviec FA, eds. Principles and Practice of Ophthalmology. Philadelphia: WB Saunders, 1994:2242.

11.06 *Retinopathy of Prematurity*

EPIDEMIOLOGY

Retinopathy of prematurity is a vasculoproliferative disorder of newborns that was previously referred to as retrolental fibroplasia. This disease is responsible for some degree of visual loss in 1300 children and for severe visual loss in 500 children each year in the United States. The disorder occurs in premature infants with low birth weights. Results from the Cryotherapy Multicenter Trial indicate that 82% of infants with birth weights less than 1 kg will have some form of retinopathy of prematurity, and that 9.3% will contract vision-threatening disease. The incidence of the disease decreases with larger birth weights; 47% of infants with birth weights between 1 and 1.25 kg will have retinopathy of prematurity, with only 2% of these patients experiencing significant visual loss.

CLINICAL FEATURES

The exact cause of retinopathy of prematurity is unknown. This disease occurs in premature infants who have a protracted hospital course and require supplemental oxygen. In the past, prolonged oxygen therapy was believed to be the causative factor for retinopathy of prematurity. Although there is a proven association between the duration of oxygen exposure and severity of this disease, the exact role of oxygen is not known. Patients with lower birth weights (< 1.25 kg) are at a greater risk for development of retinopathy than are infants who weigh more than 1.25 kg. Increased ambient light in neonatal intensive care nurseries and reduced levels of vitamin E have also been implicated as etiologic factors.

The greater susceptibility of the temporal retina to retinopathy of prematurity results from the fact that the vasculature is still developing in this region in premature infants. Retinopathy of prematurity may be diagnosed as early as 6 to 8 weeks after delivery. Clinically, the initial manifestations of retinopathy include the development of a demarcation line between the vascular and avascular retina (stage 1). Avascular retina is present anterior to this line, whereas abnormally branched and tortuous vessels are found posterior to this line. The line of demarcation progresses into a "ridge" that extends out of the plane of the retina (stage 2). Vessels may extend from the posterior surface of the retina to enter the ridge, but do not enter the vitreous. The disease is still reversible at this point. With further progression, the abnormal retinal vessels may extend into the vitreous, giving the ridge a ragged appearance. Continued growth may lead to migration of myoblasts into the vitreous, eventually forming a fibrovascular mass (stage 3). This mass may lead to partial retinal detachment (stage 4). Fluid in the subretinal space may also accumulate. Uncontrolled disease results in extensive circumferential scarring and complete retinal detachment (stage 5).

There is no effective method of treatment of retinopathy of prematurity. However, most cases are reversible. Treatment options depend on the extent of the disease and include photocoagulation and cryotherapy for severe acute retinopathy, scleral buckling for cases associated with retinal detachment, and intraocular vitreoretinal surgery for the treatment of severe cicatricial disease. Prophylactic administration of vitamin E has also been recommended for prevention and inhibiting the progression of this disease.

IMAGING FEATURES

Either computed tomography (CT) or magnetic resonance (MR) imaging may be used in patients suspected of having retinopathy of prematurity. CT may be performed to exclude calcifications and, hence, retinoblastoma. However, chronic retinopathy of prematurity occasionally may have calcifications. The imaging findings of retinopathy depend on the extent of disease. Radiographic findings characteristic of chronic changes include a noncalcified, retrolental, hyperdense mass that may be associated with partial or complete retinal detachment (Fig. 11.06-1). Approximately 80% to 90% of these retinal detachments resolve spontaneously. The eyes are often small in the late stages of the disease because of scarring of the vitreous. The MR imaging findings usually are nonspecific in mild forms of retinopathy. Fluid (hyperintense on T2-weighted images or hypointense on postcontrast T1-weighted images) may be found within the subretinal space in the early stages of disease. Persistence of the embryonic hyaloid vascular system may also be noted in some patients with retinopathy of prematurity.

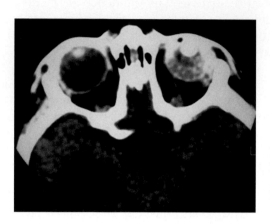

FIGURE 11.06-1.

Retinopathy of prematurity. Axial computed tomography shows small and hyperdense left globe. (With permission from Castillo M. Neuroradiology Companion. Philadelphia: JB Lippincott, 1995.)

SUGGESTED READINGS

1. Peterson RA, Hunter DG, Mukai S. Retinopathy of prematurity. In: Albert DM, Jakoviec FA, eds. Principles and Practice of Ophthalmology. Philadelphia: WB Saunders, 1994:2799.
2. Hunter DG, Mukai S, Hirose T. Advanced retinopathy of prematurity. In: Albert DM, Jakoviec FA, eds. Principles and Practice of Ophthalmology. Philadelphia: WB Saunders, 1994:782.
3. Phelps DL. Retinopathy of prematurity: neonatologist's perspective. In: Isenberg SJ, ed. The Eye in Infancy. St. Louis: CV Mosby, 1994:437.
4. Urrea PT, Rosenbaum AL. Retinopathy of prematurity: ophthalmologist's perspective. In: Isenberg SJ, ed. The Eye in Infancy. St. Louis: CV Mosby, 1994:448.

11.07 Coats Disease

EPIDEMIOLOGY

Coats disease (also known as Leber's miliary aneurysms and congenital retinal telangiectasia) is a congenital vascular anomaly involving the retina. Coats disease occurs most commonly in boys, with a peak incidence between 6 to 8 years of age. However, the disease has been reported between the ages of 4 months and 70 years. Most cases are unilateral. The etiology is unknown; however, patients older than 30 years of age at initial presentation often have hypercholesterolemia. Most cases are sporadic, although changes in the retinal vasculature similar to those present in Coats disease have been reported in patients with certain multisystem diseases, including Turner syndrome, fasciocapsulohumeral muscular dystrophy, Senior-Loken syndrome, epidermal nevus syndrome, retinitis pigmentosa, and some chromosomal abnormalities (such as deletion of chromosome 13 and pericentric inversion of chromosome 3).

CLINICAL FEATURES

Coats disease is characterized by the presence of leaking telangiectatic and aneurysmal vessels associated with a lipid-laden exudate within the retina. The abnormality is present at birth but the disease does not become symptomatic until retinal detachment occurs. Patients usually present with leukokoria, strabismus, or both. Coats disease has been classified into five stages based on clinical findings: stage I, isolated focal exudates; stage II, massive exudation; stage III, partial exudative retinal detachment; stage IV, complete retinal detachment; and stage V, secondary complications of retinal detachment. The characteristic funduscopic findings are those of retinal telangiectases, microaneurysms, arteriovenous anastomoses, and saccular outpouchings of the retinal venules. Findings on funduscopic examination depend on the extent of the disease. Localized foci or retinal telangiectasias are seen within the retinal capillary bed, primarily in the temporal quadrants in mild cases; however, more advanced cases involve all quadrants. Intraretinal exudation occurs because of abnormal permeability of the vascular endothelial cells. This results in breakdown of the blood–retinal barrier with subsequent leakage of blood components into the retinal tissue and subretinal space. Progressive leakage may lead to the accumulation of fibrin, periodic acid-Schiff (PAS)-positive deposits, cholesterol clefts, and lipid-laden macrophages. Uncontrolled, this process forms a hard exudate and eventually results in retinal detachment with resultant loss of vision. If untreated, Coats disease is progressive and may lead to exudative retinal detachment, rubeosis (formation of blood vessels on the anterior surface of the iris), cataracts, neovascular glaucoma, uveitis, and phthisis.

Surgical intervention is usually recommended in all patients except in the most mild or most severe cases. The treatment is aimed at obliterating the abnormal leaking vessels. The techniques most commonly used are photocoagulation or transscleral cryopexy. Multiple treatment sessions are often necessary. Successful surgery stabilizes visual function and prevents the development of painful glaucoma and the need for subsequent enucleation.

IMAGING FEATURES

Imaging studies should be performed if Coats disease is clinically suspected or if retinoblastoma cannot be excluded by funduscopic examination. Either magnetic resonance (MR) imaging or computed tomography (CT) may be used. CT is superior to MR imaging for excluding calcifications (Fig. 11.07-1). However, MR imaging provides superior visualization of intraocular structures. Imaging studies may not be helpful in mild forms of Coats disease. Retinal detachment is usually the main finding in advanced cases. By CT, the size of the eye is normal, although it may be slightly reduced. The vitreous contains a "wing-shaped" hyperdense retinal detachment or diffusely increased density throughout. There are no calcifications, and therefore Coats disease is indistinguishable from the rare noncalcifying retinoblastoma. Findings in Coats disease may also be indistinguishable from persistent hyperplastic primary vitreous, toxocariosis, and retinopathy of prematurity.

The presence of subretinal fluid may help in establishing the diagnosis of Coats disease. MR imaging is superior to CT for identifying subretinal fluid, which follows the configuration of the posterior globe. This fluid is hyperintense on both T1- and T2-weighted images. Contrast-enhanced MR imaging delineates the choroid, thus allowing for identification of the posterior subretinal space. The subretinal fluid has a more heterogenous MR imaging appearance than that seen in retinoblastoma, persistent hyperplastic primary vitreous, or retinopathy of prematurity because of the combination of cholesterol, PAS-positive material, hemorrhage, and scarring, all of which are present in Coats disease. Hydrogen MR spectroscopy has shown increased lipids in Coats disease.

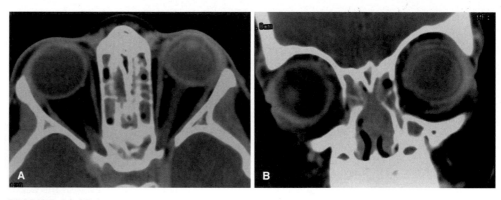

FIGURE 11.07-1.

Coats disease (presumed). **A.** Axial computed tomography (CT) shows slightly small left eye, which has a hyperdense vitreous. **B.** Coronal CT in same patient shows hyperdense vitreous to be separated from sclera by thin rim of normal-density vitreous.

SUGGESTED READINGS

1. Destro M, Gragoudas ES. Coats' disease and retinal telangiectasia. In: Principles of Ophthalmology, p. 801.
2. Mafee MF. Magnetic resonance imaging: ocular pathology. In: Newton TH, Bilaniuk LT, eds. Radiology of the Eye and Orbit. New York: Raven, 1990:3.1.

11.08   *Retinoblastoma*

EPIDEMIOLOGY

Retinoblastoma is a highly malignant tumor and is the most common intraocular tumor of childhood. This tumor accounts for 1% of all pediatric childhood deaths from cancer in the United States. Worldwide, its overall incidence is 1:20,000 live births. The tumor has no sex predilection and is responsible for 5% of childhood blindness. Although the tumor is thought to be congenital, the average age of diagnosis is 13 months. The tumor is unilateral in 70% and bilateral in 30% of patients. The nonhereditary variety usually presents at a later age, with most being diagnosed in the second year of life. These tumors are solitary and unilateral. One-third of patients have multicentric tumor in the affected eye. The hereditary form is autosomal dominant with a 90% penetrance. The gene (*Rb1* gene) has been isolated to chromosome 13, band q14. Five percent of patients have complete chromosomal deletions, whereas others have deletions within the gene that are detectable only at the DNA level.

CLINICAL FEATURES

Retinoblastomas are usually detected on physical examination. Leukokoria (white pupillary reflex) is the most common presenting sign and is caused by replacement of the vitreous humor by a white or pink mass. Other associated findings include reduced visual acuity, eye pain, and strabismus. Three percent of patients present with symptoms that simulate orbital cellulitis or endophthalmitis. Funduscopic examination reveals a creamy, pink-gray intraocular mass that may contain calcifications. The tumor may be seen anywhere along the retina, although there is a predilection for the peripheral retina (ora serrata). As the tumor enlarges, it may continue to grow within the eye, extend outside the globe, or diffusely involve the eye. The most important prognostic feature is related to tumor extension beyond the globe or involvement of the subarachnoid space.

Retinoblastomas probably derive from undifferentiated cells that are precursors of the embryonic retina. Histologically, the tumor consists of small ovoid or round cells with large nuclei and sparse cytoplasm. Some regions in the tumors show glial differentiation, whereas others consist of necrosis and calcification. The tumors may have evidence of photoreceptor differentiation, termed Flexner-Wintersteiner rosettes and fleurettes. These are doughnut-like cell structures. Rosettes without a central lumen are known as Homer-Wright rosettes.

Bilateral retinoblastomas may be associated with primitive primary intracranial tumors, the so-called "trilateral retinoblastomas." This association may in part be the result of a common neuroectodermal origin of the retina and pineal gland. Because retinoblastomas and pineoblastomas have similar histologic appearances, it is thought that similar mutations may predispose individuals to the development of both types of tumors. Although the primitive intracranial tumor usually is found in the pineal region, other parts of the brain (particularly the suprasellar region and cerebellum) may be involved, and some consider this latter constellation of findings a forme fruste of trilateral retinoblastoma.

Most retinoblastomas are treated with enucleation and irradiation. The 5-year survival rate for tumors limited to the globe approaches 92%. Useful vision in the affected eye can be preserved in 90% of patients with small tumors. Retinoblastomas with extraocular involvement have a mortality rate approaching 100%. Treated patients are at an increased risk for a second neoplasm, most commonly osteogenic sarcoma. Patients with the hereditable form of retinoblastoma are also genetically predisposed to development of a second neoplasm, and have a 500-fold to 5000-fold increased risk for development of a second neoplasm within the radiation field, and a 200-fold to 500-fold risk of a tumor developing in the soft tissues outside the radiation field. Patients with nongenetic retinoblastoma also have an increased risk for an irradiation-induced malignancy; however, this appears to be solely dose related. Overall, 10% to 15% of treated patients eventually have a subsequent malignancy, most commonly a soft tissue sarcoma.

IMAGING FEATURES   Routine computed tomography (CT) imaging in patients suspected of harboring retinoblastoma should include precontrast and postcontrast imaging of the orbits. Precontrast CT is helpful for detecting calcifications (Fig. 11.08-1A, B). Extraocular involvement of tumor can be readily detected with CT because of the low attenuation of the adjacent retrobulbar fat. Retinoblastomas present as smoothly marginated, intraocular soft tissue masses that enhance after contrast administration. Over 95% of the lesions are calcified. Calcifications may be single or scattered throughout the mass. The globe is normal in size or slightly enlarged (Fig. 11.08-1C). Although retinoblastomas grow in all directions, these tumors typically exhibit three principal growth patterns: exophytic, endophytic, and diffuse. Exophytic growth denotes spread primarily into the subretinal space, with eventual invasion of the choroid and sclera. These patients have a higher likelihood of hematogenous tumor dissemination. Invasion of the ocular venous system also predisposes the patient to distant metastases. Invasion of the optic nerve allows for tumor seeding of the subarachnoid space. Overall, 25% to 50% of patients have extraocular spread at the time of imaging. The extraocular component of the mass is rarely calcified. Endophytically spreading tumors may be associated with a better prognosis if the disease is confined to the globe. The diffuse infiltrating form of retinoblastoma rarely shows calcification. The presence of calcification is an important finding in patients suspected of having retinoblastoma (Fig. 11.08-1D). Calcification is rarely seen in other lesions mimicking retinoblastoma in patients younger than 3 years of age. In patients older than 3 years of age, optic nerve head drusen, toxocariasis, and retinopathy of prematurity may also calcify (Fig. 11.08-2). Thus, a calcified soft tissue in a child younger than 3 years of age should be considered a retinoblastoma until proven otherwise. After contrast administration, the noncalcified portions of the tumor exhibit moderate enhancement.

By magnetic resonance (MR) imaging, retinoblastomas characteristically have slightly increased signal compared to vitreous humor on T1-weighted images and are hypointense on T2-weighted images. Subarachnoid tumor seeding is better evaluated with postcontrast MR imaging. Both CT and MR imaging are helpful in the evaluation of postirradiation sarcomas (Fig. 11.08-3).

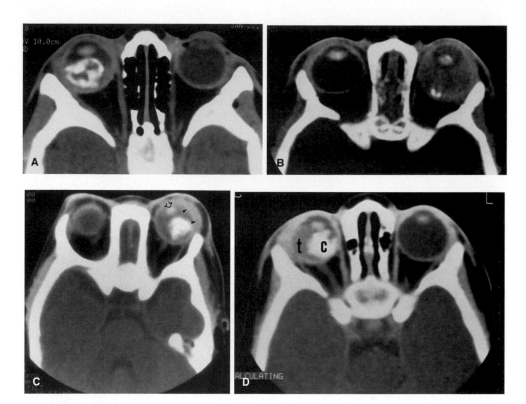

FIGURE 11.08-1.

Retinoblastoma. **A.** Axial noncontrast computed tomography (CT) shows mostly calcified retinoblastoma in right globe. Note thickening of posterior sclera but absence of retroocular extension. **B.** In a different patient, CT shows enlarged left globe containing mostly soft tissue tumor with small focus of calcification. **C.** Axial CT shows enlarged left globe with calcified retinoblastoma. There is thickening (invasion) of sclera *(arrowheads)* and medial subluxation of lens *(open arrow).* **D.** Axial CT shows partly calcified (C) and noncalcified (t) right-sided retinoblastoma. (**C** and **D** with permission from Castillo M. Neuroradiology Companion. Philadelphia: JB Lippincott, 1995.)

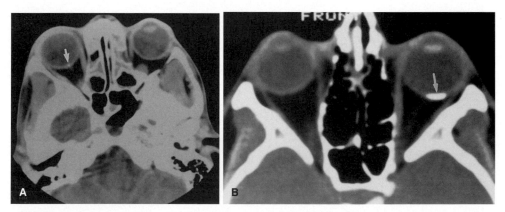

FIGURE 11.08-2.

Benign ocular calcifications. **A.** Axial computed tomography (CT) shows small calcification *(arrow)* at insertion of right optic nerve (drusen body). It may raise the optic disc and clinically simulate papilledema. **B.** Axial CT shows left choroidal osteoma *(arrow).* These lesions are unilateral or bilateral, and are more common in girls. They may represent degenerated hemangiomas and occur close to the optic disc.

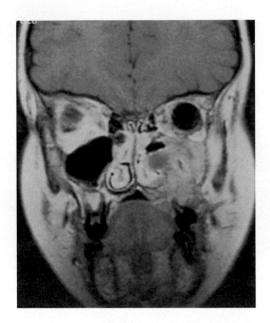

FIGURE 11.08-3.

Osteosarcoma complicating retinoblastoma. Coronal postcontrast magnetic resonance T1-weighted image shows enhancing mass in left maxillary sinus (osteosarcoma). Tumor extends medially into nasal cavity, superiorly into orbit, and inferiorly into the buccal cavity. Note left ocular prosthesis after enucleation and irradiation for retinoblastoma.

SUGGESTED READINGS

1. Sahel JA, Brini A, Albert DM. Pathology of the retina and vitreous. In: Albert DM, Jakoviec FA, eds. Principles and Practice of Ophthalmology. Philadelphia: WB Saunders, 1994:2261.
2. Stefanyszyn MA, Handler SD, Wright JE. Pediatric orbital tumors. Otol Clin North Am 1988;21:103.
3. Mafee MF. Magnetic resonance imaging: ocular pathology. In: Newton TH, Bilaniuk LT, eds. Radiology of the Eye and Orbit. New York: Raven Press, 1990:3.1.
4. Provenzale JM, Weber AL, Klintworth GK, McLendon RE. Bilateral retinoblastoma with coexistent pineoblastoma (trilateral retinoblastoma). AJNR 1995;16:157.
5. Finelli DA, Shurin SB, Bardenstein DS. Trilateral retinoblastoma: two variations. AJNR 1995;16:166.

11.09 *Hemangioma*

EPIDEMIOLOGY

Hemangiomas are common orbital lesions constituting between 10% to 15% of all orbital tumors. Capillary hemangiomas are one of the most common orbital tumors of infancy, and usually present before 6 months of age. These lesions are more common in girls.

Cavernous hemangiomas are benign vascular tumors and occur mostly in adults. Cavernous hemangiomas usually present in the third or fourth decade of life. These tumors show a distinct female preponderance.

CLINICAL FEATURES

Hemangiomas are divided into capillary (benign hemangioendothelioma) and cavernous forms. Capillary hemangiomas are believed to result from a maldevelopment of the primitive stage of vascular development. Clinically, these lesions may be diagnosed by their cutaneous manifestations. Capillary hemangiomas typically present as nonblanching, bright red, knobby masses, hence the name "strawberry hemangioma." The lesions often increase in size with crying. During the involutional stage, the lesions decrease in size and develop a bluish discoloration that eventually fades to light gray. Deep orbital lesions may occasionally be clinically occult; however, most tumors have associated cutaneous manifestations. Histologically, capillary hemangiomas are composed of endothelial and capillary proliferation with benign endothelial cells surrounding capillary-sized vascular spaces. The blood supply of orbital capillary hemangiomas is predominantly from branches of the external carotid artery.

Capillary hemangiomas undergo rapid initial growth followed by a period of stabilization. Eventually, most of these tumors regress spontaneously, with most lesions involuting by 5 to 7 years of age. Therefore, periorbital lesions that do not impair vision are treated conservatively. Aggressive treatment is indicated if progressive proptosis, visual impairment, or severe astigmatism ensues. Steroid treatment may be of some benefit in promoting tumor involution. Other treatment options include laser ablation, surgical resection, endovascular occlusion, and interferon therapy.

Cavernous hemangiomas typically present with progressive proptosis. Rarely, patients may present with acute onset of proptosis because of intratumoral hemorrhage. Impaired vision and reduced extraocular mobility may occur in large lesions or in those lesions that compress the optic nerve, extraocular muscles, or orbital apex. Symptomatic lesions may be surgically resected, whereas asymptomatic masses may be followed conservatively. On gross examination, these lesions are purplish to dark blue. Histologically, these tumors are surrounded by a distinct fibrous pseudocapsule. The internal architecture consists of multiple large (cavernous) endothelium-lined spaces. These spaces are divided into smaller compartments by septa composed of smooth muscle and collagen. Although these lesions are vascular, cavernous hemangiomas are independent of the general circulation, and communication with a major arterial supply is not present. There is stagnant vascular flow within these lesions, and focal areas of thrombosis are often present. Hemorrhage is less common than in capillary hemangioma. Enlargement of these tumors is thought to be caused by capillary proliferation into the surrounding interstitium. Cavernous hemangiomas tend to enlarge slowly, whereas capillary hemangiomas tend spontaneously to regress.

IMAGING FEATURES

Capillary hemangiomas are not routinely imaged because most spontaneously involute. Imaging may be performed to evaluate submucosal lesions and to determine the extent of large lesions. Both computed tomography (CT) and magnetic resonance (MR) imaging may be used to study capillary hemangiomas; however, MR imaging is preferred. The lesions are homogenous and their margins may be well defined or poorly delineated (Fig. 11.09-1A, B). Ill defined orbital capillary hemangiomas have a greater tendency to extend intracranially via the superior orbital fissure, optic canal, and orbital roof. Most capillary hemangiomas are extraconal, although some lesions may be intraconal (Fig. 11.09-1C). MR imaging typically demonstrates lesions of heterogenous signal intensity on noncontrast T1-weighted images, which enhance diffusely after contrast administration. Capillary hemangiomas are hyperintense on T2-weighted images. Flow voids may be present by standard spin echo techniques. Flow-sensitive techniques demonstrate these lesions to have areas of flow-related enhancement due to underlying vascular proliferation. The presence of flow voids is important because other soft tissue tumors such as rhabdomyosarcoma do not contain large vessels. Catheter angiography shows that periorbital capillary hemangiomas are supplied mostly by branches of the internal maxillary artery, whereas those affecting the parotid region are supplied by the facial arteries. Large capillary hemangiomas may demonstrate arteriovenous shunting with multiple areas of blood pooling. Transcatheter embolization may be indicated for large masses that cause disfigurement. Therapy should be directed at reducing arteriovenous shunting and reducing overall flow.

Both CT and MR may also be used to image patients with orbital cavernous hemangiomas, but MR imaging is preferred. The imaging features of orbital cavernous hemangiomas reflect their histologic composition. These lesions are usually intraconal, well defined, and oval or slightly lobular in appearance (Fig. 11.09-2). On CT, cavernous hemangiomas are hyperdense and homogenously enhance after contrast administration. Calcified phleboliths may be present. Occasionally, these lesions may extend into the extraconal space. Large lesions may remodel the surrounding bone. The MR imaging characteristics of cavernous hemangiomas include homogenous and isointense lesions on T1-weighted images. The lesions enhance markedly after contrast administration. Cavernous hemangiomas have markedly increased signal intensity on T2-weighted images. Focal areas of signal void may be present on T2-weighted images and are caused by focal deposits of hemosiderin or phleboliths. Other soft tissue malignancies may be indistinguishable from hemangiomas by both CT and MR imaging, and require biopsy (Fig. 11.09-3).

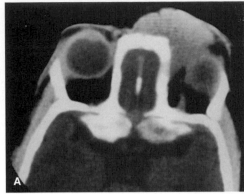
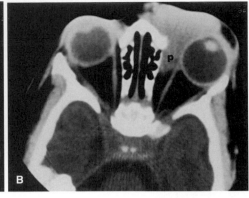

FIGURE 11.09-1.

Capillary hemangioma. **A.** Axial postcontrast computed tomography (CT) shows large enhancing mass in left periorbital region but with postseptal extension. **B.** Axial CT in same patient (at level of equator of globe) shows postseptal (p) extension and lateral displacement of globe. The tumor also extends on the nasal bridge medially. **C.** Axial postcontrast CT (different patient) shows enhancing mass in retrobulbar space. There is flattening of the posterior sclera and left-sided proptosis. The mass appears to be completely intraconal.

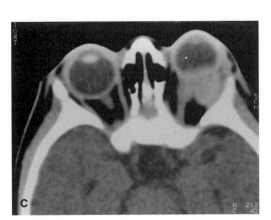

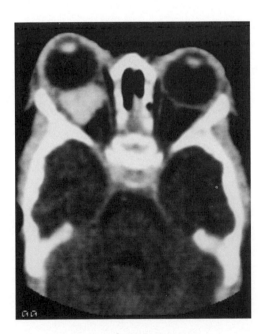

FIGURE 11.09-2.

Cavernous hemangioma. Axial postcontrast computed tomography shows enhancing mass in right intraconal space surrounding optic nerve. This type of hemangioma is more common in adults and has the same appearance as the one shown here.

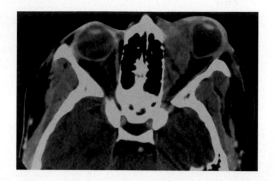

FIGURE 11.09-3.

Ewing sarcoma. Axial postcontrast computed tomography shows mostly nonenhancing mass involving left medial rectus and extraconal space, thought initially to be either hemangioma or lymphangioma. Histologic study demonstrated extraosseous Ewing sarcoma.

SUGGESTED READINGS

1. Goldberg RA, Boxrud CA, McCall LC. The orbit in infancy. In: Isenberg SJ, ed. The Eye in Infancy. St. Louis: CV Mosby, 1994:211.
2. Bilaniuk LT, Zimmerman RA, Newton RH. Magnetic resonance imaging: orbital pathology. In: Newton TH, Bilaniuk LT, eds. Radiology of the Eye and Orbit. New York: Raven Press, 1990:3.1.

11.10 *Lymphangioma*

EPIDEMIOLOGY

Orbital lymphangiomas are benign developmental lesions occurring in 3.5:100,100 individuals. They account for approximately 8% of orbital masses and are the most common vascular orbital mass in childhood. There is no gender predilection. Most are found between 1 to 5 years of age.

CLINICAL FEATURES

Orbital lymphangiomas are divided into superficial, deep, and combined lesions. Superficial lesions (including those arising in the conjunctiva) are more common than deep ones. Superficial orbital lymphangiomas are visible clinically and present in early childhood. Deep tumors may be clinically occult and are found more often in older children or young adults. Unlike capillary hemangiomas, lymphangiomas may progressively grow during childhood and result in disfigurement. Lymphangiomas have a tendency to bleed spontaneously and may result in acute or recurrent proptosis. The origin of these tumors is uncertain, but it is believed that they arise from an anlage of vascular mesenchyme that is capable of differentiating into both lymphatic and mesodermal elements. These tumors are isolated and do not communicate with adjacent normal lymphatic or vascular channels. Lymphangiomas may be histologically classified according to the size of their channels. Capillary (simple) lymphangiomas contain lymphatic channels that are normal in size. Cavernous lymphangiomas contain dilated lymphatic channels. Cystic hygromas consist of macroscopically multilobulated dilated channels. Orbital lymphangiomas are nonencapsulated, diffusely infiltrating, and composed of dysplastic lymphatic–vascular channels. They are filled with serous fluid. Because of their diffusely infiltrating nature, complete resection is often not possible. If an orbital lesion bleeds spontaneously, proptosis results and may have to be treated on an emergency basis. Conservative treatment is advocated for tumors that do not threaten the vision or are not disfiguring.

IMAGING FEATURES

Orbital lymphangiomas are multiseptated lesions with irregular and ill-defined margins (Fig. 11.10-1). They typically cross anatomic boundaries, including the orbital septum and conal fascia. These lesions are heterogenous and have both soft tissue and fluid components. The degree of enhancement after contrast administration is variable and may be ring-like. Peripheral enhancement is often present in lesions that have previously bled. Presence of blood products in different stages of degradation is typical (Fig. 11.10-2). Both computed tomography and magnetic resonance (MR) imaging may be used, but MR imaging is preferred. The presence of fluid levels is well seen by MR imaging. Fat suppression may help to differentiate methemoglobin from fat, therefore distinguishing lymphangiomas from dermoids. Calcifications may occur in the form of phleboliths. By catheter angiography, slightly increased vascularity and blush are only rarely present.

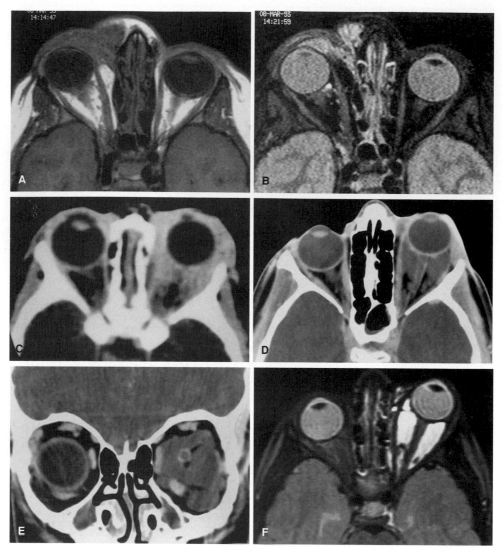

FIGURE 11.10-1.

Lymphangioma.   **A.** Axial noncontrast magnetic resonance (MR) T1-weighted image shows right superior eyelid lymphangioma extending medially but contained posteriorly by orbital septum, which is unusual because these tumors are commonly infiltrative. Note intensity of mass is identical to that of muscle. **B.** Corresponding MR T2-weighted image shows the mass to be of even higher signal intensity than fluid. **C.** Axial postcontrast computed tomography (CT; different patient) shows diffusely enhancing and infiltrating left-sided lymphangioma. The tumor involves preseptal and postseptal compartments and intraconal and extraconal spaces. **D.** Axial postcontrast CT shows cystic-appearing intraconal mass in left orbit. **E.** Coronal CT in same patient shows that lymphangioma is mostly intraconal but has extraconal components inferiorly and medially. **F.** Axial MR T2-weighted image in a different patient shows mostly hyperintense left intraconal lymphangioma with proptosis. Note that lesion contains areas of low signal intensity posteriorly, suggesting hemorrhage.

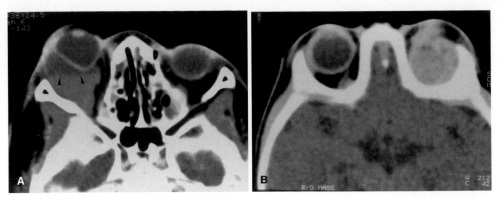

FIGURE 11.10-2.

Lymphangioma with hemorrhages.   **A.** Axial noncontrast computed tomography (CT) shows fluid level *(arrowheads)* due to hemorrhage into a right-sided retroocular lymphangioma. This appearance is typical of lymphangiomas. There is flattening of the posterior sclera and significant proptosis. **B.** Axial noncontrast CT shows hyperdense mass in left orbit. At surgery, this was a "chocolate cyst," presumably from bleeding into a lymphangioma.

SUGGESTED READING

1. Graeb DA, Rootman J, Robertson WD, Lapointe JS, Nugent RA, Hay EJ. Orbital lymphangiomas: clinical, radiologic, and pathologic characteristics. Radiology 1990; 175:417.

11.11 *Orbital Dermoid*

EPIDEMIOLOGY

Dermoids and epidermoids are the most common developmental lesions of the orbits and periorbital region, and account for 1% to 2% of all orbital masses. There is no gender predilection.

CLINICAL FEATURES

These lesions arise from sequestration of the ectoderm within adjacent suture lines; the most common suture affected is the frontozygomatic suture. Thus, most of the lesions (60%) are found in the upper outer quadrant of the orbit. Dermoids and epidermoids are both derived from the primitive germ cell layers. Epidermoids are cystic lesions lined by a layer of stratified squamous epithelium that arise from the primitive ectoderm. Dermoids arise from more than one germ cell layer and contain one or more dermal adnexal structures. Sebaceous glands, hair, or fat is commonly found in dermoids; however, they may also be purely cystic.

Most of these lesions present in childhood as subcutaneous nodules adjacent to the orbital rim, and may be fixed to the underlying periosteum. In younger children, these lesions are not usually associated with proptosis. Dermoids in older children and adults are deeper, and patients present with unilateral proptosis. Dermoids usually are isolated lesions and are not associated with other malformations. Dermoids are usually treated by simple excision. A less common type of dermoid is the epibulbar variety. Epibulbar dermoids occur on the globe and characteristically occur in the corneal limbus or at the lateral canthus. These unusual lesions may extend under the conjunctiva and along the lateral rectus muscle. These lesions often are not surgically resected because of the scarring and altered ocular motility that may result from the dissection. Epibulbar dermoids are frequently associated with hemifacial microsomia, Goldenhar syndrome, hearing loss, cleft lip or palate, upper eyelid coloboma, and ipsilateral preauricular appendages.

Occasionally dermoids may grow rapidly, raising the suspicion of an underlying lacrimal malignancy. Rupture of a dermoid may result in a granulomatous inflammatory reaction. However, most orbital dermoid lesions are clinically occult.

IMAGING FINDINGS

Computed tomography (CT) is the imaging modality of choice for evaluating patients suspected of having an orbital dermoid or epidermoid. By CT, orbital dermoids are usually well defined lesions with a low attenuation center, most commonly located in the upper outer quadrant of the orbit (Fig. 11.11-1). Imaging allows differentiating these lesions from primary lacrimal sac malignancies, which are of soft tissue density by CT. Most orbital dermoids are cystic; however, the internal appearance may vary depending on its contents. Forty percent of orbital dermoids contain fat. The presence of fat within a lesion in the superior outer quadrant of the orbit is typical for dermoids. Dermoids may contain fluid–fat levels. Dermoids often have a thick enhancing rim that is partially calcified in two-thirds of cases. Most lesions are associated with bony changes, which include smooth or irregular scalloping, thinning, sclerosis, and linear defects in the orbital bony rim.

The magnetic resonance imaging signal characteristics of dermoids are variable and depend on the contents of the lesions. Dermoids containing highly proteinaceous material have increased signal on T1- and T2-weighted images.

Lesions that contain fat have increased signal on T1-weighted images but have reduced signal intensity on standard T2-weighted images. Fat saturation may be of benefit for helping to make a diagnosis of a dermoid in this latter group of patients.

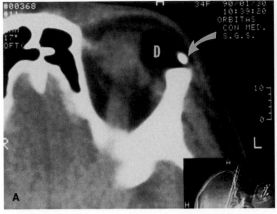 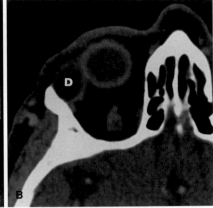

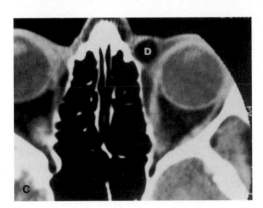

FIGURE. 11.11-1.

Orbital dermoids. **A.** Axial noncontrast computed tomography (CT) shows fatty mass (D) containing a calcification *(arrow)* in the region of the left lacrimal gland. (With permission from Castillo M. Neuroradiology Companion. Philadelphia: JB Lippincott, 1995.) **B.** Axial postcontrast CT (different patient) shows low-density (but not fatty) dermoid (D) in region of right lacrimal gland.
C. Axial CT (different patient) shows fatty rounded dermoid (D) in medial canthus of left orbit.

SUGGESTED READINGS

1. Robb R. Developmental abnormalities of the eye affecting vision in the pediatric years. In: Albert DM, Jakoviec FA, eds. Principles and Practice of Ophthalmology. Philadelphia: WB Saunders, 1994:2792.
2. Nugent RA, Lapointe JS, Rootman J, Robertson WD, Graeb DA. Orbital dermoids: features on CT. Radiology 1987;165:475.

11.12 *Staphyloma*

EPIDEMIOLOGY

Staphyloma refers to focal ectasia of the globe, believed to result from bulging of the uvea into a thinned and stretched sclera. The focal reduction in resistance of the sclera may be caused by prior infection or injury; however, heritable forms have also been reported. Staphylomas may be isolated or associated with other conditions such as glaucoma, scleritis, trauma, and infection. They are rare in children. There is no gender predilection.

CLINICAL FEATURES

Focal ectasia of a globe results either from increased intraocular pressure or abnormal compliance of the sclera, resulting in altered mechanical stress. Staphylomas may occur in various regions of the globe, and are classified as anterior (located between the ciliary body and cornea), ciliary (within the ciliary body), equatorial (at the equator of the globe), and posterior (between the equator and the optic nerve).

Myopia may be caused by an increase in the refractive power of the media (refractive myopia) or to an increase in the size of the globe (axial myopia). Staphylomas result in a reduction of vision because of an increase in the size of the globe (axial myopia). Highly myopic eyes may be unilateral or bilateral; congenital forms of myopia are usually unilateral. Highly myopic eyes have a characteristic "egg shape," with the elongation of their anteroposterior axes. This elongation is thought to be the result of a defect in the collagenous structure of the outer coat of the sclera. With advanced changes, there is a focal outward bulge of the posterior pole of the sclera, resulting in a staphyloma. The adjacent retina and choroid are also thin and bulge outward into the ectatic sclera.

Posterior staphylomas are associated with a poor visual prognosis. Thirty-four percent of patients with posterior staphylomas progress to complete blindness. The likelihood of complete visual loss increases with age. These lesions also are associated with advanced chorioretinal degeneration. These changes consist of thinning and stretching of the choroid and retina, retraction of the edge of the optic disc, resulting in exposure of the sclera (temporal crescent), posterior vitreous detachment, breaks in Bruch's membrane (lacquer cracks) which may eventually lead to scar formation, Forster-Fuchs spots, and partial or complete retinal detachment.

Contact lens wear may be helpful in patients with normal vision and low degrees of myopia. Focal scleral resection, scleral implants, or surgical reinforcement have been advocated for more advanced cases, but these procedures have limited success.

IMAGING FEATURES

Both computed tomography (CT) and magnetic resonance (MR) may be used to image patients with staphylomas. There is a focal asymmetric ocular bulge associated with thinning of the scleral uveal rim (Fig. 11.12-1). The globe may also be enlarged and elongated along the anteroposterior axis (axial myopia). There is focal protrusion of the vitreous into the staphyloma. There are no adjacent masses or significant enhancement associated with staphylomas. More advanced changes may demonstrate increased proteinaceous fluid within the vitreous, indicative of previous hemorrhage or retinal detachment.

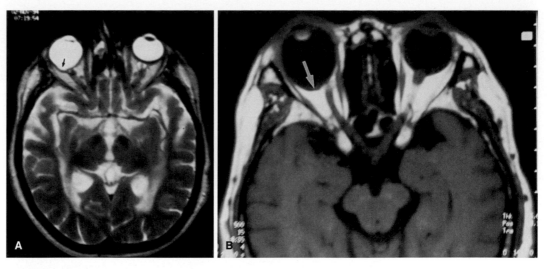

FIGURE 11.12-1.

Staphyloma.   **A.** Axial magnetic resonance (MR) T2-weighted image shows posterior protrusion of sclera *(arrow)* laterally to insertion of optic nerve at level of equator of right eye. **B.** In a different patient, MR T1-weighted image shows elongation of the anteroposterior diameter of right eye (axial myopia) with lateral staphyloma *(arrow)*. (Both figures with permission from Castillo M. Neuroradiology Companion. Philadelphia: JB Lippincott, 1995.)

SUGGESTED READINGS

1. Swayne LC, Garfinkle WB, Bennett RH. CT of posterior ocular staphyloma in axial myopia. Neuroradiology 1984;26:241.
2. Anderson RL, Epstein GA, Dauer EA. Computed tomography diagnosis of posterior ocular staphyloma. AJNR 1983;4:90.
3. Pruett RC. Pathologic myopia. In: Albert DM, Jakoviec FA, eds. Principles and Practice of Ophthalmology. Philadelphia: WB Saunders, 1994:878.
4. Smith M, Castillo M. Imaging and differential diagnosis of the large eye. Radiographics 1994;14:721.

Imaging of the Pediatric Head, Neck, and Spine
by Mauricio Castillo and Suresh K. Mukherji,
Lippincott-Raven Publishing, Philadelphia © 1996.

12
Face

12.0 *Applied Embryology of the Face*

The face may be divided into three compartments that have different origins (Fig. 12.0-1). The oral opening separates the superior face from the mandibular arch. The mandibular arch derives from first branchial arch. The second branchial arch produces the pinnae, tympanic membranes, ossicles (up to the superstructure of the stapes), styloid process, hyoid bone, cranial nerves V and VII, and muscles of mastication and facial expression. Although the development of the superior face and orbit are relatively independent, hypoplasia of the inferior face may result in lack of growth of the bony orbit and zygomatic arches.

Step 1. The Basic Structures of the Face

The superior compartment of the face is mostly formed by the frontonasal processes. The nasooptic groove separates the inferior maxillary process from the nasomedial and nasolateral processes. These two processes are separated from each other by the nasal pits. The nasal pits eventually become the nostrils. The nasooptic groove extends from the nasal pit to the medial orbital canthus, and develops into the nasolacrimal apparatus. The frontal prominence is massive and located superior to all of the previous processes.

Step 2. Formation of the Midline Face

At 6 weeks of life, the nasomedial processes merge with the frontal prominence (Fig. 12.0-2). The following structures are produced: nasal bones and cartilaginous capsule, frontal bones, central one-third of upper lip and alveolar ridge, central incisors, and primary palate. Overgrowth of the nasomedial processes results in stenosis of the piriform aperture. Inferiorly, the same nasomedial processes merge with the maxillary processes and give rise to the columella and the philtrum (Fig. 12.0-3).

Step 3. Formation of Facial Structures Off-Midline

During the fourth to eighth week, the structures located off the facial midline are formed. The nasolateral processes fuse with the maxillary processes, resulting in the nasal alae. Hypoplasia of the nasal alae produces respiratory obstruction but does not require imaging. The maxillary processes reach superiorly and fuse with the frontal prominence, giving rise to the lateral one third of the upper lip, lateral one third of the superior alveolar ridges, and the palatal shelves. The maxillary processes reach inferiorly and merge with the mandibular arches to produce the outer margins of the mouth and cheeks (anomalies at this stage result in transverse facial clefts and macrostomia). The nasooptic groove also deepens and becomes the nasolacrimal ducts (anomalous formation results in mucoceles or cysts of the ducts).

Step 4. Formation of the Upper Digestive Space

In the middle of the previous processes lies the oral placode, which forms the mouth and buccal cavity. The oral placode is a depression lined by ectoderm. This depression enlarges to become the stomodeum, which is separated from the cephalic portion of pharyngeal gut by the buccopharyngeal membrane. By the fourth week of life, this membrane dissolves, leaving behind the Waldeyer ring.

Step 5. Formation of the Nasal Spaces

During the same stage of development, the nasal pits deepen but are separated from the stomodeum and pharynx by the bucconasal plate. This plate evolves into a membrane and eventually dissolves. Persistence of the plate results in bucconasal atresia. Before the airway is established, the nasal pits form the primitive choanae. As the nasal cavity is divided into separate compartments by the descending septum, the secondary choanae are formed. Plugs of epithelium seal the secondary choanae and are resorbed later in life. The exact mechanism for choanal atresia is uncertain, but incomplete formation of the secondary choanae, lack of canalization of the plugs, or misdirection of the flow of mesodermal elements may be responsible. The palatal shelves fuse in the middle with each other (Fig. 12.0-4). Anteriorly, they fuse with the wedge-shaped primary palate. This completes the formation of the hard palate, which occurs simultaneously with the descent of the nasal septum. The posterior palatal shelves, which are devoid of cartilage, also fuse and form the soft palate. Lack of fusion of the primary palate with the palatal shelves produces an anterior cleft palate (which is usually eccentric). Lack of fusion of the palatal shelves produces a secondary cleft palate, which is usually midline. Lack of fusion of the posterior palatal shelves results in a bifid uvula, which is the mildest form of cleft palate.

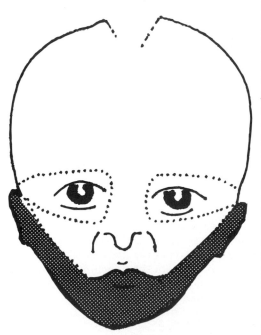

FIGURE 12.0-1.

The face is divided into three distinct sections according to their embryology. The mandibular arch *(shaded)* is derived from the first branchial arch. Note that the external and middle ears are also derived from the same arch, and therefore mandibular hypoplasia is usually accompanied by aural atresia–hypoplasia and malformed middle ear cavities and ossicles. Because the zygomas are partly derived from the mandibular arch, they may also be small in facial microsomia. Although the bony orbits *(dotted lines)* form as distinct units, their formation is influenced by the formation of the entire face, and they may therefore also be hypoplastic in facial microsomia. The midface derives from the frontonasal prominence, nasomedial and nasolateral processes, and maxillary processes. Closure of the optic vesicle and midface occur at the same time. Lack of closure of one may be related to abnormalities in closure of the other.

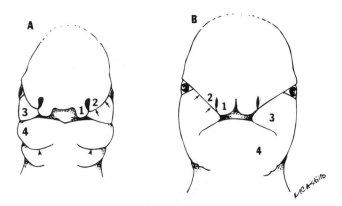

FIGURE 12.0-2.

A. The fetal face at approximately 5 weeks of age. The orbits are widely separated, and the nasooptic groove *(arrows)* extends from the medial canthus to the primitive nostril, which separates the nasomedial (1) process from the nasolateral (2) processes. Under these two processes lies the maxillary (3) process. Most of the inferior face consists of the mandibular arch (4), which in itself is separated from the neck by the hypomandibular cleft *(arrowheads).* **B.** The fetal face at approximately 7 weeks of age. The orbits have started to descend and approximate medially. The nasooptic groove *(arrows)* extends to the inferior nasal opening, which separates the nasomedial (1) and nasolateral (2) processes. Most of the lateral midface consists of the maxillary processes (3). The inferior face is formed by the massive mandibular arch (4). (With permission from Castillo M. Congenital abnormalities of the nose: CT and MR findings. AJR 1994;162:1211.)

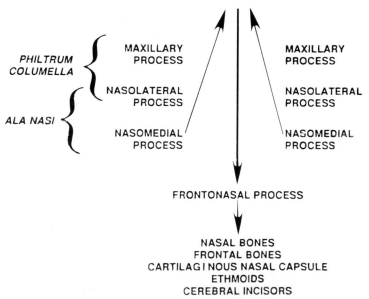

FIGURE 12.0-3.

Fusion and origin of the several processes that form the midface. Fusion of the nasomedial and nasolateral processes gives rise to the alae nasi. Fusion of the nasolateral process and the maxillary process gives rise to the philtrum and columella. Fusion of the nasomedial process and the frontal prominence gives rise to the frontonasal process, which develops into the nasal and frontal bones, cartilaginous nasal capsule, and central incisors.

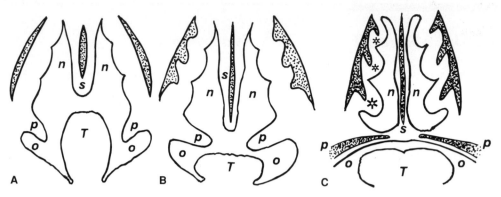

FIGURE 12.0-4.

Formation of the oral and nasal cavities. **A.** At 6 weeks of life, the oral (o) and nasal (n) cavities communicate with each other because palatal shelves (p) are very rudimentary. The nasal cavity is separated by the septum (s), which contains cartilage *(shaded area)*. The tongue (t) is large and occupies both cavities. **B.** At 8 weeks of life, the nasal septum (s) is extending inferiorly and the palatal shelves (p) medially. The tongue (t) is now relatively smaller and contained in the oral (o) cavity, which still communicates with the nasal cavity (n). **C.** At 10 weeks of life, the nasal septum (s) is fused inferiorly and in the midline with the palatal (p) shelves, forming the palate. Therefore, the nasal (n) cavities are formed and separated from the oral (o) cavity, which contains the tongue (t). The rudimentary nasal conchae (*) are now formed. The appearance of these spaces is now similar to that of an adult.

SUGGESTED READINGS

1. Hiatt JL, Gartner LP. Embryology of the head and neck. In: Textbook of Head and Neck Anatomy. New York: Appleton-Century-Crofts, 1982:57.
2. Naidich TP, Osborn RE, Bauer BS, et al. Embryology and congenital lesions of the midface. In: Som PM, Bergeron RT, eds. Head and Neck Imaging, 2nd ed. St. Louis: CV Mosby, 1991:1.

12.01 *Median Facial Cleft Syndromes*

EPIDEMIOLOGY

The incidence of these syndromes is unknown, but they represent less than 1% of all facial clefting anomalies. Most cases are sporadic, with a few familial cases reported (either autosomal recessive or dominant). Some subtypes have been reported to occur in twins.

CLINICAL FEATURES

The clinical features of these syndromes are the presence of a midline facial cleft (which may or may not be visible) and hypertelorism. All patients have hypertelorism and may or may not have a cranium bifidum occultum frontale. According to the Sedano classification, the face may be divided into four distinct types. Patients with type A have no visible cleft, no brain anomalies, and are neurologically normal (Fig. 12.01-1). Patients with type B facies have true midfacial clefts and may be divided into a low group (group A) and a high group (group B). In the low group, the cleft involves the upper lip, the palate, and occasionally the nose. It is associated with basal encephaloceles, dysgenesis of the corpus callosum, intracranial lipomas (mainly interhemispheric), and dysplasias of the optic nerve (particularly coloboma, optic pit, and megalopapilla). In the high group, the cleft involves the nose and the forehead and only occasionally the upper lip and palate. It is associated with frontoethmoidal and intraorbital cephaloceles, cranium bifidum occultum, intracranial lipomas, and dysgenesis of the corpus callosum. The eye is commonly small (microophthalmos) or absent (anophthalmos). There is a "widow's peak" hairline. This group may be familial. In the type C facies, the cleft involves the nasal alae and the patients may have any of the intracranial abnormalities described for type B. Patients with type D facies show a combination of type B and C features. Types B, C, and D may be mentally retarded. The Tessier classification may be used to map the facial clefts. Meridian 0 is located at the left nasal ala, meridian 1 in the midline nose, 6 at the lateral canthus of the right orbit, 13 at the right nasal bones, and 14 at the centroglabellar region. As such, patients with midline facial cleft syndromes harbor clefts at meridians 0, 1, 13, and 14. The mildest type of high median cleft syndrome is the isolated cranium bifidum occultum. Other abnormalities seen in children with median facial clefting include hydrocephalus, brachydactyly, clinodactyly, camptodatyly, scoliosis, preauricular skin tags, cryptorchism, tetralogy of Fallot, Klippel-Feil syndrome, Goldenhar syndrome, Crouzon syndrome, and mental retardation. Choanal atresia has also been described. The entity called "craniofrontonasal dysplasia" has been grouped separately from the median facial cleft syndromes and is more common in girls. In these patients, coronal or lambdoidal synostoses may also be present. A patient with a midline facial cleft, but with hypotelorism, has holoprosencephaly and not a median cleft syndrome. Midline clefts may also be seen in patients with septooptic dysplasia and Kalmann syndrome.

IMAGING FEATURES

In these patients, we use computed tomography (CT) to examine the face and orbits, and magnetic resonance (MR) imaging for the brain. Patients with type A facies do not require imaging. In the type B low group, CT shows a cleft in the upper lip (50%) and palate reminiscent of the common clefts (Fig. 12.01-2). CT shows defects in the base of the skull and MR imaging confirms the presence of meningoceles, meningoencephaloceles, or encephaloceles. These commonly occur through the frontobasal and sphenoid regions. The corpus callosum may be absent or dysgenetic (40%–43%), and there may be interhemispheric collections of fat, which are better evaluated with MR imaging.

The eyes show posterior outpouchings compatible with colobomas, and may be small. In the type B high group, the cleft involves the nose, which is not widely separated (Fig. 12.01-3). These clefts tend to be subtle and cause widening or notching of the nose. The eyes are widely separated and there is a defect that may include only the forehead, or may extend from the nasofrontal suture to the bregma. The defect may be very large. The eyes may be small or absent and the bony orbit may be underdeveloped. The corpus callosum may be absent or dysgenetic, and there may be interhemispheric lipomas. A cephalocele may be present under the frontal bone and rostral to the ethmoid bones. Intraorbital cephaloceles herniate through the lacrimal bone and present as medial canthal masses. The coronal and lambdoidal sutures may be prematurely closed, leading to widening of the sagittal suture and thus creating the impression that the frontal cleft continues posterior to the lambdoid fontanelle. In the type C patient, the notching involves one or both nasal alae. Inside the nose, there may be a dermal sinus tract that may be accompanied by intranasal dermoids–lipomas. The masses may extend intracranially. The nasal root is wide, and there is hypertelorism and a cranium bifidum occultum. In type D, patients have a combination of the external and intracranial features of types B and C (Fig. 12.01-4). Also, subcutaneous scalp lipomas may be present and accompanied by intracranial lipomas.

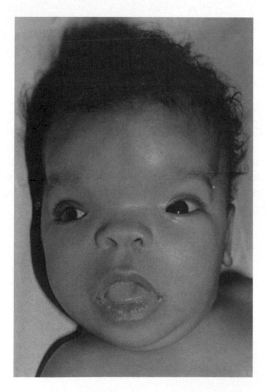

FIGURE 12.01-1.

High median cleft syndrome, type A facies, clinical features. Photograph shows child with hypertelorism and a broad nasal bridge. In general, these patients have no intracranial anomalies and are intellectually normal.

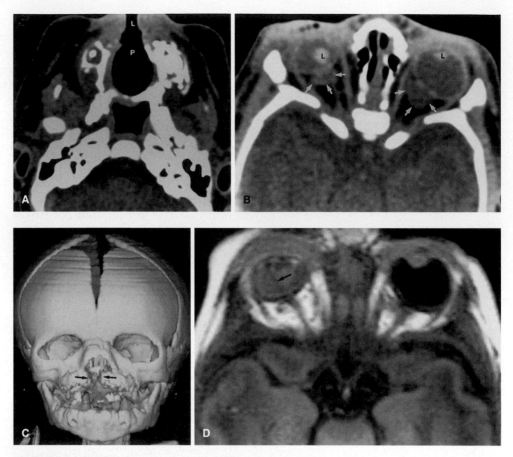

FIGURE 12.01-2.

Low median cleft syndrome, type B facies, imaging features. **A.** Axial computed tomography (CT) shows midline cleft involving upper lip (L) and palate (P). **B.** Axial CT in same child shows bilateral posterior colobomas *(arrows)* and dysplastic lenses (L). There is microophthalmia. **C.** Three-dimensional reformation of spiral CT in same child demonstrates the midline cleft *(arrows)* limited to the maxilla. **D.** Axial magnetic resonance T1-weighted image in same child suggests presence of persistent primary vitreous in right eye with a Cloquet's canal *(arrow)*. The corpus callosum was intact in this patient.

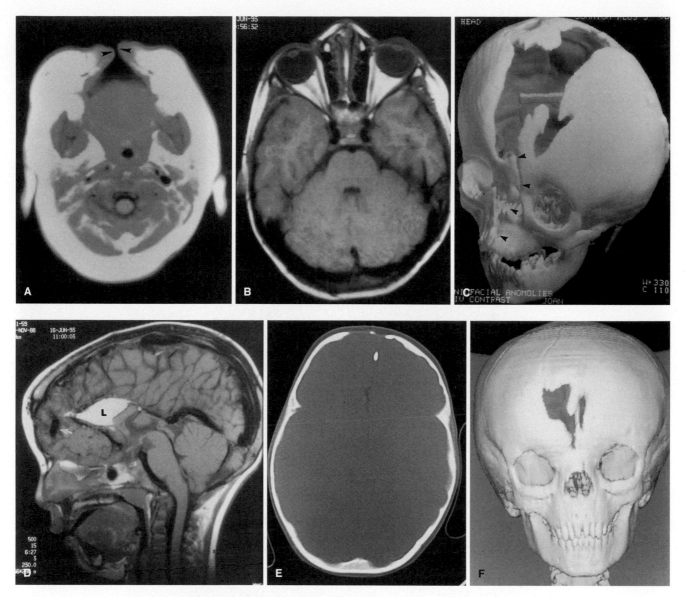

FIGURE 12.01-3.

High median cleft syndrome, type B facies, imaging features.   **A.** Axial magnetic resonance (MR) T1-weighted image shows midline cleft *(arrowheads)* involving the upper lip. **B.** Axial MR T1-weighted image in the same patient shows hypertelorism. **C.** Frontal oblique three-dimensional computed tomography (CT) reformation shows midline cleft *(arrowheads)* involving the maxilla and extending into the frontonasal area. There is a large cranium bifidum involving the entire extent of the frontal bones. A ventricular shunt is present. (With permission from Castillo M. Congenital abnormalities of the nose: CT and MR findings. AJR 1994;162:1211.) **D.** Midsagittal MR T1-weighted image in a different patient shows agenesis of the body and splenium of the corpus callosum with preservation of the genu. There is an anterior interhemispheric lipoma (L). Frontal cranium bifidum is present and there is a calcification *(arrow)* in the anterior falx cerebri. **E.** Axial CT (bone windows) in the same child shows the frontal bone defect and the calcification in the anterior falx. **F.** Frontal three-dimensional CT reformation shows the frontal bone defect and the falcine calcification. The cleft is only partially seen (because of smoothing by the algorithm) in the nasal region. There is hypertelorism.

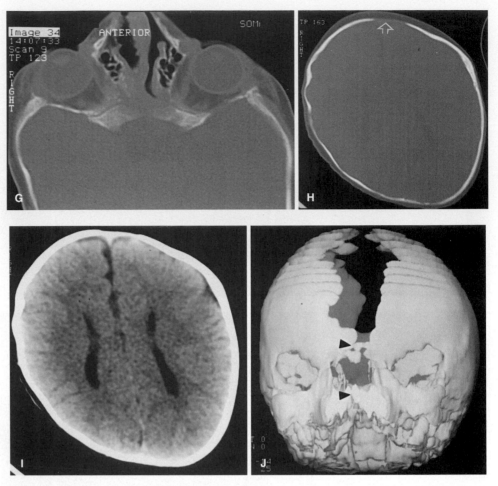

FIGURE 12.01-3. *Continued.*

G. Axial CT in a different patient shows marked hypertelorism. **H.** Axial CT in same patient shows bone defect *(arrow)* in midline of frontal bones, bicoronal synostosis, and right lambdoid synostosis with flattening of the skull. **I.** Corresponding soft tissue window settings show agenesis of corpus callosum. **J.** Three-dimensional CT reformation in same patient shows large cranium bifidum occultum, marked hypertelorism, and midline cleft *(arrowheads)* involving nasal bones and maxilla.

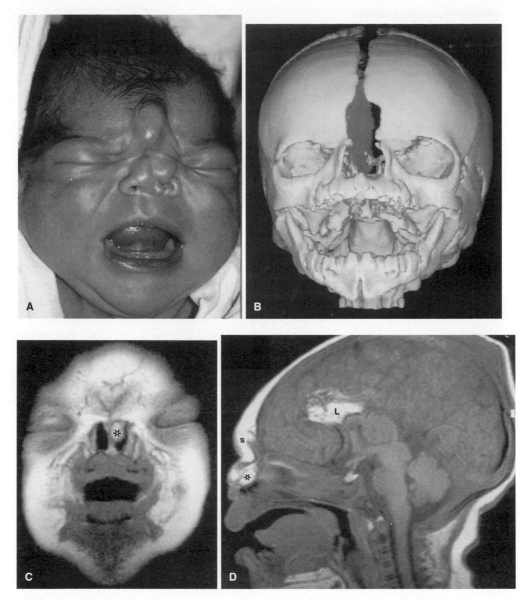

FIGURE 12.01-4.

Median cleft syndrome, type D facies, clinical and imaging features. **A.** Photograph of child shows cleft in left nasal ala and masses in nose and glabellar region. **B.** Three-dimensional computed tomography shows hypertelorism and cranium bifidum occultum frontale. **C.** Coronal magnetic resonance (MR) T1-weighted image shows left intranasal dermoid (*) of high signal intensity. **D.** Midsagittal MR T1-weighted image shows interhemispheric lipoma (L), agenesis of corpus callosum, subcutaneous lipoma (s), and intranasal dermoid (*).

SUGGESTED READING

1. Naidich TP, Osborn RE, Bauer B, Naidich M. Median cleft syndrome: MR and CT data from 11 children. J Comput Assist Tomogr 1988;12:57.

12.02 *Obstruction of the Posterior Nasal Passages*

EPIDEMIOLOGY

Stenosis or atresia of the posterior choanae occurs in 1:5000 to 8000 live births. It is more common in girls (2:1). It is seen as an isolated anomaly or associated with the following syndromes: acrocephalosyndactyly, amniotic band syndrome, gut malrotations, Antley-Bixler syndrome, CHARGE syndrome, Crouzon disease, de Lange syndrome, fetal alcohol syndrome, DiGeorge syndrome, Lenz-Majewski hyperostosis syndrome, Marshall-Smith syndrome, Schinzel-Giedion syndrome, and Treacher Collins syndrome. There is also an association with abnormalities involving chromosomes 18, 22, and X0. A familial form is also known to exist.

CLINICAL FEATURES

Fortunately, most bony choanal atresias are unilateral (unilateral to bilateral ratio, 2:1). In bilateral cases, the patients present with severe respiratory difficulty in early life. Severe bilateral stenoses behave as atresias and are treated as such. There is an inability to pass a nasogastric tube more than 3 to 4 cm into the nose despite the presence of air in the trachea and the lungs. Respiratory distress usually is aggravated by feeding (owing to closure of the mouth) and alleviated by crying. Unilateral atresias or stenoses may remain undetected until later in life. Patients with a unilateral abnormality usually present with one-sided chronic (and occasionally abundant) rhinorrhea and mild breathing obstruction. The main differential diagnosis in these older patients is that of a foreign body lodged in a nasal passage. Approximately 75% of patients with choanal abnormalities have systemic anomalies. Establishment of an oral airway is the first step needed to ensure proper breathing. Feedings may be given by gavage. Simple membranous atresias and some mild stenoses may be corrected by transnasal endoscopic perforations (including the use of laser). Bony atresias usually require oral transpalatine resection of the inferoposterior vomer and reconstruction of the choanae. Long-term placement of stents may also be used, but these patients are prone to restenosis.

IMAGING FEATURES

Computed tomography (CT) is the imaging method of choice in newborns with nasal obstruction. The examination is obtained in the supine position after the nasal passages have been suctioned clear of secretions. The CT gantry is angled 5° cephalad to the hard palate and contiguous 1 to 1.5 mm thick sections using the high-resolution bone filter are obtained. Using the CT calipers, the site of maximum stenosis of the choanae and the site of maximum width of the vomer are measured. In patients younger than 8 years of age, the vomer measures less than 0.23 cm in width and never exceeds 0.55 cm. As a general rule, the size of the posterior choanal openings is never less than 0.34 cm in children 8 years of age or younger. In cases of bony atresia or significant stenosis, the vomer is always thickened. The posteromedial maxilla is bowed inward and touches or is fused with the lateral margin of the thick vomer (Figs. 12.02-1 and 12.02-2). Ninety percent of atresias are bony and 10% are membranous. Membranous atresias are characterized by a soft tissue filling the posterior choana (Fig. 12.02-3). These membranes may be thin and strand-like, or thick and plug-like.

We have seen one case in which the posterior border of the hard palate was fused with the ventral clivus (Fig. 12.02-4). The vomer was also fused posteriorly with the clivus. The posterior choanae were malformed and the soft palate was absent. The patient presented with symptoms identical to choanal atresia. We have termed this condition "nasopharyngeal atresia" and believe it is probably a severe form of posterior bony choanal atresia.

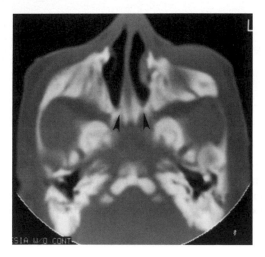

FIGURE 12.02-1.

Bony choanal atresia. Axial computed tomography shows complete bony atresia *(arrowheads)* of the posterior choanae. The posterior vomer is thick and fused laterally with the posteromedial maxilla. There is no air in the nasopharynx. (With permission from Castillo M. Congenital abnormalities of the nose: CT and MR findings. AJR 1994;162: 1211.)

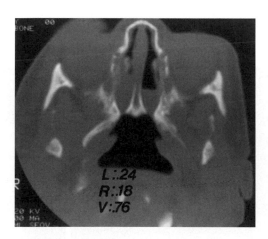

FIGURE 12.02-2.

Choanal stenosis. Axial computed tomography (CT) in a case of bilateral bony choanal stenosis with membranous atresias. The vomer is thick (0.76 cm). The right choana is markedly narrowed (0.18 cm) and the left choana is less narrowed (0.24 cm) but still stenotic. There are soft tissue plugs completely obstructing the choanae. The left side contains a fluid level probably secondary to inadequate suctioning before the CT study.

12.03 *Obstruction of the Anterior Nasal Passages*

Obstruction of the anterior nasal passages is secondary to mucoceles (cysts) of the distal nasolacrimal ducts, stenosis of the piriform aperture, or hypoplasia of the alae nasi. The incidence of these anomalies is very low. In our experience, there is no gender predilection.

Hypoplasia of the alae nasi is a clinical diagnosis for which no imaging is needed and therefore is not discussed here. Agenesis of the nose is extremely rare, and comprises absence of the nasal bones, premaxilla, and anterior nasal cavities. The nostrils are absent (Fig. 12.03-1). Surgical correction is performed after 5 years of age. Patients with bilateral distal nasolacrimal duct cysts and piriform aperture stenosis present with severe and early respiratory obstruction, similar to patients with choanal atresia–stenosis. The main difference is that a nasogastric tube may not be advanced past the anterior nasal openings in these children. The low incidence of distal nasolacrimal duct cysts is probably also secondary to their rupture and resolution as a result of forceful insertion of nasogastric tubes. Mucoceles may arise anywhere within the nasolacrimal duct. The proximal ones present as medial canthal reddish masses. The distal ones present as soft tissue masses under the inferior turbinates. These mucoceles are believed to be secondary to lack of canalization of the distal nasolacrimal ducts (Fig. 12.03-2). However, we have found chronic inflammatory changes in their walls, suggesting the possibility of in utero inflammation. This inflammation probably produces edema and obstruction of the valve of Hasner, resulting in an accumulation of retained secretions. Treatment of cysts is accomplished by endoscopic resection at their base or fenestration of their walls.

Stenosis of the piriform aperture may be seen as an isolated anomaly or with alobar or semilobar holoprosencephaly. Some patients have other abnormalities, including facial hemangiomas, clinodactyly, endocrine dysfunction, and upper teeth anomalies. In the latter, fusion of the superior central incisors into a single megaincisor may be seen. When a megaincisor is present, there is a strong association with holoprosencephaly. Stenosis of the piriform aperture without a megaincisor is almost always an isolated anomaly. Treatment of this anomaly requires resection of the anteromedial maxilla and reconstruction of the anterior nasal orifices.

In agenesis of the nose, there is a bony plate at the vestibule. The maxilla is small. The nasal cavities are small and unformed (see Fig. 12.03-1). In cases of distal nasolacrimal duct mucoceles, computed tomography (CT) shows rounded, bilateral or unilateral, homogenous soft tissue density structures in the anterior and inferior nasal passages (Fig. 12.03-3). If bilateral, these mucoceles usually are asymmetric in size. The inferior turbinates may be small and slightly displaced superiorly. In cases of unilateral mucoceles, the nasal septum may be slightly deviated toward the contralateral side. These cysts may be associated with choanal abnormalities.

By CT, patients with stenosis of the piriform aperture show thickening of the anterior and medial maxilla and narrowing of the inferior nasal passages (Fig. 12.03-4). There are no measurements for this region, and therefore the diagnosis varies according to the judgment of the radiologist. The anterior nasal septum may be thinned. In patients with a single central megaincisor, imaging of the brain, preferably with magnetic resonance, is suggested to exclude holoprosencephaly and to evaluate the integrity of the hypothalamic–pituitary axis.

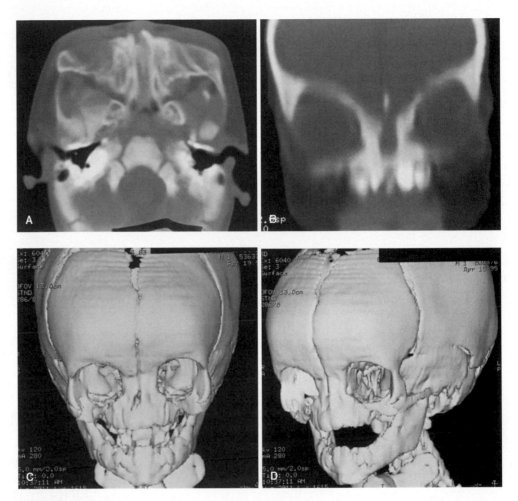

FIGURE 12.03-1.

Agenesis of the nose.   **A.** Axial computed tomography (CT) shows absent nasal cavities and small nasopharynx.   **B.** Coronal CT shows small maxilla with normal number of teeth. There is no hypotelorism.   **C.** Frontal three-dimensional CT view shows bony plate at nasal vestibule.   **D.** Oblique three-dimensional CT shows absent nasal bones and piriform aperture. A midline cleft is present in the atretic plate and is continuous superiorly with the metopic suture. (Case courtesy of I. Ihmeidan, M.D., Sparks Regional Medical Center, Fort Smith, AR.)

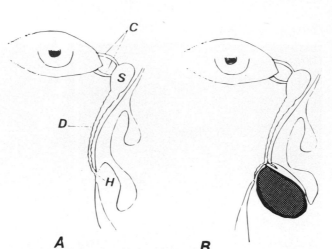

FIGURE 12.03-2.

Normal anatomy and formation of nasolacrimal duct mucoceles. A. Normal anatomy. C, canaliculi; S, lacrimal sac; D, nasolacrimal duct; H, valve of Hasner. **B.** With inflammation or lack of canalization in the region of the valve of Hasner, there is infolding of the mucosa with subsequent expansion due to retained secretions forming a fluid-filled cyst *(shaded area).* (With permission from Castillo M, Merten DF, Weissler MC. Bilateral nasolacrimal duct mucoceles, a rare cause of respiratory distress: CT findings in two newborns. AJNR 1993; 14:1011.)

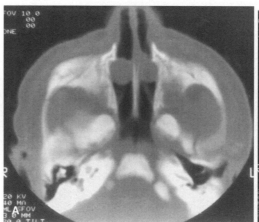
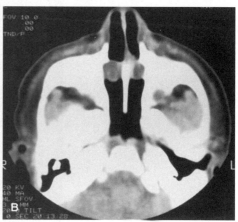

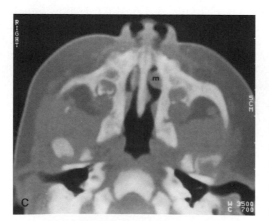

FIGURE 12.03-3.

Nasolacrimal duct mucoceles. A. Axial computed tomography (CT; bone windows) shows bilateral (right > left) rounded mucoceles in the inferior and anterior nasal passages. These cysts were arising from the distal nasolacrimal ducts. Note slight widening of the distal ducts. **B.** Same axial CT (soft tissue windows) shows the somewhat hypodense nature of these fluid-filled cysts. **C.** Axial CT in a different patient with a unilateral left-sided mucocele (m) arising from the distal nasolacrimal duct. (**A** and **B** with permission from Castillo M, Merten DF, Weissler MC. Bilateral nasolacrimal duct mucoceles, a rare cause of respiratory distress: CT findings in two newborns. AJNR 1993;14:1011.)

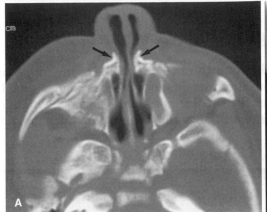

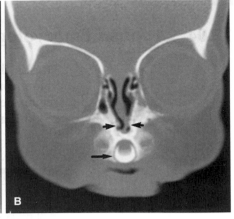

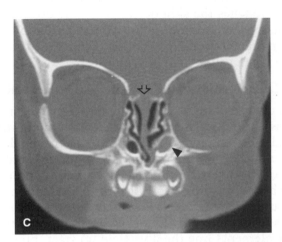

FIGURE 12.03-4.

Piriform aperture stenosis. **A.** Axial computed tomography (CT) shows severe narrowing *(arrows)* of the anterior and inferior nasal orifices due to overgrowth of the maxilla, which is bowed inward. The adjacent nasal septum is slightly thinned. **B.** Coronal CT in same patient again shows the medial overgrowth of the maxilla *(short arrows)* narrowing the anterior (piriform) nasal aperture. There is a single central megaincisor *(longer arrow)*. **C.** Coronal CT posterior to **B** shows patent foramen cecum *(open arrow)* and possible cyst *(arrowhead)* of distal left nasolacrimal duct.

SUGGESTED READINGS

1. Castillo M, Merten DF, Weissler MC. Bilateral nasolacrimal duct mucoceles, a rare cause of respiratory distress: CT findings in two newborns. AJNR 1993;14:1011.
2. Bignault A, Castillo M. Congenital nasal piriform aperture stenosis. AJNR 1994;15:877.

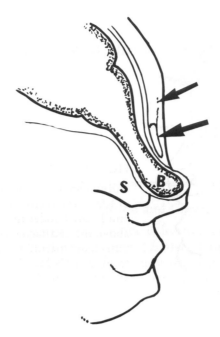

FIGURE 12.04-3.

Formation of nasoethmoidal encephalocele. The dural diverticulum in the widened prenasal space has extended and remained in contact with the skin of the nose. It contains frontal lobe (B) tissue forming an encephalocele. Encephaloceles are named by the structures that form their roof and floor. In this case of a nasoethmoidal encephalocele, the roof is the nasal bones *(large arrow)* and the floor is the cartilaginous nasal capsule (S). The frontal bone *(smaller arrow)* is fused with the nasal bones, obliterating the fonticulus frontalis.

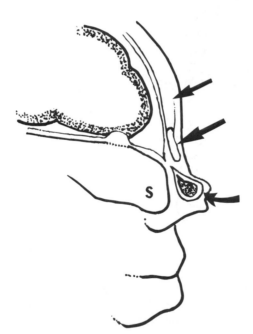

FIGURE 12.04-4.

Formation of intranasal glioma. The formation of this anomaly follows the same steps as the formation of the nasoethmoidal encephalocele, but there is closure of the medial and posterior diverticulum, severing the connection of the distal herniated brain with the frontal lobes. This results in a brain heterotopia *(curved arrow)* below the nasal bones. The frontal bones *(smaller straight arrow)* are normally fused with the nasal bones *(large straight arrow)*.

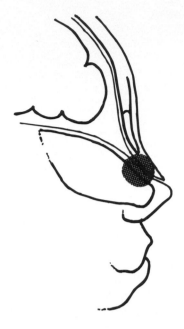

FIGURE 12.04-5.

Formation of the dermal sinus and dermoid–epidermoid. If the dural diverticulum remains too long in contact with the skin of the nose, it will drag ectoderm back with it. This ectoderm may form the lining of a dermal sinus or form masses (dermoid–epidermoid, *shaded area*) anywhere along the tract of the diverticulum.

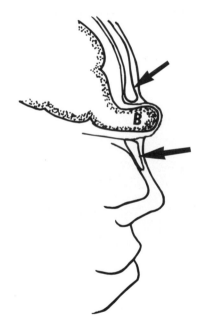

FIGURE 12.04-6.

Brain (B) herniating through a widened fonticulus frontalis. This lesion also is referred to as a frontonasal encephalocele because its roof is the frontal bones *(smaller arrow)* and its floor is the nasal bones *(large arrow)*.

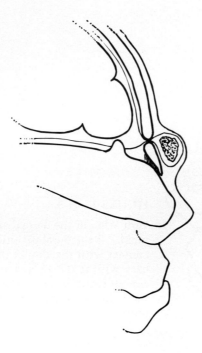

FIGURE 12.04-7.

Formation of extranasal glioma. The formation of this anomaly involves steps similar to those in the development of the frontonasal encephalocele, but note closure of the tract by fusion of the frontal and nasal bones with obliteration of the fonticulus frontalis. The connection with the frontal lobes is severed and a heterotopia of brain *(dotted region)* is sequestered outside the nasal bones.

SUGGESTED READING

1. Barkovich AJ, Vandermarck P, Edwards MSB, Cogen PH. Congenital nasal masses: CT and MR imaging features in 16 cases. AJNR 1991;12:105.

12.05 *Anomalies of the Nasofrontal Region*

EPIDEMIOLOGY

Most of these anomalies manifest as congenital midline nasal masses. They occur in approximately 1:20,000 to 40,000 live births. They are sporadic anomalies with no gender predilection.

CLINICAL FEATURES

These anomalies include masses such as encephaloceles, "nasal gliomas," dermoids–epidermoids, hemangiomas, and aberrant ethmoid sinuses. The latter two are not addressed here. These children usually present with a midline nasal mass that may be static or grow. These masses may become infected, resulting in meningitis. Anomalies without a mass are related to the presence of dermal sinuses. In these cases, repeated meningitis is common, and occasionally bilateral subfrontal intracranial abscesses may occur.

Encephaloceles may grow with the child and, if large, may be accompanied by hypertelorism. These cephaloceles tend to be isolated and not associated with systemic syndromes. They are perhaps slightly more common in boys than in girls.

"Nasal glioma" is a misnomer because most (> 60%) of them are extranasal and actually are cerebral heterotopias with no malignant potential. Extranasal gliomas do not grow. Intranasal gliomas may have a pedicle that communicates with the brain, and therefore may grow. Dermoids and epidermoids occur in approximately 50% of patients with dermal sinuses (less than 1% of all dermoids–epidermoids occur in this location). In over half of these patients, the abnormality communicates with the brain, predisposing to infections. Epidermoids are slightly more prone to infection than dermoids. In 50% of patients, only a dermal sinus is found. The anterior opening from a dermal sinus occurs with equal frequency in the glabella, nasal dorsum, nasal tip, and columella.

IMAGING FEATURES

Encephaloceles are readily demonstrated by magnetic resonance (MR) imaging. The frontal lobe herniates, and if the amount of herniated tissue is small, the appearance of the intracranial structures remains normal. Most encephaloceles (40%–60%) in this region are nasofrontal (Fig. 12.05-1). In these, the brain protrudes through a patent fonticulus frontalis. The roof of these encephaloceles is the frontal bones and the floor is the nasal bones. Approximately 30% of encephaloceles in this region are nasoethmoidal, with the roof formed by the nasal bones and the floor by the cartilaginous nasal capsule (which gives origin to the ethmoid complex; Fig. 12.05-2). The remaining encephaloceles in this region are nasolateral, protrude through the frontal process of the maxilla and the lacrimal bones into the orbits, and are occasionally bilateral. Most cephaloceles are of heterogenous signal intensity on MR T1-weighted images. On T2-weighted images, they are of intermediate intensity, with areas of higher signal probably related to gliosis or cerebrospinal fluid-filled spaces.

Over 60% of "nasal gliomas" are extranasal. They are located over the nasal bones, and MR imaging shows them to have mixed (but mostly low) signal intensity on T1-weighted images (Fig. 12.05-3). On T2-weighted images, they are commonly hyperintense, probably reflecting gliosis. Intranasal gliomas are located under the nasal bones. Nasal gliomas demonstrate soft tissue attenuation by computed tomography.

Nasal dermoids are midline and show fatty attenuation by CT (Fig. 12.05-4A,B). Normally they do not enhance. By MR imaging, they have short T1 and T2 relaxation times, reflecting their fatty nature (Fig. 12.05-4C,D). If in-

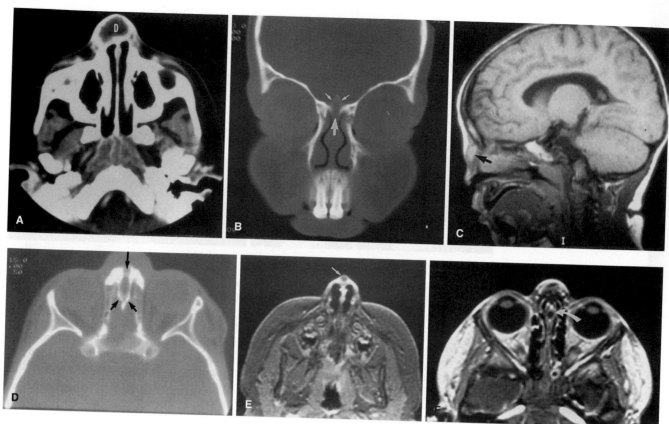

FIGURE 12.05-4.

Dermoid. **A.** Axial postcontrast computed tomography (CT) in a 5-year-old child with presumed abscess in tip of nose and concurrent meningitis. There is a hypodense dermoid (D) in the midline with surrounding thickened skin due to inflammation. **B.** Coronal CT (bone windows) in the same patient shows widened foramen cecum *(longer arrow)* and splayed crista galli *(small arrows)*. At surgery, a fibrous pedicle was found trasversing this region. **C.** Midsagittal magnetic resonance (MR) T1-weighted image (different patient) shows hyperintense mass *(arrow)* overlying nasal bones. **D.** Axial CT (bone windows) in the same patient shows tract through nasal bones *(long arrow)*, widened foramen cecum, and a crista galli that is bifid anteriorly *(short arrows)*. This dermoid had a tract communicating with the intracranial cavity. **E.** In a different patient, axial postcontrast fat-suppressed MR T1-weighted image shows midline nasal dermoid *(arrow)*. **F.** Axial MR T1-weighted image in same case shows sinus tract *(arrow)* coursing in nasal septum.

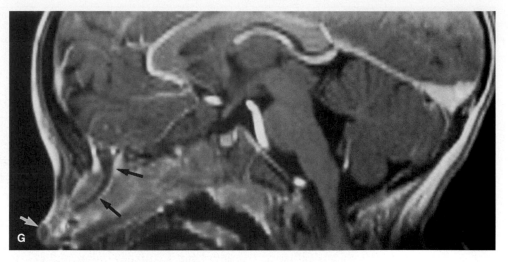

FIGURE 12.05-4. *Continued.*

G. Midline sagittal MR T1-weighted reformation shows nasal dermoid *(white arrow)* and tract *(black arrows)* extending to region of foramen cecum. (**A** with permission from Castillo M. Congenital abnormalities of the nose: CT and MR findings. AJR 1994;162:1211; **E–F** courtesy of R. McGhee, M.D., Children's Hospital, Columbus, OH.)

SUGGESTED READING

1. Barkovich AJ, Vandermarck P, Edwards MSB, Cogen PH. Congenital nasal masses: CT and MR imaging features in 16 cases. AJNR 1991;12:105.

12.06 *Common Syndromes Involving the Lower Face*

**EPIDEMIOLOGY AND
CLINICAL AND
IMAGING FEATURES**

Epidemiologic, clinical, and imaging features of the more common syndromes involving the lower face are given in Table 12.06-1.

**TABLE 12.06-1. *Epidemiologic, Clinical, and Imaging Features
of the Common Syndromes Involving the Lower Face***

Syndrome	Genetics	Clinical Features	Imaging Features
Treacher Collins syndrome	Autosomal dominant	Hypoplasia of zygomatic arches and mandible, small or absent pinnae, ear tags, down-slanted orbits	Small mastoids and middle ears, deformities of malleus and incus, aberrant course of cranial nerve VII, absent hard palate, colobomas (Fig. 12.06-1)
Crouzon disease	Autosomal dominant or sporadic	Hypoplastic maxilla, narrow or absent external auditory canals, hypertelorism, proptosis	Small middle ear cavity with deformed ossicles, craniosynostosis, hydrocephalus, absent septum pellucidum
Hemifacial microsomia	Unknown	Hypoplasia of maxilla and mandible, small pinnae, narrow or absent external auditory canals, may be confused with Goldenhar syndrome	Deformed or absent ossicles, deformed temporomandibular joint
Goldenhar syndrome	Sporadic	Hypoplasia of maxilla and mandible, deformed pinnae, preauricular skin tags, atresia of external auditory canals	Absence of ossicles, small middle ear, abnormal otic capsule, colobomas, anomalies of cervical vertebrae (Fig. 12.06-2)
Nager syndrome	Usually sporadic, some autosomal recessive	Hypoplasia of zygomatic arches and mandible, deformed pinnae	Colobomas, main differential diagnosis is Treacher Collins syndrome (Fig. 12.06-3)

In most of these syndromes, the anomalies arise from faulty development of branchial arches 1 through 4. These give rise to the lower maxilla, mandible, ears (pinnae, external canals, middle ear cavities), and the upper neck. The first branchial arch gives rise to the mandible, lower maxillary, a portion of the malleus, and the incus. The second arch gives rise to a portion of the hyoid bone, styloid process, portions of the malleus and incus, and the superstructure of the stapes. The third and fourth branchial arches develop into the upper airway and its supporting cartilages. Anomalies of the branchial apparatus therefore produce unilateral or bilateral hypoplasia of the mandible, and deformed or absent pinnae, external auditory canal, and middle ear cavity.

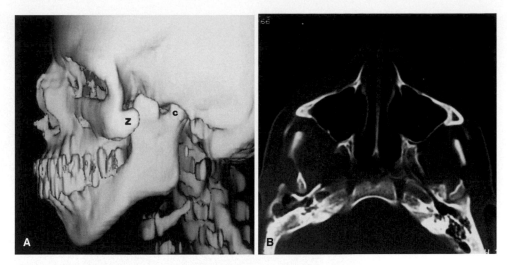

FIGURE 12.06-1.

Treacher Collins syndrome. **A.** Lateral three-dimensional computed tomography (CT) reformation of the lower face shows hypoplasia of the zygomatic arch (Z) and mild hypoplasia of the mandible. The mandibular condyle (c) is also small. The orbit is small and slanted down. The external auditory canal is absent. **B.** Axial CT of the temporal bones in the same patient shows bilateral bony atresia of the external auditory canals. The middle ear and mastoid cavities are small and the ossicles are not seen. Note hypoplastic zygomatic arches and small condyles.

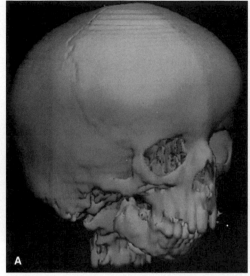

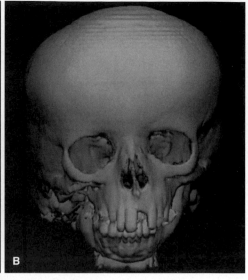

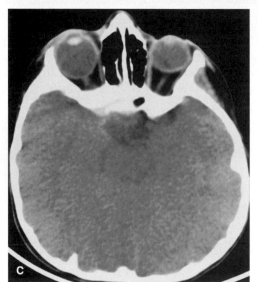

FIGURE 12.06-2.

Goldenhar syndrome. **A.** Oblique lateral three-dimensional computed tomography (CT) reformation of the face shows severe mandibular hypoplasia with absent condyle/coronoid process. The external auditory canal is present but very small. **B.** Frontal three-dimensional CT reformation in the same patient shows extreme hypoplasia of the maxilla with orbits slanted down. Note that the left hemiface is smaller than on the right side. **C.** Axial CT, same patient, shows that the left orbit and globe are smaller than on the right side. This syndrome has a similar appearance to hemifacial microsomia.

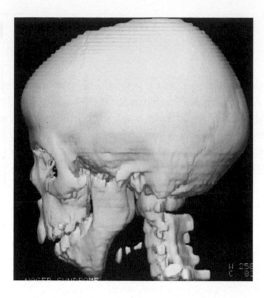

FIGURE 12.06-3.

Nager syndrome. Lateral three-dimensional computed tomography reformation shows hypoplasia of the zygomatic arch, small condyle, mild hypoplasia of the mandible, and down-slanted orbit. Note similarities with Treacher Collins syndrome (Fig. 12.06-1).

SUGGESTED READING

1. Rapin I. Children with hearing impairment. In: Swaiman KF, ed. Pediatric Neurology, 2nd ed. St. Louis: CV Mosby, 1994:1160.

12.07 *Fibrous Dysplasia*

EPIDEMIOLOGY

Fibrous dysplasia is probably one of the most common benign skeletal disorders. It is rare in children but not uncommon in adolescents. In most cases (> 70%), the disorder affects a single bone (monostotic form). The skull and face are affected in 40% to 60% of patients with the polyostotic form. The monostotic form is more common in boys, whereas the polyostotic form is more common in girls.

CLINICAL FEATURES

Clinical manifestations consist of a progressive facial, orbital, or skull deformity which begins and grows between 5 to 15 years of age. After puberty, the abnormality stabilizes. Patients commonly complain of a hard scalp mass with local pain. In cases of skull base involvement, cranial neuropathies may develop. Compression of skull base foramina tends to occur prominently at the level of the optic foramen, leading to progressive visual loss and extraocular muscle weakness. The McCune-Albright syndrome is a rare variant seen mostly in girls. It comprises unilateral polyostotic fibrous dysplasia, café-au-lait spots (commonly ipsilateral to the bone involvement), and precocious puberty. Other endocrinopathies may also be present. Cherubism is a familial form of fibrous dysplasia localized to the mandible. It is inherited as an autosomal dominant trait. It is seen commonly between ages of 18 months to 4 years.

Significant but rare complications of fibrous dysplasia include benign and malignant degeneration. Benign (cystic) degeneration refers to rapid expansion of the process by hemorrhage. Frank malignant transformation occurs in less than 0.5% of cases, mostly into osteosarcoma, chondrosarcoma, and fibrosarcoma. Malignant degeneration is more common in the face/skull, the polyostotic form, and in boys.

Histologically, the bone is replaced by dense fibrous tissues, leading to erosion, hyperostosis, deformity, and fractures. Surgery is performed for neural compression and for cosmetic improvement. Better cosmetic results are achieved after skeletal maturation is complete. Irradiation is of no value as a primary mode of treatment.

IMAGING FEATURES

The imaging features are relatively specific. Plain radiographs and computed tomography are the imaging methods of choice. The bones are thickened and sclerotic with a "ground glass" appearance. The bones may be expanded (Fig. 12.07-1A–D). Cyst-like abnormalities may also be present. Involvement of the base of the skull is commonly sclerotic. By magnetic resonance imaging, fibrous dysplasia has a heterogenous appearance on both T1- and T2-weighted images (Fig. 12.07-1E,F). There are scattered hyperintense areas within the abnormal bone. Enhancement after contrast administration is variable but commonly present (reflecting the lesion's hypervascular nature). In cherubism, the mandible is unilaterally or bilaterally, symmetrically or asymmetrically, expanded by bubbly, lucent lesions.

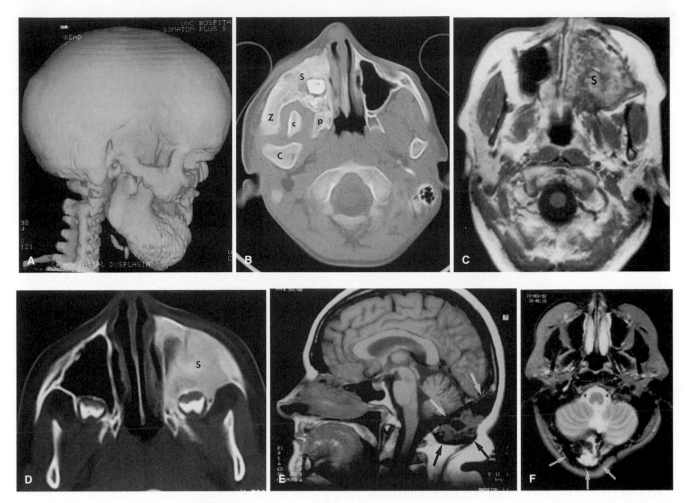

FIGURE 12.07-1.

Fibrous dysplasia. **A.** Oblique posterolateral three-dimensional computed tomography (CT) reformation in a patient with fibrous dysplasia involving the mandible (cherubism) shows marked expansion of the vertical ramus (including condyle and coronoid process) and horizontal ramus. The anterior maxilla is also involved. **B.** Axial CT (bone windows) in the same patient shows fibrous dysplasia involving the maxillary sinus (s), zygomatic arch (Z), pterygoid plates (p), coronoid process (c), and mandibular condyle (C). **C.** Axial postcontrast magnetic resonance (MR) T1-weighted image (different patient) shows heterogenous and expansile abnormality in the left maxillary sinus (S). (With permission from Castillo M. Neuroradiology Companion. Philadelphia: JB Lippincott, 1995.) **D.** Axial CT (bone windows, same patient as **C**), reveals changes typical of fibrous dysplasia in the left maxillary sinus (S). **E.** Midsagittal MR T1-weighted image in a young adult shows heterogenous and expansile area of fibrous dysplasia *(arrows)* in low occipital region. **F.** Axial MR T2-weighted image in the same patient shows that the abnormality *(arrows)* is heterogenous but mostly bright.

SUGGESTED READING

1. Casselman JW, DeJonge I, Neyt L, et al. Magnetic resonance imaging in craniofacial fibrous dysplasia. Neuroradiology 1993;35:234.

12.08 *Vascular and Lymphatic Tumors*

EPIDEMIOLOGY

Hemangiomas and vascular malformations are the most common vascular lesions of the face and neck in children. There is no hereditary predisposition, and they are almost always isolated anomalies, but some patients with syndromes (Sturge-Weber, Beckwith-Wiedemann, Klippel-Trenaunay, and Rendu-Osler-Weber syndromes) may have facial hemangiomata. They are more common in whites and girls. Lymphangiomas are less common and present earlier in life. Over half of them are present at birth, and 90% are detected before 2 years of age.

CLINICAL FEATURES

Vascular malformations of the face and neck are divided into hemangiomas (low flow) and arteriovenous malformations (high flow). Hemangiomas may be capillary or cavernous, but these two terms are no longer in vogue because they do not reflect the clinical behavior of the tumors. Hemangiomas are commonly found in the neonatal period. They are reddish, intradermal lesions occupying large areas. Some hemangiomas may grow extremely fast during the initial months of life, reflecting the endothelial proliferation that is their histologic landmark. However, 50% spontaneously involute, and the patient may be considered cured. Spontaneous involution is usually completed between 4 to 6 years of age. Involution occurs via fibrosis and fatty infiltration of the lesion. Rapidly growing lesions may produce bone changes and ulcerate, with a potential for life-threatening hemorrhages. Treatment is very difficult and usually is not indicated because the results of surgery are unpredictable. If surgery is contemplated, it should not be attempted in infancy or early childhood. Argon laser therapy is promising. Irradiation should be avoided and steroid administration is of questionable benefit.

Vascular (arteriovenous) malformations present early in life and grow with the child, only to become stable; they do not involute. Histologically, they are characterized by vascular channels lined with nonproliferative mature endothelium. If arteriovenous shunting is present, they may be clinically devastating. Endovascular embolization followed by surgical resection is often curative.

Lymphangiomas are divided into the simplex, cavernous, and cystic types. They are hypercellular tumors of lymphatic origin, and are common in the face and mouth. There is no significant skin discoloration and no pain unless they become infected. The lesions grow slowly with the child. Spontaneous regression does not occur. Surgery is indicated in small tumors, but treatment is difficult in large lymphangiomas.

IMAGING FEATURES

In our experience, magnetic resonance (MR) is the imaging method of choice because it helps to determine the exact location of the mass (Figs. 12.08-1 and 12.08-2). Hemangiomas are of homogenous and intermediate (similar to muscle) signal intensity on T1-weighted images. High T1 signal intensity may be seen and may be caused by fatty regression. On T2-weighted images, hemangiomas tend to be hyperintense and may harbor septa and some vascular flow voids (Fig. 12.08-1A). Satellite nodules are typical. All hemangiomas show moderate to marked enhancement after contrast administration (Figs. 12.08-1B and 12.08-2B, C). They should be distinguished from true arteriovenous malformations, which may be amenable to endovascular therapy (Fig. 12.08-3).

In lymphangiomas, MR imaging shows a multicystic mass on T1-weighted images. These cysts are mostly hypointense, but their walls may enhance after contrast administration. Enhancement is also seen when the lesions become infected. On T2-weighted images, lymphangiomas are hyperintense.

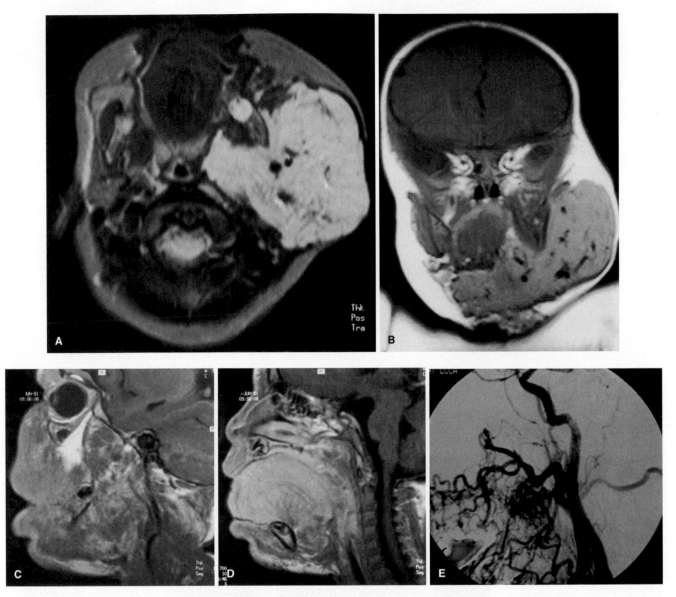

FIGURE 12.08-1.

Facial hemangioma. **A.** Axial magnetic resonance (MR) T2-weighted image shows a very large hemangioma arising in the left cheek and extending into the parapharyngeal space. Note that the mass is mostly hyperintense but contains some rather large flow voids, suggesting vessels. **B.** Coronal postcontrast MR T1-weighted image in the same patient shows that the mass enhances diffusely and homogenously. Again noted are the large flow voids, suggesting vessels. The mass extends into the submandibular space and left sublingual region. **C.** Parasagittal MR T1-weighted image in a different patient shows extensive hemangioma involving the face. **D.** Midline T1-weighted image shows hemangioma to involve and diffusely enlarge the tongue. **E.** Catheter angiogram injection into common carotid in same patient shows myriad of feeding vessels arising from external carotid artery.

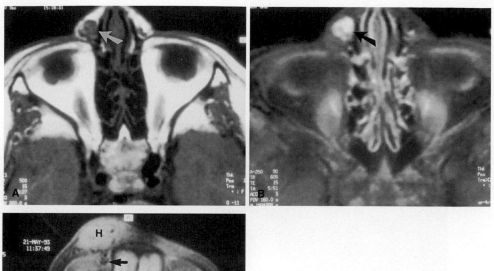

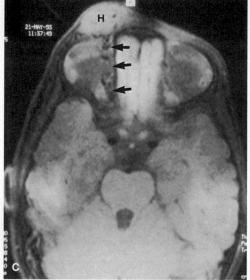

FIGURE 12.08-2.

Orbital hemangioma. **A.** Axial magnetic resonance (MR) T1-weighted image in a different patient shows small hypointense hemangioma *(arrow)* in the medial right orbital canthus. **B.** Axial postcontrast MR fat-suppressed, T1-weighted image in the same patient shows lesion *(arrow)* to enhance markedly. **C.** Axial postcontrast MR fat-suppressed, T1-weighted image in a different patient shows enhancing hemangioma (H) with associated large vessels *(arrows; veins?)* in the retrobulbar region.

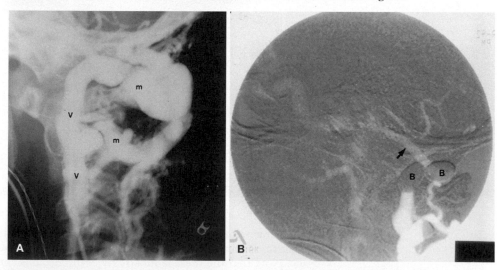

FIGURE 12.08-3.

Arteriovenous malformation. **A.** Lateral view from injection into vertebral artery (V) shows large suboccipital vascular malformation supplied by muscular branches (m). This 9-year-old boy became symptomatic after visiting an amusement park. **B.** Corresponding view after occlusion of feeding vessels with detachable balloons (B). Note preservation of flow in vertebral artery *(arrow)* with filling of basilar artery and internal carotid artery via patent posterior communicating artery.

SUGGESTED READINGS

1. Smith JK, Castillo M, Wilson JD. MR characteristics of low flow facial vascular malformations in children and young adults. Clinical Imaging, 1995;19:109.
2. Meyer JS, Hoffer FA, Barnes PD, Mulliken JB. Biological classification of soft tissue vascular anomalies: MR correlation. AJR 1991;157:559.
3. Mulliken JB, Glowacki J. Hemangiomas of vascular malformations in infants and children: a classification based on endothelial characteristics. Plast Reconstr Surg 1982;69:412.

Imaging of the Pediatric Head, Neck, and Spine
by Mauricio Castillo and Suresh K. Mukherji,
Lippincott-Raven Publishing, Philadelphia © 1996.

13
Temporal Bone

13.0 *Applied Embryology*

The ear is composed of three separate regions that are embryologically distinct; these are the external, middle, and inner ear.

EXTERNAL EAR

Step 1. Formation of the Pinna

The external ear is composed of the pinna (auricle) and the external auditory canal. The pinna arises during the fourth week of gestation from the first branchial groove and the mesoderm of the first and second branchial arches. By the sixth week, the arches have given rise to six outgrowths, termed the hillocks of His. These hillocks fuse to form the pinna by the third month of gestation.

Step 2. Formation of the External Auditory Canal

The external auditory canal is derived from the dorsal end of the first branchial groove. Between the fourth and fifth weeks of gestation, the ectoderm of the first branchial groove comes in contact with the endoderm of the first pharyngeal pouch. At 8 weeks of gestation, the initial groove formed by the first branchial pouch, also referred to as the cavum concha, deepens to form a funnel-shaped tube termed the "primary meatus." This is the precursor of the cartilaginous portion of the external auditory canal. During the ninth week of gestation, the groove deepens and comes into contact with the epithelium of the first pharyngeal pouch (tubotympanic recess). An epidermal plug (meatal plate) subsequently forms and extends from the primary meatus to the epithelium of the tubotympanic recess (primitive tympanic cavity). A core of epithelial cells within the plug begins to resorb during the 28th week of gestation. This new ectodermal tube is the precursor of the bony portion of the external auditory canal. The tympanic membrane is derived from the ectoderm of the first branchial groove, the endoderm of the tubulotympanic recess, and the mesoderm of the first and second branchial arches. Except for the tympanic ring, the external auditory canal is unossified at birth. Complete ossification occurs by the second year of life. The adult size of the external auditory canal is normally reached by 9 years of age. Normally, the outer one-third of the external auditory canal is cartilaginous, whereas the medial two-thirds is bony.

Step 3. Formation of the Mastoid Antrum

The mastoid antrum is nearly of adult size at birth but it is poorly pneumatized. A central mastoid canal is usually present at birth. Formation of the mastoid air cells occurs as a result of progressive pneumatization of the developing mastoid bone via the central mastoid canal. Pneumatization begins during the 33rd week of gestation. Pneumatization of the petrous apex is variable and begins during the 28th week of gestation.

Step 1. Formation of the Middle Ear Cavity

The middle ear consists of the tympanic cavity, three ossicles, eustachian tube, and several muscles and tendons. The middle ear cavity is formed from the expansion of the endodermally lined first pharyngeal pouch (also termed the "tubotympanic recess"). Growth begins during the third week of gestation. During the seventh week of gestation, there is a constriction of the mid-portion of the tubotympanic recess by the second branchial arch, resulting in the formation of the tympanic cavity (laterally) and the eustachian tube (medially; Fig. 13.0-1A). The epitympanum communicates with the mastoid antrum via the additus ad antrum, which is formed by expansion of the tympanic cavity during the 18th week of gestation.

Step 2. Formation of the Ossicles

The ossicles comprise the malleus, the incus, and the stapes. They arise from mesenchymal tissues adjacent to the developing middle ear cavity. The ossicles begin to form during the fourth week of gestation (Fig. 13.0-1B). They originate as cartilaginous models that reach their adult size by the 18th week of gestation. Ossification of the malleus and the incus begins at 15 weeks of gestation, whereas ossification of the stapes begins at 18 weeks of gestation (Fig. 13.0-1C). At birth, the ossicles are of adult size. The head of the malleus and body and short process of the incus derive from the dorsal cartilaginous end of the first branchial arch (Meckel's cartilage). Portions of the first branchial arch cartilage also give rise to the anterior malleolar ligament and the sphenomandibular ligament. The dorsal cartilaginous end of the second branchial arch (Reichert's cartilage) gives rise to the manubrium of the malleus, long process of the incus, and most of the stapes (head, neck, crura, and tympanic surface of the footplate). The medial surface of the stapes footplate and stapedial ligament derive from the otic capsule.

The inner ear structures are composed of the membranous labyrinth, which is covered by the bony labyrinth and is situated in the petrous portion of the temporal bone. Except for the endolymphatic sac, most of the inner ear structures are of adult size and configuration at birth.

Step 1. Formation of the Membranous Labyrinth

The membranous labyrinth consists of the utricle, saccule, semicircular canals, endolymphatic sac and duct, and cochlear duct. The inner ear originally develops from a thickening at the surface ectoderm, termed the "otic placode." This occurs on both sides of the developing rhombencephalon. During the fourth week of gestation, the otic placode invaginates into the underlying mesenchyme and forms the otic vessicle (otocyst). The mesenchyme surrounding the otocyst is the precursor of the cartilaginous capsule of the otocyst, and is termed the "otic capsule." The otocyst divides into two separate components by three folds. The dorsal utricular component gives rise to the utricle, semicircular canals, and endolymphatic duct, whereas the ventral saccular component gives rise to the saccule and cochlear duct. The utricle, saccule, and endolymphatic sac form initially during the sixth week of gestation and attain an adult configuration by 8 weeks of gestation. The duct connecting the saccule and utricle (ductus reuniens) develops at 7 weeks of gestation. The semicircular canals develop from diverticular outpouchings of the utricular portion of the developing membranous labyrinth during the sixth week of gestation. The cochlea develops from the ventral portion of the otocyst. The number of turns of the cochlea increases with progressive development. One cochlear turn is present at 7 weeks of gestation, whereas the adult configuration of $2\frac{1}{2}$ to $2\frac{3}{4}$ turns is present by the eighth week of gestation. The endolymphatic sac forms from the dorsal component of the otocyst at 6 weeks of gestation and is one of the few inner ear structures that continues to grow after birth. The hair cells and auditory sensory network are almost complete by the 26th to 28th weeks of gestation.

Step 2. Formation of the Bony Labyrinth

The bony labyrinth is formed and encloses the membranous labyrinth in three stages. The initial stage occurs between the fourth and sixth weeks of gestation and consists of condensation of the mesenchyme surrounding the membranous labyrinth. The second stage involves the formation of the bony vestibule, which encloses the perilymphatic spaces surrounding the utricle, saccule, and part of the cochlear duct. This stage also includes the development of perilymph-containing scala tympani and the scala vestibuli which surrounds the endolymph-containing cochlear duct. The third stage involves ossification of the otic capsule and begins during the 15th week of gestation. Ossification begins in 14 centers and results in formation of the petrous portion of the temporal bone. Fusion of the ossification centers is complete by the 23rd week of gestation.

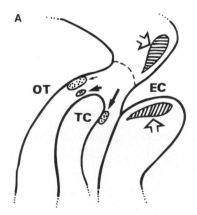

FIGURE 13.0-1.

The development of the ear apparatus. **A.** At 9 weeks of life, the otic capsule (OT) in the temporal bone is flanked laterally by the tympanic cavity (TC), which insinuates itself between the malleus *(longer arrow)* and incus *(medium arrow)*. The stapes *(small arrow)* is adjacent to the otic capsule. The external auditory canal (EC) ends blindly, and its outer walls contain the cartilaginous centers *(open arrows)*.

B

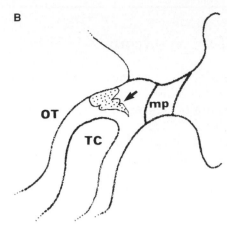

FIGURE 13.0-1. *(continued)*

B. Between the fourth and sixth weeks of life, the ossicles *(arrow)* develop. The superior aspect of the tympanic cavity (TC) expands and begins to migrate superiorly. The external auditory canal is present but occluded by the meatal plug (mp), which later becomes the meatal plate, eventually transforming into the tympanic membrane. OT, otic capsule in temporal bone.

C

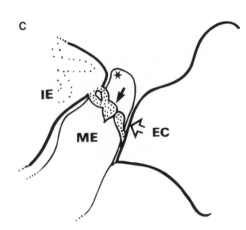

FIGURE 13.0-1. *(continued)*

C. Around the 20th week of life, the ossicles *(solid arrow)* are relatively well formed and begin to ossify. The meatal plug has thinned out, giving rise to the tympanic membrane *(open arrow)* and opening the external auditory canal (EC). The manubrium of the malleus is embedded in the tympanic membrane. The middle ear cavity is relatively well formed and its superior extension contains the attical pouches *(star)*, which later become the epitympanum. The inner ear is well formed at this stage.

SUGGESTED READINGS

1. Moore KL. The eye and ear. In: Moore KL, ed. The Developing Human: Clinically Oriented Embryology, 4th ed. Philadelphia: WB Saunders, 1988:402.
2. Kenna MA. Embryology and developmental anatomy of the ear. In: Bluestone CD, Stool SE, Scheetz MD, eds. Pediatric Otolaryngology, Vol 1. Philadelphia: WB Saunders, 1990:77.

13.01 *Large Vestibular Aqueduct Syndrome*

EPIDEMIOLOGY

Large vestibular aqueduct syndrome refers to enlargement of the bony vestibular aqueduct seen in children with sensorineural hearing loss. It is assumed to be the most commonly identifiable cause of congenital hearing loss. Approximately 1.5% of patients referred for imaging of the inner ear have an abnormally enlarged vestibular aqueduct. This syndrome is slightly more common in boys than in girls, and symptoms usually present during early childhood. Sixty percent of patients have associated malformations of the inner ear, whereas 40% of cases are isolated. Bilateral involvement is more common.

CLINICAL FINDINGS

The vestibular aqueduct is a bony canal that extends from the medial aspect of the vestibule to the posterior wall of the petrous bone. The vestibular aqueduct contains the endolymphatic duct and sac. The duct begins at the union of the utricular and saccular ducts, and therefore it is in direct communication with the membranous labyrinth. The sac is a focal dilatation of the duct, and is located in a small enlargement of the bony vestibular aqueduct. The sac participates in pressure equalization between cerebrospinal fluid (CSF) and endolymph, normal endolymph resorption, and digestion of foreign bodies. Embryologically, the endolymphatic sac arises from the primitive otocyst during the fourth week of gestation. Unlike the remainder of the membranous labyrinth, which is completely developed by the 26th week of gestation and is of adult size and configuration at birth, the endolymphatic duct and sac continue to enlarge during childhood. Enlargement of the bony vestibular aqueduct is therefore indicative of anomalous growth and development of the underlying duct and sac.

Large vestibular aqueduct syndrome is associated with congenital or early acquired deafness. Most patients have progressive high-frequency sensorineural hearing loss, but some patients may present with mixed hearing loss. The relationship between the large aqueduct and sensorineural hearing loss is controversial. The syndrome probably represents anomalous embryogenesis of the duct and sac. Because these two structures are outpouchings of the membranous labyrinth, anomalies of the duct and sac may indicate a generalized abnormality of the inner ear. Potential mechanisms responsible for hearing loss include inability to maintain normal endolymphatic pressure after increases in CSF pressure, disruption of cochlear hair cells due to reflux of hyperosmolar sac contents, and a diffuse intrinsic abnormality of the membranous labyrinth.

IMAGING FINDINGS

Computed tomography is the imaging modality of choice for evaluating patients suspected of having large vestibular aqueduct syndrome because it readily identifies the bony abnormality (Fig. 13.01-1). The diameter of the vestibular aqueduct should not exceed 1.5 mm in its posterior opening. A diameter of more than 2 mm is abnormal. In some patients, the vestibular aqueduct may not be visualized, and this is considered normal. Both temporal bones must be evaluated, given the high incidence of bilateral involvement. More than half of patients with large aqueducts have associated abnormalities of the inner ear. The most common are an enlarged and rounded vestibule, abnormal configuration of the semicircular canals (most often characterized by dilation of the ampullae of the horizontal and superior semicircular canals), and hypoplasia of the cochlea (similar to a Mondini defect). Preliminary work seems to support the observation that high-resolution fast spin echo magnetic resonance (MR) T2-weighted images show the fluid contents of the endolymphatic duct and sac. This is seen as high signal intensity in the region of the bony aqueduct. Dilation of the duct and sac is therefore also visible with MR imaging.

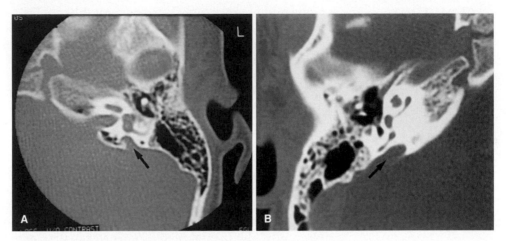

FIGURE 13.01-1.

Enlarged vestibular aqueduct. **A.** Axial computed tomography (CT) shows moderately enlarged left vestibular aqueduct *(arrow)* in patient with congenital hearing loss. **B.** In a different patient, CT shows markedly enlarged right vestibular aqueduct *(arrow)*.

SUGGESTED READINGS

1. Valvassori GE, Clemis JD. The large vestibular aqueduct syndrome. Laryngoscope 1976;88:723.
2. Swartz JD, Harnsberger HR. The otic capsule and otodystrophies. In: Imaging of the Temporal Bone, 2nd ed. New York: Thieme, 1992:192.
3. Hasso AN, Broadwell RA. Congenital anomalies. In: Som P, Bergeron RT, eds. Head and Neck Imaging, 2nd ed. St. Louis: CV Mosby, 1991:961.

13.02 *Congenital Aural Atresia*

EPIDEMIOLOGY

Congenital aural atresia is a congenital hypoplasia or aplasia of the external auditory canal that occurs in approximately 1:10,000 births. It is unilateral in 70% of cases, with the right side being affected most often. It is slightly more common in boys than girls (60% vs. 40%). Most cases are sporadic, although 14% of cases are familial. Congenital aural atresia is also associated with Treacher Collins syndrome, Crouzon disease, Klippel-Feil syndrome, and the Möbius, Duane, Vater CHARGE, and Pierre Robin syndromes.

CLINICAL FEATURES

Congenital aural atresia results from anomalous development of the first branchial groove. The first branchial groove deepens during the eighth week of gestation, forming the lateral third of the external auditory canal. The medial two-thirds of the external auditory canal develop from the meatal plate, which is a solid cord of epithelial cells extending from the lateral third of the canal to the precursor of the middle ear cavity (pharyngeal pouch endoderm). Normally, the meatal plate begins to canalize between 21st to 26th weeks of gestation. Failure of the meatal plate to canalize results in congenital aural atresia. Because the first and second branchial pouches and first pharyngeal pouches develop simultaneously, congenital aural atresia is often associated with anomalies of the middle ear and mastoid.

Patients with this disorder are diagnosed early in life and present with deformity of the auricle and no visible external auditory canal. Association of congenital aural atresia with a systemic malformation is usually a negative prognostic indicator for successful corrective surgery. Congenital aural atresia is divided into membranous and bony forms; it may also be classified into four types based on a combination of clinical evaluation, surgical findings, and the type of repair needed. Type A is a high-grade meatal stenosis limited to the cartilaginous portion of the external auditory canal. Type B is a partial atresia of both the cartilaginous and bony portions of the external auditory canal. This form of congenital aural atresia is often associated with a short or curved malleus that may be fixed to the tympanic annulus or wall of the epitympanum. A bony septum may separate the middle ear cavity into a lateral compartment that contains the malleus and incus and a medial compartment containing a normal stapes. Type C consists of a completely atretic canal with a well pneumatized tympanic cavity. There is an atretic plate that may be partial or complete. Characteristically, the malleus and incus are fused; however, the stapes is mobile. The tympanic membrane is absent. The course of the facial nerve may overlap the oval window and then proceed anteriorly within the atretic plate. Type D is complete atresia with markedly reduced pneumatization of the temporal bone. This form of congenital aural atresia is associated with anomalies of the bony labyrinth and abnormal course of the facial nerve.

Surgical correction of congenital aural atresia is the treatment of choice. Surgery should be delayed until the temporal bone is pneumatized (usually by 5 years of age). For cases of unilateral aural atresia, some recommend that surgery be delayed until adulthood, whereas others advise against surgery.

IMAGING FEATURES

Computed tomography (CT) is the modality of choice for imaging patients with congenital aural atresia (Fig. 13.02-1). CT is performed to identify the type and extent of the abnormality and to determine if the lesion is surgically correctable. The CT findings in congenital aural atresia vary with the type of anomaly. Types A and B are associated with stenosis of the external auditory canal and a normally formed middle ear cavity (Fig. 13.02-1E). Types C and D consist of thick, irregular atretic bony plates that often are associated with ossicular anomalies and an abnormal course of the facial nerve (Fig. 13.02-1A–D). The malleus and incus are malformed, fused, rotated, or absent. The head of the malleus is bulbous or amorphous and usually fused with the tegmen tympani or laterally to the bony atretic plate. The stapes usually is not involved (Fig. 13.02-1F, G). The middle ear cavity usually is small (smaller ones are correlated with poor surgical results). The oval and round windows may be hypoplastic or absent. The tympanic membrane is absent in patients with complete atresia of the external auditory canal.

Patients with complete atresia or high-grade stenosis of the external auditory canal are at increased risk for development of cholesteatoma. These cholesteatomas may either be primary (arising from epidermal inclusion cysts) or secondary. Secondary cholesteatomas, in patients with type A or B atresias, arise as a result of inhibition of normal egress (due to external canal stenosis) of desquamated epithelium.

The course of the facial nerve must be identified in all cases of congenital aural atresia. The most common variation is a more anterior location of the posterior genu and descending segment. Proper identification of the facial nerve is necessary to prevent injury to the nerve during reconstructive surgery.

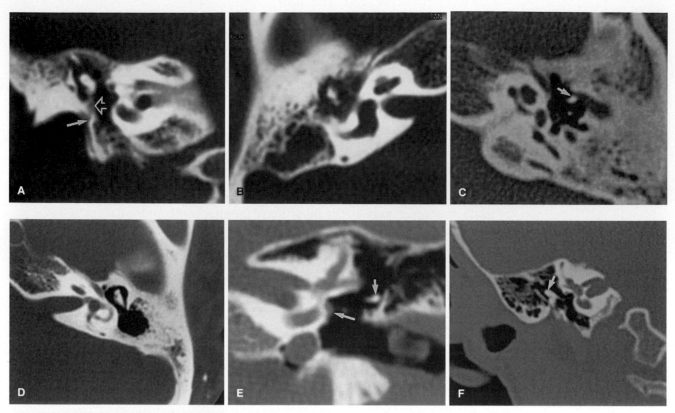

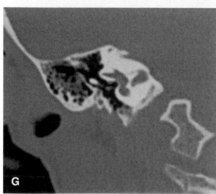

FIGURE 13.02-1.

Aural atresia and bony atresia of the external auditory canal. **A.** Coronal computed tomography (CT) shows bony plate *(solid arrow)* in fundus of external canal. The handle of the malleus *(open arrow)* is fused laterally to the atretic plate. The middle ear is partially filled with soft tissue. **B.** In same patient, axial CT shows ossicles to be dysplastic and rotated. The middle ear cavity and mastoid antrum contain soft tissue density. Note normal inner ear structures. **C.** Axial CT (different patient) shows thick atretic bone plate. The malleus *(arrow)* is rotated and fused laterally. The middle car is small and the mastoid antrum unformed. **D.** Axial CT (different patient) shows relatively normal middle ear in bony atresia of the external auditory canal. **E.** In a different patient with soft tissue atresia, the horizontal portion of the facial nerve *(larger arrow)* has an anomalous course and lies on the footplate of the stapes. The ossicles *(shorter arrow)* are fused laterally. **F.** Coronal CT in a different patient with right microtia and bony atresia (this patient's father had a similar anomaly) shows absent external canal and bony plate. The head of the malleus *(arrow)* is dysplastic and fused laterally to the atretic plate. Inner ear and facial nerve appear normal. **G.** In the same patient, the incus and stapes appear normal.

SUGGESTED READINGS

1. Swartz JD, Faeber EN. Congenital malformations of the external and middle ear: high-resolution CT findings of surgical importance. AJNR 1985;6:71.
2. Schutnecht HF. Congenital aural atresia and congenital middle ear cholesteatoma. In: Nadol JB, Schuknecht HF, eds. Surgery of the Ear and Temporal Bone. New York: Raven, 1993:263.
3. Swartz JD, Harnsberger HR. The external auditory canal. In: Imaging of the Temporal Bone. New York: Thieme, 1992:20.

13.03 *Congenital Malformations of the Inner Ear*

EPIDEMIOLOGY Inner ear malformations result from interruption of the developing ear during the first trimester of pregnancy. The arrest may be idiopathic, associated with inborn genetic errors, or caused by exposure to teratogenic agents. Genetic errors may be autosomal dominant or recessive. Malformations of the inner ear may be isolated or associated with Crouzon disease, Apert disease, Hurler syndrome, Klippel-Feil syndrome, Wildervanck syndrome, Waardenburg syndrome, Usher syndrome, Refsum syndrome, Cockayne syndrome, X-linked hypophosphatemic osteomalacia, Treacher Collins syndrome, Jervell and Lange-Nielsen syndrome, Pendred syndrome, Turner syndrome, and Alagille syndrome. Acquired causes include exposure to teratogenic agents such as ototoxic antibiotics (eg, aminoglycosides), chemical teratogens (eg, thalidomide), in utero viral infections (eg, rubella), and irradiation.

THE MALFORMED COCHLEA

Clinical Features

Patients with congenital cochlear malformations present with sensorineural hearing loss. Most inner ear malformations are bilateral and symmetric. Half of patients with unilateral demonstrable abnormalities have a hearing loss in the "unaffected" ear. The degree of hearing loss is variable and depends on the extent of underlying membranous dysplasia. In general, earlier developmental arrests result in more severe deformities and reduced hearing. Patients with inner ear malformations have a greater likelihood for development of perilymph fistulas after head trauma or after surgery. Other potential complications of inner ear malformations include recurrent meningitis and vestibular symptoms.

The Bing-Siebenmann malformation (complete membranous labyrinthine dysplasia) is an extremely rare form of total dysplasia of the membranous labyrinth. Schiebbe dysplasia (cochleosaccular dysplasia) is the most common form of inner ear malformation and is inherited as an autosomal recessive trait. It is a form of partial dysplasia of the membranous labyrinth confined to the cochlea and saccule. Schiebbe dysplasia is associated with Jervell and Lange-Nielson, Refsum, Usher, and Waardenburg syndromes. Histologically, it is characterized by a poorly differentiated organ of Corti with malformation of the tectorial membrane. There is collapse of Reissner's membrane, which deforms the scala media. The superior portion of the inner ear, including the utricle, semicircular canals, and bony labyrinth are normally formed. Patients may have preservation of low-frequency hearing and certain individuals may benefit from conventional amplification. Alexander malformation is characterized by dysplasia limited to the basal turn of the cochlea (partial membranous labyrinthine dysplasia). Patients present with familial high-frequency sensorineural hearing loss, although some are asymptomatic. Preservation of low-frequency hearing justifies the use of amplication. Michel malformation is very rare and results from complete aplasia of the membranous labyrinth. This disorder is the most severe malformation involving the osseous and membranous labyrinth. It is inherited as an autosomal dominant trait, and results from an arrest of differentiation of the otic placode during the third week of gestation. Patients present with anacusis. In cochlear aplasia, there is absence of the cochlea but relatively normal formation of the utricle, saccule, and semicircular canals. This deformity is thought to result from an arrest in development of the cochlear bud during the fifth week of gestation. Cochlear hypoplasia comprises 15% of cochlear anomalies and is more common than true aplasia. This anomaly results from an insult between the sixth and eighth weeks of gestation (which is normally a period of rapid cochlear growth). Histologically, the modiolus may be malformed or absent. Patients present with variable hearing loss that depends on the degree of development of the membranous labyrinth within the hypoplastic cochlea. The Mondini malformation is an autosomal dominant trait accounting for 50% of cochlear malformations, and is the most common type of cochlear anomaly. This malformation also occurs in a variety of systemic disorders, including Pendred, Waardenburg, Treacher Collins, and Wildervaank syndromes. Mondini malformation results from an arrest in development between the sixth and seventh weeks of gestation. Histologically, Mondini malformation is characterized by incomplete interscalar or osseous spiral lamina (incomplete septum), resulting in a confluence of the apical and middle turns of the cochlea that resembles a primitive cloacal canal. The basal turn may be normally formed. The degree of development of the organ of Corti and other auditory neural elements is variable. Hearing loss depends on the extent of underlying dysplasia involving the membranous labyrinth. The presence of some normally developed neurosensory structures justifies attempts at early rehabilitative programs, including conventional amplification. Common cavity denotes a deformity in which the vestibule and cochlea are confluent and devoid of an internal architecture. This anomaly results from an arrest in development between the fourth and fifth weeks of gestation, before the division of the otocyst into dorsal and ventral compartments. Histologically, the common cavity is ovoid or spherical, smooth walled, and contains a primordia of the membranous cavity. The overall neural population is sparse, although some cells that resemble organs of Corti may be scattered along the periphery of the cyst. Patients present with profound sensorineural hearing loss.

Imaging Features

Cochlear malformations may be divided into those that are radiographically occult and those that are radiographically demonstrable. Only 5% to 15% of congenitally deaf children have radiographically detectable abnormalities. Cochlear malformations in which computed tomography (CT) is normal are Bing-Siebenmann, Schiebbe, and Alexander dysplasias. The following cochlear malformations have abnormalities detectable by CT:

1. *Michel malformation.* There is complete absence of the cochlea, vestibule, and semicircular canals. The external and middle ear are often normally formed. Occasionally, Michel aplasia may be difficult to distinguish from labyrinthitis ossificans. However, labyrinthitis ossificans is associated with a sizeable and dense otic capsule and a deformity along the medial wall of the middle ear, indicating the presence of an obliterated lateral semicircular canal.
2. *Cochlear aplasia.* CT demonstrates an absent cochlea with partially or well formed vestibule and semicircular canals.
3. *Cochlear hypoplasia.* CT demonstrates a small cochlear bud, usually measuring 1 to 3 mm, arising from an enlarged vestibule (Fig. 13.03-1). The semicircular canals are malformed in approximately 50% of patients (Fig. 13.03-2).
4. *Mondini malformation.* CT shows a small dysplastic cochlea with absent interscalar septum. The cochlea consists of only $1\frac{1}{2}$ to $1\frac{3}{4}$ turns. Only the basal turn is normal. The vestibule may be enlarged and the semicircular canals bulbous. The lateral semicircular canal may be absent and may form a single cavity with the vestibule.
5. *Common cavity.* CT shows replacement of the vestibule and cochlea by a common cystic cavity measuring between 7 to 10 mm. This cavity is de-

void of internal structures. This malformation is also associated with malformed semicircular canals.

THE MALFORMED SEMICIRCULAR CANALS

Clinical Features

Malformations of the semicircular canals may be isolated or occur with anomalies of the membranous labyrinth. Deformities of the semicircular canals result from a failure of the vestibular anlage during the sixth week of gestation. Complete failure of development results in aplasia. Aplasia is less common than dysplasia, and is usually associated with cochlear anomalies. The superior semicircular canal reaches full development by the 19th week of gestation. It is followed by development of the posterior and lateral semicircular canals (22nd week of gestation). Deformity of the superior semicircular canal is always accompanied by malformations of the other canals.

Histologically, the utricle and saccule may be atretic, collapsed, or overtly distended. A rudimentary crista ampularis is often present. Patients present with vestibular dysfunction, although there appears to be an association with conductive hearing loss due to congenital stapes fixation. This latter association occurs because a portion of the stapes footplate is derived from the otic capsule. Alagille syndrome (arteriohepatic dysplasia) is associated with aplasia of the posterior semicircular canal, with sparing of the lateral semicircular canal.

Imaging Features

By CT, there is cystic dilation of the semicircular canals, with the lateral one being most commonly involved (Figs. 10.03-2, 10.03-3, and 13.03-3). Cystic dilation of the lateral semicircular canal may be accompanied by a dilated vestibule. It may also be an incidental finding. Dilation of both the lateral canal and the vestibule may be difficult to distinguish from a cochlear common cavity dysplasia. However, a cystic lateral semicircular canal is located posterior to the internal auditory canal, whereas a cochlear common cavity is located anterior to the internal auditory canal.

Anomalies of the semicircular canals are also associated with anomalies of the membranous labyrinth. Forty percent of patients with cochlear malformations have accompanying dysplasia of the lateral semicircular canal. The external auditory canal and the middle ear are usually normal in patients with dysplasia of the semicircular canals.

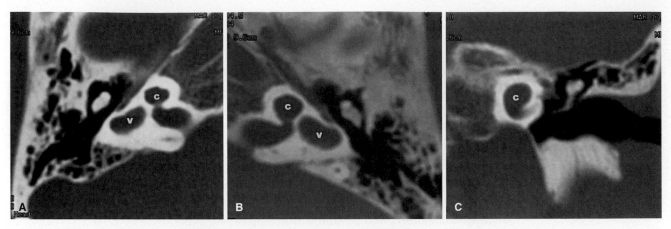

FIGURE 13.03-1.

Malformed cochlea. **A.** Axial computed tomography (CT) shows bulbous right cochlea (c) with fusion of basal and apical turns. The vestibule (v) is also enlarged. The heads of the malleus and incus appear dysplastic. **B.** Axial CT in same patient shows similar deformities involving left cochlea (c), vestibule (v), and ossicles. **C.** Coronal CT (same patient) shows dysplastic cochlea (c) devoid of its normal turns.

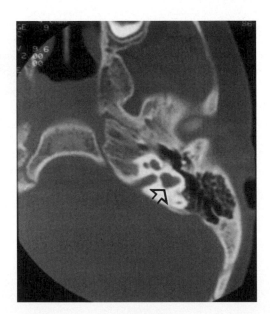

FIGURE 13.03-2.

Malformed vestibule. Axial computed tomography shows bulbous vestibule *(arrow)* that is fused with a deformed lateral semicircular canal, forming a single cavity. The cochlea is also dysplastic.

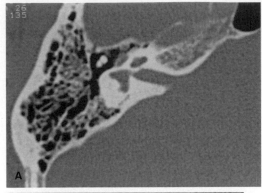
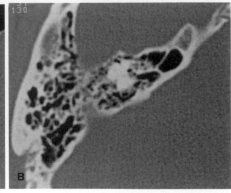
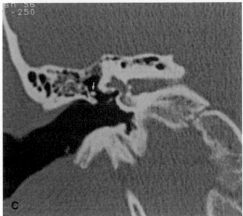

FIGURE 13.03-3.

Dysplasia of vestibule, lateral semicircular canals, and ossicles. **A.** Axial computed tomography (CT) shows almost completely absent lateral semicircular canal and somewhat ectatic vestibule. **B.** Axial CT (superior to **A**) shows absence of superior semicircular canal. **C.** Coronal CT (same patient) shows truncated lateral and superior semicircular canals. Note incus *(arrow)* fused laterally with scutum.

SUGGESTED READINGS

1. Jackler RK. Congenital malformations of the inner ear. In: Cummings CW, Frerickson JM, Harker LA, Krause CJ, Schuller DE, eds. Otolaryngology–Head and Neck Surgery, Vol 4, Ear and Skull Base. St. Louis: CV Mosby, 1993:2756.
2. Brookhauser PE. Genetic hearing loss. In: Johnson JT, Kohut RI, Pillsbury HC, Tardy ME, eds. Otolaryngology–Head and Neck Surgery, Vol 2. Philadelphia: JB Lippincott, 1993:1754.
3. Swartz JD, Harnsberger HR. The otic capsule and otodystrophies. In: Imaging of the Temporal Bone, 2nd ed. New York: Thieme, 1992:190.
4. Curtin HD. Congenital malformations of the ear. Otol Clin North Am 1988;21:317.

13.04 *Ossicular Dysplasias*

EPIDEMIOLOGY
Congenital ossicular deformities are a relatively common cause of conductive hearing loss. There is no gender predilection. They may be unilateral or bilateral. If bilateral, they have an autosomal dominant mode of inheritance. They may be isolated or occur with other ear dysplasias or systemic disorders, such as Klippel-Feil syndrome, Wildervanck syndrome, Duane retraction syndrome, Madelung dyschondrosteosis, otopalatodigital syndrome, Pyle craniometaphyseal dysplasia, Aperts disease, achondroplasia, Crouzon disease, and Paget disease.

CLINICAL FEATURES
The ossicles are formed from the primitive cartilages of the first and second branchial arches. A portion of the footplate of the stapes derives from the otic capsule. The ossicles develop between 4 to 6 weeks of gestation. The head of the malleus and body and short process of the incus derive from the dorsal end of the cartilage of the first branchial arch (Meckel's cartilage). Portions of the first branchial arch cartilage also give rise to the anterior malleolar ligament and the sphenomandibular ligament. The dorsal cartilaginous end of the second branchial arch (Reichert's cartilage) gives rise to the manubrium of the malleus, the long and lenticular processes of the incus, and most of the stapes (head, neck, crura, and tympanic surface of the footplate). The medial surface of the stapes footplate and stapedial ligament are derived from the otic capsule. The ossicles form by progressive ossification of primordium cartilaginous precursors. Cartilage models of the ossicles begin to form during the sixth week of gestation. The incus and malleus form as a single mass and separate between the eighth and ninth weeks of life, forming the malleoincudal joint. The cartilaginous models for the malleus and the incus reach adult size by 15 weeks' gestation, whereas the stapes model attains full size by the 18th week of life. Ossification of the malleus and incus begins during the 15th week of gestation, whereas stapedial ossification begins during the 18th week of gestation. The incudostapedial articulation forms between the sixth to eighth weeks of gestation. The ossicles are of adult size at birth.

The most commonly reported congenital ossicular deformity is incudostapedial disconnection, which involves anomalous articulation between the long process of the incus and the head of the stapes. Congenital anomalies of these adjacent structures are expected because both originate from Reichert's cartilage. This congenital dislocation is mostly the result of improper development of the long process of the incus. Congenital ossicular deformities are commonly associated with severe aural atresia. The malleus and incus may be dysplastic and fused. The malleus is more severely deformed than the incus. Ossicular fixation may involve any ossicle. Fixation of the malleus or incus, or both, usually occurs to the lateral wall of the epitympanum, whereas the stapes may become fused to the oval window.

Most children with ossicular dysplasias present with isolated conductive hearing loss (40–60 dB) and without prior history of infection or trauma or with aural atresia. Patients with isolated congenital ossicular dysplasias may be candidates for prostheses. The type of prosthesis depends on the extent of the abnormality and the number of ossicles involved. Potential surgical options include wire prosthesis, total ossicular replacement prosthesis, partial ossicular replacement prosthesis, and remodeling of the existing ossicular chain.

IMAGING FINDINGS
Computed tomography is the imaging modality of choice for evaluating patients suspected of having ossicular dysplasias. Incudostapedial dislocation

may be associated with absence of the stapes suprastructure. The malleus is usually normal. Congenital stapes fixation is seen as abnormal thickening of the footplate. Fixation of the malleus or incus usually involves the neck of the malleus to the lateral wall of the epitympanum or atretic plate, and is seen as lateralization of the malleus. A small fusion plate may be present between the malleus and lateral wall of the epitympanum. The alignment between the incus and the malleus is often abnormal.

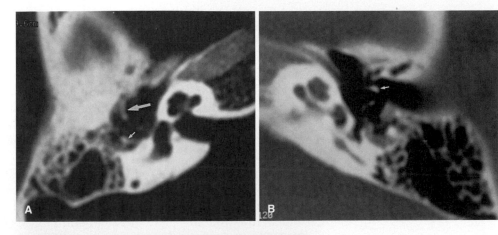

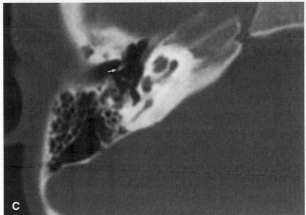

FIGURE 13.04-1.

Dysplastic ossicles.   A. Axial computed tomography (CT) in a patient with bony atresia of the external auditory canal shows handle of malleus *(large arrow)* rotated and fused laterally with atretic plate. The incus *(tiny arrow)* is dysplastic and fused posteriorly.   **B.** Axial CT (different patient) shows isolated malrotation of the malleus *(arrow)*.   **C.** Axial CT (different patient) shows rotation of manubrium *(arrow)* in patient with conductive hearing loss. No other abnormalities were present.

SUGGESTED READINGS

1. Kenna MA. Embryology and developmental anatomy of the ear. In: Bluestone CD, Stool SE, Scheetz MD, eds. Pediatric Otolaryngology, Vol 1. Philadelphia: WB Saunders, 1990:77.
2. Swartz JD, Harnsberger HR. Middle ear and mastoid. In: Imaging of the Temporal Bone, 2nd ed. New York: Thieme, 1992:105.
3. Swartz JD, Faerber EN. Congenital malformations of the external and middle ear: high-resolution CT findings of surgical import. AJNR 1985;6:71.

13.05 *Bone Dysplasias*

EPIDEMIOLOGY

Fibrous dysplasia is a progressive idiopathic anomaly of bone-forming mesenchyme. It usually presents during the first and second decades of life, and is more common in girls than in boys (3:1). Some cases are inherited, whereas others have no familial predisposition. The McCune-Albright syndrome consists of polyostotic fibrous dysplasia, precocious puberty, and cutaneous pigmentation (café-au-lait spots).

Osteogenesis imperfecta is characterized by abnormal collagen synthesis. It occurs in all races and there is no gender predilection. It may be autosomal recessive or dominant.

Osteopetrosis may be inherited as an autosomal recessive trait (severe form), intermediate recessive form (presents in older patients), or autosomal dominant (Albers-Schönberg disease). It may also be seen in patients with renal tubular acidosis and intracranial calcifications.

CLINICAL FINDINGS

Fibrous dysplasia is related to inability of osteoblasts to undergo normal maturation. This leads to disruption of the normal reparative processes after an injury to bone. Fibrous dysplasia may also be caused by an extraskeletal disorder of calcium and phosphate metabolism. Fibrous dysplasia may be classified with other similar lesions under the broad category of "fibroosseous lesions" of bone. Histologically, fibrous dysplasia is characterized by an irregular, whorled pattern of woven bone arranged within a fibrovascular stroma that replaces the normal cancellous bone. Fibrous dysplasia may involve a single bone (monostotic) or multiple bones (polyostotic). The polyostotic variety may be associated with endocrine dysfunction. Spontaneous malignant degeneration is known to occur, but, in general, is unusual. Clinical manifestations of fibrous dysplasia include pathologic fractures and bony deformities. Involvement of the temporal bone is rare, although it may occur in both the monostotic and polyostotic forms. Patients with involvement of the temporal bone present with slow, progressive, and painless swelling in the squamosal or mastoid portions of the temporal bone and the external auditory canal. Progressive cranial nerve palsies occur as a result of narrowing of the foramina in the base of the skull. Hearing loss is usually conductive and is commonly caused by progressive external auditory canal stenosis. This condition may be complicated by impingement of the ossicles by bony overgrowth or cholesteatoma formation. Sensorineural hearing loss may also occur, but is much less common than the conductive form. The treatment of fibrous dysplasia is based on the severity of the patient's symptoms. Surgical intervention usually is limited to biopsies and to the relief of functional deficits. Surgery may be beneficial for maintaining a patent external auditory canal and preserving vestibular and cochlear function. Radiation therapy is not indicated because it may increase the rate of malignant degeneration.

Congenital osteogenesis imperfecta accounts for 10% of cases and carries a high mortality. It probably results from spontaneous mutations or an autosomal pattern of inheritance. It affects the skeleton, teeth, ligaments, skin, and dura. In the tarda form, patients may have a normal lifespan. This form is probably an autosomal dominant trait. Histologically, there is a defect in extracellular bone matrix formation, abnormal collagen maturation, and reduction of osteoclastic activity. There is failure of normal lamellar bone to replace fetal bone, resulting in weak cortices. Patients may also have conductive or sensorineural hearing loss. Encroachment of the cochlea by reparative bone, hemorrhages, and microfractures may be responsible for sensorineural deafness. Structural ossicular abnormalities lead to conductive hearing loss, usually in adults. These abnormalities include fractures, resorption, and ossicular subluxations. Osteosclerotic foci are also present in the otic capsule.

Osteopetrosis results in thick, sclerotic, fragile bone that fractures easily. There is presence of calcified fetal cartilage and primitive bone, as well as failure to form medullary cavities. Patients have hepatosplenomegaly, mental retardation, and a reduced lifespan. Neurologic manifestations are secondary to compression of neural foramina by enlarging bone. Symptoms are progressive visual loss with optic atrophy, trigeminal hyperesthesia, recurrent facial palsies, and sensorineural deafness. Conductive hearing loss may be caused by ossicular involvement or overgrowth of the margins of the epitympanum, narrowing the middle ear.

IMAGING FINDINGS

Computed tomography is the imaging modality of choice for evaluating patients with dysplasias of the temporal bone. The characteristic radiographic findings in fibrous dysplasia are those of smooth bony expansion with a "ground glass" appearance. The temporal bone is enlarged, with sclerotic mastoid and petrous portions (Fig. 13.05-1). There is relative sparing of the embryologic derivatives of the otic capsule, including the cochlea, vestibule, and vestibular aqueduct. In addition, the internal auditory and facial nerve canals may be normal. This selective involvement explains why, in part, sensorineural hearing loss is an uncommon finding in patients with fibrous dysplasia. The external auditory canal may be significantly narrowed in patients with advanced disease. Cholesteatoma must be excluded in patients with high-grade canal stenosis and soft tissue masses proximal to the narrowing. The ossicles may be impinged on by adjacent bony overgrowth. The descending canal for the facial nerve may be narrowed or obliterated by this disorder.

Osteogenesis imperfecta produces diffuse demineralization of the otic capsule similar to that seen in otosclerosis. The ossicles may be dislocated or fractured. The oval and round windows may be obliterated by abnormal proliferation of bone. The paranasal sinuses are large and there is basilar invagination.

Osteopetrosis may produce thickening and sclerosis of the temporal bones and skull base with poor development of the middle ear cavities. The mastoids are underpneumatized. The ossicles and labyrinth retain a fetal configuration. Findings are similar to those seen in pyknodysostosis, Pyle disease, cleidocranial dysostosis, and Engelmann disease (Fig. 13.05-2).

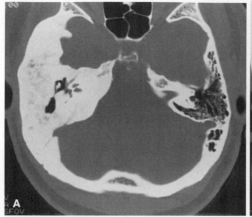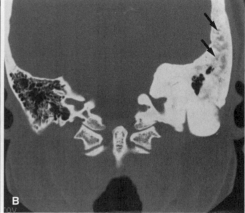

FIGURE 13.05-1.

Fibrous dysplasia. A. Axial computed tomography (CT) shows fibrous dysplasia involving the right petrous, sphenoid, and occipital bones. Note preservation of middle ear cavity, which is narrowed particularly at the level of the additus ad antrum. **B.** Coronal CT image in a different patient shows fibrous dysplasia involving the left temporal bone. Most of the mastoid air cells are obliterated and the "ground glass" matrix *(arrows)* is clearly seen. The affected bone is significantly expanded. (Cases courtesy P. Hudgins, M.D., Emory University Hospital, Atlanta, GA.)

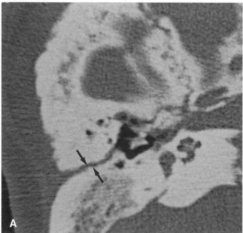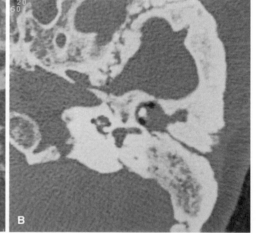

FIGURE 13.05-2.

Cleidocranial dysostosis. A. Axial computed tomography (CT) of right temporal bone shows sclerosis and expansion of bone with marked narrowing of the external auditory canal *(arrows)* and of the middle ear cavity. **B.** Axial CT of the left temporal bone at a comparable level shows similar findings, as well as soft tissue density in the middle ear cavity that was shown to be cholesteatoma.

SUGGESTED READINGS

1. Nadol JB. Manifestations of systemic disease. In: Cummings CW, Frerickson JM, Harker LA, Krause CJ, Schuller DE, eds. Otolaryngology–Head and Neck Surgery, Vol. 4, Ear and Skull Base. St. Louis: CV Mosby, 1986:3017, 3027.
2. Swartz JD, Harnsberger HR. The otic capsule and otodystrophies. In: Imaging of the Temporal Bone, 2nd ed. New York: Thieme, 1992:224.
3. May JS, Fisch U. Neoplasms of the ear and lateral skull base. In: Johnson JT, Kohut RI, Pillsbury HC, Tardy ME, eds. Head and Neck Surgery Otolaryngology, Vol 2. Philadelphia: JB Lippincott, 1993:1568.

4. Goldman AB. Collagen disease, epiphyseal dysplasias, and related conditions. In: Resnick D, Niwayama D, eds. Bone and Joint Imaging, 2nd ed. Philadelphia: WB Saunders, 1989:1020.
5. Schleuning AJ, Anderson PE. Otologic manifestations of systemic disease. In: Johnson JT, Kohut RI, Pillsbury HC, Tardy ME, eds. Head and Neck Surgery Otolaryngology, Vol 2. Philadelphia: JB Lippincott, 1993:1747.
6. McAlister WH. Osteochondrodysplasias, dysostosis, chromosomal aberrations, mucopolysaccharidoses and mucolipidoses. In: Resnick D, Niwayama D, eds. Bone and Joint Imaging, 2nd ed. Philadelphia: WB Saunders, 1989:1047.
7. Feldman F. Tuberous sclerosis, neurofibromatous, and fibrous dysplasia. In: Resnick D, Niwayama D, eds. Bone and Joint Imaging, 2nd ed. Philadelphia: WB Saunders, 1989:1227.

13.06 *Otosclerosis*

EPIDEMIOLOGY

Otosclerosis is a primary bone disease of unknown etiology unique to the otic capsule and ossicles. The disease is seen only in humans, and is predominantly transmitted as an autosomal dominant trait with variable penetrance. The variable penetrance is the result in part of foci of otosclerosis occurring in clinically silent locations. A positive family history is present in 60% of patients. Otosclerosis is more common in girls than in boys (2:1), with the clinical symptoms usually presenting in the second to third decades of life. It is bilateral in 85% of cases and is often symmetric.

CLINICAL FINDINGS

This disease manifests as a reddish hue behind an intact tympanic membrane on otologic examination that is caused by active otosclerosis occurring in the cochlear promontory. This finding is known as Schwartze's sign and is present in about 10% of patients.

Histologically, otosclerosis begins as discrete foci of abnormal bone that eventually enlarge and coalesce. There are two distinct phases of otosclerosis, the early spongiotic one and the late sclerotic one. The early phase results from replacement of normal bone by loose and spongotic bone that is immature, highly vascular, and rich in histiocytes, osteoclasts, and osteoblasts. There is resorption of bone centered along preexisting blood vessels. The late phase of the disease results from deposition of dense sclerotic bone (which is rich in collagen and has little ground substance) in areas of previous bone resorption.

Otosclerosis may occur anywhere within the temporal bone. Over 80% of cases occur in a small region located just anterior to the oval window that extends to the vicinity of the cochleariform process. This region is known as the fistula ante fenestrum and is unique in that it is the last area to undergo endochondral bone formation in the labyrinth. Thus, it may contain rests of embryonic tissue. Other sites of involvement in otosclerosis are the round window (30%–50%), isolated stapes involvement (12%), and the anteroinferior cochlea (14%).

Patients with otosclerosis characteristically present with slowly progressive conductive hearing loss. The maximum conductive hearing loss usually does not exceed 50 dB. Sensorineural hearing loss has also been described, but its exact mechanism is uncertain. Other symptoms include tinnitus, vertigo, and postural imbalance. Pregnancy worsens hearing loss in patients with otosclerosis. The treatment of otosclerosis may be either medical (using sodium fluoride) or by stapedectomy.

IMAGING FINDINGS

Computed tomography (CT) is the imaging modality of choice for evaluating patients with otosclerosis. Magnetic resonance imaging with contrast administration may show enhancement of the cochlea during the active phases of the disease. Otosclerosis is divided into two major categories, fenestral and retrofenestral. The fenestral type includes involvement of the lateral wall of the labyrinth, footplate of the stapes, oval window, round window, facial nerve canal, and cochlear promontory (Fig. 13.06-1). The retrofenestral type predominantly involves the cochlea (Fig. 13.06-2). Fenestral otosclerosis is isolated, whereas retrofenestral disease usually occurs in association with fenestral otosclerosis.

Early forms of fenestral otosclerosis present with areas of marginal demineralization. The most common CT finding in the fenestral type is a focal area of bony overgrowth anterior to the oval window. Progression of disease may lead to marginal overgrowth of the oval window, resulting in narrowing of the oval window niche. The crura and footplate of the stapes may become thickened and, in advanced cases, ankylosis of the stapediovestibular joint is present. Complete replacement of the oval window is referred to as "obliterative otosclerosis." Complete obliteration of the round window is present in only 1% of patients.

The main CT finding in retrofenestral otosclerosis is that of demineralization of the otic capsule surrounding the cochlea. However, most patients who are diagnosed with retrofenestral otosclerosis have negative CT studies. This is probably because of the fact that the bony changes occurring in the late phase of otosclerosis are indistinguishable from normal bone. Rarely, otosclerosis results in diffuse sclerosis of the bony labyrinth; however, this finding is most commonly seen in obliterative labyrinthitis or prior surgery.

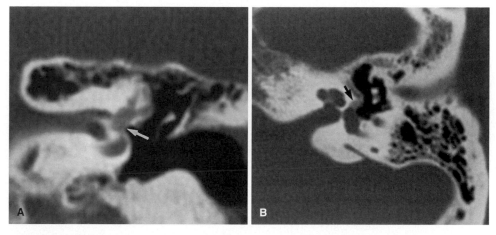

FIGURE 13.06-1.

Fenestral otosclerosis.   **A.** Coronal computed tomography (CT) shows bone covering oval window *(arrow)*. **B.** Axial CT (different patient) shows defect *(arrow)* in anterior aspect of oval window (fistula ante fenestrum).

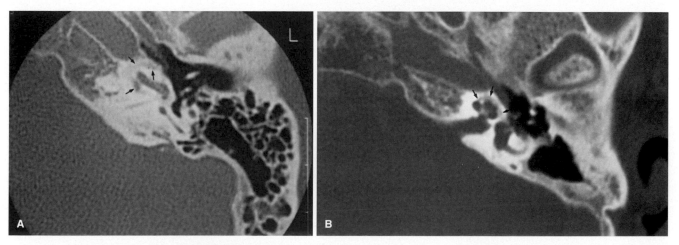

FIGURE 13.06-2.

Cochlear otosclerosis.   **A.** Axial computed tomography (CT) shows lucency *(arrows)* surrounding cochlea. **B.** Axial CT (different patient) shows prominent lucency *(arrows)* around cochlea.

SUGGESTED READINGS

1. Houck JR, Harker LA. Otosclerosis. In: Cummings CW, Frerickson JM, Harker LA, Krause CJ, Schuller DE, eds. Otolaryngology–Head and Neck Surgery, Vol 4, Ear and Skull Base. St. Louis: CV Mosby, 1986:3095.
2. Swartz JD, Harnsberger HR. The otic capsule and otodystrophies. In: Imaging of the Temporal Bone, 2nd ed. New York: Thieme, 1992:224.
3. Meyerhoff WE. Otosclerosis. In: Johnson JT, Kohut RI, Pillsbury HC, Tardy ME, eds. Head and Neck Surgery, Otolaryngology, Vol. 2. Philadelphia: JB Lippincott, 1993:1688.

13.07 *Congenital Cholesteatoma*

EPIDEMIOLOGY

Congenital (primary) cholesteatomas arise from aberrant epithelial embryonic rests and are identical to intracranial epidermoids. These lesions, unlike acquired cholesteatomas, often occur in the absence of middle ear inflammatory disease. Congenital cholesteatomas account for 2% of all middle ear cholesteatomas. The mean age of presentation is 4.5 years.

CLINICAL FEATURES

Congenital cholesteatomas occur in the middle ear, mastoid, geniculate ganglion region, petrous apex, external auditory canal, and cerebellopontine angle. The clinical presentation depends on the location of the lesion. Patients with middle ear and mastoid lesions present with conductive hearing loss. Otoscopic examination in these patients demonstrates a bulging, whitish mass behind an intact tympanic membrane. Congenital cholesteatomas may also be discovered incidentally on routine physical examination or at myringotomy. Perigeniculate and petrous apex cholesteatomas present with insidious or rapidly progressive facial nerve paralysis. Associated symptoms include sensorineural and conductive hearing loss, facial twitching, and vestibular dysfunction. Congenital cholesteatomas are associated with congenital aural atresia. Typically, the lesions are located medial to the atretic plate or a high-grade stenosis of the external canal.

Congenital cholesteatoma of the middle ear arises from an area situated at the point of epithelial transformation, located between the anterior tympanic ring and the eustachian tube. This region contains rests of stratified squamous epidermal cells whose function is to coordinate the development of the middle ear and tympanic membrane. Normally, this structure involutes at 33 weeks gestation. Persistence of this structure may lead to formation of congenital cholesteatoma in the middle ear.

Surgical management depends on the location and extent of the lesion. Congenital cholesteatoma isolated to the middle ear may be removed transtympanically or via a canal wall-up mastoidectomy. Perigeniculate or petrous apex lesions may require a middle cranial fossa or transsphenoidal approach.

IMAGING FEATURES

Computed tomography (CT) is the imaging study of choice for these patients. On CT, cholesteatomas present as focal soft tissue density masses that displace or erode adjacent bony structures (Fig. 13.07-1). Lesions localized to the middle ear cavity and near the oval window are suggestive of congenital rather than acquired cholesteatomas. In most cases, however, it is difficult to distinguish between both types of cholesteatomas. Lesions located in the middle ear and geniculate ganglion region have a tendency to grow along the facial nerve course. Identification of this common spread pattern is important to ensure complete surgical resection and to avoid damage to the nerve during surgery. The status of the ossicles must be determined because erosion dictates the need for ossicular reconstruction. Large perigeniculate and petrous apex lesions may extend into the middle cranial fossa and insinuate themselves between the dura and the floor of the middle cranial fossa. Identification of this spread pattern is important for complete removal and is easier on contrast-enhanced magnetic resonance (MR) imaging. Extension into the middle cranial fossa also places the patient at higher risk for postoperative cerebrospinal fluid leak unless dural grafting is performed. MR imaging may demonstrate the presence of congenital cholesteatoma but is unable to demonstrate bony detail. On MR imaging, the lesions demonstrate decreased signal intensity on T1-weighted images and increased signal intensity on

T2-weighted images. No appreciable enhancement is present after contrast administration. Enhancement after surgery is suggestive of granulation tissue rather than cholesteatoma. Contrary to cholesterol cysts, congenital cholesteatomas are hypovascular and do not contain blood products.

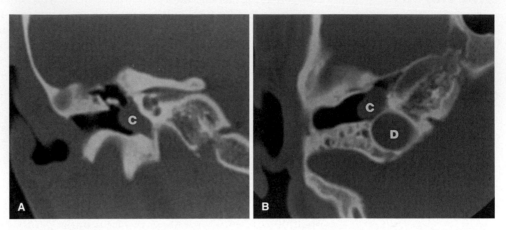

FIGURE 13.07-1.

Congenital cholesteatoma of middle ear. **A.** Coronal computed tomography (CT) shows focal rounded soft tissue mass (C) in medial and inferior middle ear cavity. **B.** Axial CT in same patient shows congenital cholesteatoma (C) in hypotympanic cavity. Note jugular bulb diverticulum (D).

SUGGESTED READINGS

1. Chole RA. Acute and chronic infection of the temporal bone including otitis media with effusion. In: Cummings CW, Frerickson JM, Harker LA, Krause CJ, Schuller DE, eds. Otolaryngology–Head and Neck Surgery, Vol. 4, Ear and Skull Base. St. Louis: CV Mosby, 1986:2963.
2. Swartz JD, Harnsberger HR. Middle Ear and Mastoid, 2nd ed. New York: Thieme, 1992:208.
3. Schutnecht HF. Congenital aural atresia and congenital middle ear cholesteatoma. In: Nadol JB, Schuknecht HF, eds. Surgery of the Ear and Temporal Bone. New York: Raven, 1993:263.

13.08 *Acquired Cholesteatoma*

EPIDEMIOLOGY

The exact incidence of acquired cholesteatoma is unknown, but approximately 4.2 of 100,000 yearly hospital discharges are for cholesteatoma. Acquired cholesteatomas are more common in boys and men, and tend to present in patients younger than 30 years of age. Acquired cholesteatomas tend to be more aggressive in children. There appears to be a hereditary predisposition, with an increased incidence in patients with cleft palate. It is also more common in patients with ruptured tympanic membranes and those with tympanoplasty tube placement.

CLINICAL FEATURES

Otoscopic evaluation shows a pearly white mass located in the middle ear cavity. Patients often present with progressive conductive hearing loss and otorrhea. A sensorineural component may be present if the cholesteatoma has invaded the otic capsule. Because cholesteatomas consist of debris within a closed space, they are prone to recurrent or superimposed infection. Purulent discharge may be seen in infected cholesteatomas. The most common organisms include *Pseudomonas aeruginosa* and *Bacteroides* species.

Histologically, acquired cholesteatomas consist of desquamated keratinizing squamous epithelial lining of the external auditory canal. The term "cholesteatoma" is misleading given the fact that the lesion is not a neoplasm and contains no cholesterol. There are four major theories regarding the pathogenesis of acquired cholesteatomas. The "invagination theory" is the most commonly accepted one. It proposes that eustachian tube dysfunction resulting in negative middle ear pressure and small retraction pockets in the pars flaccida of the tympanic membrane that prevent the egress of desquamated squamous lining. Failure of normal epithelial migration results in accumulation of keratinized debris in the posterosuperior quadrant of the tympanic membrane. The mass eventually extends into medial aspect of the epitympanum (Prussak's space), resulting in a cholesteatoma. The "epithelial invasion theory" postulates that the presence of small perforations in the tympanic membrane allow migration of keratinizing squamous epithelium from the surface of the tympanic membrane into the middle ear cavity. The "basal cell hyperplasia theory" suggests an alteration of the basal lamina of the pars flaccida that allows invasion of subepithelial tissues by proliferating columns of epithelial cells. The "squamous metaplasia theory" postulates that epithelial cells of the middle ear cavity are pleuripotential and may undergo squamous metaplasia when stimulated by an inflammatory process. Occasionally, acquired cholesteatomas begin in the pars tensa of the tympanic membrane and are referred to as "secondary acquired cholesteatoma." The mass usually begins in the posterior mesotympanum (particularly the sinus tympani) and often results in ossicular destruction.

The treatment for acquired cholesteatoma is surgical debridement. Ossicular reconstruction may be necessary in cases with advanced ossicular destruction. Cholesteatoma that extends into the roof of the epitympanum may result in herniation of intracranial contents into the middle ear cavity, requiring dural reconstruction at surgery. Cholesteatoma may erode the lateral semicircular canal, resulting in a perilymphatic fistula. Involvement of the facial nerve results in facial paralysis, which occurs in 1.1% of patients. Other complications include temporal lobe abscess, dural sinus thrombosis, and automastoidectomy.

IMAGING FEATURES

The role of imaging is mainly that of evaluating the extent of disease and the presence and amount of bone erosion. The classic appearance of cholesteatoma is that of a mass in Prussak's space (attic cholesteatomas) (Fig. 13.08-1A). The diagnosis of cholesteatoma is made by the presence of a focal mass within the middle ear cavity that displaces or erodes bone. The long process of the incus is the most common site of erosion, followed by the body of the incus and the head of the malleus (Fig. 13.08-1B). The status of the stapes should be determined in all cases because it determines the need for ossicular replacement. Erosion of the scutum is a relatively late finding. Bone erosion is present in 50% of cholesteatomas. A focal middle ear mass that does not erode or displace bone is only suggestive, and not typical for cholesteatoma. Magnetic resonance (MR) imaging has been shown to be of some benefit in differentiating cholesteatoma from granulation tissue. Granulation tissue enhances after contrast administration, whereas cholesteatoma demonstrates only ring or little enhancement. Upward growth may lead to erosion of the tegmen tympani and dural extension. Such extension may lead to cerebrospinal fluid leaks and herniation of the temporal lobe through the bony defect. MR imaging is beneficial in these patients. Other complications include labyrinthine fistula (most commonly involving the lateral semicircular canal) and spread along the facial nerve. The most commonly involved areas are the tympanic segment and posterior genu.

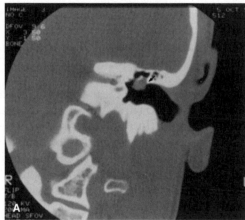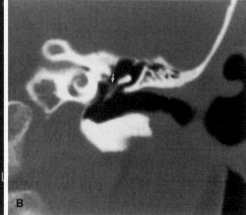

FIGURE 13.08-1.

Acquired cholesteatoma. **A.** Coronal computed tomography (CT) shows soft tissue mass in region of pars flaccida and extending into Prussak's space. There is erosion of the scutum *(arrow)*. (With permission from Castillo M. Neuroradiology Companion. Philadelphia: JB Lippincott, 1995.) **B.** Coronal CT in a different patient shows soft tissue mass *(arrow)* eroding long process of the incus (early cholesteatoma).

SUGGESTED
READINGS

1. Chole RA. Acute and chronic infection of the temporal bone including otitis media with effusion. In: Cummings CW, Frerickson JM, Harker LA, Krause CJ, Schuller DE, eds. Otolaryngology–Head and Neck Surgery, Vol. 4, Ear and Skull Base. St. Louis: CV Mosby, 1986:2963.
2. Swartz JD, Harnsberger HR. Middle Ear and Mastoid, 2nd ed. New York: Thieme, 1992:208.

13.09 Acute Mastoiditis

EPIDEMIOLOGY

Acute mastoiditis is an acute bacterial infection of the mastoid portion of the temporal bone. It occurs most commonly in children with a history of recurrent ear infections. Acute mastoiditis most commonly results as a sequela of acute otitis media. Occasionally, acute mastoiditis may be associated with chronic otitis media, cholesteatoma, leukemia, infectious mononucleosis, sarcomatous lesions of the temporal bone, and Kawasaki disease. The incidence of mastoiditis and its complications has significantly decreased as a result of timely antibiotic therapy.

CLINICAL FEATURES

Symptoms and signs include fever, tenderness, swelling, and pain over the mastoid process, proptosis of the auricle, and sagging of the superior external canal skin. Acute mastoiditis may occur without abnormalities of the tympanic membrane and middle ear in 10% to 20% of cases. Acute mastoiditis may be difficult to differentiate from severe external otitis with retroauricular extension.

Acute mastoiditis results from prolonged inflammation and resultant hyperemia of the mucoperiosteum in the air spaces of the temporal bone. Persistent inflammation leads to edema, which results in obstruction and sequestration of infection. Infection of the middle ear may spread to the mastoid air cells via the aditus ad antrum. Obstruction of the aditus ad antrum allows infection within the mastoid cavity to accumulate under pressure, resulting in osteoclastic resorption, replacement of the periosteal bone and calcified trabeculae with noncalcified woven bone. This stage of evolution is referred to as coalescent mastoiditis. The most common causative organisms include a mixed culture of aerobes and anaerobes (different from those responsible for acute otitis media). The most commonly isolated anaerobic organisms are gram-positive cocci and bacilli, and gram-negative bacilli. The most common aerobic organisms are group A beta-hemolytic streptococci, *Staphylococcus aureus*, and *Proteus mirabilis*.

Uncomplicated acute mastoiditis is treated with antibiotics, which should be continued until fever and inflammation resolve. Surgery is reserved for uncomplicated cases that fail to respond to antibiotic therapy or cases with associated complications. Complications include subperiosteal abscess, facial nerve paralysis, suppurative labyrinthitis, meningitis, epidural or brain abscess, dural sinus thrombosis, and otitic hydrocephalus.

IMAGING FEATURES

Computed tomography is the preferred modality for imaging patients with uncomplicated acute mastoiditis. Intravenous contrast administration is helpful for determining the extent of the inflammatory process. Magnetic resonance (MR) imaging aids in patients with facial nerve paralysis and in those suspected of having intracranial extension. MR venography may be used if venous sinus thrombosis is suspected.

Computed tomography findings in early acute mastoiditis are nonspecific and consist of mucosal thickening in the mastoid air cells (Fig. 13.09-1A). Proper treatment results in aeration of these air cells. Persistent infection leads to demineralization and resorption of the trabeculae and eventually results in a single cavity (coalescent mastoiditis) (Fig. 13.09-1B). Acute mastoiditis may result in subperiosteal abscesses. Abscesses that break through the mastoid and extend into the deep portion of the sternocleidomastoid muscle are referred to as Bezold abscesses. Intratemporal extension of the phlegmonous process may lead to suppurative labyrinthitis, serous labyrinthitis, or perilymph fistula. Facial nerve involvement may result from intratemporal extension or spread of the inflammatory process into the infratemporal fossa, thereby involving the facial nerve as it exits the stylomastoid foramen. Extension of the phlegmonous process to the posterior wall of the temporal bone places patients at risk for dural venous sinus thrombosis, meningitis, empyema, and intracranial abscess. "Otitic hydrocephalus" is a rarely used term that refers to patients with acute mastoiditis who present with signs and symptoms of increased intracranial pressure probably due to acute cortical venous thrombosis. Patients with aerated petrous apices are at risk for development of petrositis. This is referred to as Gradenigo syndrome, and includes sixth cranial nerve palsy, pain in the distribution of the fifth cranial nerve, and middle ear discharge. Neoplasias of the middle ear may be initially confused with acute mastoiditis (Fig. 13.09-1C).

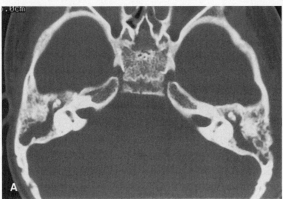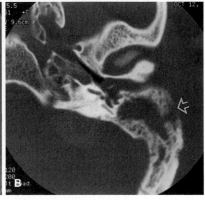

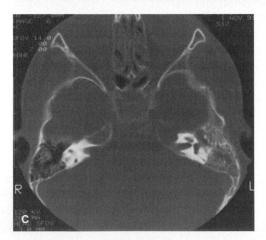

FIGURE 13.09-1.

Acute mastoiditis. **A.** Axial computed tomography (CT) shows soft tissue opacification of both middle ears and mastoid air cells. (Case courtesy of L. Fordham, University of North Carolina, Chapel Hill, NC.) **B.** Axial CT shows abnormal soft tissues in middle ear and mastoid antrum, which has been diffusely eroded. Note lytic defect (arrow) involving lateral aspect of mastoid bone. **C.** Axial CT of rhabdomyosarcoma of the left temporal bone, which produced changes similar to those seen in otomastoiditis, both clinically and radiographically. (With permission from Castillo M, Pillsbury HC. Rhabdomyosarcoma of the middle ear: imaging features in two children. AJNR 1993;14:730.)

SUGGESTED READINGS

1. McKenna MJ, Eavey RD. Acute mastoiditis. In: Nadol JB, Schuknecht HF, eds. Surgery of the Ear and Temporal Bone. New York: Raven, 1993:145.
2. Swartz JD, Harnsberger HR. Middle ear and mastoid. In: Imaging of the Temporal Bone, 2nd ed. New York: Thieme, 1992:105.

13.10 *Labyrinthitis*

EPIDEMIOLOGY

Labyrinthitis is an inflammation of the inner ear that may occur in adults and children. Viral labyrinthitis due to prior mumps or measles is a significant cause of progressive sensorineural hearing loss in children.

CLINICAL FINDINGS

Labyrinthitis may be classified based on the substance or tissue that enters the perilymphatic space, and includes serous, suppurative, and chronic forms. Labyrinthitis may occur as a result of a noxious agent directly entering the perilymph (tympanogenic) or from spread to the inner ear from infected cerebrospinal fluid (CSF) or meninges (meningogenic). The meningogenic form is more commonly bilateral, whereas the tympanogenic form affects only one ear. This inflammatory process may involve the endolymph, perilymph, or bony labyrinth. The inner ear may be involved as the sole target, or involved secondary to a systemic process.

Acute toxic (serous) labyrinthitis refers to invasion of the inner ear by viruses, bacterial toxins, or toxic chemical products (ototoxic drugs). Common viruses that invade the inner ear include mumps, measles, varicella-zoster, and cytomegalovirus. Suppurative labyrinthitis implies invasion of the perilymph by bacteria. Chronic labyrinthitis results from soft tissue entering the inner ear and is most commonly caused by cholesteatoma. The inciting soft tissue may be squamous epithelium or granulation or fibrous tissue.

Experimental data suggest that labyrinthitis may also be caused by diffusion of toxins and enzymes into the inner ear. Patients with Mondini malformations, a previous history of stapes footplate fracture, or a fistulous communication between the middle and inner ear are at increased risk for development of labyrinthitis from direct extension of toxins. One of the most common causes of direct communication between the middle and inner ear is a fistula of the horizontal semicircular canal caused by cholesteatoma. In addition, infections may spread from the CSF spaces into the inner ear through the cochlear and vestibular nerves.

Histologically, labyrinthitis results in development of serofibrinous precipitates and inflammation in the round window membrane and components of the organ of Corti. Progression of disease leads to diffuse neuroepithelial degeneration, including destruction of cochlear hair cells.

Symptoms depend on the severity of the underlying inflammatory process. Serous or toxic labyrinthitis presents with slowly progressive high-frequency hearing loss and vertigo. Suppurative labyrinthitis is fulminant compared to serous labyrinthitis. Suppurative labyrinthitis should be suspected in patients with acute or chronic middle ear infections who present with sudden or rapid hearing loss and severe vertigo. Underlying meningitis should be suspected in patients who are febrile. The clinical presentation of chronic labyrinthitis is variable. Those caused by fistulas will become symptomatic with manipulation. Ninety percent of these patients have vestibular symptoms. Prompt initiation of proper antibiotic therapy may improve or totally reverse hearing loss. Surgery may be indicated for patients with underlying cholesteatoma. Meningogenic suppurative labyrinthitis improves after treatment of underlying meningitis.

IMAGING FEATURES

Computed tomography (CT) and magnetic resonance (MR) are complementary imaging studies for evaluating patients with suspected labyrinthitis. CT permits evaluation of middle and inner ear structures and defines the extent of underlying mucosal thickening or cholesteatoma. MR imaging after contrast administration shows abnormal enhancement of the seventh and eighth cranial nerves and the membranous labyrinth, indicating an ongoing inflammatory process (Fig. 13.10-1). There are no characteristic CT findings for uncomplicated serous or suppurative labyrinthitis. Long-standing inflammation may lead to replacement of the membranous and bony labyrinth by fibrous or osseous tissues, and is referred to as labyrinthitis ossificans (Fig. 13.10-2). This appearance is nonspecific and represents an end-stage healing process that results from chronic serous or suppurative labyrinthitis. Intracochlear bone formation is often detected with CT; however, soft tissue obliterative labyrinthitis is not seen on CT (Fig. 13.10-3). In these cases, MR imaging may be useful. Loss of normal hyperintensity on T2-weighted images within the membranous labyrinth is suggestive of obliterative labyrinthitis. Contrast-enhanced MR imaging is helpful in evaluating children with acute or progressive sensorineural hearing loss. Abnormal enhancement of the inner ear structures is present with active inflammation, but may also be seen after surgery.

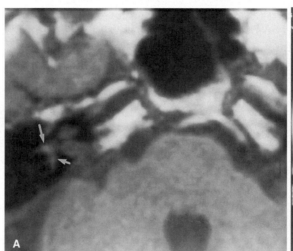
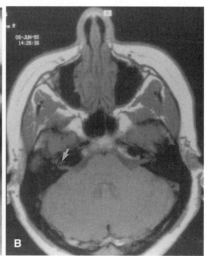

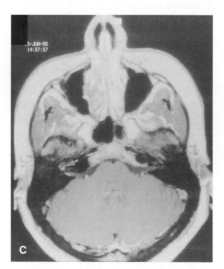

FIGURE 13.10-1.

Acute labyrinthitis. **A.** Axial noncontrast magnetic resonance (MR) T1-weighted image shows high signal intensity in right vestibule *(larger arrow)* and an ampulla *(smaller arrow)* of a semicircular canal, suggesting the presence of hemorrhage. In the absence of trauma (as was the case in this patient), the findings may be caused by hemorrhagic viral infection. **B.** In a different patient, precontrast axial MR T1-weighted image shows normal signal intensity in right cochlea *(arrow).* **C.** Corresponding postcontrast image shows enhancement of cochlea *(arrow)* and of VII–VIII nerve complex in fundus of internal auditory canal compatible with a viral inflammation.

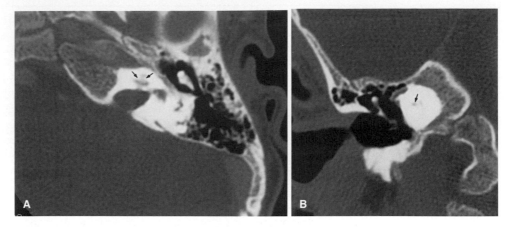

FIGURE 13.10-2.

Obliterative labyrinthitis. **A.** Axial computed tomography (CT) shows almost complete bony obliteration of middle and apical cochlear turns *(arrows)*. The basal turn is also partially ossified. **B.** Coronal CT shows nonspecific, almost complete bony obliteration of cochlea with only a small residue of cochlea present *(arrow)*.

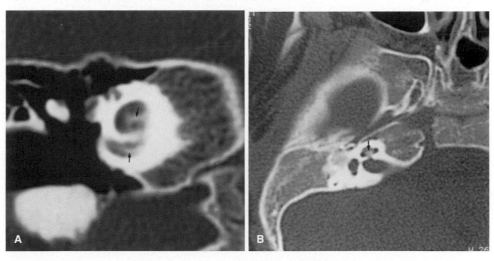

FIGURE 13.10-3.

Intracochlear bone formation. **A.** Coronal computed tomography (CT) shows intracochlear bone formation *(arrows)* in configuration of modiolus of basal and upper turns. **B.** Axial CT (different patient) shows intracochlear ossification *(arrow)* involving basal turn. This appearance is more prominent than that of the normal modiolus.

SUGGESTED
READINGS

1. Neely JG. Complications of infections. In: Cummings CW, Frerickson JM, Harker LA, Krause CJ, Schuller DE, eds. Otolaryngology–Head and Neck Surgery, Vol. 4, Ear and Skull Base. St. Louis: CV Mosby, 1986:3000.
2. Swartz JD, Harnsberger HR. The otic capsule and otodystrophies. In: Imaging of the Temporal Bone, 2nd ed. New York: Thieme, 1992:214.

13.11 *Perilymph Fistulas*

EPIDEMIOLOGY

Perilymph fistulas are anomalous communications between the inner and middle ear cavities resulting in leakage of perilymph into the middle ear. These fistulas may be congenital or acquired. Congenital forms often are associated with developmental dysplasias of the cochlea (Mondini dysplasias), vestibule, and semicircular canals. The prevalence of congenital perilymph fistulas in children with unexplained hearing loss is approximately 6%. Acquired fistulas may be the result of prior surgery, infection, trauma, or tumor.

CLINICAL FINDINGS

Perilymph fistulas should be suspected in patients who present with sudden sensorineural hearing loss in the setting of recent exertion, head trauma, or barotrauma. Patients may also complain of fluctuating hearing loss, tinnitus, ataxia, or episodic vertigo. At times, the clinical presentation may be indistinguishable from Meniere disease. Perilymph fistulas should be suspected in children who present with recurrent meningitis after middle ear infections. The diagnosis should also be suspected in patients in whom labyrinthitis or sensorineural hearing loss develops after otitis media.

The exact cause for idiopathic perilymph fistulas is controversial. Lack of a window membrane may allow direct communication between the inner and middle ear cavities. Entry of air into the inner ear (pneumolabyrinth) through a rent in the round or oval window may disrupt the normal basilar membrane mechanism, leading to hearing loss. Sudden increases in cerebrospinal fluid or middle ear pressures may also predispose patients to the development of perilymph fistulas. Fluctuations in pressure may cause tears in the intracochlear membrane in addition to tears in the round and oval window, all of which allow mixing of perilymph and endolymph with subsequent cochlear dysfunction.

Perilymph fistulas are associated with congenital deformities of the inner ear and stapes. The presence of fistulas should be suspected in patients with known congenital ear malformations who present with sudden onset of one or more of the symptoms described earlier.

Acquired perilymph fistulas occur after stapedectomy or are associated with middle ear cholesteatoma. Patients with subluxation of a stapes prosthesis, which allows egress of perilymph, may present with new sensorineural hearing loss along with violent episodes of vertigo. Cholesteatomas may erode the lateral semicircular canal or may directly extend through the oval or round windows into the inner ear, resulting in fistulas.

The treatment of idiopathic fistulas or those associated with congenital ear dysplasias is initially conservative and spontaneous resolution may occur. Exploratory tympanotomy with grafting of the oval or round windows is recommended in those patients who, under conservative management, show persistence or worsening of symptoms. The treatment of acquired forms of perilymph fistulas is directed toward the inciting factor.

IMAGING FINDINGS

Computed tomography (CT) is the modality of choice for imaging patients suspected of having perilymph fistulas. CT of patients with idiopathic fistulas is often negative. A small fluid collection located adjacent to the oval or round window is typical but only seldom identified. The possibility of perilymph fistula may be suggested in patients who, in the proper clinical setting, present with unexplained middle ear effusions. The presence of a pneumolabyrinth is strongly suggestive of underlying fistula. Congenital malformations of the stapes are also associated with an increased risk for development of perilymph fistulas. An important role of imaging is to identify patients with underlying conditions who are at risk for development of fistulas and to exclude other causes for the patient's symptoms. The bony covering over the lateral semicircular canal and the margins of the oval and round windows must be carefully evaluated in patients with middle ear cholesteatoma. Erosion of the bony covering of the inner ear by cholesteatoma is typical of underlying fistulas (Fig. 13.11-1). The position of a stapes prosthesis must be assessed in patients who have undergone previous stapedectomy or have a total ossicular replacement prosthesis. These procedures require drilling a small hole in the oval window to allow proper fixation of the prosthesis. Subluxation or nonvisualization of a prosthesis by CT is strongly suggestive of perilymph fistula in patients with proper symptomatology.

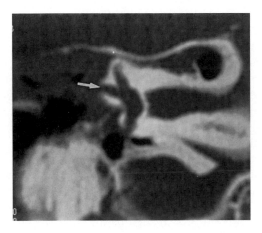

FIGURE 13.11-1.

Perilymph fistula. Coronal computed tomography shows erosion of bony covering *(arrow)* of lateral semicircular canal secondary to erosion by large acquired cholesteatoma.

SUGGESTED READINGS

1. Gulya AJ. Perilymphatic fistulas. In: Nadol JB, Schuknecht HF, eds. Surgery of the Ear and Temporal Bone. New York: Raven, 1993:307.
2. Swartz JD, Harnsberger HR. The otic capsule and otodystrophies. In: Imaging of the Temporal Bone, 2nd ed. New York: Thieme, 1992:208.

13.12 *Cochlear Implantation*

EPIDEMIOLOGY

Cochlear implants are now considered an accepted mode of rehabilitation for certain people with profound sensorineural hearing loss. Cochlear implants attempt to replace a nonfunctional inner ear hair cell transducer system by converting mechanical sound into electrical signals that can then be transmitted to the cochlear nerve. This technique may be used in both the pediatric and adult populations.

CLINICAL FINDINGS

Most cases of sensorineural hearing loss result from degeneration of hair cells within the organ of Corti. These hair cells normally convert mechanical energy into electrical signals to be carried by the cochlear nerve. Several studies suggest that the limiting factor determining the degree of sensorineural hearing loss is the number of spiral ganglion cells present within the organ of Corti. Surgically implanted devices bypass the hair cells and directly stimulate the spiral ganglion cells.

There are two major forms of cochlear implant devices. Single-channel devices provide limited-frequency information, predominantly in the lower frequency ranges (below 500 Hz). Multichannel devices are more commonly used than single-channel implants and stimulate a variety of different locations within the cochlea, therefore providing more complex sound analysis. The multichannel devices consist of external and internal components. Specific components include an intracochlear electrode, stimulator, receiver, headset, and microphone. A canal wall-up mastoidectomy is initially performed to provide access to the round window. The electrode is then inserted into the scala tympani, either through the round window or through an anteroinferior cochleostomy. The electrode is then advanced a variable distance (20–24 mm for a multichannel device and 5 mm for a single-channel device) in an apical direction. The round window or cochleostomy is then sealed with a graft.

Potential candidates in the pediatric age group must meet several criteria. First, the patients must be in good general health and physically able to undergo general anesthesia. Patients should have bilateral profound sensorineural hearing loss (in excess of 95 dB). Hearing loss may be idiopathic or the result of previous viral or bacterial labyrinthitis or ototoxic medication. Congenital malformations of the cochlea (Mondini type), with the exception of Michel dysplasia (cochlear agenesis), are not contraindications for cochlear implantation. The minimum age for eligible patients is 2 years. This allows for improved aeration of the mastoid antrum and aids in determining that affected patients have not benefited from using a hearing aid.

IMAGING FINDINGS

The imaging modality of choice for the preoperative evaluation for patients who are candidates for cochlear implants is computed tomography (CT). The routine postoperative evaluation of the position of the implant is best evaluated with plain films (Fig. 13.12-1). CT may be helpful in identifying the exact location of the electrode (Fig. 13.12-2). The cochlea should be of normal configuration and should not contain calcifications. Narrowing of the basal turn may prevent electrode insertion. With an abnormal cochlea there is a 90% risk of incomplete or difficult electrode insertion and a 70% chance of limited electrode insertion. The degree of aeration of the mastoid air cells and the presence of a high-riding jugular bulb or other aberrant vascular structures are important to identify before surgery. Special attention should be given to the patency of the round window and the size of the facial recess. The entire course of the facial nerve should be normal. Cochlear implants are contraindicated in patients with agenesis of the cochlea (Michel dysplasia) or in patients with a narrow internal auditory canal (which suggests absence of the ipsilateral cochlear nerve). The value of cochlear implants in patients with other dysplasias of the inner ear is controversial. Other radiographically identifiable conditions that may preclude the use of cochlear implants are active otosclerosis and bilateral acoustic schwannomas (neurofibromatosis type II). Middle ear infection must be treated before surgery to prevent infection of the implanted device. The value of cochlear implants in patients with the enlarged vestibular aqueduct syndrome is under investigation.

Labyrinthitis ossificans is not an absolute contraindication for cochlear implantation, but advanced cases may limit the type and length of the electrode and reduce overall benefits from the procedure. Soft tissue obliteration of the inner ear structures may be seen with high-resolution magnetic resonance T2-weighted images as reduction of signal intensity in the cochlea, vestibule, and semicircular canals and may indicate replacement of the normal endolymph and perilymph, which may potentially preclude cochlear implantation.

After implantation the electrode should be distant from the course of the facial nerve; otherwise it may damage it. The electrode should be contained within the cochlea, although occasionally it may be malpositioned with its tip in the cerebellopontine angle cistern, exiting via an enlarged cochlear aqueduct or the widened fundus of the internal auditory canal (Fig. 13.12-3). These implants do not function properly.

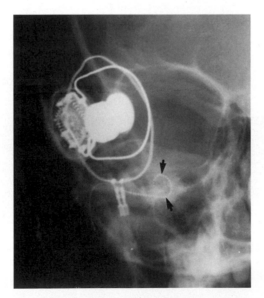

FIGURE 13.12-1.

Normally positioned cochlear implant, plain radiograph. Frontal radiograph shows multichannel electrode entering inner and coiling in basal turn of cochlea *(arrows)*. The electrode array contains 22 markers corresponding to channels. The first 10 serve to stiffen the electrode. Optimal results are achieved when 12 markers lie in the cochlea. A shallow insertion occurs with less than 12 channels and a deep insertion occurs when more than 12 markers are inside the cochlea.

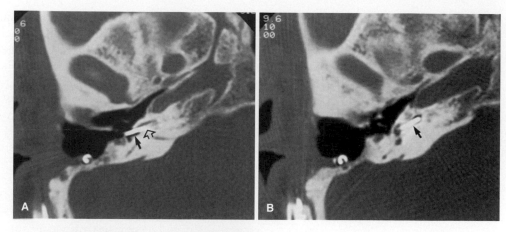

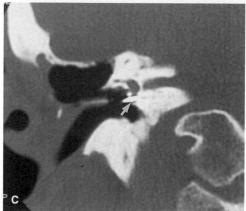

FIGURE 13.12-2.

Normally positioned cochlear implant, computed tomography (CT). **A.** Axial CT shows mastoidectomy and electrode going into the cochlea *(open arrow)* via the round window *(solid arrow)*. **B.** In same patient, the electrode is well positioned within the basal turn of the cochlea *(arrow)*. **C.** Coronal CT shows electrode traveling through the round window *(arrow)*.

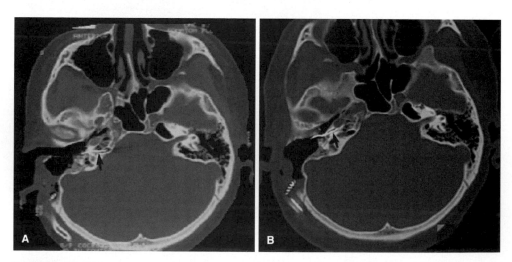

FIGURE 13.12-3.

Malpositioned cochlear implant. **A.** Axial computed tomography shows electrode *(arrow)* in region of cochlear aqueduct. **B.** Corresponding image obtained immediately after repositioning shows electrode in basal turn of cochlea *(arrow)*.

SUGGESTED READINGS

1. Swartz JD, Harnsberger HR. The otic capsule and otodystrophies. In: Imaging of the Temporal Bone, 2nd ed. New York: Thieme, 1992:242.
2. Miyamoto R. Cochlear implants. In: Johnson JT, Kohut RI, Pillsbury HC, Tardy ME, eds. Head and Neck Surgery Otolaryngology, Vol. 2. Philadelphia: JB Lippincott, 1993:1850.
3. Nadol JB. Cochlear implantation. In: Nadol JB, Schuknecht HF, eds. Surgery of the Ear and Temporal Bone. New York: Raven, 1993:315.
4. Johnson MH, Hasenstab S, Seicshnaydre MA, Williams GH. CT of postmeningitic deafness: observations and predictive value for cochlear implants in children. AJNR 1995;16:103.
5. Shpizner BA, Holliday RA, Roland JT, et al. Postoperative imaging of the multichannel cochlear implant. AJNR 1995;16:1517.

13.13 *Temporal Bone Fractures*

EPIDEMIOLOGY

Temporal bone fractures are classified according to their course relative to the long axis of the temporal bone Longitudinal ones are most common, and account for 80% of temporal bone fractures; transverse ones account for 20% of temporal bone fractures. However, in reality, many fractures are a combination of both types and cannot be reliably classified.

CLINICAL FEATURES

Longitudinal fractures follow a course that parallels the long axis of the petrous pyramid. These fractures result from a blow to the temporoparietal region and may be isolated or continuations of linear skull fractures. The fractures follow the long axis of the petrous bone and extend through the middle ear cavity in the region of the incudomalleolar joint and the anterior genu of the facial nerve. They then extend medially and course lateral to the canal for the internal carotid artery, to terminate in the vicinity of the foramen spinosum. Patients present with symptoms of basilar skull fracture. Despite the force of the injury, patients may not lose consciousness. Hemotympanum is commonly present and may be associated with perforation of the tympanic membrane and blood in the external auditory canal. Longitudinal fractures are often associated with ossicular fractures or subluxations. The facial nerve is injured in 25% to 35% of patients. This injury occurs along the tympanic portion of the facial nerve, between the geniculate ganglion and the posterior genu. Many facial palsies are transient and resolve spontaneously. This is believed to be caused by resolution of edema involving the nerve that compresses it along its descending course.

Transverse fractures have a course perpendicular to the long axis of the petrous bone. These injuries result from severe trauma to the frontal or occipital regions and often present with loss of consciousness, and may be fatal. The anteroposterior direction of the force results in fractures that begin in the region of the foramen magnum or jugular foramen and course perpendicular to the long axis of the temporal bone. These fractures characteristically extend into the region of the internal auditory canal, cochlea, and vestibule. Injuries to the internal auditory canal (and its contents) and to the inner ear result in immediate sensorineural hearing loss and vertigo. One-half of patients have facial paralysis. Facial nerve palsy is commonly permanent. Conductive hearing loss may also be present with transverse fractures, but it is more common with longitudinal fractures. Bleeding from the external auditory canal, hemotympanum, and perforation of the tympanic membrane are less common with transverse fractures than with longitudinal ones. Decompressive surgery or intravenous steroid administration may be warranted in certain instances to help preserve facial nerve function.

IMAGING FEATURES

Computed tomography is the imaging method of choice. Most temporal bone fractures are associated with ipsilateral opacification of the mastoid air cells. Internal carotid artery dissection may result from extension of fractures into the carotid canal. Catheter angiography may be indicated in patients with fractures extending into the carotid canal and acute onset of blindness or focal neurologic deficits. The course and status of the facial nerve must be determined in all cases. Reversible causes of facial nerve palsy such as hematomas or bone fragments compressing the facial nerve should be identified. A variety of ossicular abnormalities may result from temporal bone fractures. These abnormalities range from mild subluxations to complete fractures. Subluxation of the incudostapedial joint is the most common posttraumatic derangement.

Disruption of the incudomalleolar joint is the most readily identifiable ossicular subluxation (Fig. 13.13-1). The status of the tegmen tympani and tegmen mastoideum should be determined in each patient. Extension of fractures to these areas increases the patient's risk for recurrent meningitis and cerebrospinal fluid leaks (Fig. 13.13-2). The inner ear must be carefully studied in patients with acute sensorineural hearing loss or vertigo (Fig. 13.13-3). A fracture through the bony labyrinth indicates irreversible hearing loss. Delayed or fluctuating sensorineural hearing loss and persistent vertigo are suggestive of a posttraumatic perilymph fistula. Air within the vestibule (pneumolabyrinth) is strong evidence of direct communication between the middle ear/mastoid cavity and the labyrinth. In children, extensive longitudinal fractures may completely separate the petrous apex from adjacent temporal bone This has been termed "floating cochlea" and is associated with acute sensorineural hearing loss and paralysis of the abducens and facial nerves.

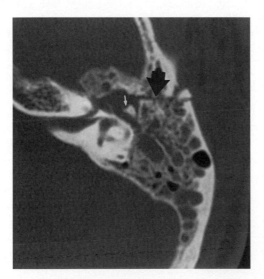

FIGURE 13.13-1.

Longitudinal fracture. Axial computed tomography shows longitudinal fracture *(large arrow)* that has extended into the ossicles. Note that the head of the malleus is not present and the incus *(tiny arrow)* appears "naked" (incudomalleal dislocation).

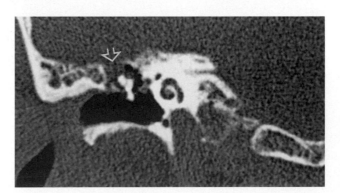

FIGURE 13.13-2.

Fracture with encephalocele. Coronal computed tomography shows fracture *(arrow)* in tegmen tympani with soft tissue (proven to be brain) protruding into epitympanic cavity.

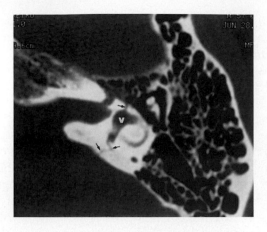

FIGURE 13.13-3.

Transverse fracture. Axial computed tomography shows transverse fracture *(arrow)* extending through the vestibule (v).

SUGGESTED READINGS

1. Parisier SC. Injuries of the ear and temporal bone. In: Bluestone CD, Stool SE, Scheetz MD, eds. Pediatric Otolaryngology, Vol. 1. Philadelphia: WB Saunders, 1990:578.
2. Swartz JD, Harnsberger HR. Trauma. In: Imaging of the Temporal Bone, 2nd ed. New York: Thieme, 1992:247.

13.14 *Neoplasms of the Temporal Bone*

EPIDEMIOLOGY

Tumors arising in the temporal bones constitute 0.4% of all pediatric neoplasms. Rhabdomyosarcoma is the most common mesenchymal tumor of the temporal bone. Only 7% of rhabdomyosarcomas occur in the temporal bone. They may arise de novo or be secondary to previous irradiation. The mean age of presentation is 6.1 years with a second peak occurring between 15 to 20 years of age. These tumors are more common in white males. Metastases may involve the temporal bone in children, but are rare. Lymphoproliferative disorders involve the temporal bones in 16% to 35% of children with lymphoma or leukemia. Histiocytosis X refers to a group of diseases characterized by proliferation of lipid-laden macrophages, giant cells, and eosinophils. Temporal bone involvement is seen mostly in patients younger than 12 years of age. Exostoses of the external auditory canal seldom present before 10 years of age and are associated with cold water entering the external auditory canal (swimmer's ear). These lesions are more common in boys than girls (3:1) and are often bilateral.

CLINICAL FEATURES

The initial symptoms of temporal bone tumors are nonspecific and, because of their rarity, most are diagnosed late in the course of the disease. Plexiform neurofibromas, mesenchymal tumors, and sarcomas are associated with growing tissues and are more commonly found in regions of the temporal bone adjacent to active growth centers. These areas include suture lines, the tympanic annulus, soft tissue components of the external auditory canal, and the auricle. Tumors rarely occur in areas that undergo no significant growth after birth, such as the inner ear and tympanic membrane. Another hypothesis that may explain the development of tumors in the temporal bones relates to trapping of other tissues during development. This hypothesis is supported by the presence of arachnoid villi, neural and salivary gland tissues, and primitive neuroectoderm in the temporal bones. These heterotopic tissues may be the precursors for many tumors.

Rhabdomyosarcomas represent 80% of tumors in children. Thirty to 50% arise in the nasopharynx, orbits, sinuses, and middle ear. Rhabdomyosarcomas are divided into three histologic forms: embryonal, alveolar, and sarcoma botryoides (pleomorphic). The embryonal type is most common. Symptoms are nonspecific and may mimic chronic otitis media. Other symptoms are pain, swelling, bloody otorrhea, and focal neurologic deficits. Tumors are often extensive at time of diagnosis. Although the survival rate has improved with new treatment modalities, the long-term prognosis is still poor. The treatment of choice consists of a combination of surgical debulking, irradiation, and chemotherapy.

Primary tumors that have been reported to metastasize to the temporal bones are renal cell and adenoid cystic carcinoma, sarcomas, and carcinomas. Obviously, these are very uncommon in children.

The most common symptoms when the temporal bones are involved by lymphoma or leukemia are sensorineural hearing loss, facial paralysis, and vertigo. On physical examination there may be ulceration, hemorrhage, and diffuse mucosal thickening of the external auditory canal and middle ear cavity.

Histiocytosis X includes Letterer-Siwe disease, Hand-Schüller-Christian disease, and eosinophilic granuloma. Although Letterer-Siwe disease (disseminated visceral involvement) presents in infants, temporal bone involvement is extremely rare. Temporal bone involvement is not unusual with Hand-Schüller-Christian disease (disseminated bony involvement) and with eosinophilic granuloma (solitary bony involvement). The clinical presentation is nonspecific, often leading to a delayed diagnosis. The most common symptoms are otitis media and externa, otorrhea, pain, and postauricular swelling. Cranial nerve involvement is rare but may occur. The most common finding on physical examination is polypoid granulation tissue in the external auditory canal with erosion of underlying bone. Treatment for lesions in the temporal bones consists mainly of irradiation.

A variety of other tumors involving the pediatric temporal bone have been described. Glomus tympanicum or jugulotympanicum are unusual in children except in the presence of von Hippel-Lindau syndrome. Tumors of neurogenic origin are seen in patients with neurofibromatosis, and should be considered when these patients present with retrocochlear hearing loss (Fig. 13.14-1). Although Ewing sarcoma is the second most common primary bone malignancy in children, it is rare in the temporal bones. Cartilaginous tumors of the temporal bones are extremely unusual in children. Exostoses are benign bony masses commonly occurring in suture lines of the external auditory canal.

IMAGING FEATURES

Both computed tomography (CT) and magnetic resonance (MR) imaging probably are needed for the correct staging of malignancies involving the temporal bone. Rhabdomyosarcomas present as aggressive soft tissue masses with bone destruction (Fig. 13.14-2). These lesions enhance after contrast administration and may contain a necrotic center. On MR images, the tumors are often hypointense on T2-weighted sequences, suggesting their hypercellular nature. The imaging features of metastases are those of aggressive soft tissue masses, often with destruction of bone. MR is the modality of choice for imaging patients suspected of having temporal bone involvement by lymphoma or leukemia. These disorders present as abnormal enhancement and thickening of meninges or cranial nerves. Rarely, they produce focal soft tissue masses and bone destruction. CT is ideal to evaluate patients with histiocytosis X, and shows lytic lesions with well defined margins that may contain an enhancing soft tissue component. The lesions may be single or multiple and bilateral.

Exostoses of the external auditory canal are smooth bony overgrowths occurring in its bony portion (Fig. 13.14-3). They may be sessile or pedunculated. As with other exostoses, the cortex of the lesion is continuous with the cortex of the adjacent external auditory canal. These lesions are well defined and are not associated with soft tissue masses or bone destruction.

Hemangiomas may involve the internal auditory canal or the course of the facial nerve (Fig. 13.14-4). These tumors are typically bright on noncontrast MR T1-weighted images and enhance after contrast administration.

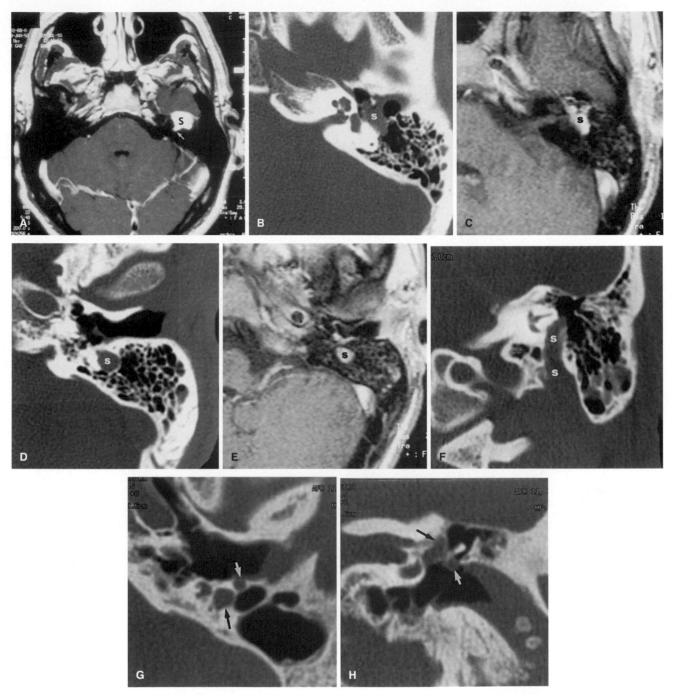

FIGURE 13.14-1.

Facial nerve schwannomas. **A.** Axial postcontrast magnetic resonance (MR) T1-weighted image shows enhancing mass (S) in region of geniculate ganglion with tail of tumor *(arrow)* projecting into fallopian canal. **B.** Axial computed tomography (CT; different patient) shows soft tissue mass (s) in region of horizontal portion of the facial nerve. **C.** Corresponding postcontrast MR T1-weighted image shows mass (s) to enhance markedly. **D.** Axial CT (same patient) shows mass (s) enlarging the descending portion of the facial nerve. **E.** Corresponding postcontrast MR T1-weighted image shows mass (s) to enhance. **F.** Coronal CT in same patient shows tumor (s) producing expansion of descending portion of left facial nerve. **G.** Axial CT in a different patient with neurofibromatosis type I shows tumor involving the descending portion of the facial nerve *(black arrow)* as well as the chorda tympani nerve *(white arrow)*. **H.** Coronal CT in the same patient shows tumor involving the horizontal portion of the facial nerve *(black arrow)* and the chorda tympani nerve *(white arrow)* lateral to the incus.

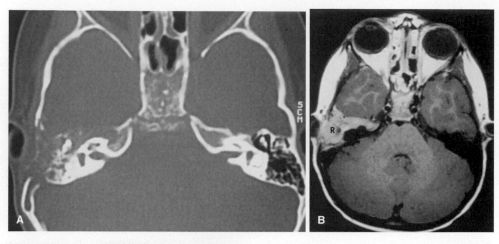

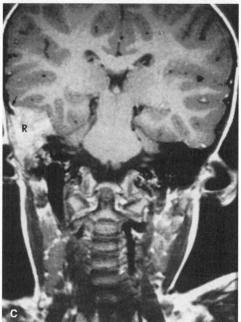

FIGURE 13.14-2.

Rhabdomyosarcoma. **A.** Axial computed tomography shows destruction of the right middle ear and mastoid. **B.** Axial postcontrast magnetic resonance T1-weighted image in same patient shows enhancing mass (R) involving most of the right temporal bone. **C.** Coronal postcontrast T1-weighted image (same patient) shows enhancing mass (R) extending intracranially and displacing brain upward. There is a small "tail" *(arrow)* of dural enhancement, suggesting tumor invasion.

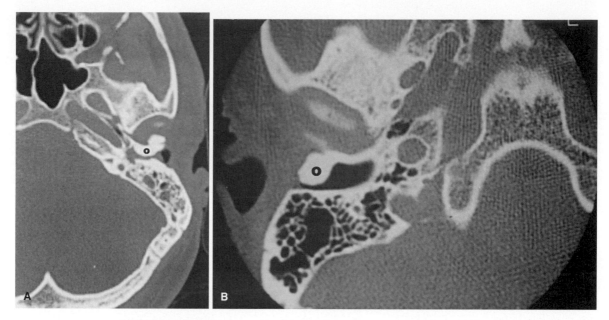

FIGURE 13.14-3.

Swimmer's ear. **A.** Axial computed tomography (CT) shows osteoma (o) producing marked narrowing of external auditory canal. The middle ear and mastoid are opacified with soft tissue. **B.** Axial CT (different patient) shows large osteoma (o) at meatus of the external canal, markedly narrowing it.

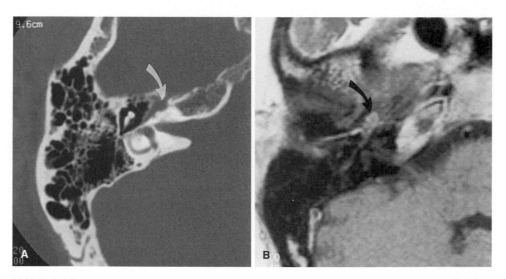

FIGURE 13.14-4.

Hemangioma. **A.** Axial computed tomography shows enlargement in region of geniculate ganglion *(arrow)*. **B.** Noncontrast magnetic resonance T1-weighted image shows mass *(arrow)* to be bright, which is typical of hemangiomas in this location and in the internal auditory canal.

SUGGESTED READINGS

1. Swartz JD, Harnsberger HR. Middle ear and mastoid. In: Imaging of the Temporal Bone, 2nd ed. New York: Thieme, 1992:105.
2. Stram JR. Tumors of the ear and temporal bone. In: Bluestone CD, Stool SE, Scheetz MD, eds. Pediatric Otolaryngology, Vol. 1. Philadelphia: WB Saunders, 1990:597.

Imaging of the Pediatric Head, Neck, and Spine
by Mauricio Castillo and Suresh K. Mukherji,
Lippincott-Raven Publishing, Philadelphia © 1996.

14

Paranasal Sinuses

14.0 *Applied Embryology*

The paranasal sinuses originate as outpouchings of the primitive nasal fossa. The sites of origin of epithelial recesses become the ostia of the developing sinuses. At birth, the primitive tubular recesses may be present; however, most of the pneumatization occurs after birth. Because the paranasal sinuses arise from the primitive nasal fossa, their mucosal lining is pseudostratified columnar ciliated epithelium, which contains mucous and serous glands.

Step 1. Development of the Maxillary Sinuses

The maxillary sinuses develop as outpouchings of the lateral walls of the ethmoid infundibula and are first evident at the 70th day of life. The mucosal recesses of the maxillary sinuses attain a relatively greater size than any other sinus primordia during fetal life, and are initially located in the region of the middle meatus between the lateral walls of the nasal cavity and the inferior turbinates. At birth, the primitive maxillary sinuses consist of fairly well developed tubular sacs measuring 8 mm in anteroposterior diameter and 4 mm in width (Fig. 14.0-1A). Pneumatization and growth of the maxillary sinuses occur at a slow rate; the growth rate of the maxillary sinuses has been estimated at 2 mm vertically and 3 mm longitudinally per year (Fig. 14.0-1B). Growth of the maxillary sinuses accelerates after 7 years of age. The sinuses expand into the region of the infraorbital nerves by 5 years of age and extend to the zygomatic processes of the mandible by 7 years of age. The maxillary sinuses reach their adult size by 15 years of age (Fig. 14.0-1C). They drain via the primary ostia into the ethmoid infundibula. Drainage passes then through the hiatus semilunaris into the middle meatus.

Step 2. Development of the Ethmoid Sinuses

The ethmoid sinuses develop from evaginations of the primitive nasal cavity during the fourth month of life. The ethmoid air cells are anatomically divided into anterior, middle, and posterior groups. Physiologically, the anterior group consists of the anterior and middle ethmoid air cells and the posterior group of the posterior ethmoid air cells. A fourth group of cells develops dorsal to the posterior ethmoid air cells and is referred to as the postreme air cells. The anterior air cells develop from an area inferior to the attachment of the middle tubinates, whereas the posterior ethmoid air cells develop superior to the middle turbinates. The anterior group develops from three areas in the middle meatus and is subdivided into infundibular, frontal, and bular cells. The infundibular and frontal cells give rise to the frontal recesses, a portion of the frontal sinus, ethmoid infundibula, anterior ethmoid air cells, and agger nasi cells. The agger nasi cells are located ventral to the anterior insertion of the middle turbinates. The primitive bular cells give rise to the middle ethmoid air cells, which contain the ethmoid bullae. The ethmoid bullae are well aerated, middle ethmoid air cells sometimes referred to as accessory conchae. The posterior ethmoid air cells arise from the superior meatus. Thus, the anterior and middle air cells drain into the middle meatus, whereas the posterior air cells drain into the superior meatus.

The ethmoid air cells are relatively well formed at birth and grow rapidly thereafter. They reach adult size and shape by mutual compression and unequal expansion. They reach adult size between 12 to 14 years of age.

Step 3. Development of the Frontal Sinus

The frontal sinus develops from the ventral and cephalic ends of the middle meatus in an area termed the "frontal recesses." Because the frontal recesses develop from primitive anterior ethmoid air cells, the drainage of the frontal sinus is via the anterior aspects of the infundibula into the middle meatus. Alternatively, the frontal sinus may drain directly into the anterior ethmoid air cells.

The development of the frontal sinus occurs by direct extension of the frontal recesses from one or more anterior ethmoid air cells or from the ventral ends of the ethmoid infundibula. Variations in development of the frontal sinus explain its inconstant drainage. In addition, the frontal recesses may be tortuous, preventing intranasal cannulation.

The frontal sinus is absent at birth and appears after the first year of life. The frontal sinus grows vertically at a rate of 1.5 mm per year. It fails to develop in 4% of the population. Adult size is reached after puberty, but there may be a small amount of growth during adulthood.

Step 4. Development of the Sphenoid Sinus

The sphenoid sinus arises from paired evaginations of the posterior primitive nasal cavity during the fourth month of life. During the first years of life, the mucosal evaginations of the developing sphenoid sinus become surrounded by the posterior portion of the cartilaginous nasal capsule, which may be ossified ("ossicle of Bertin"). During the fourth year of life, the rudimentary sphenoid sinus invaginates into the sphenoid bone and its pneumatization begins. Arrested pneumatization in the infantile position is termed the "conchal" type. This form is characterized by a thick bony plate separating small bilateral compartments, and is present in 2.5% of the population. The "presellar" type is characterized by pneumatization into the anterior aspect of the sella turcica and is present in 10% of the population. Pneumatization of the tuberculum sella is referred to as the "sellar" type. Pneumatization may extend under the floor of the sella and involve the lateral recesses of the sphenoid bone or the pterygoid plates.

The rate growth of the sphenoid sinus averages 0.25 mm per year in its posterior direction (Fig. 14.0-2). The sphenoid sinus is the first of all the paranasal sinuses to reach adult configuration (between 10–12 years of age). Drainage of the sphenoid sinus is relatively constant and occurs via the sphenoethmoid recesses into the superior meatus.

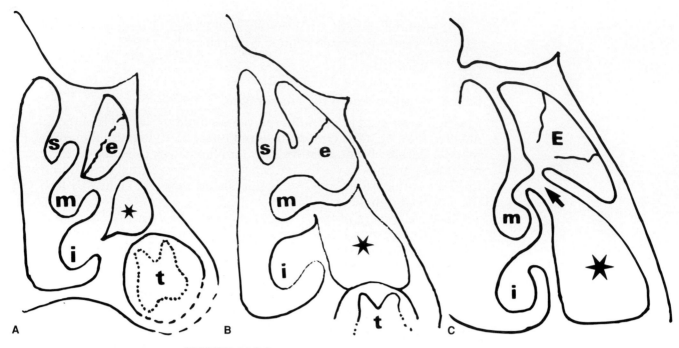

FIGURE 14.0-1.

Development of the maxillary and ethmoid sinuses. **A.** Diagram illustrating coronal cross-section of sinuses at 38 days of life. The superior (s), middle (m), and inferior (i) turbinates are present. The maxillary sinus *(star)* is present and immediately superior to the tooth bud (t). Rudimentary anterior and middle ethmoid cells (e) are present. **B.** At 3 years of age, the ethmoid sinuses (e) are well developed. The maxillary sinus *(star)* has grown inferiorly but still abuts the root of the teeth (t). s, superior turbinate; m, middle turbinate; i, inferior turbinate. **C.** At 10 years of age, the sinonasal cavities have an adult configuration. The anterior and middle ethmoid sinuses (E) drain via the ostiomeatal complex, together with the maxillary sinus *(star)*. Arrow, infundibulum; m, middle turbinate; i, inferior turbinate.

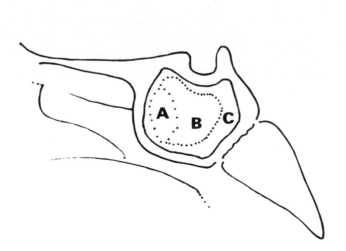

FIGURE 14.0-2.

Development of the sphenoid sinus. Diagram of sphenoid sinus in sagittal projection. The presellar portion (A) of the sphenoid bone is pneumatized by 6 years of age. By 10 years of age, pneumatization (B) has extended under the sella. C, pneumatization of adult sphenoid sinus. On magnetic resonance imaging, pneumatization is preceded by fatty replacement of active marrow. In children, the presellar (A) sphenoid sinus configuration is most common; however, in adults it is the least common type. Sellar pneumatization (C) is very uncommon in young children.

SUGGESTED READINGS

1. Fairbanks DF. Embryology and anatomy. In: Bluestone CD, Stool SE, Scheetz MD, eds. Pediatric Otolaryngology, Vol. 1. Philadelphia: WB Saunders, 1990:605.
2. Zimmerman AA. Development of the paranasal sinuses. 1938;27:7893.
3. Som PM. Sinonasal cavity. In: Som PM, Bergeron RT, eds. Head and Neck Imaging, 2nd ed. St. Louis: Mosby Year Book, 1990:60.
4. Scuderi AJ, Harnsberger HR, Boyer RS. Pneumatization of the paranasal sinuses: normal features of importance to the accurate interpretation of CT scans and MR images. AJR 1993;160:1101.
5. Aoki S, Dillon WP, Barkovich AJ, Norman D. Marrow conversion before pneumatization of the sphenoid sinus: assessment with MR imaging. Radiology 1989;172: 373.

14.01 *Allergic Rhinosinusitis*

EPIDEMIOLOGY

Allergic rhinosinusitis is the most common of all allergic disorders. It affects over 20 million people in the United States. Its prevalence in the general population is 10%, with a peak incidence in postadolescent teenagers. This incidence remains stable in the young and gradually decreases with age. Before adolescence, allergic rhinosinusitis is more common in boys, whereas girls are affected more commonly after adolescence. A familial predisposition is likely.

CLINICAL FEATURES

Allergic rhinosinusitis is characterized by presence of eosinophils in stained smears of nasal secretions. Definitive diagnosis is based on identification of allergic-specific immunoglobulin E (IgE) by a variety of skin tests or in vitro IgE measurements.

Symptoms of allergic rhinosinusitis occur at any age, but children rarely demonstrate significant symptoms before 2 years of age. Symptoms include sneezing, rhinorrhea, postnasal drainage, nasal obstruction, and itching of respiratory membranes. Symptoms vary from season to season and may differ at various times of night and day. Persistent disease may result in infraorbital tissue congestion ("allergic shiners"). Treatment is based on three primary considerations. The most effective treatment is avoidance of inciting allergens. If total avoidance of inciting allergens is not possible, pharmacotherapy is an alternative. First-line medications include antihistaminics, decongestants, and sodium cromolyn. Persistent disease may be treated with steroids or specific forms of immunotherapy.

IMAGING FEATURES

Diagnosis of allergic rhinosinusitis is a clinical one based on elevated IgE levels and identification of inciting agents. The role of imaging is to define extent of disease and detect complications. Computed tomography is the imaging modality of choice. Imaging findings are variable and depend on the extent of disease. The sinuses may be normal or their mucosa may be minimally thickened. More commonly, there is polypoid mucosal thickening in all sinuses. The paranasal sinuses are completely opacified with advanced disease (Fig. 14.01-1). Air-fluid levels may be present in patients with superimposed acute bacterial or viral infections. Mucoceles may develop in patients with long-standing mucosal thickening. Focal areas of increased attenuation may be present within the mucosal thickening that represent dessicated secretions or superimposed fungal colonization (Fig. 14.01-2). Allergic rhinosinusitis usually does not result in polyp formation.

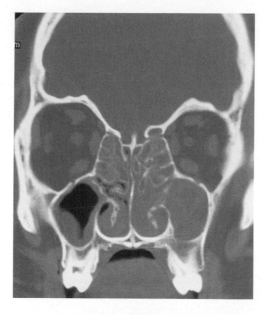

FIGURE 14.01-1.

Allergic rhinosinusitis. Coronal computed tomography shows complete opacification of both ethmoid sinuses and left maxillary sinus. There is mucosal thickening in the right maxillary sinus. The ethmoid septa and conchae are thin.

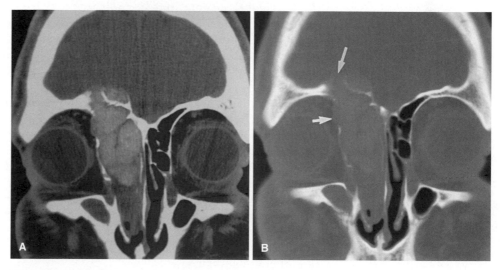

FIGURE 14.01-2.

Allergic rhinitis with superimposed fungus infection. **A.** Coronal computed tomography (CT) shows expansile mass high density (mucocele) involving right ethmoids with erosion of bone superiorly. The right maxillary sinus is opacified. **B.** Corresponding bone windows CT shows bone erosion in medial orbital wall *(short arrow)* and roof *(longer arrow)* of right ethmoids. At surgery, polyps and *Aspergillus* were found.

SUGGESTED READINGS

1. Fireman P. Allergic rhinitis. In: Bluestone CD, Stool SE, Scheetz MD, eds. Pediatric Otolaryngology, Vol. 1. Philadelphia: WB Saunders, 1990:793.
2. Mabry RL. Allergic rhinitis. In: Johnson JT, Kohut RI, Pillsbury HC, Tardy ME, eds. Head and neck surgery–otolaryngology, Vol. 1. Philadelphia: JB Lippincott, 1993: 290.
3. Friedman RA, Harris JP. Sinusitis. Annu Rev Med 1991;14:471.

14.02 *Sinusitis*

EPIDEMIOLOGY

Sinusitis, an inflammation of mucosa in the paranasal sinuses, is the most common health care complaint in the United States, affecting more than 31 million people per year. Sinusitis affects both genders and occurs in all age groups. The disease may be isolated or occur in patients with predisposing factors such as malnutrition, chronic steroid therapy, diabetes, immune deficiencies, cystic fibrosis, immotile cilia syndromes, chemotherapy, and blood dyscrasias.

CLINICAL FEATURES

Sinusitis may be classified into three separate forms based on pathologic findings. Acute suppurative sinusitis lasts from 1 day to 4 weeks. Subacute suppurative sinusitis is a reversible infection that lasts between 4 weeks and 3 months. Chronic suppurative sinusitis results from inadequately treated acute sinusitis and lasts longer than 3 months. Chronic sinusitis is unusual in patients younger than 16 years of age unless there is an underlying abnormality such as diabetes, aplastic anemias, cystic fibrosis, or immotile cilia syndrome (Fig. 14.02-1) Acute and subacute sinusitis are usually treated with antibiotics; surgical treatment may be indicated for chronic sinusitis.

Pathogens causing sinusitis differ based on the age of patients. Organisms commonly cultured in children with acute sinusitis are *Streptococcus pneumoniae, B catarrhalis, Hemophilus influenzae,* and *Streptococcus pyogenes,* whereas in adults, common organisms are *S pneumoniae, Staphylococcus aureus, S pyogenes,* and *H influenzae.* Organisms most often cultured from chronic sinusitis are different from those present in acute sinusitis, and include *H influenzae, Streptococcus viridans,* and various anaerobes. Diagnosis of sinusitis is a clinical one based on history and physical examination. Clinical presentation depends on location and duration of infection. The most common presenting symptoms in acute sinusitis are headache or pain over the infected sinus. Patients often have nasal obstruction with mucopurulent discharge, which may be associated with symptoms such as fever, lethargy, and malaise. Characteristic findings on physical examination are erythema and edema of sinus mucosa, active discharge, and edema of the turbinates. Tenderness to palpation over the acutely inflamed sinuses is strongly indicative of acute sinusitis.

Patients with chronic sinusitis present with nasal obstruction associated with mucopurulent discharge. Facial pain and constitutional symptoms are typically absent.

IMAGING FEATURES

Diagnosis of sinusitis is based on history and physical examination. The purpose of imaging is to evaluate extent of mucosal thickening. Extent of disease is best evaluated with computed tomography (CT).

Correlation between sinus mucosal thickening and active infection in children is questionable, especially before 2 years of age. Mucosal thickening may normally be seen in these young patients as a result of crying or "redundant" (loose) mucosa. Therefore, imaging findings should be interpreted in light of the clinical history and physical examination. The terms "acute" and "chronic" sinusitis do not describe imaging findings, and should be used only in the appropriate clinical context.

Imaging findings in sinusitis range from mild or moderate polypoid mucosal thickening to complete sinus opacification. The attenuation of mucosa varies with its degree of hydration. Watery secretions are of low CT attenuation and dessicated secretions are of increased CT attenuation. Areas of increased CT attenuation may indicate fungal colonization (usually aspergillosis). Mucosal thickening may also be detected with magnetic resonance (MR) imaging; however, this technique lacks bony detail. MR imaging signal intensity characteristics of mucosal thickening vary with the degree of hydration. Acutely inflamed mucosa is of low signal intensity on T1-weighted images and is hyperintense on T2-weighted images. Infection leads to submucosal edema and enhancement of mucosa with contrast. Chronic secretions are often dessicated, resulting in gradual reduction of T2 signal intensity, which may eventually progress to complete loss of T2 signal intensity (Fig. 14.02-2). Loss of T2 signal intensity may also be seen in fungal colonization.

Fluid levels are suggestive of acute sinusitis in patients who have not sustained recent trauma or are intubated (Fig. 14.02-3). In the traumatized patient, fluid levels usually are caused by hemorrhage (especially in the presence of fractures) or obstruction of drainage. Fluid levels may also be present in the maxillary sinuses after sinus lavage and may persist for 4 days after this procedure. Fluid levels in ethmoid sinuses are rare and usually associated with trauma, nasal intubation, or acute infection. Sphenoid sinus fluid levels are most often seen after nasal intubation (Fig. 14.02-4). Patients presenting with complete opacification or a fluid level in the sphenoid sinus must be evaluated for an obstructing lesion of the nasal cavity or nasopharynx, or fractures of the base of the skull. Patients with acute sphenoid sinusitis are at increased risk for intracranial infection and thrombosis of the cavernous sinuses. Fluid levels in the frontal sinus in nontraumatized children are a medical emergency because of the risk of empyema formation, which may occur within 48 to 72 hours after the onset of sinusitis. Infection may spread from the frontal sinus into the anterior cranial fossa via emissary veins without demonstrable bone erosion. Symptomatic patients should undergo contrast-enhanced CT or MR imaging to exclude intracranial involvement.

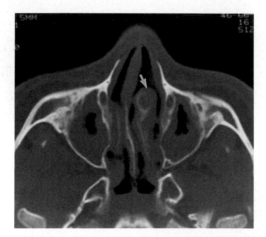

FIGURE 14.02-1.

Kartagener syndrome. Axial computed tomography shows marked thickening of the mucosa in both maxillary sinuses and an opacified concha bullosa in left middle turbinate *(arrow)* because of immotile cilia in this patient with situs inversus.

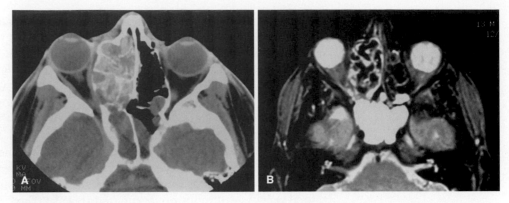

FIGURE 14.02-2.

Dessicated secretions. **A.** Axial computed tomography (CT) shows expansion of right ethmoid complex, which contains secretions of high density (no fungus found at surgery, but only dry, tenacious secretions). The medial right orbital wall is bowed outward. The sphenoid sinus contains secretions of lower density. **B.** Axial magnetic resonance T2-weighted image in same patient shows that the expanded right ethmoid complex contains multiple areas of signal void that could be misinterpreted as air without knowledge of CT findings. These represent dry secretions. Note hydrated (high signal intensity) secretions in sphenoid sinus.

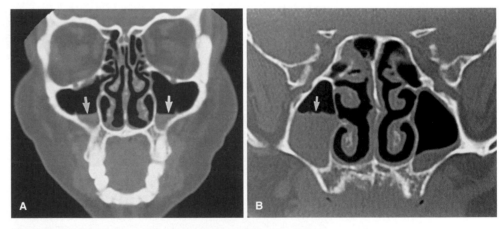

FIGURE 14.02-3.

Acute maxillary sinusitis. **A.** Coronal computed tomography (CT) shows fluid levels *(arrows)* in both maxillary sinuses. The patient was tender over this region and had a fever. The ostiomeatal complexes appear normal. **B.** Coronal CT in different patient shows fluid level *(arrow)* in right maxillary sinus and mucosal thickening in left maxillary and right ethmoid sinuses.

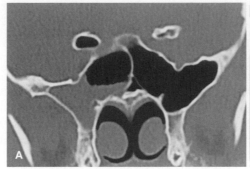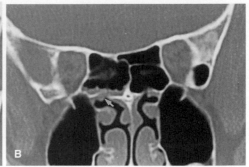

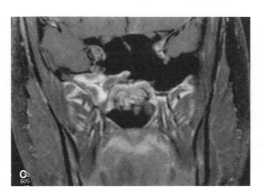

FIGURE 14.02-4.

Sphenoid sinusitis. **A.** Coronal computed tomography shows fluid level in right-sided compartment of sphenoid sinus. **B.** Coronal slice anterior to **A** shows small polyp (endoscopically confirmed) obstructing right sphenoethmoid recess. This polyp is responsible for the sinusitis. **C.** Coronal magnetic resonance (MR) fat-suppressed postcontrast T1-weighted image shows mucosal thickening in right lateral compartment of sphenoid sinus. Note that MR imaging allows for separation of enhancing superficial mucosa from low–signal-intensity submucosal edema.

SUGGESTED READINGS

1. Facer GW, Kern EB. Sinusitis: current concepts and management. In: Johnson JT, Kohut RI, Pillsbury HC, Tardy ME, eds. Head and Neck Surgery–Otolaryngology, Vol. 1. Philadelphia: JB Lippincott, 1993:366.
2. Som PM. Sinonasal cavity. In: Som PM, Bergeron RT, eds. Head and Neck Imaging, 2nd ed. St. Louis: Mosby Year Book, 1990:114.
3. Dillon WP, Som PM, Fullerton GD. Hypointense MR signal in chronically inspissated sinonasal secretions. Radiology 1990;174:73.
4. Som PM, Dillon WP, Fullerton GD, Zimmerman RA, Rajagopalan B, Maron Z. Chronically obstructed sinonasal secretions: observations on T1 and T2 shortening. Radiology 1989;172:515.

14.03 *Orbital Complications of Sinusitis*

EPIDEMIOLOGY

Approximately 60% of orbital disorders are infectious in origin. Most orbital infections are of sinus origin. Other causes of orbital infection include trauma, foreign bodies, and spread from facial infection or septicemia. Orbital complications arising from sinus infections may occur in any age group, but are most commonly seen in children and in immunocompromised patients.

CLINICAL FEATURES

Orbital complications resulting from sinonasal infections include periorbital cellulitis, periorbital cellulitis with chemosis, orbital cellulitis, subperiosteal abscess, orbital abscess, and cavernous sinus thrombosis. These complications typically result from direct extension of infection into the bony orbit. Children are especially prone to such extension because of thinner sinus walls (especially the lamina papyracea), larger communicating vascular foramina, porous bones, and open suture lines.

Ethmoid sinusitis most commonly leads to orbital complications. Obstruction of ethmoid sinus drainage results in accumulation of inflammatory debris. Persistently increased pressure leads to interruption of the periosteal blood supply, producing necrosis of the lamina papyracea. Infection may also spread via emissary veins. Congestion of venous outflow results in erythema and edema of the eyelids. Because the inflammation is anterior to the orbital septum, this stage is referred to as "preseptal" orbital cellulitis. Progression of disease may lead to chemosis. Untreated, this process may result in edema and inflammation under the periosteum of the medial orbital wall (subperiosteal phlegmon) and become "postseptal" cellulitis. Subperiosteal abscesses represent pus within such phlegmonous collections. True orbital cellulitis represents inflammation of the retrobulbar fat. Orbital cellulitis and subperiosteal abscess frequently coexist. Intraorbital abscesses may result from direct spread of subperiosteal abscesses or progression of orbital cellulitis. Progression of abscesses may lead to thrombosis of the superior ophthalmic veins, which may result in cavernous sinus thrombosis.

Periorbital cellulitis with or without chemosis may be successfully treated with antibiotics. Clinically, differentiation between a subperiosteal abscess (postseptal) and orbital cellulitis (preseptal) may be difficult. Both entities present with fever, eyelid tenderness, proptosis, and reduction in extraocular motility. Orbital cellulitis without abscess usually responds to antibiotics, whereas subperiosteal abscesses require surgical drainage. Some physicians may choose to drain a symptomatic subperiosteal phlegmon that does not respond to antibiotics. Intraorbital abscesses require surgical drainage.

IMAGING FINDINGS

Contrast-enhanced computed tomography (CT) is the imaging modality of choice. CT and magnetic resonance (MR) imaging findings in periorbital cellulitis (preseptal cellulitis) are those of edema and thickening of the eyelids, which may extend to the nasolabial fold. This thickening is anterior to the orbital septum, which is a reflection of periosteum and check ligaments of the eyelids. Subperiosteal phlegmon is characterized by diffuse mucosal thickening of an ethmoid sinus that extends through the lamina papyracea into the medial aspect of the orbit, producing lateral displacement of the medial rectus muscle and resulting in proptosis (Fig. 14.03-1). The normal fat plane between the muscle and the medial orbital wall disappears. Findings of subperiosteal abscess are similar to those of a phlegmon except that an abscess contains fluid density instead of the soft tissue density characteristic of a phlegmon (Figs. 14.03-2–14.03-4). The lamina papyracea may be intact even in the presence of an abscess. Orbital cellulitis is characterized by stranding or increased density of the retrobulbar fat. The sclera may be thickened. Presence of a fluid collection within the orbit is indicative of orbital abscess.

Because the orbital complications of sinusitis are difficult to differentiate on a clinical basis alone, imaging is important. CT should also be performed in patients who present with periorbital cellulitis and who do not respond to antibiotics within 24 hours, and in patients suspected of having orbital cellulitis, subperiosteal phlegmon/abscess, or orbital abscess. MR imaging is ideal if cavernous sinus thrombosis is suspected (Fig. 14.03-5).

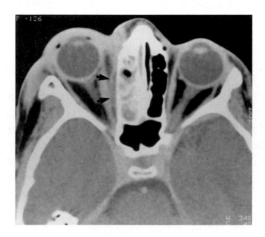

FIGURE 14.03-1.

Subperiosteal phlegmon. Axial postcontrast computed tomography shows soft tissue density collection *(arrows)* under thickened periosteum of right medial orbital wall. Note adjacent ethmoid sinusitis and swollen right medial rectus muscle.

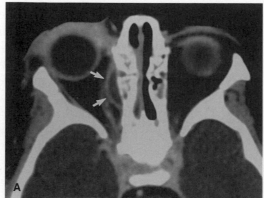
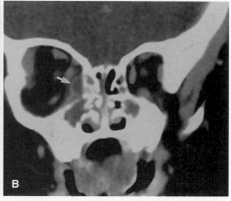
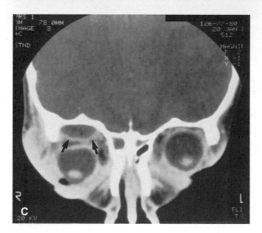

FIGURE 14.03-2.

Subperiosteal abscess. **A.** Axial postcontrast computed tomography (CT) shows low-density (pus) collection *(arrows)* under thick periosteum of right medial orbital wall. There is adjacent ethmoid sinus opacification, right proptosis, and preseptal swelling. **B.** Coronal CT in same patient clearly shows right medial abscess *(arrow)* surrounded by thick periosteum. **C.** Coronal postcontrast CT in a different patient shows subperiosteal abscess *(arrows)* in roof of right orbit secondary to frontal sinusitis. (With permission from Castillo M. Neuroradiology Companion. Philadelphia: JB Lippincott, 1995.)

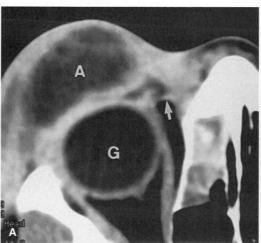
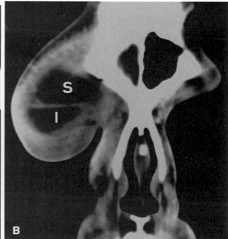

FIGURE 14.03-3.

Eyelid abscess. **A.** Axial postcontrast computed tomography (CT) shows large eyelid abscess (A) secondary to right ethmoid sinusitis. Infection is contained anteriorly by orbital septum *(arrow).* G, globe. **B.** Coronal CT in same patient shows abscess involving the right superior (S) and inferior (I) eyelids.

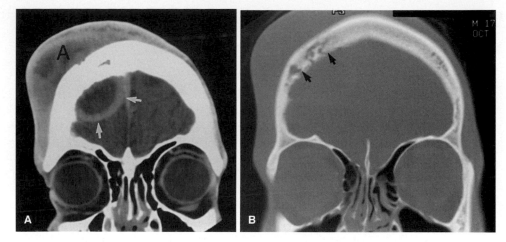

FIGURE 14.03-4.

Frontal abscess. **A.** Coronal postcontrast computed tomography (CT) in a patient with previously treated frontal sinusitis shows large abscess involving scalp (A) and extending intracranially *(arrows)* **B.** CT (bone window settings) in the same patient shows erosion *(arrows)* of skull.

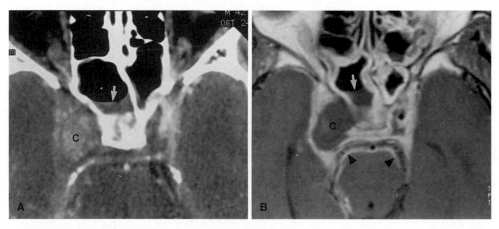

FIGURE 14.03-5.

Thrombosis of cavernous sinus. **A.** Axial postcontrast computed tomography in patient with sphenoid sinusitis (note fluid level, *arrow*) shows clot (C) expanding right cavernous sinus and bowing outward its lateral wall. **B.** Corresponding postcontrast magnetic resonance T1-weighted image shows clot (C) in right cavernous sinus and enhancement of pial surface of brain stem *(arrowheads)* due to meningitis. Fluid level *(arrow)* in right sphenoid compartment is again noted, as is mucosal thickening in left compartment.

SUGGESTED READINGS

1. Mafee MF, Schatz CJ. Complications of nasal and sinus infections. In: Bluestone CD, Stool SE, Scheetz MD, eds. Pediatric Otolaryngology, Vol. 1. Philadelphia: WB Saunders, 1990:746.
2. Som PM. Orbit. In: Som PM, Bergeron RT, eds. Imaging of the Head and Neck, 2nd ed. St. Louis: Mosby Year Book, 1990:781.

14.04 Cysts and Polyps

EPIDEMIOLOGY

Cysts and polyps arising in the paranasal sinuses result from inflammatory sinusitis. Polyps are secondary to allergy and inflammation and often occur in the older pediatric age group. There is no gender preference. Antrochoanal polyps are a specific form of nasal polyp and are the most common benign sinus tumor in children. These lesions extend from the antrum of a maxillary sinus to the nasal cavity and may continue into the posterior choanae, causing nasal obstruction. They account for 4% to 6% of all nasal polyps. Most are unilateral, but bilaterality is seen in 30% to 40% of patients. Fifteen to 40% of patients with antrochoanal polyps have a history of allergies.

CLINICAL FEATURES

There are two forms of cysts involving the paranasal sinuses: serous and mucous retention cysts. Serous cysts arise from accumulation of fluid in submucosal layers of sinus mucosa, whereas retention cysts result from obstruction of seromucinous glands. They are most common in the maxillary sinuses.

Polyps are the most common expansile lesion of the sinonasal cavities and arise from infiltration of mucosal stroma by eosinophils and polymorphonuclear leukocytes, resulting in thickening and edema. Polyps are associated with allergies, vasomotor rhinitis, infectious rhinosinusitis, cystic fibrosis, diabetes mellitus, aspirin intolerance, and nickel exposure. Nasal polyps in a prepubescent patient are unusual and often associated with metabolic or immunologic abnormalities. Such patients should be tested for immunoglobulin and sweat chloride levels. Small polyps may resolve with conservative therapy (antibiotics and allergic desensitization). Occasionally, cysts and polyps become large enough to obstruct the drainage of the involved sinus. Treatment in these cases is surgical excision. Antrochoanal polyps are routinely excised via a Caldwell-Luc approach. Up to one-third of these lesions recur if incompletely excised.

IMAGING FEATURES

Computed tomography (CT) is the imaging modality of choice for evaluating patients with sinus cysts and polyps. There are no imaging features that help to distinguish polyps from retention cysts. Both lesions are often asymptomatic and may be found incidentally on imaging studies. By CT, these lesions are homogeneous, soft tissue density masses with smooth, outwardly convex margins. (Figs. 14.04-1 and 14.04-2). Cysts and polyps have magnetic resonance imaging characteristic similar to those of inflamed mucosa. They are of low to intermediate signal intensity on T1-weighted images and of increased signal intensity on T2-weighted images, a finding that reflects high water and low protein contents. Cysts and polyps may be single or multiple. If multiple, they may be unilateral or bilateral. An enlarging cyst or polyp may mimic an air-fluid level radiographically. Polyps may be expansile and extend into the nasal cavity or intracranial cavity. Expansile polyps may erode bone and may be indistinguishable from mucoceles or primary neoplasms. Definitive diagnosis may be possible only by biopsy. Antrochoanal polyps extend from the antrum of the maxillary sinus through the ostium and into the nasal cavity (Fig. 14.04-3). Large polyps may extend through the posterior choanae into the oropharynx.

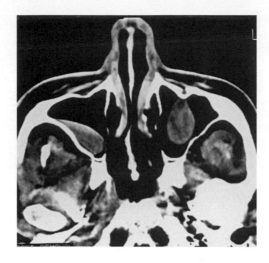

FIGURE 14.04-1.

Retention cysts.   Axial computed tomography shows masses of low density in both maxillary sinuses compatible with mucous retention cysts.

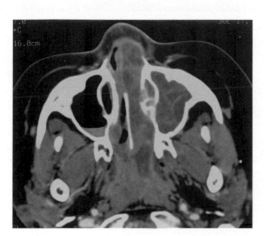

FIGURE 14.04-2.

Nasal polyps.   Axial postcontrast computed tomography shows polypoid mucosal thickening in left maxillary sinus and polyps completely filling the left nasal passages. Small fluid level is present in right maxillary sinus. The bony walls of both maxillary sinuses (left > right) are thick and sclerotic, suggesting chronicity.

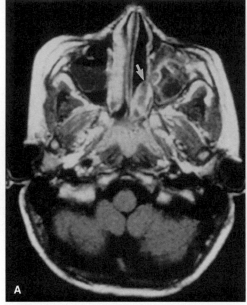

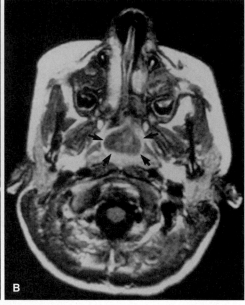

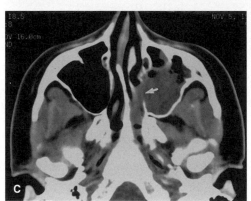

FIGURE 14.04-3.

Antrochoanal polyp. **A.** Postcontrast axial magnetic resonance (MR) T1-weighted image shows complex mass filling the left maxillary sinus and protruding via the middle meatus *(arrow)* into the posterior nasal cavity. There is a low-intensity mucous retention cyst in the right maxillary sinus. **B.** Axial postcontrast MR T1-weighted image inferior to **A** shows that the polyp fills the left posterior nasal cavity and protrudes through the posterior choana into the nasopharynx *(arrows).* Note the cnhancement of mucosa covering the mass. **C.** Axial computed tomography in a different patient shows polyp filling left maxillary sinus and extending via middle meatus *(arrow)* in posterior left nasal cavity.

SUGGESTED READINGS

1. Rabuzzi DD, Hengerer AS. Complications of nasal and sinus infections. In: Bluestone CD, Stool SE, Scheetz MD, eds. Pediatric Otolaryngology, Vol. 1. Philadelphia: WB Saunders, 1990:745.
2. Som PM. Sinonasal cavity. In: Som PM, Bergeron RT, eds. Head and Neck Imaging, 2nd ed. St. Louis: Mosby Year Book, 1990:129.
3. Weissman JL, Tabor EK, Curtin HD. Sphenochoanal polyps: evaluation with CT and MR imaging. Radiology 1991;178:145.
4. Som PM, Lawson W, Lidov MW. Simulated aggressive skull base erosion in response to benign sinonasal disease. Radiology 1991;180:755.

14.05 *Mucoceles*

EPIDEMIOLOGY

"Mucocele" is defined as a completely opacified and expanded paranasal sinus. It is the most common expansile mass in the sinuses. Mucoceles are most common in adults, but may also be seen in children. When present in children, an underlying obstructing mass or predisposing systemic disorder (eg, cystic fibrosis and immotile cilia syndrome) must be excluded.

CLINICAL FEATURES

Mucoceles are caused by obstruction of the sinus ostia or draining ducts. Obstruction of draining pathways prevents egress of secretions. The bony walls of the sinus expand to accommodate the steadily increasing intrasinus pressure caused by trapped secretions. Characteristic clinical and imaging features develop after chronic obstruction. Histologically, the lesions are retained mucous secretions surrounded by a rim of cuboidal epithelium. Pathologically, mucoceles are indistinguishable from polyps and retention cysts. However, the clinical and imaging findings between mucoceles and retention cysts are distinct.

Mucoceles occur in the frontal sinus (60%), ethmoid sinus (25%), maxillary sinus (10%), and sphenoid sinus (5%). Clinical findings depend on location, size, and extent of the mucocele. Findings include proptosis, intraorbital mass, frontal bossing, nasal obstruction, and nasal voice. Although sphenoid mucoceles are the least common, they have the highest incidence of complications because of their proximity to neural and vascular structures. Infected mucoceles ("pyomucoceles") of the sphenoid sinus predispose patients to septic cavernous sinus thrombosis, epidural abscesses, and meningitis.

Treatment of mucoceles is surgical. Frontal sinus mucoceles may be resected via frontal osteotomy with fat obliteration of the sinus. Ethmoid and sphenoid mucoceles are best treated via external ethmoidectomy. Surgical drainage of sphenoid lesions may be difficult because of proximity of optic nerves.

IMAGING FEATURES

For the evaluation of suspected mucoceles, we prefer computed tomography (CT) because of its superior visualization of bone detail. By CT, mucoceles are low-attenuation or soft–tissue-density masses arising in a nonaerated sinus. The involved sinus is smoothly expanded (Figs. 14.05-1–14.05-3). Bone surrounding large mucoceles may be hard to visualize, making a differentiation between a mucocele and a neoplasm difficult. The diagnosis of mucocele may be suggested if the patient has a history of cystic fibrosis or immotile cilia syndrome. Mucoceles may contain focal areas of high attenuation indicative of either dessicated secretions or fungal colonization (Fig. 14.05-3B). Mucoceles may also occur within a localized compartment of a sinus caused by an intrasinus septum. This appearance is very rare.

Magnetic resonance (MR) imaging findings of mucoceles depend on their water and protein contents. Lesions with high water content are hypointense on T1-weighted images and hyperintense on T2-weighted images (Fig. 14.05-1D, E). Progressive dessication of secretions and increasing protein content leads to slight hyperintensity on T1-weighed images and low T2 signal intensity. Mucoceles in the frontal sinus expand it and eventually erode its posterior wall. MR imaging is helpful in differentiating mucocele from adjacent brain. Mucoceles may also extend into the orbits, giving an appearance of multiple globes and proptosis. Infected mucoceles of the frontal and sphenoid sinuses are at increased risk for producing empyema, brain abscess, meningitis, and cavernous sinus thrombosis. Imaging should be performed with intravenous contrast and must include the brain and cavernous sinuses. MR imaging is superior to CT for detecting leptomeningeal involvement and cavernous sinus thrombosis.

It is not possible to differentiate a retention cyst or polyp from an early mucocele or tumor that has not expanded the sinus walls. Thus, the finding of a polypoid soft tissue lesion in an otherwise normal sinus is best described as "polypoid mucosal thickening" rather than a specific disease entity.

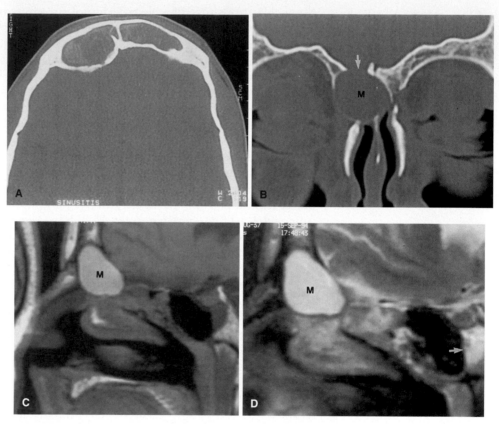

FIGURE 14.05-1.

Frontal mucocele. **A.** Axial computed tomography (CT) shows opacified frontal sinus with expansion of right-sided compartment. The posterior wall is thin and the mucocele contains subtle areas of high density suggesting dessicated secretions or superimposed fungal infection. **B.** Coronal CT in a different patient shows frontal mucocele (M). Note that medial wall is very thin and superior wall has been eroded. **C.** Midsagittal magnetic resonance (MR) T1-weighted image in same patient shows mucocele (M) to have high signal intensity, probably reflecting high proteinaceous contents. **D.** Corresponding MR T2-weighted image shows mucocele (M) to have high signal intensity, reflecting hydrated contents. Note fluid level *(arrow)* in dependent sphenoid sinus.

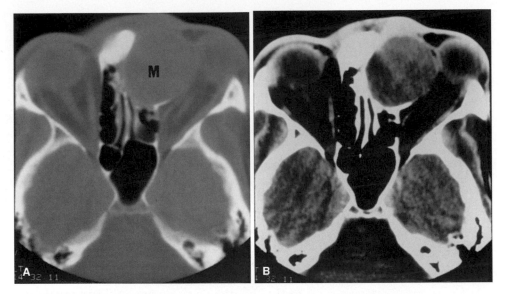

FIGURE 14.05-2.

Ethmoid mucocele. **A.** Axial computed tomography (CT) shows expansion of anterior and middle left ethmoids by mucocele (M). (With permission from Castillo M. Neuroradiology Companion. Philadelphia: JB Lippincott, 1995.) **B.** Corresponding CT using soft tissue window settings shows mucocele to be of low density.

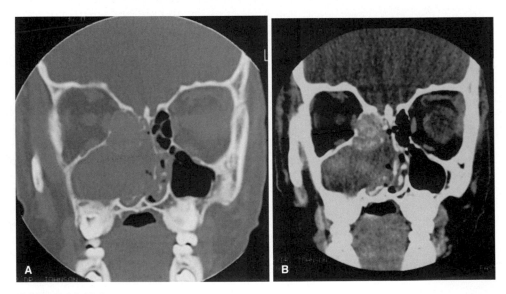

FIGURE 14.05-3.

Maxillary mucocele. **A.** Coronal computed tomography shows expansion of right maxillary and ethmoid sinuses. The nasal septum is bowed to the left. **B.** Corresponding soft tissue window setting shows areas of high density within mucoceles (especially in ethmoid one) that were related to *Aspergillus* infection.

SUGGESTED READINGS

1. Rabuzzi DD, Hengerer AS. Complications of nasal and sinus infections. In: Bluestone CD, Stool SE, Scheetz MD, eds. Pediatric Otolaryngology, Vol. 1. Philadelphia: WB Saunders, 1990:750.
2. Som PM. Sinonasal cavity. In: Som PM, Bergeron RT, eds. Head and Neck Imaging, 2nd ed. St. Louis: Mosby Year Book, 1990:150.

14.06 *Fungal Diseases*

EPIDEMIOLOGY

Fungal disorders affecting the sinonasal cavities include nonaggressive colonization, allergic fungal sinusitis, mycetoma formation, and invasive and fulminant forms that occur in immunocompromised patients. Fungal diseases occur equally in male and female patients and affect all age groups.

CLINICAL FEATURES

The most common fungal disease is allergic rhinitis secondary to fungal antigens. It involves 15% to 30% of adults with sinusitis and is less common in children. The incidence of atopy to specific fungal antigens in patients with chronic sinusitis is approximately 52%. This reaction corresponds to type 1 Bell and Coombs hypersensitivity and occurs in immunocompetent hosts. Clinical findings may mimic those of "hay fever." The most common precipitating molds are *Alternaria, Aspergillus, Candida, Mucor, Penicillium, Hormodendrum,* and *Cladosporium.* Treatment of allergic fungal rhinitis is similar to that of allergic rhinosinusitis and initially consists of avoidance and environmental control of molds. If this is not successful, pharmacotherapy (decongestants, antihistamines, sodium cromolyn, and topical steroids) and immunotherapy may be indicated.

When allergic fungal sinusitis occurs in children and young adults it is analogous to allergic bronchopulmonary aspergillosis. The reaction is a combination of types I and III Bell and Coombs hypersensitivity. Patients usually have asthma or other atopy and present with protracted symptoms involving more than one sinus. The disease is characterized by eosinophilia and increased levels of serum immunoglobulin E. Histologically, secretions contain degenerated eosinophils and Charcot-Leyden crystals. Fungi may be present without invasion of adjacent mucosa. This noninvasive form of fungal disease may be treated medically or surgically. Surgery consists of debridement and drainage of the sinuses via external ethmoidectomy, although some suggest an endoscopic approach. Systemic steroids may be used in recurrent disease. Antifungal medications are not commonly used for noninvasive disease.

Mycetomas may occur in patients with a normal immune status. Their incidence is unknown. They may mimic chronic or recurrent sinusitis. Mycetomas may arise from a variety of genera, the most common being *Aspergillus.* The disease is noninvasive and most often results from colonization of the paranasal sinuses. The maxillary sinus is most frequently involved. Patients may be asymptomatic or present with foul-smelling chronic nasal discharge. Treatment of mycetomas is surgical resection. Systemic steroids are usually not indicated.

Fulminant and invasive fungal sinusitis is potentially life threatening and usually seen in immunocompromised patients. Fulminant disease may progress rapidly and result in intracranial extension and death. The most important immune deficiencies that predispose patients to this aggressive form of fungal disease are severe neutropenia and T-cell deficiency. The population at risk includes patients with hematologic malignancies, AIDS, congenital immunodeficiencies, organ transplants, and chronic steroid and chemotherapy. Other predisposing conditions include uncontrolled diabetes, desert climates, chronic bacterial infection, osteomeatal obstruction, malnutrition, and chronic renal failure. The most commonly implicated fungi are zygomycetes, ascomycetes, and mucoracea (rhinocerebral mucormycoses). The disease becomes established after inhalation of spores. These aggressive organisms may erode bone and invade blood vessels, resulting in endothelial damage, ischemia, thrombosis, and infarction. Uncontrolled disease may invade the orbits, cavernous sinuses, skull base, and brain. On physical examination, there is black crusting and necrotic tissue overlying the turbinates, sinuses, and palate. Patients with intracranial extension may present with cranial nerve deficits, visual loss, or hemiparesis. Treatment consists of antifungal pharmacoptherapy and surgical debridement.

IMAGING FEATURES

Computed tomography (CT) is the preferred modality for imaging patients with noninvasive forms of fungal sinus disease (Fig. 14.06-1). Patients suspected of having fulminant fungal sinus disease may benefit from having both CT and magnetic resonance (MR) imaging. MR imaging is helpful to evaluate leptomeningeal and intracranial extension.

Noninvasive disease may present with nonspecific sinus disease characterized by polypoid mucosal thickening. It is often bilateral in patients with allergic fungal sinusitis and unilateral in cases of superimposed fungal colonization. Fungal disease may result in mucocele formation. Fluid levels are uncommon in patients with fungal sinusitis. Fungal sinus disease may be suggested by presence of focal areas of increased CT attenuation within the paranasal sinuses (Fig. 14.06-1B). These areas of increased attenuation are caused by deposition of calcium salts (calcium phosphate and calcium sulfate) and heavy metals in mycetomas. However, focal areas of increased attenuation may also be caused by dessicated secretions. Mycetomas may also be suggested by presence of a high-attenuation mass that is separated from the sinus wall by mucosa. MR imaging findings are more specific. Affected sinuses demonstrate isointense to decreased signal intensity on T1-weighted images and markedly reduced signal on T2-weighted images. Reduction in T2 signal intensity is caused by the presence of calcium and ferromagnetic elements (including iron and manganese). The quantity of ferromagnetic substances is greater in fungal infections as opposed to bacterial infections. The cavernous sinuses may thrombose and show high T1 signal intensity on precontrast images and low-intensity filling defects after contrast administration. In these cases, the superior ophthalmic veins are prominent and the presence of prominent cortical and deep medullary veins may indicate venous hypertension. Arterial infarctions, due to invasion of vessel walls (especially with mucormycosis), may also occur.

Invasive fungal disease shows soft tissue masses with bone erosion and extension into the face or intracranial cavity (Fig. 14.06-2). Aggressive fungal infections may be indistinguishable from tumor, with the exception that mycetomas tend to be of low T2 signal intensity, whereas tumors tend to be isointense to brain or hyperintense. A history of altered immunity is helpful in making the diagnosis. However, tissue sampling may be necessary for final diagnosis.

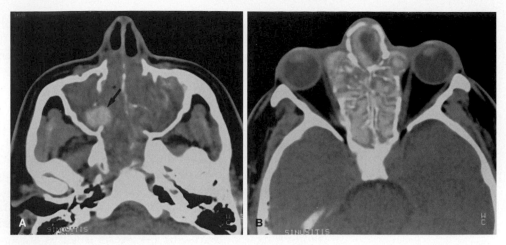

FIGURE 14.06-1.

Polyposis and aspergillosis. **A.** Axial computed tomography (CT) shows filling of both maxillary sinuses and nasal cavity (including nasopharynx) by soft tissue (polyps). The posterior walls of the maxillary sinuses are thick, compatible with a chronic inflammatory process. The right maxillary sinus contains a mycetoma *(arrow).* **B.** Axial CT above **A** shows expansion of ethmoid and frontal sinuses by polyposis, which contains multiple areas of high density that proved to be *Aspergillus* infection. There is secondary hypertelorism.

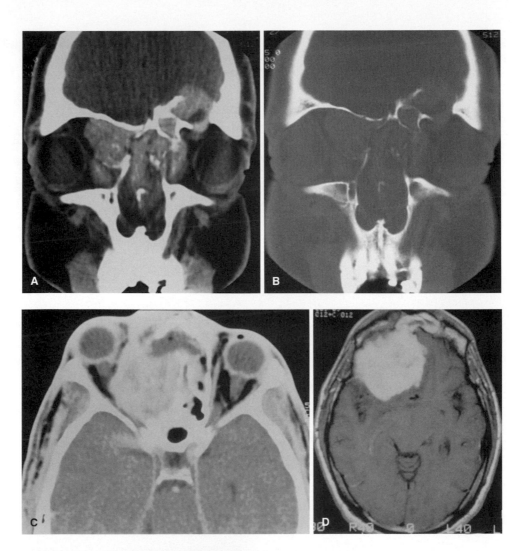

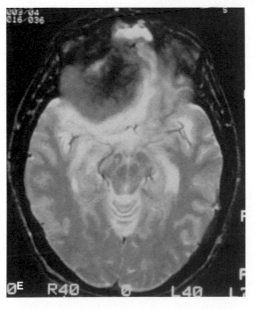

FIGURE 14.06-2.

Aggressive polyposis with superimposed aspergillosis. **A.** Coronal computed tomography (CT) shows high-density masses in nasal cavity and frontal sinus extending into left anterior cranial fossa and both orbits. **B.** Corresponding bone window settings CT shows extensive bone erosion involving the superior and left aspect of the frontal sinuses and medial orbital walls. **C.** In a different patient, axial CT shows hyperdense mass expanding the right ethmoid complex and eroding bone. **D.** Axial postcontrast magnetic resonance (MR) T1-weighted image in same patient shows large aspergilloma invading the brain. **E.** Corresponding MR T2-weighted image shows aspergilloma to be of low signal intensity and surrounded by edema.

SUGGESTED
READINGS

1. Corey JP, Romberger CF, Shaw GY. Fungal diseases of the sinuses. Otolaryngol Head Neck Surg 1990;103:1012.
2. Som PM. Sinonasal cavity. In: Som PM, Bergeron RT, eds. Head and Neck Imaging, 2nd ed. St. Louis: Mosby Year Book, 1990:142.
3. Zienrich SJ, Kennedy DW, Malat J, et al. Fungal sinusitis: diagnosis with CT and MR imaging. Radiology 1988;169:439.
4. Kopp W, Fotter R, Steiner H, Beaufort F, Stammberger H. Aspergillosis of the paranasal sinuses. Radiology 1985;156:715.
5. Gamba JL, Woodruff WW, Djang WT, Yeates AE. Craniofacial mucormycosis: assessment with CT. Radiology 1986;160:207.

14.07 *Juvenile Angiofibroma*

EPIDEMIOLOGY

Juvenile angiofibromas are the most common benign tumors of the nasopharynx and account for 0.05% of all head and neck neoplasms. The lesions are highly vascular and typically present in adolescents, almost always boys. Gender predilection is so strong that sex chromosome analysis of female patients with juvenile angiofibromas is recommended.

CLINICAL FEATURES

Patients present with nasal obstruction and recurrent epistaxis. Other symptoms include rhinolalia, facial swelling, deformities of the hard and soft palate, nasal voice, nasal discharge, serous otitis media, headache, anosmia, and proptosis.

Juvenile angiofibromas arise from anomalous growth of the soft tissue and vascular structures within the sphenopalatine foramina. The site of origin explains their characteristic growth pattern. Lesions arising in the sphenopalatine foramen have access to various locations through preexisting pathways. Tumors may grow into the posterior nasal cavity or maxillary sinuses superiorly via the sphenoethmoid recesses into the sphenoid sinus. Tumors may also grow into adjacent pterygopalatine fossae, gaining access to infratemporal fossae and orbital apices. Tumors may grow directly into cavernous sinuses or middle cranial fossae.

Treatment of juvenile angiofibromas is controversial. Small lesions may be treated with surgery. Preoperative embolization is effective in decreasing tumor vascularity. Large lesions associated with skull base destruction may be treated with a combination of irradiation and surgery. Recurrence is commonly seen in tumors that are incompletely treated. Radiation may be indicated in large masses. Some tumors involute spontaneously.

IMAGING FEATURES

The tumors are highly vascular. Biopsy is not recommended because of risk of bleeding. Diagnosis is on clinical and imaging findings. Both computed tomography (CT) and magnetic resonance (MR) may be used. CT allows evaluation of bony changes, whereas MR imaging allows visualization of flow voids (reflecting vascularity) and invasion of the sinuses and intracranial structures (Fig. 14.07-1).

Juvenile angiofibromas are slow growing and not commonly associated with bone erosion. They show smooth bone remodeling, particularly along the borders of the pterygopalatine fossae. Advanced tumors that have extended in the orbits, cavernous sinuses, or infratemporal fossae may show bone destruction. Invasion of maxillary or ethmoid sinuses occurs in 30% of patients, and intracranial extension in 5% to 10% of patients.

The diagnosis of juvenile angiofibroma may be suggested on radiographs by presence of a soft tissue mass in the nasopharynx bowing the posterior wall of a maxillary sinus anteriorly. On CT, the lesions are solid, enhancing masses centered in a sphenopalatine foramen. Most of the lesions are associated with remodeling of adjacent bone. The differential diagnosis includes lymphoma, nerve sheath tumors, fibrous histiocytomas, and lymphoepithelioma. MR imaging is helpful in further characterizing the lesions. Typical MR imaging features include multiple intratumoral flow voids, indicative of enlarged feeding arteries. Tumors have intermediate signal intensity on T1-weighted images and variable signal intensity on T2-weighted images.

Angiographically, juvenile angiofibromas are highly vascular and show arteriovenous shunting (Fig. 14.07-2). Major supply is by the internal maxillary and ascending pharyngeal arteries. However, large tumors may parasitize any branches of the external carotid artery. Occasionally, supply from the contralateral external carotid artery may be present. Intracavernous or intracranial extension may be determined angiographically by parasitization of flow from the internal carotid artery. Arteriovenous malformations may have similar imaging features (Fig. 14.07-3).

After successful irradiation, juvenile angiofibromas demonstrate reduction in size and number of flow voids. They rarely involute completely with irradiation alone. Thus, presence of residual mass after irradiation does not indicate treatment failure.

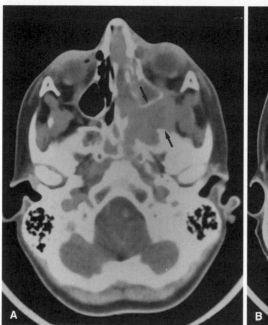
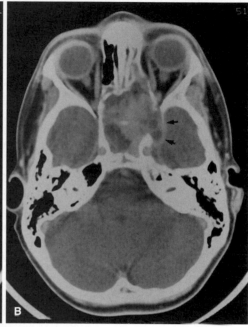
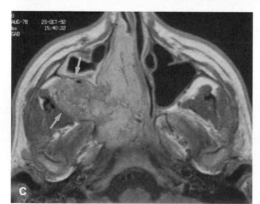

FIGURE 14.07-1.

Angiofibroma. A. Axial postcontrast computed tomography (CT) shows dense mass arising in left pterygopalatine fossa *(arrows),* which is markedly expanded. Mass also fills the left nasal cavity. **B.** Axial CT in same patient showing tumor invading the sphenoid sinus and the left cavernous sinus *(arrows).* **C.** Axial postcontrast magnetic resonance T1-weighted image in different patient shows large and enhancing angiofibroma expanding pterygopalatine fossa *(between arrows)* and extending into nasopharynx and right-sided nasal passages.

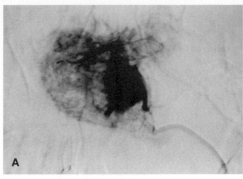 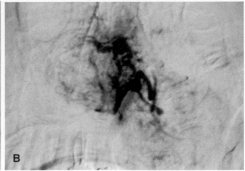

FIGURE 14.07-2.

Angiogram of angiofibroma. **A.** Lateral subtraction view from contrast injection of internal maxillary artery shows intense vascular blush in juvenile angiofibroma. **B.** Corresponding image after particulate embolization shows considerable reduction of blush. Embolization was terminated at this stage because of back reflux.

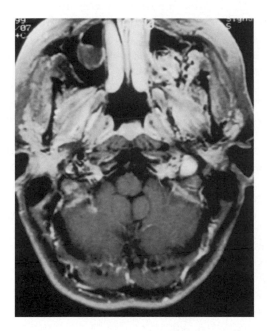

FIGURE 14.07-3.

Arteriovenous malformation of maxillary sinus. Axial postcontrast magnetic resonance T1-weighted image shows enhancing mass in left maxillary sinus with extension into retroantral space. The mass contains multiple flow voids and proved to be an arteriovenous malformation and not a neoplasia.

SUGGESTED READINGS

1. Stanievich JF, Lore JM. Tumors of the nose, paranasal sinuses and nasopharynx. In: Bluestone CD, Stool SE, Scheetz MD, eds. Pediatric Otolaryngology, Vol. 1. Philadelphia: WB Saunders, 1990:175.
2. Som PM. Sinonasal cavity. In: Som PM, Bergeron RT, eds. Head and Neck Imaging, 2nd ed. St. Louis: Mosby Year Book, 1990:175.

14.08 *Sinus Tumors*

EPIDEMIOLOGY   Benign and malignant neoplasms of the paranasal sinus in children are unusual. Benign tumors in the maxillary sinuses usually occur after 6 years of age. Lesions of fibroosseous origin (particularly fibrous dysplasia) or dental origin are the most common benign sinus tumors in children. Malignancies are very rare and represent less than 5% of tumors in the pediatric age group. There is no gender predilection.

CLINICAL FINDINGS   Fibrous dysplasia is the most common of the fibroosseous lesions of the sinuses. Ossifying fibroma is a fibroosseous lesion that consists of highly cellular fibrous and osseous stroma. Unlike fibrous dysplasia, which consists of woven bone, ossifying fibromas consist of lamellar bone. Ossifying fibromas have a greater propensity for aggressive growth and tend to recur frequently after surgery.

Odontogenic lesions may involve the sinuses in children. A dentigerous cyst is a form of odontogenic tumor arising from the developing enamel and surrounding the crown of an unerupted tooth. These lesions occur in children during the second decade of life and may be associated with Gorlin syndrome. Adenomatoid odontogenic tumors (adenomeloblastomas) are benign lesions most commonly seen in girls between 10 to 20 years of age. These lesions are a hamartoma or bony overgrowth of odontogenic tissues. They are usually found in the maxillary incisor/cuspid area and are associated with impacted teeth. Fibromyxomas are a group of several fibrous variants of myxomas that include nonossifying fibromas, desmoplastic fibromas, and odontogenic fibromas. In children, these lesions occur during the second decade of life. In the sinuses they may be locally aggressive. Fibromyxomas have a high rate of recurrence if incompletely resected.

Giant cell granulomas and giant cell tumors (osteoclastomas) occur in the mandible and maxilla and may extend into the paranasal sinuses. Clinically, these lesions are indistinguishable from each other and present with painless swelling, palpable palatal and maxillary mass, and facial asymmetry. Both lesions are slow growing and may destroy bone. The lesions have a tendency to recur if incompletely excised.

Lesions of mesenchymal origin such as hemangiomas may also occur in the paranasal sinuses. These lesions may intermittently bleed and may also invade adjacent bone.

The most frequent malignant tumors involving the paranasal sinuses are rhabdomyosarcoma and undifferentiated carcinoma. Other primary tumors include transitional cell carcinoma, squamous cell carcinoma, adenocarcinoma, osteosarcoma, fibrosarcomas, lymphomas, Ewing sarcoma, and chondrosarcomas. Children who have undergone prior radiotherapy are at risk for development of a malignancy within the treated area. Patients treated for retinoblastoma with irradiation are at increased risk for development of osteosarcoma of the maxillary sinuses. In children, metastases to the paranasal sinuses are most commonly neuroblastoma. Malignancies of the paranasal sinuses present with nonspecific symptoms that may be indistinguishable from benign masses or inflammation. Some malignant lesions are characterized by rapid progression of disease before diagnosis. Bone destruction and neurologic abnormalities are indicative of malignancy.

IMAGING FEATURES   Computed tomography is helpful in determining bone erosion as well as the presence of calcifications within a sinus mass. Magnetic resonance imaging is ideal to outline extension into adjacent soft tissue and intracranial cavity. Therefore, in most patients, both imaging modalities are needed.

Fibrous dysplasia presents with a so-called "ground-glass" appearance and commonly replaces and expands an entire sinus (Fig. 14.08-1). Sudden expansion can be caused by bleeding into the lesion. Ossifying fibromas are expansile lesions that contain large zones of fibrous tissue (more than in fibrous dysplasia) (Fig. 14.08-2). Dentigerous cysts present low-density, expansile lesions surrounding the crown of unerupted teeth (Fig. 14.08-3). The cyst may be unilocular or multilocular and may involve neighboring teeth. In Gorlin syndrome (basal cell nevus syndrome), they are multiple and images of the brain show prominent dural calcifications. Fibromyxomas are expansile lesions that often contain foci of calcification. These lesions occasionally demonstrate bone destruction. Giant cell granulomas and giant cell tumors are indistinguishable from each other when they involve the paranasal sinuses. Both lesions have a lytic bone pattern with areas of destruction and soft tissue masses. Hemangiomas are typically well demarcated and enhance with contrast. Small calcifications are occasionally present (phleboliths).

Rhabdomyosarcomas and other highly malignant lesions present as an aggressive lesion with bone destruction and often local nodal metastases (Fig. 14.08-4). In our experience, all sarcomas of the face enhance after contrast administration. Osteosarcomas often contain calcifications and show spiculated periosteal reaction (Fig. 14.08-5). Chondrosarcomas also contain calcifications and tend to occur near or at synchondroses. Metastases from neuroblastoma produce expansion of bone that appears permeated and always has associated enhancing soft tissue masses. Aggressive soft tissue sarcomas usually present with nonspecific imaging features (Figs. 14.08-6 and 14.08-7).

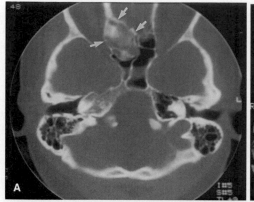

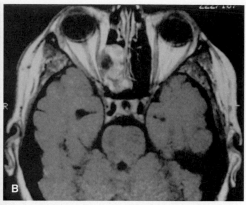

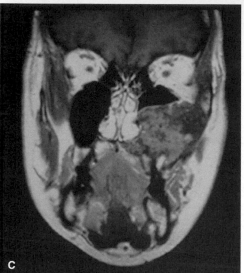

FIGURE 14.08-1.

Fibrous dysplasia. **A.** Axial computed tomography shows typical "ground-glass" appearance of fibrous dysplasia *(arrows)* involving (and expanding) the right posterior ethmoid sinuses. **B.** Corresponding postcontrast magnetic resonance (MR) T1-weighted image shows abnormality to enhance. Note that zone of sclerosis seen anteriorly in **A** appears as an area of low signal intensity on this image. **C.** Coronal postcontrast MR T1-weighted image in a different patient shows fibrous dysplasia involving left maxillary sinus and hard palate. The sinus is expanded.

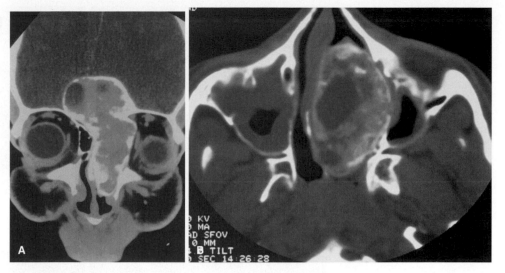

FIGURE 14.08-2.

Ossifying fibroma.   A. Coronal postcontrast computed tomography (CT) shows expansile lesion involving left nasal cavity and ethmoid sinuses and protruding into anterior cranial fossa. The lesion is mostly hyperdense and is surrounded by a rim of bone. **B.** Axial CT in a different patient shows left intranasal ossifying fibroma with expansion of cavity. Fibrous dysplasia of the turbinates has an identical appearance.

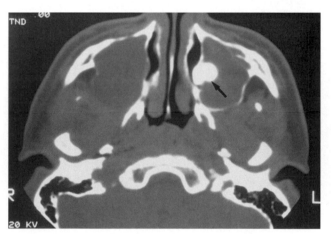

FIGURE 14.08-3.

Dentigerous cysts in Gorlin syndrome.   Axial computed tomography shows expansile lesions in both maxillary sinuses. The posterior wall of the right-sided one is eroded. The left-sided one contains a remnant of a tooth *(arrow)*. Similar cysts were present in the mandible, and a skull radiograph showed dural calcifications.

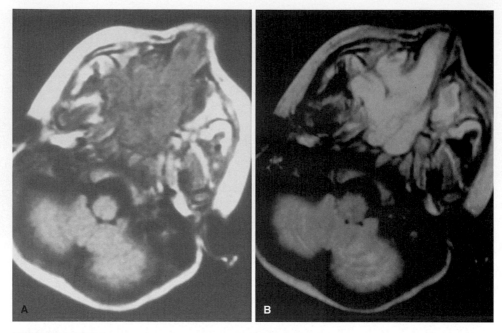

FIGURE 14.08-4.

Rhabdomyosarcoma. **A.** Axial noncontrast magnetic resonance (MR) T1-weighted image shows soft tissue mass (isointense to muscle) filling nasal cavities, maxillary sinuses, and nasopharynx. **B.** Corresponding MR T2-weighted image shows the mass to be hyperintense.

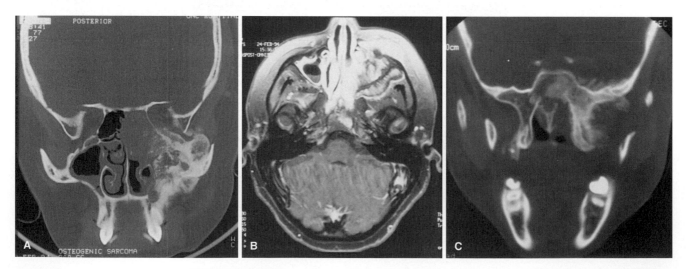

FIGURE 14.08-5.

Osteosarcoma. **A.** Coronal computed tomography (CT) shows osteosarcoma of left maxillary sinus with soft tissue component extending into nasal cavity and left ethmoid sinuses. Note sclerotic bone formation with this sinus mass and a spiculated periosteal reaction. **B.** Axial postcontrast magnetic resonance fat-suppressed T1-weighted image in same patient shows mass in left maxillary sinus and nasal cavity to enhance. Note thickening of posterior wall of involved maxillary sinus and extension into the retroantral fat pad. **C.** Coronal CT in a different patient with an osteosarcoma arising in vicinity of sphenoid sinus shows sclerotic bone formation in sinus extending into floor of left middle cranial fossa and pterygoid plates.

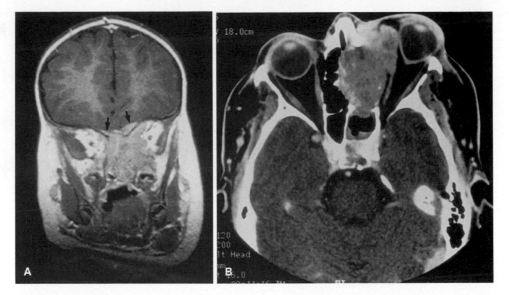

FIGURE 14.08-6.

Esthesioneuroblastoma.   **A.** Coronal postcontrast magnetic resonance T1-weighted image shows enhancing mass in nasal cavities extending into left maxillary sinus and orbit. Note dural invasion *(arrows)*.   **B.** Axial postcontrast computed tomography in a different patient shows mass in left ethmoids eroding medial wall of the orbit with extraconal invasion. Note proptosis and compressive deformity of left eye.

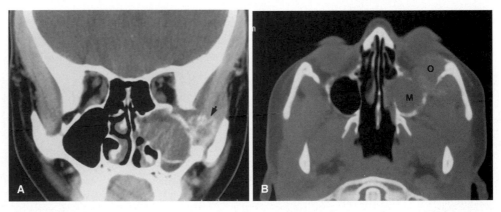

FIGURE 14.08-7.

Ewing sarcoma.   **A.** Coronal postcontrast computed tomography (CT) shows mass in left maxillary sinus with erosion of the lateral wall and extension into soft tissues. Extrasinal portion of the tumor is calcified *(arrow)*.   **B.** Axial CT (bone window settings) shows sarcoma filling superior recess of maxillary sinus (M), erosion of the anterior wall with extension into the orbit (O), and erosion of the lateral wall with periosteal reaction.

SUGGESTED READINGS

1. Schramm VL. Inflammatory and neoplastic masses of the nose and paranasal sinus in children. Laryngoscope 1979;89:1887.
2. Som PM. Sinonasal cavity. In: Som PM, Bergeron RT, eds. Head and Neck Imaging, 2nd ed. St. Louis: Mosby Year Book, 1990:195.
3. Stainevich JF, Lore JM. Tumors of the nose, paranasal sinuses, and nasopharynx. In: Bluestone CD, Stool SE, Scheetz MD, eds. Pediatric Otolaryngology, Vol. 1. Philadelphia: WB Saunders, 1990:780.

Imaging of the Pediatric Head, Neck, and Spine
by Mauricio Castillo and Suresh K. Mukherji,
Lippincott-Raven Publishing, Philadelphia © 1996.

15
The Neck

SECTION A. ■ AIRWAY

SECTION B. ■ SOFT TISSUES

SECTION A   AIRWAY

15A.0 *Applied Embryology*

The larynx comprises supraglottic, glottic, and infraglottic components. The supraglottic larynx is irrigated and innervated by the superior laryngeal artery and nerve. Lymphatic drainage is via deep cervical nodes (groups II–IV). The glottic and subfraglottic larynx are supplied by branches of the inferior laryngeal artery and nerve and the recurrent laryngeal nerve. Lymphatic drainage is via pretracheal and peritracheal nodes.

Step 1. The Subglottic Larynx

The infraglottic larynx is the oldest portion and is primarily concerned with ventilation. The supraglottic larynx forms later and primarily has a vocal function. The vocal cords are the last to appear. The respiratory system develops from an elongated outpouching of the primitive pharynx during the fourth week of life. Development is first noted by formation of the laryngotracheal groove (groove of furcula), which is located on the ventral wall of the primitive pharynx caudal to the fourth pharyngeal pouch. This groove along the floor of the pharynx will give rise to supraglottic and glottic structures. The laryngotracheal groove elongates in a rostrocaudal direction to form the laryngotracheal diverticulum, which is ventral to the primitive foregut. The diverticulum is the precursor of the trachea and bronchi. With continued growth, the diverticulum becomes surrounded by splanchnic mesenchyme and its distal segments form the primitive lung buds. Proximally, the diverticulum separates from the primitive pharynx by the formation of longitudinal furrows (tracheoesophageal folds) that develop during the fourth week of life (Fig. 15A.0-1A). These tracheoesophageal folds develop on both sides of the diverticulum at its union with the primitive pharynx. These folds grow medially and fuse to form the tracheoesophageal septum during the seventh week of life (Fig. 15A.0-1B). The tracheoesophageal septum separates the foregut into a ventral respiratory portion and a dorsal digestive portion. The ventral respiratory portion is termed the laryngotracheal tube and is the precursor of the larynx, trachea, lungs, and bronchi (Fig. 15A.0-1C). Incomplete division of the foregut into respiratory and digestive portions results in tracheoesophageal fistulas. Unequal partitioning of the foregut into trachea and esophagus causes tracheal stenosis and atresia.

Step 2. Supraglottic and Glottic Larynx

The supraglottic larynx forms from mesenchyme surrounding the laryngotracheal groove. During the fifth to sixth weeks of life, the opening of the laryngotracheal groove (laryngeal aditus) is modified by rapid proliferation of the pharynx (Fig. 15A.0-2A). The anterior mass derives from the hypobranchial eminence and fourth branchial arch and is the precursor of the epiglottis (Fig. 15A.0-2B,C). The two lateral masses are the anlage for the aryepiglottic folds and arytenoid cartilages. Rapid proliferation of these structures results in temporary occlusion of the laryngeal lumen. Recanalization occurs during the 10th week of life. The true and false vocal cords and the laryngeal ventricle form during recanalization. Incomplete recanalization results in laryngeal atresia, subglottic stenosis, and laryngeal webs.

Step 3. The Laryngeal Framework

The arytenoid and corniculate cartilages derive from the fourth branchial arch and begin as the arytenoid swellings surrounding the laryngeal aditus. The vocal processes are formed at the beginning of the third month of life in association with the thyroid cartilage and vocal ligament.

The cricoid cartilage derives from the sixth branchial arch and develops into two cartilaginous centers. The anterior ring of the cricoid cartilage fuses by the sixth week of life, whereas the posterior ring fuses by the seventh week of life. Fusion of the posterior aspect of the cricoid cartilage is aided by the advancing tracheoesophageal septum. Arrest in development of the tracheoesophageal septum prevents fusion of the posterior cricoid cartilage and results in laryngotracheoesophageal cleft.

The epiglottis derives from the floor of the pharynx and the fourth branchial arch. The floor of the pharynx also gives rise to the cuneiform cartilages.

The thyroid cartilage develops from the fourth branchial arches. The cartilage develops as two lateral plates that fuse in the midline and are united by a membrane. Formation is usually completed by the 10th week of life.

The hyoid bone derives from the second and third branchial arches. The second arch cartilage forms the lesser cornua and a part of the body of the hyoid bone, whereas the third arch cartilage forms the greater cornu and remaining body.

Step 4. The Laryngeal Muscles

The intrinsic laryngeal muscles initially appear in the larynx as an intrinsic ring of mesenchyme derived from the sixth branchial arch. These muscles are innervated by the recurrent laryngeal nerve. The cricothyroid muscle arises from the ventral portion of the inferior constrictor muscle, which is a derivative of the fourth branchial arch. The cricothyroid muscle is innervated by the superior laryngeal nerve. The intrinsic muscles are first recognized by the seventh week of life.

The extrinsic strap muscles derive from an epicardial ridge of primitive infrahyoid muscle mass. All muscles arising from this anlage are supplied by the hypoglossal nerve.

A   B   C

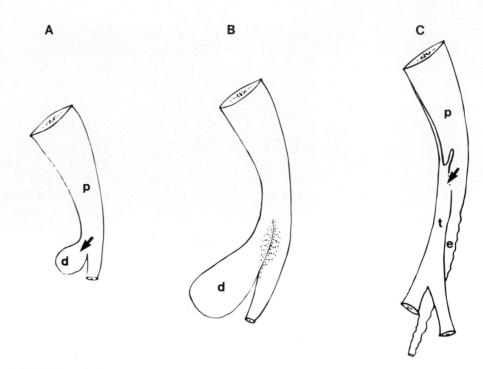

FIGURE 15A.0-1.

Development of tracheoesophageal septum.   **A.** At 4 weeks of life, the pharynx (p) communicates with the laryngotracheal diverticulum (d) via the primitive glottis *(arrow)*, whose walls are the tracheoesophageal folds. **B.** The laryngotracheal diverticulum (d) elongates and the tracheoesophageal folds approximate medially and fuse, forming the tracheoesophageal septum *(dotted region)*. **C.** At 5 weeks of life, the laryngotracheal tube (t) is well formed, communicates with the pharynx (p) via the laryngeal aditus *(arrow)*, and ends in the primitive bronchi. The esophagus (e) is now present.

A   B   C

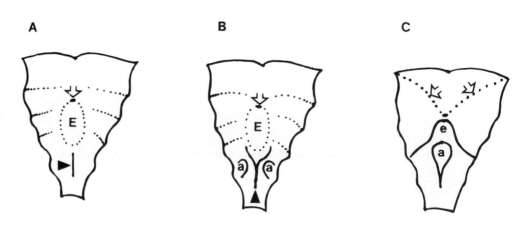

FIGURE 15A.0-2.

Development of the larynx (view from posterior into pharyngeal inner surface).   **A.** At 4 weeks of life, the laryngotracheal groove *(arrowhead)* is present inferior to the hypobranchial eminence (E). Note foramen cecum *(open arrow)*. **B.** At 6 weeks of life, the primitive glottis *(arrowhead)* is flanked by the arytenoid swellings (a) and is inferior to the hypobranchial eminence (E). Open arrow, foramen cecum. **C.** At 10 weeks of life, the laryngeal aditus (a) is well formed, as is the epiglottis (e). The palatine tonsils and terminal sulcus *(open arrows)* of the tongue are present.

SUGGESTED READINGS

1. Moore KL. The respiratory system. In: Moore KL, ed. The Developing Human: Clinically Oriented Embryology, 4th ed. Philadelphia: WB Saunders, 1988:207.
2. Spector GJ. Developmental anatomy of the larynx. In: Ballenger JJ, ed. Diseases of the Ear, Nose and Throat. Philadelphia: Lea and Febiger, 1985:369.
3. Hast MH. Developmental anatomy of the larynx. In: Gardner J, ed. Scientific Foundations of Otolaryngology. London: Heineman Medical, 1976:369.

15A.01   *Stenosis of the Subglottis and Trachea*

EPIDEMIOLOGY

Subglottic stenosis is defined as luminal narrowing below the true vocal cords and above the base of the cricoid cartilage. It may be congenital or result from prior prolonged intubation or laryngeal trauma. It is the most common anomaly requiring tracheostomy in patients younger than 1 year of age. Its incidence is increased in patients with Down syndrome. There is no gender predilection. Tracheal stenosis is associated with tracheoesophageal fistulas, pulmonary hypoplasia, and anomalies of the great vessels.

CLINICAL FEATURES

The diameter of the normal subglottic lumen in full-term infants varies from 4.5 to 5.5 mm, and in premature newborns is approximately 3.5 mm. Congenital subglottic stenosis occurs when the subglottic lumen is less than 3.5 mm in diameter in full-term infants and less than 3 mm in prematures.

Congenital subglottic stenosis results from failure or inadequate recanalization of laryngeal lumen after the completion of normal epithelial fusion at the end of the third month of life. The degree of stenosis depends on the amount of recanalization and ranges from laryngeal atresia to webs and stenoses. Subglottic stenosis is considered to be congenital when there is no previous history of intubation or trauma. The diagnosis is difficult to substantiate because it is not known how many patients who require intubation actually had underlying subglottic stenosis that was aggravated by intubation.

Congenital subglottic stenosis may be membranous or cartilaginous. The membranous form is circumferential and presents as soft tissue thickening in the subglottic region. Histologically, this thickening is caused by increased fibrous connective tissue and hyperplastic mucous glands. Membranous stenosis occurs 2 to 3 mm below the undersurface of the true vocal cords and may extend to the trachea. The cartilaginous form is caused by an abnormally formed cricoid cartilage. The cricoid is thickened and deformed, resulting in a plate of cartilage on its inner surface. This cartilaginous shelf extends posteriorly, causing a stenosis. Subglottic stenosis may also be caused by a trapped first tracheal ring. Tracheal stenosis may be generalized, funnel-shaped, or segmental. The main bronchi usually are of normal size. Segmental stenosis occurs anywhere in the trachea. Stenosis is caused by abnormal cartilage that completely encircles the trachea. The normal horseshoe-shaped cartilages are replaced by complete or near-complete rings. The membranous posterior wall is absent and the trachea is rigid.

Patients with subglottic stenosis present within the first year of life with signs of airway obstruction. Symptoms are often exacerbated by infections involving the upper respiratory tract that produce mucosal edema. Diagnosis is based on endoscopic findings of circumferential narrowing in the subglottic region. Stenosis may be localized to the subglottic region or extend to the trachea. The full extent of narrowing may at times be difficult to determine by endoscopy alone. Over 40% of patients have a history of difficult intubation. The natural course of congenital subglottic stenosis is different from that of acquired subglottic stenosis; therefore, it is important to differentiate between them. Most patients with subglottic stenosis improve with progressive growth of the larynx. In patients who have small larynxes, acquired stenosis may develop from prolonged intubation. A tracheostomy may be required if a 3.5-mm endoscope cannot be easily passed through the affected region. Most children with congenital subglottic stenosis who require airway control may be decanulated by the second to third year of life. Alternatively, an anterior cricoid split may be beneficial in patients with severe respiratory compromise. Acquired subglottic stenosis usually is more severe and often requires aggressive, long-term management. Symptoms may also be those of croup or bronchiolitis. Endoscopy confirms the diagnosis, but is risky. The residual lumen usually is less than 3 mm and the tracheal walls are rigid. The prognosis is poor.

Symptoms of patients with tracheal stenosis include cough, persistent wheezing, stridor, and intermittent cyanosis.

IMAGING FEATURES

Subglottic stenosis may be seen as narrowing of the air column on frontal and lateral radiographs of the neck. Computed tomography (CT) is the imaging modality of choice if the extent of the narrowing cannot be fully appreciated by endoscopy. By CT, subglottic stenosis is seen as circumferential soft tissue thickening below the true vocal cords. This abnormal soft tissue thickening may extend to the trachea, resulting in narrowing. Segmental stenosis usually measures between 1 to 1.5 cm in length. It does not enhance after contrast administration. Because the trachea is not calcified in young children, the cricoid cartilage is not well seen by CT, the exact location of the abnormality may be difficult to determine, and it is not possible to separate membranous from cartilaginous stenoses. The full extent of the involved area should be determined and the diameter of the air column at the level of the most severely affected area should be measured.

Tracheal stenosis is readily evaluated with CT. The lumen usually measures less than 3 mm (Figs. 15A.01-1 and 15A.01-2A–C). The cartilages are not seen because they are not calcified. Three-dimensional reconstruction is helpful in visualizing the abnormality (Fig. 15A.01-2D).

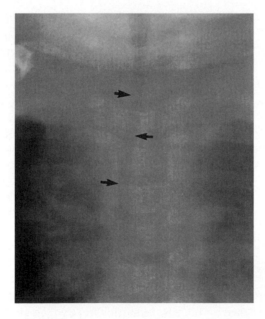

FIGURE 15A.01-1.

Diffuse tracheal stenosis. Frontal radiograph shows diffuse narrowing *(arrows)* of tracheal air column.

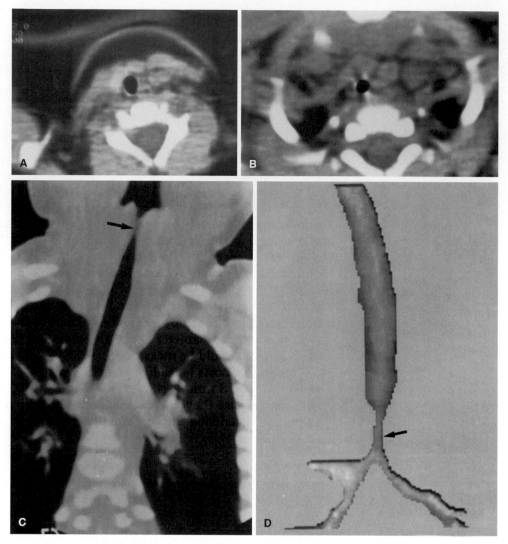

FIGURE 15A.01-2.

Segmental tracheal stenosis. **A.** Axial computed tomography (CT) shows normal tracheal lumen. **B.** Axial CT slice below **A** shows reduction of tracheal lumen compatible with stenosis, which in this case was secondary to a complete tracheal ring. Note that rings are not calcified and therefore not visible. (Cases courtesy of D. Merten, University of North Carolina, Chapel Hill, NC.) **C.** Direct coronal CT shows focal glottic/subglottic stenosis *(arrow)*. (Case courtesy of J. Lucaya, M.D., Institut Catala de la Salut, Hospital Universitari Materno-infantil Vall d'Hebron, Barcelona, Spain.) **D.** Three-dimensional reformation from magnetic resonance imaging data set in a child with a low vascular ring shows focal stenosis *(arrow)* of distal trachea. (Case courtesy of E. R. Bank, M.D., Egleston Children's Hospital, Atlanta, GA.)

SUGGESTED READINGS

1. Cotton RT, Reilly JS. Congenital malformations of the larynx. In: Bluestone CD, Stool SE, Scheetz MD, eds. Pediatric Otolaryngology, Vol. 2. Philadelphia: WB Saunders, 1990:1126.
2. Cotton RT, Andrews TM. Laryngeal stenosis. In: Johnson JT, Kohut RI, Pillsbury HC, Tardy ME, eds. Head and Neck Surgery–Otolaryngology, Vol. 1. Philadelphia: JB Lippincott, 1993:658.
3. Curtin HC. The larynx. In: Som PM, Bergeron RT, eds. Head and Neck Imaging, 2nd ed. St. Louis: CV Mosby, 1991:669.
4. Myer CM, Cotton RT. Congenital abnormalities of the larynx and trachea and man-

agement of congenital malformations. In: Paparella MM, Shumrick DA, Gluckman JL, Meyeroff WL, eds. Otolaryngology, Vol. 3, 3rd ed. Philadelphia: WB Saunders, 1991:1991.

5. Benjamin B. Congenital disorders of the trachea. In: Cummings CW, Frerickson JM, Harker LA, Krause CJ, Schuller DE, eds. Otolaryngology and Head and Neck Surgery, Vol. 3. St. Louis: CV Mosby, 1993:2294.

6. Loeff DS, Filler RM, Vinograd I, et al. Congenital tracheal stenosis: a review of 22 patients from 1965–1987. J Pediatr Surg 1988;23:744.

15A.02 *Laryngeal Atresia and Webs*

EPIDEMIOLOGY

Laryngeal atresia is a rare condition that, in most instances, if not immediately recognized, is incompatible with life. Most patients with laryngeal atresia are stillborn. Occasionally, patients with tracheoesophageal fistulas that are large enough to permit ventilation may survive the perinatal period. Laryngeal atresia is often associated with other congenital anomalies.

Laryngeal webs are rare lesions resulting from incomplete canalization of the embryonic larynx during the seventh to eighth weeks of life. These webs are part of a continuum of congenital abnormalities that vary from laryngeal atresia to subglottic stenosis. Laryngeal webs are associated with other congenital anomalies. One-third of patients have an abnormality of the respiratory tract, the most common being subglottic stenosis. The incidence of associated anomalies increases with the severity of laryngeal webs.

CLINICAL FEATURES

Patients with laryngeal atresia attempt respiratory movements but are unable to ventilate their lungs. Cyanosis rapidly develops after clamping of the umbilical cord. Attempts to intubate them are unsuccessful. Tracheostomy is necessary to prevent death. Laryngoscopy and bronchoscopy should be performed. Management of laryngeal atresia depends on the extent of the atretic segment. Occasionally, a small-bore bronchoscope may be passed in patients with a short atretic segment. More extensive atresia requires tracheotomy or insertion of a large-bore catheter or needle distal to the atretic segment.

Seventy-five percent of laryngeal webs are located at the true vocal cords. These lesions are most often located at the anterior commissure. Webs may also occur in the posterior commissure, resulting in interarytenoid fixation. Laryngeal webs may also involve the supraglottic and subglottic larynx.

Endoscopically, laryngeal webs appear as soft tissue membranes extending across the laryngeal air column. The thickness of the web is variable and ranges from a thin membrane to a thick, fibrous band. Larger webs produce greater airway obstruction. The peripheral portion of the webs usually is thicker than their free margins, which are concave and sharply outlined.

Patients with laryngeal webs are usually symptomatic at birth and present with signs of airway obstruction, including a weak cry, aphonia, respiratory distress, and cyanosis. Stridor is unusual. Some patients may present later in life with symptoms simulating recurrent or atypical croup.

Treatment of laryngeal webs depends on their thickness. Thin webs may be treated with endoscopic lysis using carbon dioxide laser or knife. Patients with large webs producing severe respiratory distress may require intubation or tracheostomy. Thick webs may also require an open laryngeal procedure. Laryngeal dilation is often required to prevent recurrence after the initial procedure.

IMAGING FEATURES

Patients with laryngeal atresia are seldom imaged because they are stillborn. Those in whom this anomaly is recognized and treated promptly may be imaged initially with radiographs. Radiographs show abrupt termination of the air column. Severe stenosis behaves (and is treated) identically to atresia and shows marked dilation of the hypopharynx superior to the narrowing. Computed tomography (CT) allows for exact determination of the cross-sectional diameter of residual lumen. Residual lumen of less than 2 mm in diameter may be considered atresia for practical purposes (Fig. 15A.02-1).

In patients with laryngeal webs, lateral radiographs provide adequate initial information. Webs are seen as shelves of soft tissue located immediately inferior to the true vocal cords or at the level of the anterior commissure. The vocal cords may be fixed. The radiographic findings are similar to those seen in croup or vocal cord paralysis. The hypopharynx is distended and there is narrowing in the region of the web on inspiration. On expiration, the subglottic airway is distended and the region of the web remains narrowed. Sagittal and coronal reformations of spiral CT provide valuable information regarding the thickness of the webs.

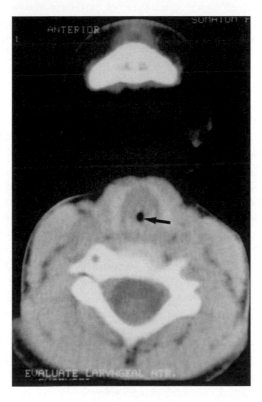

FIGURE 15A.02-1.

Tracheal atresia. Axial computed tomography shows severe narrowing *(arrow)* of tracheal lumen; in this case down to 2 mm, which behaves clinically the same as atresia and is treated as such.

SUGGESTED READINGS

1. Myer CM, Cotton RT. Congenital abnormalities of the larynx and trachea and management of congenital malformations. In: Paparella MM, Shumrick DA, Gluckman JL, Meyeroff WL, eds. Otolaryngology, Vol. 3, 3rd ed. Philadelphia: WB Saunders, 1991:2220.
2. Benjamin B. Congenital disorders of the larynx. In: Cummings CW, Frerickson JM, Harker LA, Krause CJ, Schuller DE, eds. Otolaryngology and Head and Neck Surgery, Vol. 3. St. Louis: CV Mosby, 1993:1846.
3. John SD, Swischuk LE. Stridor and upper airway obstruction in infants and children. RadioGraphics 1992;12:625.
4. MacPherson RI, Leithiser RE. Upper airway obstruction in children: an update. RadioGraphics 1985;5:339.

15A.03 *Esophageal Atresia and Tracheoesophageal Fistula*

EPIDEMIOLOGY   Tracheoesophageal fistula and esophageal atresia are congenital malformations characterized by abnormal communication between the esophagus and trachea. It occurs in 1:3000 to 4000 of births and is found within 24 hours of birth in 85% of cases. One-third of patients are born premature. It is more common in boys. Coexisting anomalies are present in 50% of patients. The best known patterns of anomalies are referred to by the acronyms VATER (vertebral defects, imperforate anus, tracheoesophageal fistula, radial and renal dysplasia) and VACTERL (vertebral, anal, cardiac, tracheal, esophageal, renal, and limb deformities). Other coexisting anomalies include Down syndrome and atresias of the gastrointestinal tract (including duodenal atresia). Cardiovascular anomalies include patent ductus arteriosus, ventricular septal defect, and right-sided aortic arch. Patients with tracheoesophageal fistula have an increased incidence of tracheomalacia.

CLINICAL FEATURES   These abnormalities result from anomalous separation of the primitive foregut into trachea and esophagus due to a failure of complete formation of the tracheoesophageal septum, which normally separates the respiratory and digestive systems. The developmental error occurs between the fourth to fifth weeks of life.

Tracheoesophageal fistulas are divided into type I, isolated esophageal atresia (5%–10%); type II (proximal fistula—1%), esophageal atresia with an upper fistula connecting the proximal blind-ending esophageal pouch with the trachea, with no communication with the distal esophagus; type III (distal fistula—85%), esophageal atresia with a blind-ending upper pouch and a fistula connecting the trachea with the distal pouch; type IV (proximal and distal fistulas—2%), esophageal atresia with separate fistulas from the trachea communicating with both the proximal and distal esophageal segments; and type V (H-type—6%), direct communication between esophagus and trachea. Type V is the one without esophageal atresia (Fig. 15A.03-1).

Patients with tracheoesophageal fistulas present with drooling, cough, respiratory distress, and choking, all of which are exacerbated by feeding. Other symptoms are recurrent pneumonias, gaseous abdominal distention, and failure to thrive. Failure to pass a nasogastric tube into the stomach is characteristic of these anomalies, although a tube may be passed into the stomach in the H-type (V) fistula. The treatment of tracheoesophageal fistulas is surgical repair. The type of repair depends on the type of fistula and the distance between the proximal and distal ends of the esophagus.

IMAGING FEATURES   Radiographs demonstrate lack of air in the stomach in patients with complete esophageal atresia (Fig. 15A.03-2A,B). The presence of gas in abdominal viscera in patients with esophageal atresia indicates a communication between the trachea and the distal esophageal pouch. A coiled nasogastric tube in the proximal esophagus is indicative of underlying atresia. Air may be injected into the nasogastric tube to visualize better the proximal pouch on radiographs (Fig. 15A.03-2C,D). Care must be taken not to perforate the proximal pouch or advance the tube into the bronchial tree, as could occur in proximal tracheoesophageal fistula. Contrast may be injected into the proximal esophageal pouch to confirm the diagnosis of atresia and to identify a fistula (Fig. 15A.03-2E). Contrast in the esophagus also aids in determining the side of the aortic arch and excluding the possibility of pharyngeal pseudodiverticulum. The patient should be placed in the lateral decubitus position with the head slightly elevated before administration of contrast. Initially, an 8-Fr polyethylene feeding tube is placed in the distal esophagus. Barium should be administered under pressure while slowly withdrawing the tip of the feeding tube. Only 0.5 to 1.0 mL of aqueous barium suffices. The patient is then turned prone and horizontal beam fluoroscopy allows visualization of barium opacifying the ventral esophageal wall, thus maximizing visualization of fistulas (Fig. 15A.03-3). Computed tomography (CT) and magnetic resonance imaging may be used to evaluate associated anomalies. CT may at times be helpful in identifying patients with obliquely oriented fistulas.

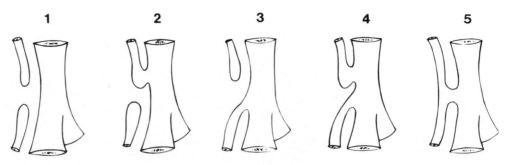

FIGURE 15A.03-1.

Different types of esophageal atresia and fistulas. 1, Blind-ending proximal and distal esophageal pouches; 2, proximal fistula with blind-ending distal pouch; 3, blind-ending proximal pouch and distal fistula; 4, proximal and distal fistulas; 5, H-type fistula.

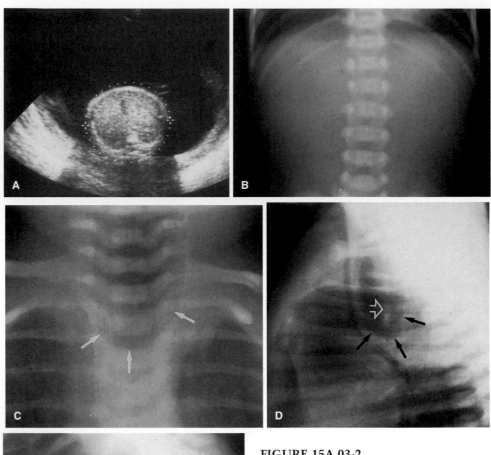

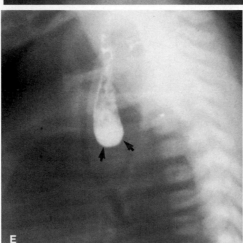

FIGURE 15A.03-2.

Type I esophageal atresia. **A.** In utero sonogram shows increased amniotic fluid and absent stomach bubble. **B.** Immediately after birth, frontal radiograph of the abdomen confirms absent gas in stomach. **C.** Frontal radiograph of the upper thorax shows dilated and blind-ending proximal esophageal pouch *(arrows)*. **D.** Lateral radiograph of upper thorax after insertion of nasogastric tube. The tube *(open arrow)* is coiled in the proximal esophageal pouch *(solid black arrows)*, which is distended. **E.** Lateral radiograph after instillation of radiopaque contrast clearly delineates the proximal esophageal pouch *(arrows)*. Trachea is bowed anteriorly. (Case courtesy of D. Merten, University of North Carolina, Chapel Hill, NC.)

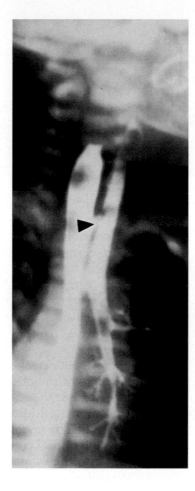

FIGURE 15A.03-3.

Type V tracheoesophageal fistula. Oblique radiograph after barium swallow shows short communication *(arrowhead)* between upper esophagus and trachea. Contrast has "spilled" in tracheobronchial tree. (Case courtesy of D. Merten, University of North Carolina, Chapel Hill, NC.)

SUGGESTED
READING

1. Kirks DR, Caron KH. Gastrointestinal tract. In: Kirks DR, ed. Practical Pediatric Imaging Diagnostic Radiology of Infants and Children, 2nd ed. Boston: Little, Brown, 1991:744.

15A.04 *Laryngotracheoesophageal Cleft*

EPIDEMIOLOGY

Laryngotracheoesophageal clefts are rare congenital anomalies resulting in abnormal communication between the larynx, trachea, and esophagus. Thirty percent of fetuses show polyhydramnios. It is associated with other congenital abnormalities with 20% of patients. There is no gender predilection.

CLINICAL FEATURES

Laryngotracheoesophageal clefts result from lack of development of the tracheoesophageal septum at approximately 35 days of life. The absence of the septum inhibits proper formation and fusion of the cricoid cartilage. This results in a communication between the larynx and pharynx. The anomalous communication may be localized to the posterior aspect of the cricoid cartilage or be more extensive, involving the entire common wall between the trachea and esophagus.

Patients present early in life with feeding difficulties and respiratory distress. Patients with very small clefts may be asymptomatic. Affected individuals often have choking and coughing episodes during feeding, and cyanosis. Other symptoms include stridor, recurrent aspirations, and voice abnormalities.

Diagnosis is made by endoscopy. An endotracheal tube should be placed at time of endoscopy to separate the edges of the cleft. Every attempt should be made at endoscopy to determine the extent of the cleft.

The surgical management of this anomaly is directed toward controlling airway function and preventing aspiration. The endotracheal tube maintains airway patency initially. In extensive clefts, tracheotomy tubes may migrate over the superior edge of the defect into the esophageal lumen, resulting in respiratory arrest. The type of surgical closure depends on the length and extent of the defect.

IMAGING FEATURES

Chest radiographs may show parenchymal opacities consistent with aspiration pneumonia. The diagnosis of laryngotracheoesophageal cleft is confirmed with esophagography demonstrating contrast material extending from the esophagus into the trachea (Fig. 15A.04-1). The esophogram is best performed using barium with the patient placed in prone position. The roles of computed tomography and magnetic resonance imaging have not been defined.

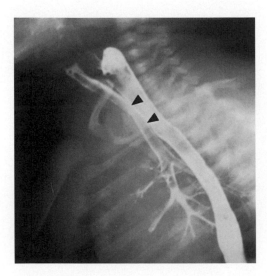

FIGURE 15A.04-1.

Tracheoesophageal cleft. Oblique radiograph after barium swallow shows large communication *(arrowheads)* between the middle and anterior esophagus and trachea. (Case courtesy of L. Fordham, University of North Carolina, Chapel Hill, NC.)

SUGGESTED READINGS

1. Cotton RT, Reilly JS. Congenital malformations of the larynx. In: Bluestone CD, Stool SE, Scheetz MD, eds. Pediatric Otolaryngology, Vol. 2. Philadelphia: WB Saunders, 1990:1127.
2. Myer CM, Cotton RT. Congenital abnormalities of the larynx and trachea and management of congenital malformations. In: Paparella MM, Shumrick DA, Gluckman JL, Meyeroff WL, eds. Otolaryngology, Vol. 3, 3rd ed. Philadelphia: WB Saunders, 1991:2222.
3. Pillsbury HC, Fischer ND. Laryngotracheoesophageal cleft: diagnosis, management and presentation of a new diagnostic device. Arch Otol 1977;103:735.

15A.05 *Laryngomalacia (Congenital Flaccid Larynx)*

EPIDEMIOLOGY

Laryngomalacia is the most common congenital laryngeal abnormality, accounting for 60% of laryngeal problems in newborns. It is the most common cause of stridor in infants. This condition usually presents during the first few weeks of life. Laryngomalacia is often benign and self-limited, resolving within 6 months to 2 years of age. It frequently coexists with other abnormalities of the larynx. There is no gender predilection.

CLINICAL FEATURES

The exact cause of laryngomalacia is unknown, but certain anatomic abnormalities predispose patients to development of this disease. These anomalies include: 1) an enlongated epiglottis that curls upon itself ("omega"-shaped epiglottis), 2) foreshortened aryepiglottic folds, and 3) bulky arytenoids that tend to prolapse into the airway with inspiration. Laryngomalacia may also be caused by poor neuromuscular control, resulting in inadequate muscular support of the cartilaginous framework of the epiglottis with increased compliance of the supraglottic tissues. This lack of neuromuscular control may be caused by delayed development of neuromuscular pathways.

Patients present with inspiratory stridor, which is not present at birth but begins during the first few days to weeks of life. The stridor is of variable intensity and is aggravated with crying, feeding, and other periods of excitement or activity. Stridor is worse when patients are lying on their back or with their head flexed. Patients are not cyanotic and have a normal cry. Laryngomalacia is only rarely associated with dyspnea or difficulty swallowing.

Definitive diagnosis is made by direct endoscopic examination. Characteristic findings include a narrowed and elongated epiglottis, which may curve upon itself, with long, floppy, and redundant aryepiglottic folds; prominent arytenoids; and a deep interarytenoid cleft. During inspiration, the supraglottic structures collapse into the lumen of the airway, resulting in a slit-like opening.

Laryngomalacia is often a self-limited condition that resolves spontaneously (usually by 18 months of age). Symptoms are improved by placing the child in a prone position with the head hyperextended. Surgical intervention is necessary only in patients who fail spontaneously to improve or have persistent symptoms of sleep apnea, cor pulmonale, feeding difficulties, or failure to thrive.

IMAGING FEATURES

Frontal and lateral radiographs and fluoroscopy are the imaging modalities of choice for patients suspected of having laryngomalacia. Computed tomography may be helpful for detecting the presence of associated laryngeal anomalies, including subglottic or tracheal stenosis. Characteristic radiographic findings include anterior bowing and inferior displacement of the aryepiglottic folds during inspiration (Fig. 15A.05-1). The epiglottis and hyoid bone may also be positioned lower than normal because of an imbalance between the suprahyoid and infrahyoid strap muscles. The hypopharynx and valecullae are dilated because of intermittent airway obstruction. At fluoroscopy, the epiglottis and aryepiglottic folds prolapse into the airway during inspiration and also vibrate. The valleculae and hypopharynx are distended.

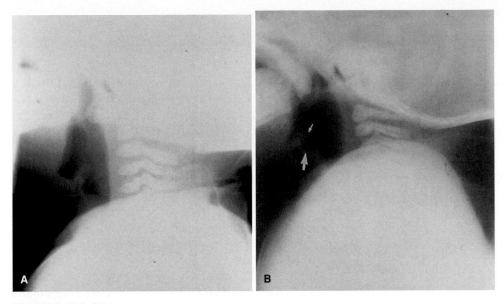

FIGURE 15A.05-1.

Laryngomalacia. **A.** Expiratory lateral view of upper airway shows normal configuration. **B.** During inspiration, the epiglottis *(smaller arrow)* folds back posteriorly upon itself and the aryepiglottic folds *(larger arrow)* prolapse anteriorly. The hypopharynx is distended. (Case courtesy of B. Specter, University of North Carolina, Chapel Hill, NC.)

SUGGESTED READINGS

1. Benjamin B. Congenital disorders of the larynx. In: Cummings CW, Frerickson JM, Harker LA, Krause CJ, Schuller DE, eds. Otolaryngology and Head and Neck Surgery, Vol. 3. St. Louis: CV Mosby, 1993:1840.
2. Myer CM, Cotton RT. Congenital abnormalities of the larynx and trachea and management of congenital malformations. In: Paparella MM, Shumrick DA, Gluckman JL, Meyeroff WL, eds. Otolaryngology, Vol. 3, 3rd ed. Philadelphia: WB Saunders, 1991:2217.
3. Cotton RT, Reilly JS. Congenital malformations of the larynx. In: Bluestone CD, Stool SE, Scheetz MD, eds. Pediatric Otolaryngology, Vol. 2. Philadelphia: WB Saunders, 1990:1122.

15A.06 *Tracheomalacia*

Tracheomalacia is an abnormality of the tracheal wall resulting in weakness and softening of supporting cartilage and abnormal widening of the posterior wall. It occurs independently of laryngomalacia, but may be associated with it. Tracheomalacia usually presents in infants. There is no gender predilection.

CLINICAL FEATURES
Tracheomalacia is divided into primary and secondary forms. Primary tracheomalacia presents in premature or term infants who are otherwise healthy or who have dyschondroplasia or bronchomalacia. Secondary tracheomalacia is associated with anatomic anomalies resulting from extrinsic compression of the trachea. Tracheal weakening is often limited to the area of compression. External compression is caused by the innominate artery, pulmonary sling, double aortic arch and other vascular rings, bronchogenic cyst, duplication cyst, teratoma, abscess, cystic hygroma, hemangioma, and other benign or malignant neoplasms. The secondary form also occurs in patients with tracheoesophageal fistulas. Tracheomalacia is the most common cause of respiratory problems after surgical repair of tracheoesophageal fistulas. Structural changes in tracheomalacia are partly the result of a deficiency in the tracheal cartilages. The cartilaginous tracheal rings are abnormally shaped and of a consistency predisposing to collapse and accumulation of secretions. Collapsibility of the trachea increases during expiration.

Patients present with inspiratory and expiratory stridor, barking cough, wheezing, recurrent respiratory infections, and difficulty clearing endobronchial secretions. Patients frequently attempt to hyperextend their neck to compensate for the underlying abnormality. Occasional attacks of apnea also occur. Respiratory or cardiac arrests ("dying spell") are very rare.

Diagnosis is based on endoscopic findings, which include widening of the posterior membranous wall. The trachea lacks its usual firmness and its anterior and posterior walls appose each other during respiration and coughing, resulting in a reduction of the tracheal lumen.

Tracheomalacia is usually self-limited. Most children with primary tracheomalacia spontaneously improve by 2 years of age. Patients with episodes of acute respiratory arrest may require surgical intervention. The treatment of secondary tracheomalacia involves alleviating the cause of extrinsic compression. Outcome depends on the extent and severity of damage to the trachea.

IMAGING FEATURES
The initial imaging studies performed in these patients should be radiographs and fluoroscopy of the airway. Radiographs show narrowing of the tracheal air column. The lumen of the trachea decreases by more than 50% during inspiration in patients with tracheomalacia (Fig. 15A.06-1). Dynamic magnetic resonance (MR) imaging using a cine loop mode performed during the respiratory cycle in sagittal and axial planes may prove beneficial for evaluating these patients. Real-time axial imaging may be especially helpful for evaluating the degree of tracheal collapse during expiration, and may be accomplished with MR imaging or spiral computed tomography (CT).

Computed tomography is also useful and shows an abnormally formed, oval-shaped trachea with reduced sagittal diameter (Fig. 15A.06-2). Focal areas of dystrophic calcification may be present within tracheal cartilages, and their presence helps confirm the diagnosis of tracheomalacia. The length of the affected region is assessed by noting the extent of the misshaped and deformed trachea.

Imaging also plays an important role in patients suspected of having secondary tracheomalacia. Contrast-enhanced CT is optimal for evaluating the possibility of compressive lesions. MR imaging may be helpful in certain instances because of its multiplanar and angiographic capabilities. Catheter angiography may eventually be necessary in cases secondary to anomalies of the great vessels.

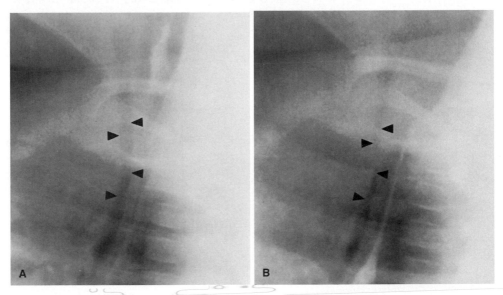

FIGURE 15A.06-1.

Tracheomalacia, fluoroscopy. **A.** Oblique spot film during expiration shows normal tracheal air column *(arrowheads).* **B.** Corresponding inspiratory view shows marked collapse of tracheal air column *(arrowheads).* (Case courtesy of B. Specter, University of North Carolina, Chapel Hill, NC.)

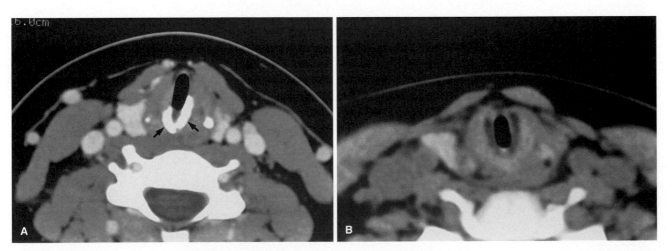

FIGURE 15A.06-2.

Tracheomalacia, computed tomography (CT). **A.** Axial postcontrast CT shows marked reduction of the lateral tracheal diameter. The cricoid cartilage *(arrows)* has dystrophic calcification and has assumed a "V" shape because of collapse. **B.** Axial CT in a different patient with tracheomalacia shows reduced lateral tracheal diameter and slight flattening of posterior tracheal wall. In this case, there are no dystrophic calcifications. (Case courtesy of D. Merten, University of North Carolina, Chapel Hill, NC.)

SUGGESTED READINGS

1. Benjamin B. Congenital disorders of the trachea. In: Cummings CW, Frerickson JM, Harker LA, Krause CJ, Schuller DE, eds. Otolaryngology and Head and Neck Surgery, Vol. 3. St. Louis: CV Mosby, 1993:2290.
2. Myer CM, Cotton RT. Congenital abnormalities of the larynx and trachea and management of congenital malformations. In: Paparella MM, Shumrick DA, Gluckman JL, Meyeroff WL, eds. Otolaryngology, Vol. 3, 3rd ed. Philadelphia: WB Saunders, 1991:2224.
3. Cotton RT, Reilly JS. Congenital malformations of the larynx. In: Bluestone CD, Stool SE, Scheetz MD, eds. Pediatric Otolaryngology, Vol. 2. Philadelphia: WB Saunders, 1990:1130.

15A.07 *Vocal Cord Paralysis*

EPIDEMIOLOGY

Vocal cord paralysis is the second most common developmental laryngeal anomaly, accounting for 10% of all congenital laryngeal abnormalities. Some cases are associated with an underlying lesion. Hereditary causes of bilateral vocal cord paralysis are extremely rare.

CLINICAL FEATURES

The etiology of vocal cord paralysis differs depending on whether the abnormalities are unilateral or bilateral. Unilateral paralysis is often caused by a peripheral lesion and requires evaluation of the entire course of the ipsilateral recurrent laryngeal nerve. Common causes of congenital unilateral vocal cord paralysis are ventricular septal defect, tetralogy of Fallot, and patent ductus arteriosus. Unilateral paralysis may follow surgical repair of tracheoesophageal fistulas or congenital heart defects. Bilateral vocal cord paralysis is secondary to meningomyelocele, hydrocephalus, Chiari malformations, bulbar palsy, traumatic birth delivery, intracranial hemorrhage, encephalocele, or dysgenesis of the nucleus ambiguus.

Vocal cord paralysis may be unilateral or bilateral, but unilateral left-sided paralysis is more common. Most cases are diagnosed soon after birth, although unilateral paralysis may go undiagnosed in some infants. Patients with unilateral vocal cord paralysis present in the newborn period with a weak cry, intermittent cyanosis, aspiration of pharyngeal secretions, and choking during feedings. Stridor and other symptoms of respiratory distress are rare. Bilateral vocal cord paralysis presents with acute respiratory distress and a high-pitched inspiratory stridor that is aggravated by agitation. These patients have a normal cry and significant dysphagia produced by pharyngeal incoordination secondary to multiple cranial nerve abnormalities. They also are prone to development of recurrent aspiration pneumonias.

The diagnosis of vocal cord paralysis is reliably made by flexible fiberoptic endoscopy. Most patients with unilateral abnormalities require no airway support. Patients who aspirate may benefit from a medialization procedure, either direct injection of polytetrafluorethylene (Teflon) or an external medialization procedure. Occasionally, patients with unilateral vocal cord paralysis will improve spontaneously. Patients with bilateral abnormalities may require intubation and eventual tracheostomy. Tracheostomy may be necessary in patients with progressive stridor and airway obstruction, and in patients with recurrent aspiration.

IMAGING FEATURES

We prefer computed tomography (CT) for imaging patients with vocal cord paralysis. Contrast administration is necessary to opacify the vascular structures and allow detailed study of the course of the recurrent laryngeal nerves. Magnetic resonance imaging is superior to CT for evaluation of patients in whom the abnormality is thought to reside in the brain stem. Fluoroscopy may be helpful for evaluation of vocal cord motion. The role of imaging is that of detecting underlying lesions, which may occur anywhere from the brain stem (nucleus ambiguus) to the mediastinum. The nucleus ambiguus lies in the upper medulla, anterior to the floor of the fourth ventricle, and posterior to the inferior olivary complex. High signal intensity on T2-weighted images at this level suggest lesions involving it. The course of the vagus and the recurrent laryngeal nerves needs to be imaged in all cases of unexplained vocal cord paralysis. The vagus nerves descend in the carotid sheaths into the mediastinum. The right recurrent laryngeal nerve hooks around the right subclavian artery, whereas the left one hooks around the ligamentum arteriosum.

CT is helpful for evaluating patients who have undergone Teflon injection into a true vocal cord in an attempt to medialize it (Fig. 15A.07-1). Imaging in these patients allows for evaluation of both the position of the true vocal cord as well as its Teflon implant. Migration of the implant is easily detected with CT.

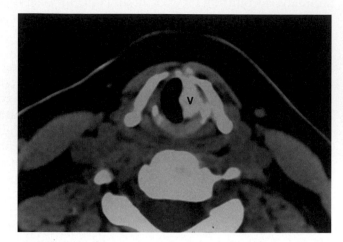

FIGURE 15A.07-1.

Vocal cord palsy after Teflon medialization. Axial computed tomography shows high density and medial position of left true vocal cord (V) after injection of Teflon for treatment of congenital idiopathic vocal paralysis.

SUGGESTED READINGS

1. Benjamin B. Congenital disorders of the larynx. In: Cummings CW, Frerickson JM, Harker LA, Krause CJ, Schuller DE, eds. Otolaryngology and Head and Neck Surgery, Vol. 3. St. Louis: CV Mosby, 1993:1845.
2. Myer CM, Cotton RT. Congenital abnormalities of the larynx and trachea and management of congenital malformations. In: Paparella MM, Shumrick DA, Gluckman JL, Meyeroff WL, eds. Otolaryngology, Vol. 3, 3rd ed. Philadelphia: WB Saunders, 1991:2219.

15A.08 *Laryngeal Cysts*

EPIDEMIOLOGY   Laryngeal cysts denote a variety of air- or fluid-filled cysts, including laryngo-celes and saccular cysts. Laryngoceles and laryngeal cysts may be seen in all ages. Laryngeal cysts are a well known cause of stridor in infants and children. There is no gender predilection.

CLINICAL FEATURES   Both laryngoceles and saccular cysts represent abnormal dilation of the laryngeal saccule. A laryngocele is distinguished from a saccular cyst in that the former has a persistent communication with the ventricle, whereas the latter is isolated from the ventricle. The laryngeal ventricle is the air-containing space between the true and false vocal cords. Laryngeal saccules arise from the anterior roof of the ventricle and normally maintain a small communication with the ventricle. Saccules rise vertically between the false vocal cords, the base of the epiglottis, and the thyroid cartilage. In infants, saccules may extend as high as the level of the thyrohyoid membrane. The surface of the saccules contains 60 to 70 mucous glands and their openings. Located along the medial and lateral aspects of the saccules are delicate muscles that act to compress the sacules and express their secretions onto the vocal cords. A crescentric mucous fold located at the orifice of the saccules helps direct secretions along the posterior aspect of the vocal cords.

Laryngoceles are abnormal dilations or diverticula that communicate with the laryngeal ventricle. These lesions may be filled with air or mucus, and are classified as internal, external, or mixed. Laryngoceles are considered internal when they are confined to the interior of the larynx and limited to the endolaryngeal structures of the larynx. External laryngoceles extend through the thyrohyoid membrane into the soft tissue of the neck. This extension usually occurs through the membrane via its natural openings for the superior laryngeal arteries. Laryngoceles with both internal and external components are considered mixed. Laryngoceles may be unilateral or bilateral, and may become infected during upper respiratory tract infections. Laryngoceles may be congenital or acquired. In children, they are congenital; in adults, there is an increased association of laryngoceles with glottic tumors.

Saccular cysts (congenital cysts) are fluid-filled dilations of the saccules that do not communicate with the laryngeal lumen. These cysts may be congenital or acquired. Congenital forms result from simple atresia of the saccular orifice. Acquired saccular cysts arise from complete occlusion and isolation of cysts secondary to inflammation, tumor, and trauma. There are two forms of saccular cysts. Lateral saccular cysts extend posterior and superior into the false vocal cords and aryepiglottic folds. Anterior saccular cysts extend medial and posterior between the true and false vocal cords into the laryngeal lumen.

Laryngopyoceles are infected (pus-containing) laryngoceles and saccular cysts. Ductal cysts (mucus retention cysts) result from retention of mucus within the glands in the submucosa of the larynx. These cysts may occur anywhere in the larynx and may also involve the vallecula. These cysts are smaller than laryngoceles and saccular cysts, usually measuring less than 1 cm in diameter. However, they may become large enough to obstruct the airway.

Symptoms depend on the size and extent of the lesion. Children present with inspiratory stridor, intercostal retractions, and episodes of cyanosis. Patients may have an intermittent hoarseness, aphonia, or muffled cry. Associated anomalies include laryngomalacia and vocal cord paralysis. At endoscopy, saccular cysts and laryngoceles appear as rounded, submucosal, soft tissue masses involving pyriform sinuses, aryepiglottic folds, pyriform sinuses, glottis, and hypopharynx. The lesions are mucosal and have a characteristic bluish hue. Large lesions may obstruct the laryngeal lumen. The diagnosis of laryngocele is confirmed when a lesion inflates and deflates at endoscopy. Treatment of saccular cysts in children is by needle aspiration. Unroofing may be necessary in recurrent cysts. Treatment of laryngoceles consists of surgical removal. Biopsies of the orifice of laryngoceles and saccular cysts should be taken to exclude the presence of an underlying neoplasm.

IMAGING FEATURES   Both computed tomography (CT) and magnetic resonance (MR) imaging may be used to evaluate patients with laryngeal cysts. CT is preferred in children. Spiral CT may be especially helpful in studies that are initially limited by motion artifact.

It may be difficult to separate a laryngocele from a saccular cyst by imaging alone. On plain films, laryngeal cysts present as soft tissue masses within the glottic and supraglottic region. The presence of air within the lesion indicates that the mass communicates with the airway, and suggests a laryngocele. On CT and MR imaging, these lesions show as smoothly marginated soft tissue masses (Fig. 15A.08-1). The internal characteristics of a laryngeal cyst are those of a fluid-filled mass (Fig. 15A.08-2). The internal attenuation and signal characteristics vary according to the protein content of the secretions or the presence of gas (Fig. 15A.08-3). Highly proteinaceous fluid is of increased attenuation on CT and increased signal intensity on T1-weighted MR images. Laryngoceles typically extend along the paraglottic fat planes and may extend superiorly into the preepiglottic fat. Extension of the mass through the thyrohyoid membrane suggests an external component. Noninfected laryngeal cysts do not enhance with contrast. Focal-enhancing areas, especially those located at the base of the lesions, suggest underlying neoplasm.

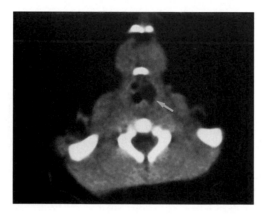

FIGURE 15A.08-1.

Saccular laryngeal cyst.   Axial computed tomography shows cyst *(arrow)* in left supraglottic larynx, probably arising at level of vallecula. (Case courtesy of W. Nemzek, M.D., University of California, Davis, CA.)

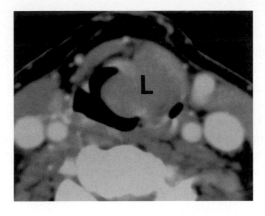

FIGURE 15A.08-2.

Mixed laryngocele. Axial computed tomography shows a fluid-filled laryngocele (L) simulating a soft tissue mass. There are intralaryngeal and extralaryngeal components.

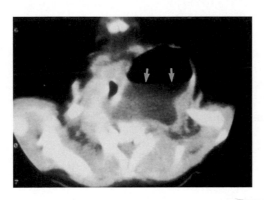

FIGURE 15A.08-3.

External laryngocele. Axial computed tomography shows a very large left-sided external laryngocele in a newborn. The sac contains a fluid level *(arrows)* and displaces the trachea.

SUGGESTED READINGS

1. Hollinger LD, Rarnes DR, Smid LJ, Holinger PH. Laryngocele and saccular cysts. Arch Otolaryngol 1978;87:675.
2. Doengan JO, Strife JL, Seid AB, Cotton RT, Dunbar JS. Internal laryngocele and saccular cysts in children. Ann Otol Rhinol Laryngol 1980;89:408.
3. Curtin HC. The larynx. In: Som PM, Bergeron RT, eds. Head and Neck Imaging, 2nd ed. St. Louis: CV Mosby, 1991:667.
4. Lewis C, Castillo M, Patrick E, Sybers R. Symptomatic external laryngocele in a newborn: plain radiograph and CT findings. AJNR 1990;11:10020.

15A.09 *Subglottic Hemangioma*

EPIDEMIOLOGY

Airway hemangiomas occurring in young children may be located anywhere in the larynx, but have a predilection for the subglottic region. They present during the first year of life (85% of hemangiomas present before 6 months of age). Subglottic hemangiomas are more common in girls and have a left-sided predominance. However, they may arise on the right side of the larynx or be bilateral. Cutaneous hemangiomas coexist with subglottic hemangiomas in 50% of patients.

CLINICAL FEATURES

Patients present with airway obstruction and inspiratory or biphasic stridor. Continued tumor growth may cause significant airway obstruction. Symptoms include stridor, dyspnea, cyanotic episodes, hoarseness, cough, and difficulty feeding. Symptoms are exacerbated by excitement, crying, or respiratory tract infections. Occasionally, acute respiratory distress occurs.

The diagnosis of subglottic hemangioma is made at endoscopy. Typical appearance is that of a red or blue submucosal mass in the subglottis. The mass is compressible and may extend into the posterior commissure or upper trachea.

Histologically, the lesions are of the capillary type. Subglottic hemangiomas may contain both capillary and cavernous elements, although the capillary variety is predominant. Most subglottic hemangiomas involute spontaneously, although some lesions persist and may enlarge. Tracheostomy may be necessary in patients with respiratory obstruction. Treatment includes carbon dioxide laser excision and steroids. Irradiation is not appropriate given the risk for malignant transformation.

IMAGING FEATURES

Diagnosis of subglottic hemangioma is based on direct visualization of the lesion. The lesions usually are promptly treated, and no imaging studies are obtained in most patients. Radiographs of the neck may show a soft tissue mass extending into and narrowing the tracheal air column, especially below the level of the vocal cords (Fig. 15A.09-1). This narrowing tends to be asymmetric. Occasionally, subglottic hemangioma may present as concentric narrowing rather than an endophytic mass. Computed tomography and magnetic resonance (MR) imaging may be beneficial to define the extent of the mass. On cross-sectional imaging, these lesions present as enhancing polypoid soft tissue masses that extend into the airway. Phleboliths may occasionally be present in larger lesions. They have similar signal intensity to muscle on precontrast T1-weighted MR images, and enhance after contrast administration. On T2-weighted images, they are of high signal intensity and contain areas of signal void that are related to large vessels or calcifications.

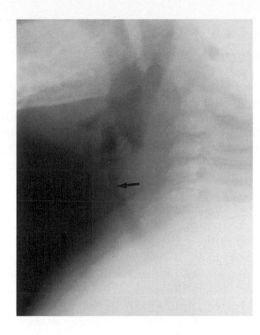

FIGURE 15A.09-1.

Subglottic hemangioma. Lateral radiograph shows soft tissue density mass *(arrow)* arising from posterior subglottic tracheal wall and compressing air column. (Case courtesy of D. Merten, University of North Carolina, Chapel Hill, NC.)

SUGGESTED READINGS

1. Pransky SM, Seid AB. Tumors of the larynx, trachea and bronchi. In: Bluestone CD, Stool SE, Scheetz MD, eds. Pediatric Otolaryngology, Vol. 2. Philadelphia: WB Saunders, 1990:1218.
2. Curtin HC. The larynx. In: Som PM, Bergeron RT, eds. Head and Neck Imaging, 2nd ed. St. Louis: CV Mosby, 1991:654.
3. Vasquez E, Enriquez G, Castellote A, et al. US, CT, and MR imaging of neck lesions in children. RadioGraphics 1995;15:105.

15A.10 *Juvenile Laryngeal Papillomatosis*

EPIDEMIOLOGY

Squamous papillomas are the most common laryngeal tumors in children. Multiple papillomas are referred to as juvenile laryngeal papillomatosis, and although they may be seen in both children and adults, they are more common in children. This lesion is usually detected before 3 years of age and may become symptomatic during the first year of life. The age of presentation is related to the amount and location of tumor(s), hormonal influence, and incubation time. There is no gender predilection.

CLINICAL FEATURES

Laryngeal papillomas are caused by the human papilloma virus, which is a DNA virus that induces epithelial proliferation. Viruses types 6 and 11 have been identified as the subtypes responsible for juvenile laryngeal papillomatosis. Virus type 6C is the most common subtype, and is associated with extensive and severe disease. Juvenile laryngeal papillomatosis is associated with condylomata acuminatum (maternal genital warts). This association is strengthened by the fact that viruses types 6 and 11 are also responsible for 90% of genital warts. The DNA sequences of viruses isolated from laryngeal papillomas and condylomata acuminatum are indistinguishable. In addition, laryngeal papillomatosis is rare in patients delivered by cesarean section.

Patients present with airway obstruction. Symptoms include hoarseness, stridor, recurrent croup, or a change in voice quality. Although histologically benign, laryngeal papillomas may be life threatening because of obstruction of the airway. Acute respiratory distress is unusual because laryngeal papillomas result in gradual airway narrowing.

Laryngeal papillomas tend to involve the true vocal cords. Supraglottic or subglottic extension is common. Tracheal involvement may be as high as in 26% of cases, and results from "seeding" of viral particles (especially during airway manipulation). Therefore, tracheostomies may increase the likelihood of distal spread. Distal spread may also result in multiple lung nodules, which may cavitate. Esophageal papillomas may also be found.

On physical examination, laryngeal papillomas are pink or red, irregular, pedunculated, exophytic, nodular masses that vary in size. Histologically, they consist of a vascular core of connective tissue covered by stratified squamous epithelium with abnormal keratinization.

Laryngeal papillomatosis has an unpredictable course and may spontaneously regress, respond partially to treatment, or progress. Malignant transformation in chronic disease is exceptional. Treatment includes medical therapy (antibiotics, hormones, interferon, steroids, antiviral agents, and various antimetabolites), irradiation, and surgery (including carbon dioxide laser resection).

IMAGING FEATURES

Diagnosis is based on endoscopic findings and biopsy. Both computed tomography (CT) and magnetic resonance imaging may be used for evaluating the extent of disease in the glottic region. Spiral CT is helpful because of reduced imaging time. CT is also the modality of choice for evaluating pulmonary disease.

Laryngeal papillomatosis is characterized by nodular soft tissue masses involving the trachea (Fig. 15A.10-1). There may be distention of the oropharynx above the soft tissue masses. On CT, the lesions appear as multiple, endophytic, nodular soft tissue masses that narrow the airway. Lesions may enhance after contrast administration. Pulmonary findings consist of multiple, bilateral, parenchymal nodules that may be solid or cavitary (Fig. 15A.10-1C). These lesions may result in consolidation or atelectasis. Cavities are thin-walled, may contain fluid levels, and are prone to recurrent infections. Enlarging solid lesions are suggestive of malignant transformation.

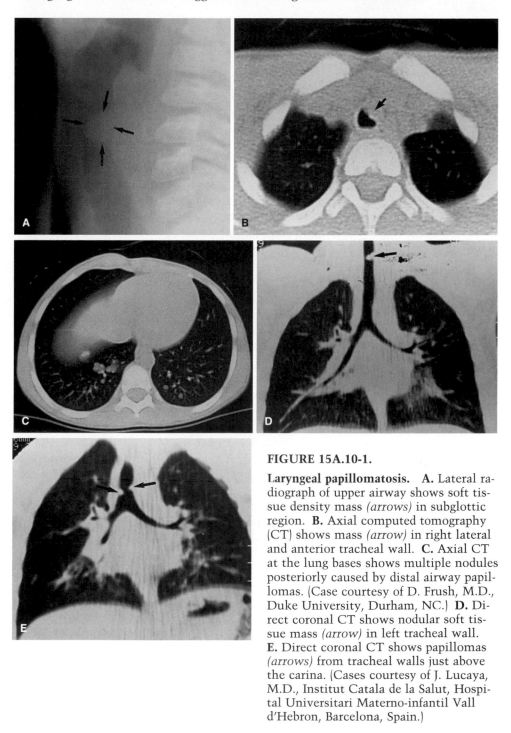

FIGURE 15A.10-1.

Laryngeal papillomatosis. **A.** Lateral radiograph of upper airway shows soft tissue density mass *(arrows)* in subglottic region. **B.** Axial computed tomography (CT) shows mass *(arrow)* in right lateral and anterior tracheal wall. **C.** Axial CT at the lung bases shows multiple nodules posteriorly caused by distal airway papillomas. (Case courtesy of D. Frush, M.D., Duke University, Durham, NC.) **D.** Direct coronal CT shows nodular soft tissue mass *(arrow)* in left tracheal wall. **E.** Direct coronal CT shows papillomas *(arrows)* from tracheal walls just above the carina. (Cases courtesy of J. Lucaya, M.D., Institut Catala de la Salut, Hospital Universitari Materno-infantil Vall d'Hebron, Barcelona, Spain.)

SUGGESTED READINGS

1. Pransky SM, Seid AB. Tumors of the larynx, trachea and bronchi. In: Bluestone CD, Stool SE, Scheetz MD, eds. Pediatric Otolaryngology, Vol. 2. Philadelphia: WB Saunders, 1990:1215.
2. Kramer SS, Wehnut WD, Stocker JT, Kashima H. Pulmonary manifestations of juvenile laryngotracheal papillomatosis. AJR 1985;144:687.

15A.11 *Tumors*

EPIDEMIOLOGY

Tumors of the larynx and trachea are unusual malignancies in children. The most common lesions in children are laryngeal papillomatosis and hemangiomas. This discussion focuses on less common benign and malignant lesions.

CLINICAL FEATURES

Neurogenic tumors may occur in the larynx (Fig. 15A.11-1). They are most common in patients with neurofibromatosis type I. These lesions are often multiple and are associated with other cutaneous and systemic manifestations of the disease. The lesions often involve the arytenoid cartilage regions or aryepiglottic folds. Tumors of neural crest cell origin may also involve the larynx or trachea. Granular cell tumors are slow-growing masses most commonly seen in young girls (Fig. 15A.11-2). These lesions are usually located in the glottic and subglottic regions. They grow slowly and are treated with local excision. Multiple recurrences may require partial or total laryngectomy. Paragangliomas of the larynx are most often seen in patients with Von Hippel-Lindau syndrome or neurofibromatosis type I. These lesions characteristically arise from the paired inferior paraganglia located between the inferior horns of the thyroid cartilage and the cricoid cartilage. A characteristic clinical finding is pain referred to the ipsilateral ear that is aggravated by swallowing. This symptom resolves after removal of the lesion. These lesions are highly vascular and may result in significant hemorrhage if biopsies are taken.

Tumors may also arise from major and minor salivary glands. Malignant tumors include mucoepidermoid carcinoma, adenoid cystic carcinoma, adenocarcinoma, and acinic cell carcinoma (Fig. 15A.11-3). Benign lesions of salivary gland origin include pleomorpic adenomas (Fig. 15A.11-4). These lesions are more common in adults. Most laryngeal malignancies are squamous cell carcinomas (Fig. 15A.11-5). In children, these lesions are slightly more common in boys than girls (3:2). Benign mesenchymal tumors include fibromas, fibromatoses, and angiomas. Their malignant counterparts are spindle cell carcinomas, fibrosarcomas, and rhabdomyosarcomas (Fig. 15A.11-6).

Symptoms depend on location and size of the lesions. Symptoms caused by lesions in the glottic and subglottic regions include hoarseness, dysphagia, and dyspnea (Fig. 15A.11-7). Supraglottic lesions present with dysphagia, muffled voice, dyspnea, and a sensation of tightness or fullness in the throat. Tracheal tumors present with dyspnea, stridor, and wheezing. Large masses may cause acute respiratory obstruction. Symptoms suggestive of malignancy include referred pain, progressive loss of cranial or peripheral nerve function, and enlarging neck masses suggesting nodal involvement. Diagnosis is made by endoscopy in most cases. Treatment depends on histology and extent of tumor at time of presentation.

IMAGING FEATURES

Its multiplanar capabilities and excellent soft tissue contrast make magnetic resonance (MR) imaging the preferred technique for evaluating patients with airway masses. Computed tomography (CT) is also very helpful, especially in patients with airway compromise who cannot tolerate MR imaging (Fig. 15A.11-7). Imaging findings usually are nonspecific. CT typically shows soft tissue endolaryngeal masses extending into the airway. Large, aggressive soft tissue masses extending into the extralaryngeal soft tissues are highly suggestive of malignancy. The vertical extent of glottic lesions is best demonstrated with MR imaging obtained in coronal and sagittal planes. Both benign and malignant tumors enhance with contrast. The presence of reduced T2 signal intensity suggests fibrous components or increased cellularity. Both CT and MR imaging may be used to detect cartilage and tracheal wall invasion. MR imaging may be superior to CT in this aspect because in children the cartilages and rings are calcified.

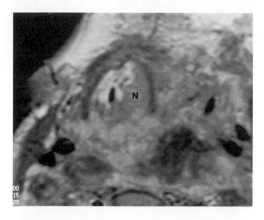

FIGURE 15A.11-1.

Neurofibroma. Axial postcontrast magnetic resonance T1-weighted image in a patient with neurofibromatosis type I shows neurofibroma (N) involving left true vocal cord. Note extensive plexiform neurofibromata in neck.

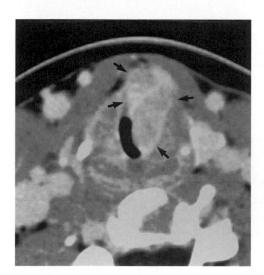

FIGURE 15A.11-2.

Granular cell tumor. Axial postcontrast computed tomography shows enhancing tumor *(arrows)* that had been resected twice previously. Note that this tumor, which is submucosal in origin, has now extended into the endolaryngeal space and out into the extralaryngeal soft tissues.

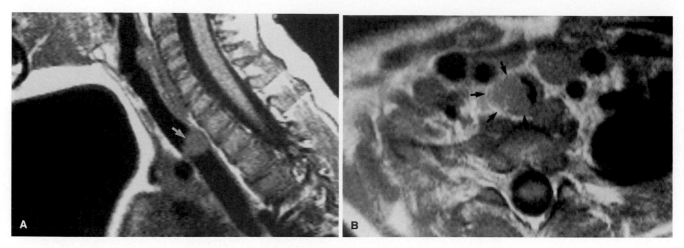

FIGURE 15A.11-3.

Mucoepidermoid carcinoma. **A.** Sagittal noncontrast magnetic resonance (MR) T1-weighted image shows endolaryngeal mass *(arrow)*. **B.** Axial noncontrast MR T1-weighted image shows mass *(arrows)* arising from tracheal mucosa and almost completely occluding airway.

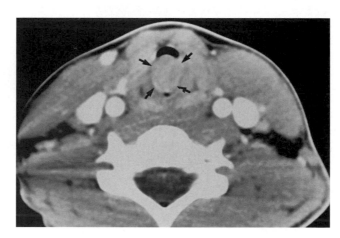

FIGURE 15A.11-4.

Pleormophic adenoma. Axial postcontrast computed tomography shows well marginated endolaryngeal mass *(arrows)* almost completely occluding tracheal lumen.

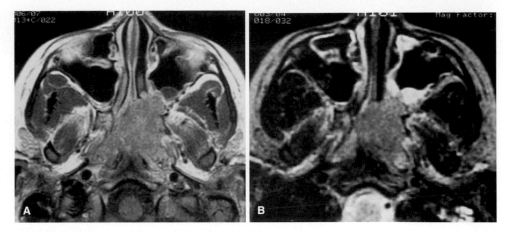

FIGURE 15A.11-5

Lymphoepithelioma. **A.** Axial postcontrast magnetic resonance T1-weighted image shows moderately enhancing mass in posterior nasopharynx. **B.** Corresponding T2-weighted image shows the mass to be somewhat hypointense, which is the typical appearance of highly cellular malignant tumors in this region.

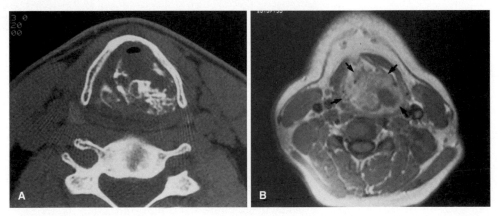

FIGURE 15A.11-6.

Sarcoma. **A.** Axial computed tomography (bone window settings) shows mass arising from cricoid cartilage. Note that this chondrosarcoma contains multiple calcifications and almost completely effaces the airway. **B.** In a different patient, postcontrast magnetic resonance T1-weighted image shows a synovial cell sarcoma *(arrows)* to enhance and contain some central low intensity, suggesting necrosis.

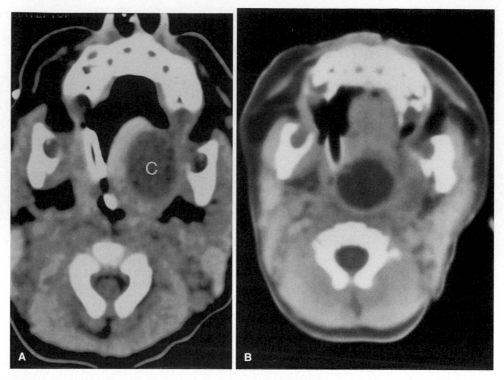

FIGURE 15A.11-7.

Benign epithelial cysts of the oropharynx. **A.** Axial computed tomography (CT) in child with respiratory distress shows cystic mass (C) arising from left lateral oropharyngeal wall. **B.** Axial noncontrast CT in a different patient shows well defined cyst in posterior oropharynx arising from the posterior wall.

SUGGESTED READINGS

1. Pransky SM, Seid AB. Tumors of the larynx, trachea and bronchi. In: Bluestone CD, Stool SE, Scheetz MD, eds. Pediatric Otolaryngology, Vol. 2. Philadelphia: WB Saunders, 1990:1220.
2. Thawley S. Cysts and tumors of the larynx. In: Paparella MM, Shumrick DA, Gluckman JL, Meyeroff WL, eds. Otolaryngology, Vol. 3, 3rd ed. Philadelphia: WB Saunders, 1991:2310.
3. Mukherji SK, Castillo M, Rao V, Weissler M. Granular cell tumors of the subglottic region of the larynx: CT and MR findings. AJR 1995;164:1492.

15A.12 *Epiglottitis*

EPIDEMIOLOGY

Epiglottitis is a systemic disease with supraglottic involvement as a major abnormality. It usually occurs between 2 to 4 years of age, although its incidence is increasing in younger patients. There is no gender predilection.

CLINICAL FEATURES

Epiglottitis is the regional manifestation of septicemia due to *Hemophilus influenzae* type B infection. Newborns are protected because of immunity to capsular antigens acquired from the mother. This passive immunity disappears by 3 months of age and the child's immune system does not produce similar antibodies until 3 to 4 years of age. This window of diminished antibody levels explains the high incidence of *H influenzae* infections in this age group.

Patients with epiglottitis characteristically present with high fever and respiratory obstruction. These children are often sitting upright, drooling, and have inspiratory stridor. The onset of symptoms is often acute, often over a 2- to 6-hour period. On examination, the epiglottis is swollen and cherry-red in appearance. The aryepiglottic folds are swollen and the supraglottic airway is narrowed. Secretions are thick and tenacious. Patients are prone to acute laryngospasm and obstruction during forced inspiration, and every attempt should be made not to excite the child during initial evaluation. Affected children require nasotracheal or orotracheal intubation under anesthesia. Tracheostomy is not recommended. Cephalosporins are the drugs of choice at many institutions.

IMAGING FEATURES

Lateral radiographs of the neck should be performed in patients suspected of having epiglottitis. There is no role for computed tomography and magnetic resonance imaging in these patients, and these studies may be life threatening because placing the patient in a supine position further reduces the caliber of the airway.

Findings on radiographs include a diffusely thickened epiglottis, which is often two to three times the size of a normal one (Figs. 15A.12-1 and 15A.12-2). The aryepiglottic folds and false vocal cords are also thickened. There may be dilation of the oropharynx if the supraglottic larynx is narrowed. Epiglottis abscesses are extremely rare (Fig. 15A.12-3).

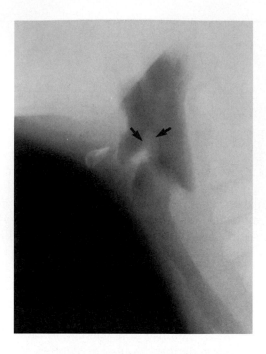

FIGURE 15A.12-1.

Normal epiglottis. Lateral radiograph shows normal epiglottis *(arrows)*.

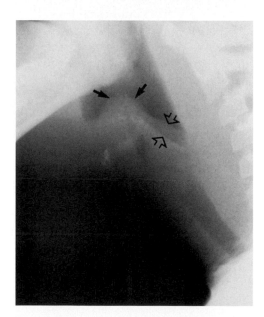

FIGURE 15A.12-2.

Epiglottitis. Lateral radiograph shows thickened ("thumb-like") epiglottis *(solid arrows)* and edema of aryepiglottic folds *(open arrows)*. (Case courtesy of D. Merten, University of North Carolina, Chapel Hill, NC.)

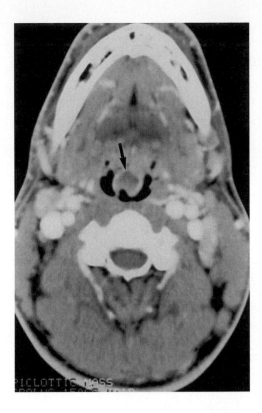

FIGURE 15A.12-3.

Epiglottis abscess. Axial postcontrast computed tomography shows low-density mass *(arrow)* in epiglottis that proved to be an abscess. The differential diagnosis is a benign epithelial cyst, neurofibroma, or teratoma.

SUGGESTED READING

1. Jones KR, Pillsbury HC. Infections and manifestations of systemic disease of the larynx. In: Cummings CW, Frerickson JM, Harker LA, Krause CJ, Schuller DE, eds. Otolaryngology and Head and Neck Surgery, Vol. 3. St. Louis: CV Mosby, 1993: 1854.

15A.13 *Croup (Laryngotracheitis)*

EPIDEMIOLOGY

Croup is a viral infection of the upper respiratory tract most often occurring in children between 1 to 3 years of age. Croup frequently occurs during winter and is more common in boys. It usually lasts between 3 to 7 days.

CLINICAL FEATURES

Croup is most often caused by infection with parainfluenza 1 or 2 and influenza A viruses. Patients present with a barking cough and stridor. The infection results in diffuse edema of the mucosa in the subglottic region and trachea. Two anatomic characteristics of the subglottic area make this area crucial for respiration in children. First, the subglottic region is the narrowest portion of the respiratory tract in children younger than 3 years of age. Second, the subglottis is the only portion of the upper respiratory tract that is surrounded completely by cartilaginous rings. Thus, the lumen of the subglottis is easily compromised by edema. Severe croup may progress to complete laryngeal obstruction. Stridor at rest occurs when greater than 80% of the subglottic lumen is narrowed.

Air humidification is the primary mode of treatment. Racemic epinephrine and steroids are beneficial. Tracheostomy is reserved for patients who are unresponsive to medical management. Indications for direct airway control include increasing blood carbon dioxide levels and decreasing neurologic status. Croup is labeled atypical if it lasts more than 7 days or occurs in infants younger than 1 year of age.

IMAGING FEATURES

The imaging method of choice for evaluating patients suspected of having croup are frontal and lateral radiographs of the neck. Imaging serves to confirm the diagnosis of croup and to exclude other causes of stridor, such as foreign bodies.

Characteristic radiographic findings include loss of normal subglottic angles, resulting in a "steeple-shaped" or "wine-bottle" configuration of the subglottic region on frontal films (Figs. 15A.13-1 and 15A.13-2). Lateral radiographs reveal indistinctness of soft tissues in the glottic region. An ill-defined haziness is present at the soft tissue–air interphases between the glottic and subglottic regions. Dilation of pyriform sinuses and ballooning of the pharynx may be present.

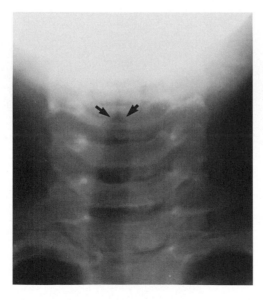

FIGURE 15A.13-1.

Normal airway. Frontal radiograph shows "shoulder-like" appearance *(arrows)* of normal subglottic region.

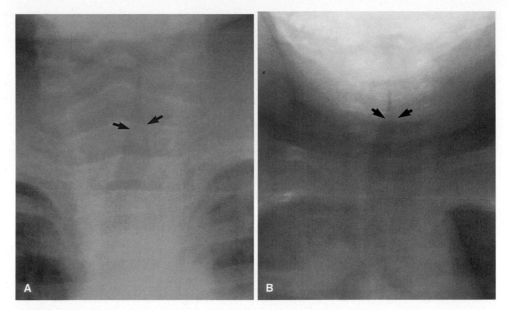

FIGURE 15A.13-2.

Croup. **A.** Frontal radiograph shows smooth tapering *(arrows)* of subglottic region secondary to mucosal edema. **B.** In a different patient with croup, frontal radiograph shows tapered *(arrows)* subglottic region, also known as "steeple" or "wine-bottle" sign. (Cases courtesy of D. Merten, University of North Carolina, Chapel Hill, NC.)

SUGGESTED READING

1. Jones KR, Pillsbury HC. Infections and manifestations of systemic disease of the larynx. In: Cummings CW, Frerickson JM, Harker LA, Krause CJ, Schuller DE, eds. Otolaryngology and Head and Neck Surgery, Vol. 3. St. Louis: CV Mosby, 1993: 1854.

15A.14 *Trauma*

Laryngotracheal trauma is uncommon in children but potentially life threatening. Trauma may involve the supraglottis, glottic, and infraglottic regions of the airway.

Most cases of laryngeal trauma involve the subglottic region and upper trachea. The glottic region (true vocal cords, arytenoid, and thyroid cartilages) is the second most common location. Injuries of supraglottic structures (false vocal cords, aryepiglottic folds, epiglottis, and hyoid bone) are rare in children. This is because in children the larynx is at a higher position than in adults, and the mandible protects it against crush injuries involving the anterior neck. With age, the larynx descends in the neck, and the incidence of supraglottic injuries increases.

Laryngotracheal trauma is divided into internal and external injuries. The causative factors and demographics are different for each type of injury. Internal trauma most commonly occurs in children younger than 12 years of age. Most of such injuries are caused by prolonged endotracheal intubation. Injuries result from denuding of the laryngeal mucosa, chronic irritation, and pressure necrosis. Traumatic intubation may also result in dislocation of arytenoid cartilages. Other causes of internal injury are ingestion of caustic substances (toxic chemicals, smoke inhalation) and aspiration of foreign bodies. Healing and reepithelialization of the injured laryngeal mucosa result in scarring and fibrosis. Severe scarring may narrow the airway and reduce vocal cord mobility. Damage caused by prolonged intubation may be localized to the posterior commissure or subglottic regions and result in diffuse fibrosis of the larynx and trachea. Stenosis caused by tracheotomy is located 1 to 2 cm distal to the tracheostomy stoma. Ingestion of toxic substances results in diffuse edema of the larynx, trachea, and esophagus, resulting in stricture formation. Affected patients present with stridor, hoarseness, cough, dyspnea, and difficulty clearing secretions. Stenosis caused by prolonged intubation may develop immediately after extubation or may be delayed by as much as 90 days. Treatment of the injuries occurring from internal trauma depends on the extent of the damaged segment. Localized granulomas may be resected using laser excision. Partial or circumferential subglottic and tracheal stenoses may require more aggressive treatment. Patients who are unresponsive to repeated dilatations may require open surgical repair.

The most common cause of external injuries to the larynx and trachea is motor vehicle accidents. Tracheal injuries account for 1% of traffic fatalities, with 30% of injured patients succumbing within the first hour after the accident. Three percent to 11% of motor vehicle accident victims have tracheal injuries at autopsy. Other causes include gunshot and stab wounds. Such injuries are more common in older children.

Internal trauma results in tracheal tears or transections, complete laryngotracheal disruption, fracture or dislocation of laryngeal cartilages (thyroid, arytenoid, cricoid), and hematomas. Severe forms of trauma are often associated with injuries to one or both recurrent laryngeal nerves, or esophageal lacerations. Tracheal trauma may accompany injury to the esophagus, cervical spine, and brachiocephalic vessels. There are several proposed mechanisms for internal trauma. In blunt trauma, the larynx is crushed between an object and the rigid spine, resulting in fracture of cartilages or rupture of the membranous tracheal wall. Tracheal injuries may also result from severe hyperextension of the cervical spine, producing a marked increase in intraluminal pressure, which results in lacerations or transections. Patients with injuries resulting from blunt or penetrating trauma present with respiratory obstruction, respiratory difficulties (stridor, wheezing, retractions), hoarse or muffled voice, subcutaneous emphysema, hemoptysis, and odinophagia. Physical examination reveals neck or chest contusions and lacerations with loss of the normal prominence of the cricoid and thyroid prominence.

Treatment of these injuries is initially directed at stabilizing the airway. Emergent intubation may be necessary in patients with significant trauma. Laryngeal injuries consisting of hematomas may be managed conservatively. Extensive injuries with disruption of the laryngeal architecture require open surgery. Functional results may be obtained if injuries are reduced within 3 to 7 days after the injury. Delay increases the likelihood of scarring and chronic laryngeal stenosis.

IMAGING FEATURES

Infants and young children with internal acute or chronic laryngeal injuries are best imaged with computed tomography (CT). Findings of granulation tissue or scarring resulting from prolonged intubation include partial or circumferential soft tissue thickening involving the subglottic region or trachea. Deformity of the air column or dystrophic calcification of the cricoid cartilage or tracheal rings is suggestive of associated laryngomalacia or tracheomalacia.

In the setting of acute external trauma, radiographs provide evidence of laryngeal injuries. Findings include diffuse swelling, subcutaneous air, fracture or displacement of the hyoid bone, and opacification of the lung parenchyma. Foreign bodies may also be present. Complete laryngotracheal separation is suggested by malalignment or step-off of the tracheal air column or elevation of the hyoid bone or both. Most of these patients are not imaged because of the high mortality of this injury. CT is the study of choice in patients with external laryngeal trauma. CT demonstrates the integrity of the laryngeal skeleton. Characteristic findings include diffuse edema of endolaryngeal and exolaryngeal structures. Focal or diffuse hemorrhage may be present throughout the injured region (Fig. 15A.14-1). CT provides information regarding the degree of airway compromise due to edema or hematoma. Severe trauma may produce disruption of the thyroepiglottic ligaments, resulting in subluxation of the epiglottis. Subcutaneous air indicates airway laceration. Severe trauma may be associated with subluxations, fractures, and dislocations of the hyoid bone. Lack of cartilage calcification makes it difficult to evaluate these structures in young children. Severe laryngeal trauma may also result in fractures and dislocations of the thyroid cartilage. Thyroid cartilage fractures are horizontal or vertical (Fig. 15A.14-2). Vertical fractures are best detected with CT because they are perpendicular to the acquisition plane. Comminuted and displaced fractures of the thyroid cartilage provide no support for the true and false vocal cords, resulting in reduced vocal function. The arytenoid cartilages are more likely to dislocate than fracture. When dislocation occurs, the arytenoids are displaced anterior and superior with respect to their normal position. Subluxation of the cricoarytenoid joints is seen as an abnormal articulation between the arytenoid and cricoid cartilages. Displacement of the arytenoid cartilages is often associated with foreshortening and paramedian positioning of the involved true vocal cord, which may be indistinguishable from vocal cord paralysis. The cricoid cartilage is the foundation of the larynx, and its status after severe trauma is one of the most important prognostic factors regarding function of the larynx. Fractures of the cricoid cartilage usually are associated with a reduced likelihood of regaining normal laryngeal function. Cricoid fractures result in deformity and collapse of the cricoid ring, which is manifested by deformity of the airway. Severe crush injuries may result in comminution of the anterior and posterior portions of the cricoid, causing its two halves to "spring" apart. Resultant migration of fragments into the airway may cause respiratory compromise.

Contrast esophagography may be necessary in patients suspected of having esophageal perforation (Figs. 15A.14-3 and 15A.14-4). Evaluation of the aorta may be indicated in patients with external laryngeal injuries associated with severe chest trauma or in some patients with stab wounds.

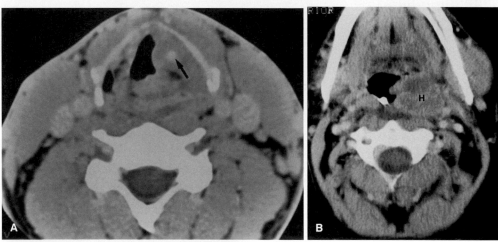

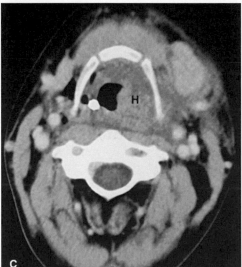

FIGURE 15A.14-1.

Hematomas. A. Axial computed tomography (CT) after upper airway trauma shows swelling of left true vocal cord region, which also contains a focal area of increased density *(arrow)* compatible with hematoma. The inner border of the vocal cord is in an abnormally medial position. **B.** Axial CT after blunt trauma shows hematoma (H) in left parapharyngeal space with compression of the airway. There is a left masseter muscle hematoma. **C.** Axial CT in same patient shows hematoma extending down into the left paralaryngeal space and compressing the airway. There is also a hematoma in the left submandibular region.

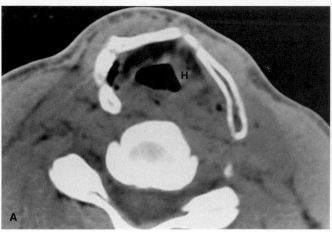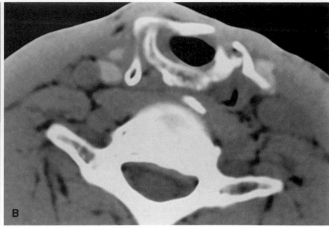

FIGURE 15A.14-2.

Tracheal injury with fractures. **A.** Axial computed tomography (CT) shows comminuted fractures of thyroid cartilage. Note increased and localized density in left paraglottic fat (H), indicating hematoma. **B.** Axial CT (below **A**) in same patient shows collapse of thyroid cartilage due to fractures and irregularly shaped left cricoid, also secondary to fracture. The tracheal air column has lost its normal shape and is flat in its anteroposterior diameter.

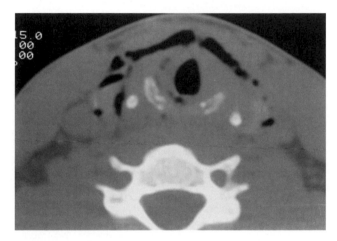

FIGURE 15A.14-3.

Tracheal perforation. Axial computed tomography shows air dissecting soft tissue planes secondary to tracheal perforation.

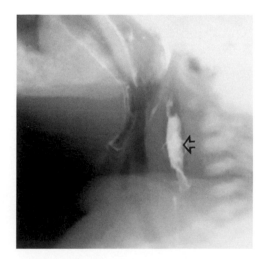

FIGURE 15A.14-4.

Iatrogenic injury. Lateral radiograph after barium swallow shows abnormal collection of contrast *(open arrow)* in precervical region secondary to pharyngeal perforation after intubation. (Case courtesy of D. Merten, University of North Carolina, Chapel Hill, NC.)

SUGGESTED READINGS

1. Alonso WA. Injuries of the lower respiratory tract. In: Bluestone CD, Stool SE, Scheetz MD, eds. Pediatric Otolaryngology, Vol. 2. Philadelphia: WB Saunders, 1990:1178.
2. Mancuso AA, Hanafee WN. Larynx and hypopharynx. In: Computed Tomography and Magnetic Resonance of the Head and Neck, 2nd ed. Baltimore: Williams & Wilkins, 1985:269.
3. Curtin HC. The larynx. In: Som PM, Bergeron RT, eds. Head and Neck Imaging, 2nd ed. St. Louis: CV Mosby, 1991:667.
4. Stark P. Congenital anomalies of the trachea. In: Radiology of the Trachea. Stuttgart: Thieme, 1991:13.

15B.0 *Applied Embryology*

The anatomic structures of the face and neck predominantly derive from the branchial apparatus on the 15th day of life. The branchial apparatus consists of six paired arches separated on their outer surface by five paired ectodermal clefts. On their inner surface, the arches are separated by five paired endodermally derived pharyngeal pouches (Fig. 15B.0-1A). The external branchial clefts are lined with flat epithelium, whereas the internal pharyngeal pouches are lined with columnar epithelium. Each branchial cleft is transiently in contact with a corresponding pharyngeal pouch, forming a double-layered membrane termed the "closing membrane." The ectodermal and endodermal layers of each membrane are soon separated by migrating mesodem. Only the first closing membrane persists and forms the tympanic membrane. Each component of the branchial apparatus is the precursor for various anatomic structures of the extracranial head and neck. By the end of the fourth week of life, four well defined pairs of arches are visible. The fifth and sixth arches are rudimentary. Each arch is composed of a central core of mesoderm and is lined externally by ectoderm and internally by endoderm. Each arch contains a characteristic central cartilage, blood vessel, muscle elements, and nerve. The cartilaginous, vascular, and muscular elements associated with each arch are derived from the mesoderm affiliated with that arch. The nerve is derived from the developing brain and not from the adjacent mesoderm. The branchial apparatus typically disappears between the fourth to sixth weeks of life.

Step 1. The First Branchial Apparatus

The first branchial arch divides into maxillary and mandibular processes. The mesenchymal core of the mandibular division forms a cartilaginous bar known as Meckel's cartilage. The dorsal aspect of Meckel's cartilage forms the majority of the malleus and incus. The ventral aspect gives rise to the anterior malleolar ligament, sphenomandibular ligament, and a portion of the mandibular cartilaginous primordium. Other derivatives of the first branchial arch include the muscles of mastication, tensor veli palatini, tensor tympani, and anterior belly of the digastrics. All receive innervation from the mandibular division of the trigeminal nerve.

The dorsal portion of the first branchial cleft forms the external auditory canal and the middle portion forms the cavum conchae. The ventral portion does not significantly contribute to normal structures; however, incomplete obliteration of the ventral groove results in residual ectopic ectodermal rests (first branchial cleft cysts). The auricle, although not a direct derivative, forms around the superficial opening of the first branchial cleft.

The first pharyngeal pouch is the precursor of the eustachian tube, tympanic cavity, and the mastoid air cells (Fig. 15B.0-1B). The tympanic membrane arises from the branchial plate, which results from apposition of invaginating walls of the adjacent first branchial cleft and pharyngeal pouch. As the mandible and face develop, the mandible and its associated muscles migrate ventrally and inferiorly, whereas the pinna migrates dorsolaterally. This migration may allow anomalous cell rests or unobliterated sinuses to assume the characteristic morphology and position of first branchial anomalies.

Step 2. The Second Branchial Apparatus

The cartilage of the second branchial arch (Reichert's cartilage) appears between the 45th to 48th days of life and gives rise to several bony structures of the head and neck. Its ventral portion forms the lesser cornu and superior portion of the hyoid bone. The dorsal portion gives rise to several temporal bone structures, including portions of the ossicles, middle ear, and styloid process. A portion of the cartilage between the hyoid bone and styloid process involutes and forms the stylohyoid ligament. Muscles that derive from mesoderm of the second arch and innervated by the facial nerve include the posterior belly of the digastric, stylohyoid, stapedius, and superficial muscles of facial expression. With continued growth, the second branchial arch extends caudally and overlaps with the second, third, and fourth branchial clefts, thus forming the cervical sinus.

The second pharyngeal pouch is largely obliterated by the development of the palatine tonsil; however, a portion of this pouch may persist as the intertonsillar cleft. The surface endoderm of the pouch continues to proliferate and forms the surface epithelium lining the crypts of the palatine tonsil. The mesenchyme of the pouch gives rise to the lymphatic nodules within the palatine tonsil.

The second branchial cleft forms the palatine tonsils. The ventral portion of the cleft gives rise to the tonsillar fossa and the palatine tonsil. The dorsal portion of the cleft is incorporated into the eustachian tube. The cleft is eventually covered by the caudal growth of the second arch, thereby forming the cervical sinus. Persistent remnants of the cervical sinus and second branchial cleft are the precursors of anomalies associated with the second branchial apparatus.

Step 3. The Third Branchial Apparatus

The cartilage of the third branchial arch forms the lower body and greater horns of the hyoid bone. The musculature derived from the third branchial arch is limited to the stylopharyngeus muscle, which is supplied by the glossopharyngeal nerve. The mucosa covering the posterior one-third of the tongue also derives from the third arch. The palatopharyngeus muscle and portions of skin over the carotid artery may also be third arch derivatives. The third branchial cleft is normally obliterated by overgrowth of the second branchial arch.

The communication between the developing pharynx narrows into a duct that normally degenerates. The pouch expands and forms an embryonic structure composed of a hollow ventral component and a solid dorsal bulbar component. By the sixth week of life, the dorsal bulbar component differentiates into the inferior parathyroid glands. The hollow ventral component migrates medially and fuses to form the bilobed thymus. The primordia of the parathyroid and thymus glands lose their communication with the pharynx and migrate inferiorly. The parathyroid glands separate from the thymus and are normally found on the dorsal surface of the thyroid gland. The thymus continues its descent into the upper mediastinum. Occasionally, the inferior parathyroid glands migrate inferiorly and are found at the lower poles of the thyroid gland or within the thorax in close proximity to the thymus.

Step 4. The Fourth to Sixth Branchial Apparatuses

The fourth through sixth branchial arches form various laryngeal cartilages and muscles. Portions of the skin of the neck also derive from the fifth and sixth branchial arches.

The fourth pharyngeal pouch forms dorsal and ventral components. Its dorsal portion develops into the superior parathyroid glands, which eventually migrate caudally to rest along the dorsal surface of the thyroid gland. These glands are located superiorly to the pair derived from the third pouch. The ventral portion of the fourth pouch forms the ultimobranchial body, which subsequently fuses with the thyroid gland. These arise from neural crest cells that have previously migrated into the branchial apparatus. The ultimobranchial body gives rise to the parafollicular cells (C cells), which produce calcitonin. The fifth pharyngeal pouch is incorporated into the fourth pouch and may, in part, contribute to the formation of the ultimobranchial body.

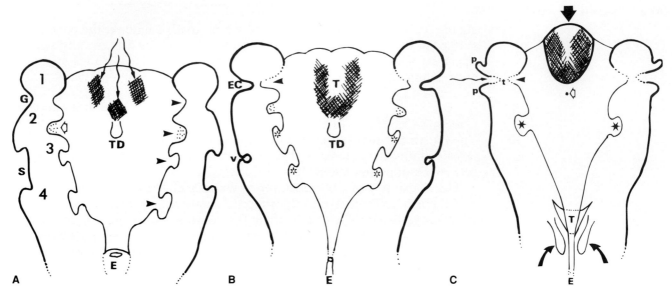

FIGURE 15B.0-1.

Development of the branchial apparatus.   A. At 5 weeks of life there are four (1–4) sequential branchial arches that laterally contain the first branchial groove (G) and the cervical sinuses (S). Medially are the four pharyngeal pouches *(arrowheads)*; note that the second one contains the primordia *(open arrow)* for the palatine tonsils. The tongue buds *(wavy arrows)* are located superior to the thyroid diverticulum (TD). E, esophagus. **B.** At 6 weeks of life, the first branchial groove has deepened to form the external auditory canal (EC) and the cervical sinus has closed into a vesicle (v). The first pharyngeal pouch becomes the tubotympanic recess *(arrowhead)*. The parathyroids *(asterisks)* begin to develop. The tongue buds are confluent (T). TD, thyroid diverticulum; E, esophagus. **C.** Between the seventh and eighth weeks of life, the pinnae (p) are forming. The external auditory canal *(wavy arrow)* deepens and is separated from the tympanic cavity *(arrowhead)* by the rudimentary tympanic membrane (t). The palatine tonsils *(stars)* are well formed, as is the thyroid (T). The thymus *(curved arrows)* begins its descent into the upper chest. At the base of the tongue *(large solid arrow)* lies the foramen cecum *(open arrow)*. E, esophagus.

SUGGESTED READINGS

1. Moore KL. The branchial apparatus and the head and neck. In: Moore KL, ed. The Developing Human: Clinically Oriented Embryology, 4th ed. Philadelphia: WB Saunders, 1988:170.
2. Smoker WRK, Harnsberger HR, Reede DL, Holliday RA, Som PM, Bergeron RT. The neck. In: Som PM, Bergeron RT, eds. Head and Neck Imaging, 2nd ed. St. Louis: CV Mosby, 1991:498.
3. Batsakis JG. Cysts, sinuses, and "coeles." In: Tumors of the Head and Neck, 2nd ed. Baltimore: Williams & Wilkins, 1979:514.

15B.01 *First Branchial Anomalies*

EPIDEMIOLOGY

First branchial anomalies are an uncommon group of lesions (cysts, sinuses, and fistulas) that result from abnormal embryogenesis of the first branchial apparatus. They account for approximately 8% of all branchial complex anomalies, are more common in children than in adults, and usually present before 10 years of age. These lesions appear more often on the left side than the right side. Girls are affected twice as often as boys. These anomalies are isolated or seen in patients with congenital syndromes (ie, Crouzon's disease), ossicular malformations, and congenital epidermoids.

CLINICAL FEATURES

First branchial anomalies may be classified as type 1 and type 2. In Arnot's classification, type 1 defects are derived from buried cell rests of the first branchial cleft, resulting in cyst or sinus formation within the parotid gland with a predilection for its lower portion. These lesions are lined by squamous epithelium with subepithelial lymphoid tissue and usually present as painful masses or discharging sinuses in the region of the parotid gland. Type 2 defects result from incomplete closure of the branchial cleft. These lesions present in childhood as cysts or sinuses in the anterior triangle of the neck and may communicate with the external auditory canal. In a different classification scheme (Work's classification), type 1 anomalies are ectodermally lined cysts anterior or inferior to the pinna, continuous with a tract running parallel to and possibly communicating with the external auditory canal. These lesions end in a cul-de-sac or bony plate at the level of the mesotympanum. Type 2 anomalies consist of both ectodermal and mesodermal elements extending from the angle of the mandible to the vicinity of the membranous external auditory canal. The external sinus opens adjacent to the hyoid bone near the angle of the mandible. At surgery, many of the lesions are simply parotid cysts with sinus or cul-de-sac extending to the external auditory canal.

Clinically, first branchial anomalies present as masses in the periparotid, perimandibular, and suprahyoid neck regions. Type 1 lesions are often asymptomatic. Type 2 lesions have a greater likelihood of being asymptomatic, and often present as painful, enlarging masses in the region of the parotid tail. Type 2 lesions may be associated with a draining sinus tract that typically is situated below the angle of the mandible. Occasionally, patients may present with otalgia or recurrent otitis media that is refractory to medical therapy. This is caused by a fistulous tract communicating the anomaly with the external auditory canal. Surgical resection is the treatment of choice.

IMAGING FEATURES

Computed tomography (CT) is the study of choice for evaluating patients suspected of having a first branchial anomaly. Type 1 lesions are easily detected by both CT and magnetic resonance (MR) imaging. However, fistulous tracts presenting in type 2 lesions are best seen with coronal CT.

Type 1 lesions appear as thin-rimmed unilocular cysts located within the substance of the parotid gland (Fig. 15B.01-1). The rim does not enhance significantly after contrast administration. Type 1 lesions are typically located in the pretragal portion of the parotid gland. Other lesions that may mimic a type 1 lesion include retention cysts, sialocoeles, and lymphoepithelial cysts of the parotid gland. Less commonly, benign and malignant neoplasms of the parotid gland and necrotic intraparotid lymph nodes may mimic the appearance of a first branchial anomaly.

Type 2 lesions are elongated, multilobular cysts extending from the undersurface of the external auditory canal and coursing through the parotid gland.

Occasionally, these lesions involve the parapharyngeal space. The fistulous communication with the external auditory canal is best seen on thin-section coronal CT images (Fig. 15B.01-2). The internal CT density of the cyst varies with its protein content. Pure cystic lesions are of low density and are hypointense on MR T1-weighted images and hyperintense on T2-weighted images. Lesions with superimposed infection have a thick, enhancing wall and higher protein content. Their attenuation on CT and signal intensity on MR T1-weighted images is increased.

The course of the facial nerve in these anomalies is variable and must be determined before surgery. The lesions may be deep or superficial to the facial nerve. Occasionally, a lesion may encircle the intraparotid facial nerve. It should be remembered that between the seventh to eighth weeks of life the parotid gland migrates cranially and dorsally to rest caudal and ventral to the ear. Concurrently, the facial nerve and its muscular innervations migrate anteriorly. These migrations and the progressive elongation of the mandible result in different positions of first branchial anomalies with respect to the facial nerve.

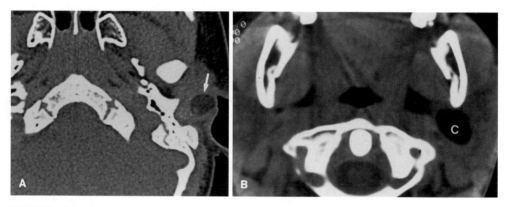

FIGURE 15B.01-1.

Type 1 first branchial anomaly.   **A.** Axial computed tomography (CT) shows cyst *(arrow)* within the parotid gland just inferior to external auditory canal.   **B.** Axial CT in a different patient shows intraparotid branchial cleft cyst (C).

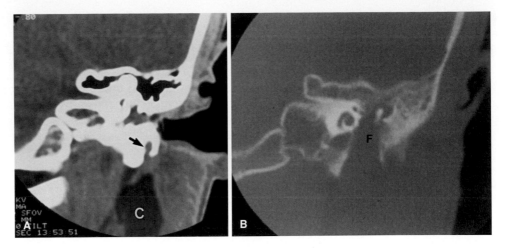

FIGURE 15B.01-2.

Type 2 first branchial anomaly. **A.** Coronal computed tomography (CT) shows intra-parotid cyst (C) in fistulous tract *(arrow)* into the external auditory canal. **B.** In a different patient, axial CT (bone window settings) shows large fistulous tract (F) that communicated between the first branchial cleft cyst and the middle ear cavity, which is opacified.

SUGGESTED
READINGS

1. Mukherji SK, Tart RP, Slattery WH, Stringer SP, Benson MT, Mancuso AA. Evaluation of first branchial anomalies by CT and MR. J Comput Assist Tomogr 1993;17: 576.
2. Arnot JS. Defects of the first branchial cleft. S Afr J Surg 1971;9:93.
3. Work WP. Newer concepts of first branchial cleft defects. Laryngoscope 1972;82: 1581.

15B.02 *Second Branchial Anomalies*

EPIDEMIOLOGY

Lesions of the second branchial complex constitute 95% of all branchial abnormalities. Anomalous development may result in the formation of a cyst, sinus, or fistula. Cysts are most common and usually present between 10 to 40 years of age. In children, cysts are most often seen before 10 years of age. There is no gender predilection.

CLINICAL FEATURES

Branchial cysts result from incomplete obliteration of the epithelial-lined cervical sinus. Complete isolation of the persistent cervical sinus results in a second branchial cyst. The usual position of these lesions is high in the lateral neck along the anterior border of the sternocleidomastoid muscle (Fig. 15B.02-1). These cysts may occur anywhere along the developmental path of the second branchial complex and can occur as high as the tonsillar fossa at the level of the hyoid bone. The most common location is lateral to the jugular vein at the level of the carotid bifurcation. These lesions are typically lateral to the hypoglossal and glossopharyngeal nerves. Occasionally, these lesions may extend medially between the internal and external carotid arteries.

Histologically, branchial cysts are characteristically thin-walled lesions lined by stratified squamous epithelium with lymphoid tissues deep to the lining membrane. The lesions may occasionally show chronic inflammation. These cysts are filled with a turbid, yellowish fluid that may contain cholesterol crystals. Occasionally, branchial cysts are lined by a respiratory epithelium. Carcinomas occurring in branchial cysts are extremely rare.

Branchial cysts are classified in four types (Bailey's classification). Type 1 cysts are superficial lesions located along the anterior border of the sternocleidomastoid muscle and beneath the superficial cervical fascia. Type 2 are the most common form, and represent deeper lesions resting on the carotid sheath. These lesions must be carefully resected because they are adherent to underlying vessels. Type 3 cysts pass medially between the internal and external carotid arteries and extend inward toward the lateral wall of the pharynx. Occasionally, type 3 cysts extend to the skull base. Type 4 comprises cysts that are lined by columnar epithelium.

Clinically, these lesions present as fluctuant masses at the angle of the mandible and deep to the anterior border of the sternocleidomastoid muscle. The lesions are usually painless and moveable. Branchial cysts are treated with surgical excision. The likelihood of adherence to surrounding structures is increased if the cysts have been chronically infected. Preoperative antibiotics should be administered if the cyst is acutely infected.

A sinus arising from the second branchial apparatus arises from a communication between an incompletely obliterated cervical sinus and the skin. Clinically, these lesions present as a dimple or pigmented spot along the anterior border of the sternocleidomastoid muscle. The fistulous opening is usually at the level of the hyoid bone or lower. The lesions frequently discharge mucoid secretions, which may increase if infected. These lesions are also treated by surgical excision. The full extent of the lesion should be evaluated with a sinogram. Sinus tracts follow the course of the second branchial complex and tend to course between the carotid bifurcation. Surgical dissection is often aided by filling the sinus tract with methylene blue at the time of surgery.

Second branchial groove fistulas develop when the second branchial groove communicates with the second branchial pouch. The result is a fistula with an internal opening at the tonsilar fossa, often adjacent to the posterior pillar, and an external opening along the anterior border of the sternocleidomastoid muscle. The fistula courses inferiorly from the tonsillar fossa and is lateral to cranial nerves IX and XII. The tract then passes between the internal and external carotid arteries and pierces the platysma muscle. The lining of the fistulous tract is stratified epithelium along its external portion and columnar epithelium along its internal course. These lesions often present with discharge of a clear, yellow mucoid secretion. The tract is prone to recurrent infection; however, some lesions may be completely asymptomatic. Treatment is surgical excision.

IMAGING FEATURES

The study of choice for imaging patients with branchial cysts is either computed tomography (CT) or magnetic resonance (MR) imaging. Direct injection of radiopaque, water-soluble contrast into the external orifice should be performed in patients with a sinus or fistula. Direct opacification of a cyst or sinus is essential before surgical resection because it provides valuable information regarding the extent of the lesion and its relation to adjacent structures. CT may be helpful in certain instances after opacification of the tract to better determine its course.

We prefer CT as the initial imaging modality, but MR imaging may be helpful for evaluating complex lesions because of its multiplanar capabilities. On CT, these lesions present as thin-walled cysts most often located along the anterior aspect of the sternocleidomastoid muscle (Fig. 15B.02-2). Typically, the lesions show very little peripheral contrast enhancement. The presence of a thicker enhancing rim may be evidence of prior infection. Reticulation of the surrounding subcutaneous fat may be present with infection. Type 2 cysts are deep and abut the carotid artery sheath (Fig. 15B.02-3). The sternocleidomastoid muscle is displaced posteriorly or posterolaterally. The internal characteristics of the lesions vary. Chronically infected cysts may contain fluid of increased CT attenuation because of higher protein content. Branchial cysts may also contain internal septations. On MR, these lesions are cystic and of low signal intensity on T1-weighted images and high signal intensity on T2-weighted images. However, the MR signal intensity may vary depending on the protein content of the cyst. Highly proteinaceous fluid may have increased T1 signal intensity. Enhancement and thickening of the wall depends on prior infection. Demonstration of the course of the fistulous tract requires injection of iodinated contrast material into the cyst.

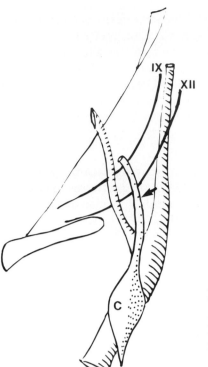

FIGURE 15B.02-1.

Second branchial arch anomaly. The cyst (c) is lateral to the common carotid artery, and its superior fistulous tract *(arrow)* courses between the carotid artery bifurcation and lateral to cranial nerves IX and XII.

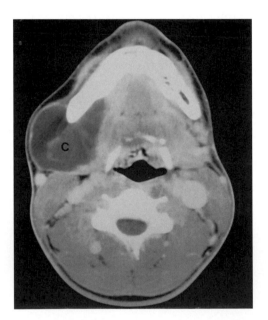

FIGURE 15B.02-2.

Type 1 second branchial cleft cyst. Axial postcontrast computed tomography shows cyst (C) in region of angle of mandible but extending medially into the sublingual space. Laterally, the lesion is limited by the platysma muscle. The cyst is anterior to the sternocleidomastoid muscle and separate from the carotid artery. The cyst contains some inner septations.

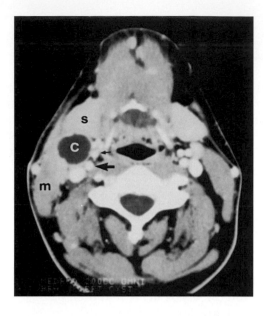

FIGURE 15B.02-3.

Type 2 second branchial cleft cyst. The cyst (C) is located posterior to the submandibular gland (s), anterior to the sternocleidomastoid muscle (m), and abuts the internal *(larger arrow)* and external *(smaller arrow)* carotid arteries.

SUGGESTED READINGS

1. Karmody CS. Developmental abnormalities of the neck. In: Bluestone CD, Stool SE, Scheetz MD, eds. Pediatric Otolaryngology, Vol. 2. Philadelphia: WB Saunders, 1990:1308.
2. Reede DL, Holliday RA, Som PM, Bergeron RT. Nonnodal pathologic conditions of the neck. In: Som PM, Bergeron RT, eds. Head and Neck Imaging, 2nd ed. St. Louis: CV Mosby, 1991:536.
3. Batsakis JG. Cysts, sinuses, and "coeles." In: Tumors of the Head and Neck, 2nd ed. Baltimore: Williams & Wilkins, 1979:518.
4. Mancuso AA, Hanafee WN. The neck. In: Computed Tomography and Magnetic Resonance of the Head and Neck, 2nd ed. Baltimore: Williams & Wilkins, 1985: 181.

15B.03 *Third and Fourth Branchial Anomalies*

EPIDEMIOLOGY

Congenital anomalies of the third and fourth branchial complexes are extremely rare lesions. Fistulas from both the third and fourth branchial complexes communicate with the hypopharynx. Because the third and fourth pouches also give rise to the parathyroid glands and thymus, anomalous embryogenesis may result in a multisystem disease (ie, DiGeorge's anomaly) or an isolated anomaly.

CLINICAL FEATURES

Defects arising from the third branchial complex are extremely unusual. These defects may result in squamous epithelium-lined cysts in the region of the laryngeal ventricle. A fistula of third branchial origin begins in the skin covering the anterior border of the sternocleidomastoid muscle or, rarely, in skin covering the posterior surface of the sternocleidomastoid muscle (Fig. 15B.03-1). The tract ascends in the carotid sheath between the common carotid artery and the vagus nerve and then passes posterior to the internal and external carotid arteries. The fistula then courses between the IX and XII cranial nerves. Eventually, it penetrates the thyrohyoid membrane between the hyoid bone and the internal branch of the superior laryngeal nerve to communicate with the pyriform sinus.

Isolated third branchial lesions are epithelial-lined cysts located in the lateral compartment of the neck. A sinus opening may not be present. Fistulous tracts arising from the fourth branchial complex are even less common than anomalies of the third branchial apparatus. The lesions are more frequently found on the right side than the left (9:1). The opening of the fistulous tract is located along the anterior border of the sternocleidomastoid muscle. The tract then hooks inferiorly around the aorta on the left side and the subclavian artery on the right side (similar to the recurrent laryngeal nerves; Fig. 15B.03-2). Both ascend anterior to the common carotid artery in close association with the recurrent laryngeal nerves up to the level of the hypoglossal nerves. The tracts loop over the hypoglossal nerves and pass deep to the internal carotid artery. The tracts remain inferior to the superior laryngeal nerves. The tracts penetrate the thyrohyoid membrane caudal to the internal branch of the superior laryngeal nerves and eventually communicate with the hypopharynx near the apex of the pyriform sinus.

DiGeorge's anomaly is related to abnormal embryogenesis of the third and fourth branchial pouches and results in aplasia or hypoplasia of the parathyroid glands and thymus. This disorder is usually sporadic, although autosomal dominant and recessive forms are known to exist. DiGeorge's anomaly is associated with a variety of malformations, including cardiovascular malformations, genitourinary anomalies, micrognathia, hypertelorism, bifid uvula, high-arched palate, CHARGE and fetal alcohol syndromes, diabetic mothers, and mothers inadvertently treated with retinoic acid during pregnancy. These patients present with hypocalcemia and reduced parahormone levels and have an isolated T-cell deficiency, although some, also have a deficiency in immunoglobulin production.

IMAGING FEATURES

A fistulogram performed with water-soluble contrast is the study of choice for evaluating patients with fistulas arising from malformations of the third and fourth branchial apparatuses (Fig. 15B.03-3). Computed tomography (CT) or magnetic resonance (MR) imaging is of limited value because the small fistulous tract may not be detected. CT performed after opacification of the tract may be beneficial. The diagnosis of an isolated third branchial cleft cyst may be suggested by CT or MR imaging (Fig. 15B.03-4). The lesions are located in the lateral compartment of the neck, posterior to the common carotid artery and jugular vein. They may extend inferiorly to the level of the thyroid gland. There is no significant enhancement of the cyst wall. The overlying sterno-cleidomastoid muscle is displaced laterally by the lesion. The lesions may be difficult to differentiate from a well delineated lymphangioma. Histologic examination is necessary for confirmation of the diagnosis.

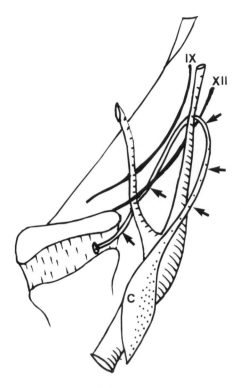

FIGURE 15B.03-1.

Third branchial anomaly. The cyst (c) is located lateral to the common carotid artery and the tract *(arrows)* courses upward dorsal to the internal carotid artery. The tract extends between cranial nerves IX and XII, posterior to the external carotid artery, and pierces the thyrohyoid membrane.

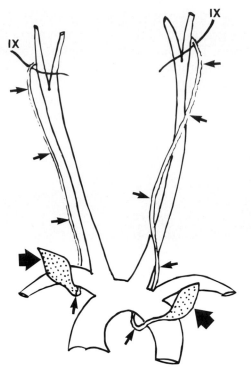

FIGURE 15B.03-2.

Fourth branchial anomalies. The cysts *(large arrows)* are situated anterior and inferior to the subclavian arteries. On the left, the tract *(small arrows)* hooks under the aorta and travels anterior to the common carotid artery, and hooks again on the IX cranial nerve to travel posterior to the internal carotid artery. On the right, the tract *(small arrows)* hooks under the subclavian artery and travels anterolaterally to the common carotid artery. The tract then hooks on the IX cranial nerve and travels posterior to the internal carotid artery.

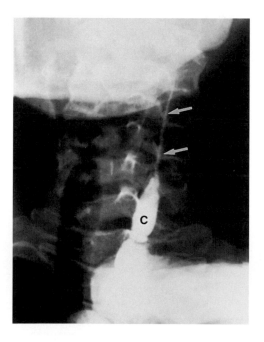

FIGURE 15B.03-3.

Third branchial anomaly, fistulogram. Oblique view from fistulogram shows filling of cyst (C) and fistulous tract *(arrows)* superiorly.

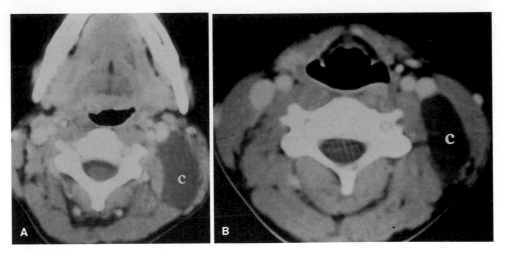

FIGURE 15B.03-4.

Third branchial cleft cyst. **A.** Axial postcontrast computed tomography (CT) shows cyst (c) located posterior to the left jugular vein. **B.** Axial CT in same patient shows that cyst (c) extends inferiorly to mid-neck and laterally displaces the sternocleidomastoid muscle.

SUGGESTED
READINGS

1. Himalstein MR. Branchial cysts and fistulas. Ear Nose Throat J 1980;59:47.
2. Reede DL, Holliday RA, Som PM, Bergeron RT. Nonnodal pathologic conditions of the neck. In: Som PM, Bergeron RT, eds. Head and Neck Imaging, 2nd ed. St. Louis: CV Mosby, 1991:536.
3. Hong R. Immunity, allergy, and diseases of inflammation. In: Behrman RE, Kleigman RM, Nelson WE, Vaughan VC, eds. Nelson's Textbook of Pediatrics, 14th ed. Philadelphia: WB Saunders, 1992:552.
4. DiGeorge A. Hypoparathyroidism. In: Behrman RE, Kleigman RM, Nelson WE, Vaughan VC, eds. Nelson's Textbook of Pediatrics, 14th ed. Philadelphia: WB Saunders, 1992:1432.
5. Benson MT, Dalen K, Mancuso AA, Kerr HH, Cacciarelli AA, Mafee MF. Congenital anomalies of the branchial apparatus: embryology and pathologic anatomy. Radiographics 1992;12:943.

15B.04 *Tornwaldt (Thornwaldt) Cyst*

EPIDEMIOLOGY

Tornwaldt cysts are benign developmental lesions in the nasopharynx. Their incidence in autopsy series is 4%. The peak age of incidence is 15 to 30 years of age. There is no gender predilection.

CLINICAL FEATURES

Tornwaldt cysts represent anomalous embryogenesis of the cephalic end of the notochord. During development, the notochord descends into the nasopharynx in the region of the pharyngeal bursa (pouch of Luschka). When a focal adherence develops between the notochord and the overlying ectoderm, a small portion of the nasopharyngeal mucosa is carried along with the notochord as it ascends into the developing skull base. This results in a cyst or tract between the longus colli muscles that is surrounded by nasopharyngeal mucosa. Histologically, these cysts are lined by squamous epithelium. Cyst fluid is highly proteinaceous and often contains debris.

Tornwaldt cysts are commonly asymptomatic and incidentally found on imaging studies. Occasionally, patients present with halitosis, foul taste, or persistent nasal discharge. On endoscopic examination, these cysts are submucosal lesions that are nontender to palpation. However, they may become infected and form an abscess in the retropharyngeal space. Asymptomatic cysts require no treatment. Symptomatic or infected cysts are drained, usually via an intraoral approach.

IMAGING FEATURES

We prefer magnetic resonance (MR) imaging for evaluating patients suspected of having Tornwaldt cysts. Typical findings are a well delineated, thin-walled, cystic lesion usually measuring 2 to 10 mm in diameter (Figs. 15B.04-1 and 15B.04-2). Their MR signal intensity is increased on T1- and T2-weighted images. The increased T1 signal intensity is the result of the presence of highly proteinaceous fluid. Tornwaldt cysts typically do not enhance after contrast administration. On computed tomography (CT), these cysts appear as submucosal rounded lesions in the posterior nasopharynx. The high protein content of the cyst may result in increased CT attenuation. By CT, Tornwaldt cysts may mimic other soft tissue masses. In patients with prominent adenoid tissue, the cyst may not be visualized completely. MR imaging is helpful in these patients.

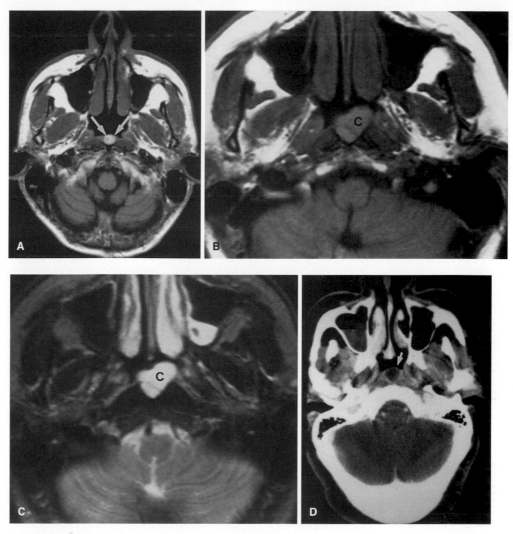

FIGURE 15B.04-1.

Tornwaldt cyst. **A.** Axial noncontrast magnetic resonance (MR) T1-weighted image shows well defined cyst *(arrows)* between the longus colli muscles. Its contents are hyperintense, reflecting high protein contents. **B.** Axial noncontrast MR T1-weighted image in a different patient shows slightly hyperintense cyst (C), which is large and eccentric in location. **C.** Corresponding T2-weighted image shows cyst (C) to be hyperintense and contain a septation. **D.** Axial postcontrast computed tomography shows low-density cyst *(arrow)* covered by thin and enhancing mucosa.

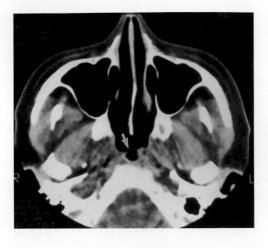

FIGURE 15B.04-2.

Ruptured Tornwaldt cyst. Axial computed tomography in a patient complaining of posterior nasal discharge shows rounded cavity *(arrow)* in the posterior nasopharynx compatible with spontaneously ruptured cyst.

SUGGESTED
READING

1. Dillon WP. The pharynx and oral cavity. In: Som PM, Bergeron RT, eds. Head and Neck Imaging, 2nd ed. St. Louis: CV Mosby, 1991:431.

15B.05 *Dermoid Cyst*

EPIDEMIOLOGY

The term "dermoid cyst" identifies a variety of lesions arising in the extracranial head and neck. These include epidermoid, dermoid, and teratoid cysts. About 7% of dermoid cysts occur in the head and neck region. Most of these lesions (65%) occur in orbital and nasal regions, whereas 24% arise in the oral cavity. Epidermoid cysts are present at birth. True dermoid cysts are present in infancy but are not identified until the second or third decades of life. There is no gender predilection.

CLINICAL FEATURES

The various lesions denoted under the terms "dermoid cysts" are histologically distinct. Epidermoid cysts, which are the most common of these lesions, are encapsulated by a fibrous wall and lined by simple squamous epithelium. They have no adnexal structures. Dermoid cysts are epithelial lined and contain a variety of structures derived from mesoderm such as hair, sebaceous glands, and fat. Teratoid cysts are the least common of these lesions and are lined by simple stratified squamous epithelium or respiratory-like ciliated epithelium. These lesions contain cheesy, keratinaceous material that is protein rich.

One hypothesis proposes that dermoid cyst arise from epithelium trapped in an unusual location due to traumatic implanatation or anomalous development. Trapping of ectodermal elements during fusion of the lateral processes of the mandible and tuberculum may result in floor-of-mouth dermoids. A second hypothesis suggests that dermoid cysts represent heterotopias or choristomatic cysts. Dermoid cysts in the oral cavity arise in the floor of the mouth and are midline lesions; however, it is not uncommon for large lesions to lateralize. Occasionally, dermoid cysts may be located on the dorsum of the tongue, or the hard and soft palates. Clinical presentation depends on their location with respect to the mylohyoid muscle. Sublingual dermoids are centered above the mylohyoid muscle and present as submucosal masses in the floor of the mouth. These lesions may elevate the tongue and interfere with glutination, and may be confused clinically with a ranula. Submental dermoid cysts are centered below the mylohyoid muscle and present as an external swelling situated above the hyoid bone. Occasionally, these lesions may extend to the thoracic inlet.

On physical examination, dermoids have a doughy texture and may demonstrate pitting after palpation. The lesions are not fixed to the tongue or hyoid bone, and, unlike thyroglossal duct cysts, do not move when the tongue is protruded. Treatment is surgical excision with the specific approach based, in part, on the position of the lesion with respect to the mylohyoid muscle. Lesions situated above the mylohyoid may best be resected by an intraoral approach, whereas those lesions located inferior to the mylohyoid muscle benefit from a direct approach.

IMAGING FEATURES

Both computed tomography (CT) and magnetic resonance (MR) imaging may be used to evaluate patients with dermoid cysts. The lesions are cystic midline lesions located within the floor of the mouth (Fig. 15B.05-1). On CT, the presence of fat attenuation within the lesion is pathognomonic of a true dermoid cyst. Dermoids are sharply demarcated and may have a thin enhancing rim. Bone erosion or remodeling is an unusual finding. On MR imaging, dermoids usually have signal characteristics that reflect their cystic nature. Occasionally, a dermoid containing highly proteinaceous fluid or fat may demonstrate increased T1 signal intensity and low T2 signal intensity. The multiplanar capabilities of MR are helpful in defining the exact location of the lesions with respect to mylohyoid muscle.

Epidermoids may be off the midline or near it (Fig. 15B.05-2). By CT, they appear as well marginated, nonenhancing masses of low density. By MR imaging, they may have signal intensities similar to that of water, or be of high signal intensity on both the T1- and T2-weighted images.

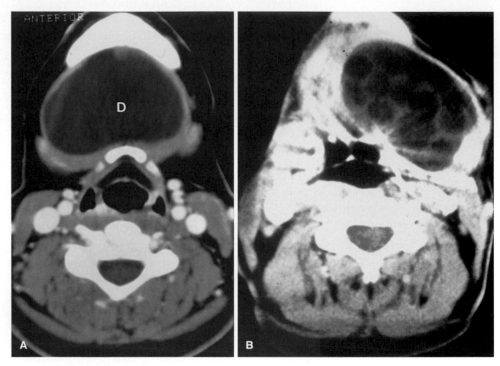

FIGURE 15B.05-1.

Dermoid. **A.** Axial postcontrast computed tomography (CT) shows cystic-appearing dermoid (D) in the floor of the mouth. **B.** Axial postcontrast CT in a different patient shows multiseptated dermoid in floor of mouth. Many of these lesions have components above and below the mylohyoid muscle, and determining their exact location requires coronal imaging with CT or magnetic resonance imaging.

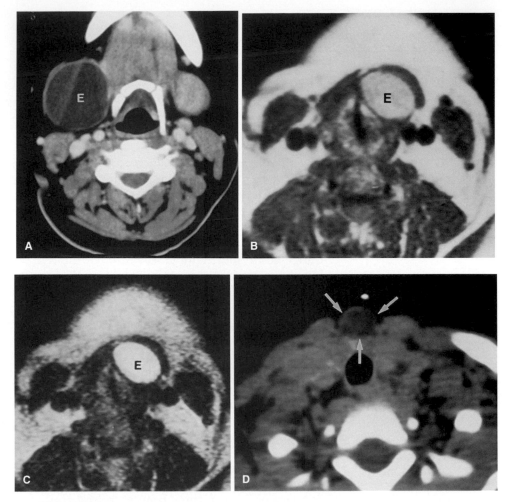

FIGURE 15B.05.2.

Epidermoid. **A.** Axial postcontrast computed tomography (CT) shows cystic-appearing mass (E) in right submandibular space. **B.** Axial noncontrast magnetic resonance (MR) T1-weighted image shows bright epidermoid (E) superficial to larynx and deep to strap muscles. **C.** Corresponding MR T2-weighted image shows epidermoid (E) to be bright. **D.** Axial noncontrast CT in a different patient shows midline, low-density epidermoid *(arrows)* in the low neck. (Cases courtesy of M. Benson, M.D., Macomb Hospital, Warren, MI.)

SUGGESTED READINGS

1. Batsakis JG. Teratomas of the head and neck. In: Tumors of the Head and Neck, 2nd ed. Baltimore: Williams & Wilkins, 1979:226.
2. Reede DL, Holliday RA, Som PM, Bergeron RT. Nonnodal pathologic conditions of the neck. In: Som PM, Bergeron RT, eds. Head and Neck Imaging, 2nd ed. St. Louis: CV Mosby, 1991:544.
3. Vogl TJ, Steger W, Ihrler S, Ferrera P, Grevers G. Cystic masses in the floor of the mouth: value of MR imaging in planning surgery. AJR 1993;161:183.

15B.06 *Thyroglossal Duct Cyst*

EPIDEMIOLOGY

Thyroglossal duct cysts are congenital lesions that develop from remnants of the thyroid anlage. They may present in all ages but are more common in children, in whom they are the most common midline neck mass. There is no gender predilection.

CLINICAL FEATURES

The thyroid is the first endocrine gland to appear in the fetus, around the 24th day of life. The thyroid arises from an endodermal thickening in the floor of the primitive pharynx at the midline of the tongue base. This area, known as the foramen cecum, is located posterior to the circumvallate papillae. The thyroid gland descends as a result of elongation and growth of the fetal tongue. The developing gland migrates inferiorly as a bilobed diverticulum. The thyroid gland passes through the tongue musculature and the mylohyoid muscle into the neck. During its descent it forms an epithelial-lined tube termed the thyroglossal duct. The cartilage of the second branchial arch (Reichert's cartilage), which gives origin to the hyoid bone, grows forward in close proximity to the descending thyroglossal duct. The final relationship between the hyoid bone and thyroglossal duct is variable. The duct courses anterior to the hyoid bone and then loops around its inferior surface, where it then extends upward by a short distance, either directly piercing it or along its inner surface. The duct then continues down along the strap muscles and thyrohyoid membrane. The duct terminates at the superior border of the thyroid gland. Migration of the thyroid gland is complete by the eighth week of life. Involution of the thyroglossal duct occurs between the eighth to tenth weeks of life. Failure of involution of the thyroglossal duct predisposes to formation of cysts. Cyst formation is caused either by inflammatory changes stimulating secretion of fluids within the duct remnants, or by persistent drainage of fluids formed from secretory epithelium into the area of the foramen cecum, which then become trapped within the duct. Fistulas result from infection, cyst rupture, or as a complication of surgery. Overall, fistulous communication of a thyroglossal duct cyst with the skin is uncommon.

Thyroglossal duct cysts may arise anywhere along the course of migration of the embryonic thyroglossal duct and thyroid gland. Most lesions (65%) occur below the hyoid bone (Fig. 15B.06-1). Twenty percent of lesions are suprahyoid in location, and 15% are located at the level of the hyoid bone. Seventy-five percent of lesions are midline masses, although occasionally they may be paramedian.

Clinically, they present as nontender, mobile, midline masses. They are 2 to 4 cm in diameter at initial presentation and progressively enlarge. These cysts may show rapid growth as a result of associated upper respiratory tract infection. Because thyroglossal duct cysts are often attached to the tongue or hyoid bone, they move when the tongue is protruded. Most thyroglossal duct cysts are benign. Carcinomas may coexist in less than 1% of cysts, and are usually incidental findings at surgery (Fig. 15B.06-2). Malignancies arise from ectopic thyroid tissue, and 85% of them are papillary carcinomas.

Treatment of choice is surgical resection. The Sistrunk procedure is the method of choice and involves complete removal of the cyst and its tract from the tongue base to the superior border of the thyroid gland. The central portion of the hyoid bone and cuff of the tongue base are included in this resection. Complete resection using the Sistrunk procedure is associated with a 3% recurrence rate, whereas the recurrence rate is significantly increased if the lesions are only locally excised (Fig. 15B.06-3).

IMAGING FINDINGS

Both computed tomography (CT) and magnetic resonance (MR) imaging may be used to evaluate patients suspected of having a thyroglossal duct cyst, but we recommend CT as the initial modality. Contrast-enhanced CT should be performed from the soft palate to the inferior aspect of the thyroid gland.

On CT, thyroglossal duct cysts present as a unilocular or multilocular cystic masses with peripheral enhancement (Fig. 15B.06-1). Recurrent infection may increase their intrinsic attenuation and result in thickening of the enhancing rim. The lesion may extend from the tongue base to the superior portion of the thyroid gland. The cyst may be anterior, posterior, or encompass the hyoid bone. A midline cleft in the hyoid bone may be visible. Below the hyoid bone, the cysts are centered in the strap muscles. The superior margin of the lesion may consist of only a small tract. Knowledge of the entire extent of the lesion is necessary for presurgical planning. By MR imaging, the cysts appear as fluid-containing lesions that are of low to intermediate signal intensity on T1-weighted images and increased signal intensity on T2-weighted images. Ectopic thyroid tissue may be found anywhere along the path of descent of the thyroid gland. Scintigraphy is more sensitive than MR imaging or CT for localizing rests of ectopic thyroid tissue.

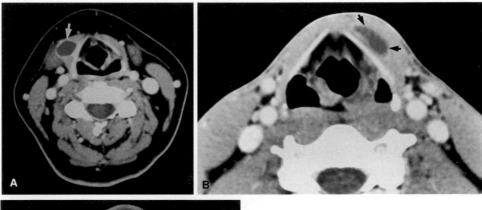

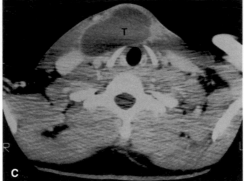

FIGURE 15B.06-1.

Thyroglossal duct cyst. **A.** Axial postcontrast computed tomography (CT) shows cystic lesion *(arrow)* with enhancing rim in right strap muscles. **B.** Axial postcontrast CT in a different patient shows smaller thyroglossal duct cyst *(arrows)* in left strap muscles. **C.** Axial postcontrast CT in a different patient shows large cyst (T) above superior aspect of thyroid gland.

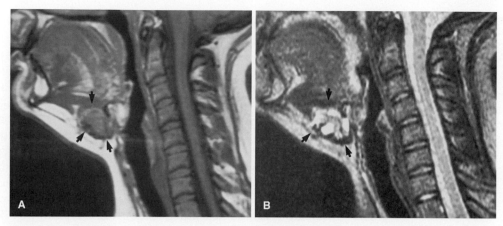

FIGURE 15B.06-2.

Carcinoma in thyroglossal duct cyst. **A.** Midsagittal noncontrast magnetic resonance (MR) T1-weighted image shows suprahyoid soft tissue mass *(arrows).* **B.** Corresponding MR T2-weighted image shows complex pattern of signal intensity in this lesion *(arrows).*

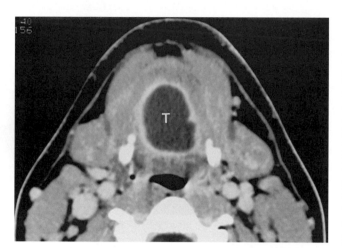

FIGURE 15B.06-3.

Recurrent thyroglossal duct cyst. Axial postcontrast computed tomography in a patient who had undergone prior resection of cyst in region of strap muscles, but not resection of the thyroglossal duct tract, shows a cystic mass (T) in posterior tongue surrounded by a relatively thick and enhancing rim.

SUGGESTED READINGS

1. Karmody CS. Developmental abnormalities of the neck. In: Bluestone CD, Stool SE, Scheetz MD, eds. Pediatric Otolaryngology, Vol. 2. Philadelphia: WB Saunders, 1990:1313.
2. Pincus RL. Congenital neck masses and cysts. In: Johnson JT, Kohut RI, Pillsbury HC, Tardy ME, eds. Head and Neck Surgery Otolaryngology, Vol. 1. Philadelphia: JB Lippincott, 1993:754.
3. Reede DL, Holliday RA, Som PM, Bergeron RT. Nonnodal pathologic conditions of the neck. In: Som PM, Bergeron RT, eds. Head and Neck Imaging, 2nd ed. St. Louis: CV Mosby, 1991:532.
4. Moore KL. The branchial apparatus and the head and neck. In: Moore KL, ed. The Developing Human: Clinically Oriented Embryology, 4th ed. Philadelphia: WB Saunders, 1988:184.

15B.07 *Lymphangioma*

EMBRYOLOGY

Lymphangiomas are congenital lesions resulting from faulty embryogenesis of the lymphatic system. They occur with equal frequency in boys and girls. Sixty-five percent of lesions are noted at birth, and 80% and 90% at 1 and 2 years of age, respectively. Ten percent of lesions present in adults. The extracranial head and neck is the site of occurrence in 75% of cases. Lymphangiomas are associated with Turner syndrome, Noonan syndrome, fetal alcohol syndrome, familial pterygium syndrome, distichiasis–lymphedema syndrome, and various chromosomal aneuploidies.

CLINICAL FEATURES

There are two main hypotheses to explain embryogenesis of the lymphatic system. The *centripetal* one states that lymphatic channels develop from rests of primitive mesenchyme and eventually communicate with the venous system. The *centrifugal* one is most widely accepted, and states that lymphatic primordia develop as direct outpouchings from the large central veins located in different regions of the body. These primordia develop into lymphatic vessels that grow into the surrounding mesenchyme and form a complicated network. The lymphatic system develops between the sixth to seventh weeks of life and is characterized by six paired primary lymph sacs that arise from the venous system. These consist of two jugular sacs arising near the junction of the anterior cardinal vein (future internal jugular vein), two iliac sacs, one retroperitoneal sac, and one cisterna chyli. Some sacs temporarily lose their connection with adjacent veins and become blind sacs. Under normal circumstances, these blind sacs later regain a venous connection. At 7.5 weeks of life, the jugular sacs connect with the recently formed paired axillary sacs to form the juguloaxillary complex. Between 8 to 9 weeks of life, there is rapid peripheral growth of the juguloaxillary complex, resulting in formation of a complex network of lymphatic vessels that extends cranially and dorsolaterally. The main juguloaxillary trunk communicates with the venous system at the confluence of the internal and external jugular veins. At 9 weeks of life, the primordia that will form the thoracic duct are present. These primordia anastomose with the left juguloaxillary complex and are continuous inferiorly with the cisterna chyli, forming the thoracic duct. By 10 weeks of life, one continuous lymphatic network has formed with its branchings paralleling the venous system. The juguloaxillary complex predominantly drains the neck and face. The axillary portion drains the thoracic inlet and axillae.

Lymphangiomas occur from a drainage defect of lymphatic channels into the venous system. This results in progressive enlargement of isolated lymphatic spaces due to accumulation of lymph. Early malformations involve the primitive jugular, subclavian, and axillary sacs and result in formation of cystic hygromas. These lesions, which occur in soft areolar tissues separated by wide fascial planes, are sharply demarcated, round, or oval lesions. Lesions composed of smaller channels occur peripherally during late embryogenesis. These malformations grow distally along narrower fascial planes and insinuate themselves along vessels and nerves. Thus, lymphatic malformations occurring in areas rich in neurovascular structures, such as the cheeks and lips, tend to contain more angiomatous components and smaller cystic spaces than cystic hygromas. The degree of obstruction and distention of the draining channels is important in the patient's prognosis. Diffuse lymphangiectasia is incompatible with life. Reestablishment of communications between the lymphatic and venous systems results in the reduction of edema and redundant overlying skin. This sequence of events is typical in patients with Down syndrome.

Lymphangiomas are classified into three forms based on the size of the anomalous lymphatic spaces. Cystic hygromas are the most common form and consists of a honeycomb of dilated lymphatic spaces lined by a single layer of flat endothelium. These lesions are often solitary and may occur in the presence of an otherwise normal lymphatic system. Seventy-five percent occur in the neck and have a predilection for the posterior compartments. Cavernous lymphangiomas are composed of mildly to moderately dilated lymphatic spaces, of a size intermediate between cystic hygromas and capillary hemangiomas. The lesions are situated in the oral cavity or salivary glands. Cavernous lymphangiomas are subcutaneous lesions that tend to penetrate adjacent muscular and neurovascular structures without destroying them. Their peripheral location and subcutaneous spread suggests a defect during the later phase of lymphatic development (9–10 weeks of life). Capillary hemangiomas (lymphangioma simplex) are composed of a network of small, thin-walled channels that are the size of normal capillaries. It is the least common form of lymphangioma. The lesions are located predominantly within the epidermis and occur anywhere throughout the body. Because of their superficial location, capillary hemangiomas are thought to form latest in development.

Lymphangiomas present as painless neck masses anywhere in the extracranial head and neck. Cystic hygromas present as soft, doughy, compressible masses in the posterior triangle of the neck. Facial lesions are more likely to be cavernous or capillary lymphangiomas and tend to enlarge with the growth of the child. This growth represents excess secretions from endothelial lining, but may also be related to endothelial proliferation. Complications include disfigurement, respiratory compromise, and recurrent infections. Surgical resection is the treatment of choice. Well defined cystic hygromas are easily resected. Lesions extending over several anatomic areas are difficult to resect and prone to recurrence. Such patients may require multiple surgeries.

IMAGING FEATURES

Both computed tomography (CT) and magnetic resonance (MR) may be used to image patients with lymphangiomas. We prefer CT for patients with lesions confined to the neck. For extensive lesions, we complement the CT with MR imaging.

It may be possible to differentiate cystic hygromas from capillary and cavernous lymphangiomas by CT. Cystic hygromas are sharply demarcated, low-attenuation lesions devoid of visible walls (Fig. 15B.07-1). They have a tendency to occur in the posterior compartment of the neck. Large lesions may be multilobular, have mass effect, and displace the carotid artery sheath and sternocleidomastoid muscle. Atrophy or invasion of this muscle is seen with cystic hygromas. Partially resected or repeatedly infected lesions may have enhancing walls or internal septations. Capillary or cavernous lymphangiomas may be found throughout the head and neck but tend to occur in the face and oral cavity (Fig. 15B.07-2). By CT, these lesions are of heterogeneous density and insinuate themselves between normal structures. Their angiomatous components enhance after contrast administration. They spread along fascial planes and may involve many compartments of the suprahyoid neck (Fig. 15B.07-3).

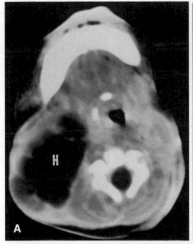

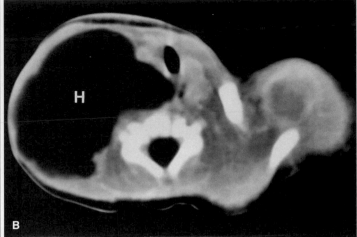

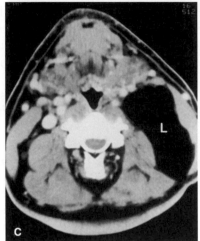

FIGURE 15B.07-1.

Cystic hygroma. **A.** Axial computed tomography (CT) shows large cystic mass (H) in the posterior triangle in the right neck. (With permission from Castillo M. Neuroradiology Companion. Philadelphia: JB Lippincott, 1995.) **B.** Axial CT at level of low neck in same patient shows inferior continuation of large cystic hygroma (H). **C.** Axial CT in a different patient shows low-attenuation mass (L) in left posterior triangle that measures −90 Hounsfield units; this is not a cyst but a lipoma. Note similarity with **A.**

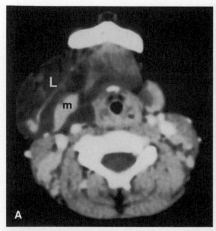

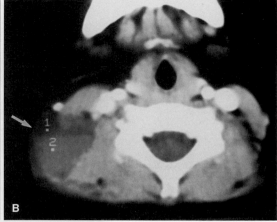

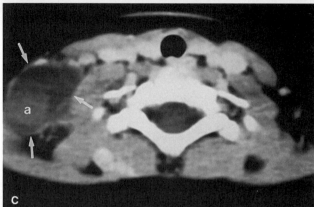

FIGURE 15B.07-2.

Lymphangioma. A. Axial computed tomography (CT) shows infiltrative lymphangioma (L) superficial to the platysma muscle and lateral and medial to the sternocleidomastoid muscle (m). **B.** Axial postcontrast CT in a different patient shows lymphangioma *(arrow)* in posterior triangle of right neck with dependent high-density (2) fluid level and low-density (1) supernatant, compatible with intratumoral hemorrhage. **C.** Axial CT in same patient shows inferior extent of lesion *(arrows)*, which contains an area (a) of slightly higher density probably related to clot or angiomatous components.

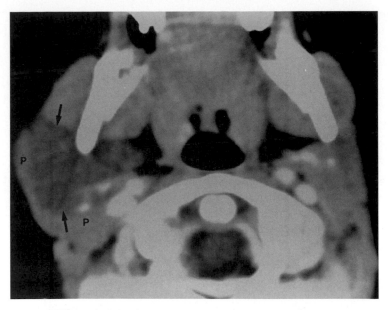

FIGURE 15B.07-3.

Intraparotid lymphangioma. Axial postcontrast computed tomography shows cystic mass *(arrows)* in right parotid gland (P). The mass involves both the superficial and deep lobes of the parotid gland.

SUGGESTED READINGS

1. Zadvinski DP, Benson MT, Kerr HH, et al. Congenital malformations of the cervicothoracic lymphatic system: embryology and pathogenesis. RadioGraphics 1992;12: 1175.
2. Batsakis JG. Vasoformative tumors. In: Tumors of the Head and Neck, 2nd ed. Baltimore: Williams & Wilkins, 1979:518.
3. Reede DL, Holliday RA, Som PM, Bergeron RT. Nonnodal pathologic conditions of the neck. In: Som PM, Bergeron RT, eds. Head and Neck Imaging, 2nd ed. St. Louis: CV Mosby, 1991:537.
4. Mulliken JB. Vascular malformations of the head and neck. In: Mulliken JB, Young AE, eds. Vascular Birthmarks: Hemangiomas and Malformations. Philadelphia: WB Saunders, 1988:301.

15B.08 *Ranula*

EPIDEMIOLOGY

Ranulas (mucoceles, pseudocysts) are cystic lesions in the floor of the mouth that result from obstruction of sublingual or minor salivary glands. The obstruction is thought to be congenital in origin. Ranulas occur in any group, but are more common in children and young adults. There is no gender predilection.

CLINICAL FEATURES

There are two types of ranulas. Simple ranulas are most common and consist of lesions contained within the floor of the mouth. These lesions are paramedian in location, usually in the sublingual gland region. Diving ranulas, either plunging or complex, arise from a ruptured simple ranula. These lesions extend inferiorly below the mylohyoid muscle, either over its free margin or directly through it.

Ranulas present as mucosal-covered masses in the floor of the mouth and may have a "frog-belly" appearance. These masses are cystic and have a transluscent bluish hue. Ranulas may occasionally rupture, expulsing a viscid fluid into the mouth. Diving ranulas present as painless, fluctuant, soft tissue neck masses. Most diving ranulas are located above the hyoid bone, although large lesions may extend into the thoracic inlet and mediastinum. Simple and diving ranulas do not contain an epithelial lining. Secreted mucus is extravasated into the floor of the mouth and dissects along fascial planes. Histologically, recently formed ranulas consist of mucin and histiocytes (mucocytes) surrounded by vascularized connective tissue. Long-standing ranulas consist of a cyst with a wall composed of vascularized connective tissue. The treatment of ranulas depends on their type. Simple ranulas are treated by marsupialization. Removal of the ipsilateral sublingual gland is associated with fewer recurrences. Diving ranulas may require widespread dissection of the floor of the mouth and the neck, depending on their extent.

IMAGING FEATURES

Computed tomography (CT) and magnetic resonance (MR) imaging may be used to evaluate patients with ranulas. MR imaging is helpful to localize the most inferior extent of a diving ranula and in identifying the mylohyoid muscle. Both CT and MR should be performed after contrast administration.

By CT, simple ranulas are well defined, low-attenuation, unilocular lesions confined to the floor of the mouth (Fig. 15B.08-1A,B). Simple ranulas conform to the fascial boundaries of the sublingual space and are bordered laterally by the mylohyoid muscle and medially by the genioglossus and geniohyoid muscles. Large ranulas have a mass effect, resulting in medial displacement of the latter muscles. The walls of the ranulas are thin, often imperceptible, and usually do not enhance after contrast administration. Complex ranulas extend into the submandibular or parapharyngeal space. Ranulas that have been repeatedly infected or have had prior surgery may contain septations or have an enhancing wall. The MR imaging appearance of ranulas is that of cystic lesions of low to intermediate signal intensity on T1-weighted images and increased signal intensity on T2-weighted images (Fig. 15B.08-1C,D). The T1 signal intensity may vary depending on the protein content of the lesion. The differential diagnosis includes dermoid, epidermoid, lymphangioma, hemangioma, and lateral thyroglossal duct cyst. The diagnosis of a ranula may be suggested if a cystic lesion with an imperceptible wall is found to be confined to the sublingual space.

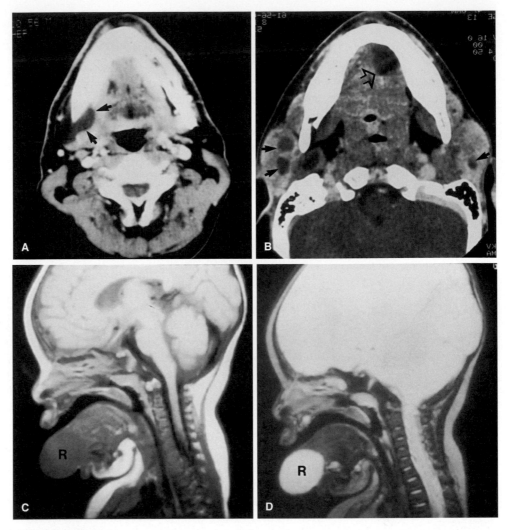

FIGURE 15B.08-1.

Ranula. **A.** Postcontrast computed tomography (CT) shows ranula *(arrows)* in right floor of the mouth. **B.** Axial postcontrast CT shows ranula *(open arrow)* in left anterior floor of the mouth and bilateral parotid cysts *(small arrows)* in a young patient with AIDS. **C.** Midsagittal magnetic resonance (MR) T1-weighted image shows ranula (R) in tip of tongue in a 5-month-old child. Presumably the lesion arises from obstruction of a minor salivary gland. **D.** Corresponding MR T2-weighted image shows ranula (R) to be hyperintense. (**C** and **D** with permission from Silverstein MI, Castillo M, Hudgins PA, Hoffman JC. MR imaging of intralingual ranula in a child. J Comput Assist Tomogr 1990;14:672.)

SUGGESTED READINGS

1. Gonzalez C. Tumors of the mouth and pharynx. In: Bluestone CD, Stool SE, Scheetz MD, eds. Pediatric Otolaryngology, Vol. 2. Philadelphia: WB Saunders, 1990:964.
2. Som PM. Salivary glands. In: Som PM, Bergeron RT, eds. Head and Neck Imaging, 2nd ed. St. Louis: CV Mosby, 1991:318.
3. Batsakis JG, McClathchy KD. Cervical ranulas. Ann Otol Rhinol Laryngol 1988;97: 561.
4. Coit WE, Harnsberger HR, Osborn AG, Smoker WRK, Stevens MH, Lufkin RB. Ranulas and their mimicks: CT evaluation. Radiology 1987;163:211.

15B.09 *Retropharyngeal Space Infection*

EPIDEMIOLOGY Retropharyngeal space infections occur almost exclusively in children younger than 6 years of age. However, its incidence has been noted to be increasing in older patients. It is more common in boys than girls (2:1). Infections in the retropharynx result from involvement of an area whose primary lymphatic drainage is to the retropharyngeal lymph nodes. These sites include the sinonasal tract, throat, tonsils, middle ears, and odontogenic disease. Occasionally, retropharyngeal infections may occur from direct innoculation as a result of trauma.

CLINICAL FEATURES The retropharyngeal space is a potential space situated between the middle and deep layers of the deep cervical fascia. Its anterior boundary is formed by the middle layer of the deep cervical fascia (visceral fascia) and its posterior boundary is formed by the alar layer of the deep cervical fascia. Laterally, it is limited by the carotid sheath. The retropharyngeal space extends from the skull base to the level at which the alar fascia fuses with the visceral fascia (C7–T2). A second potential space found posterior to the retropharyngeal space is referred to as the "danger space." This space is bounded anteriorly by the alar fascia and posteriorly by the prevertebral fascia. Superiorly, it extends to the skull base and inferiorly it is continuous with the posterior mediastinum. Because of this communication, infections involving the danger space may extend into the posterior mediastinum. Infections that involve the retropharyngeal space may enter the danger space because of their close proximity. By imaging, it is difficult to determine if an infection is located within the true retropharyngeal space or in the danger space. Therefore, mediastinal extension must be excluded in all patients. The retropharyngeal space contains fat and lymph nodes. The retropharyngeal lymph nodes are divided into lateral and medial groups. The lateral group consists of one to three nodes situated medial to the carotid artery sheath. The lateral group lies on the longus colli and longus capitus muscles behind the posterior pharyngeal wall. These lymph nodes usually extend from the skull base to C3. The medial lymph node group is inconstant and located near the midline. These nodes are located at the level of C2, although they may extend inferiorly to the C6 level. The afferent drainage of the retropharyngeal lymph nodes is from the nasopharynx, oropharynx, palate, nasal cavity, paranasal sinuses, middle ear, and eustachian tube. All of these are potential sites of infection that may extend into the retropharyngeal space. The efferent drainage is to the high internal jugular nodes (group 2).

Patients with retropharyngeal space infection present with underlying infection of the upper aerodigestive tract, which may be indistinguishable from meningitis. Symptoms include fever, chills, odynophagia, sore throat, dysphagia, nausea, vomiting, respiratory distress, and neck pain and stiffness. On physical examination, patients may be drooling and diaphoretic. Bulging of the posterior oropharyngeal wall is characteristic.

Retropharyngeal space abscesses result from infection spreading to the retropharyngeal lymph nodes, which enlarge, undergo suppuration, and develop liquefaction. Eventual rupture of purulent material contained within retropharyngeal nodes into the retropharyngeal space results in an abscess. Because of widespread use of antibiotics, the disease usually is diagnosed and treated before the development of abscesses. True retropharyngeal abscesses are now more likely caused by penetrating trauma of the oropharynx or nasopharynx, direct spread from vertebral osteomyelitis or discitis, or result from previous surgery. Treatment is surgical drainage by intraoral or open procedures, depending on the size of the abscess and clinical stability of the patient. Early imaging of retropharyngeal infections before formation of true retropharyngeal space abscesses that shows enlarged nodes with low-attenuation centers is indicative of suppurative retropharyngeal adenitis. Suppurative retropharyngeal adenitis consisting of a single lateral retropharyngeal lymph node measuring less than 2 cm and containing central liquefaction may be managed with antibiotics alone (personal communication, A. Mancuso, M.D., University of Florida, Gainesville, FL). Although traditionally it has been accepted that only 10% to 15% of retropharyngeal space infections resolve with medical therapy alone, recent experience suggests that 40% to 50% of patients can be successfully treated without the need for surgical drainage. Successfully treated patients show clinical improvement within 24 to 48 hours.

IMAGING FEATURES   The initial diagnostic evaluation of patients suspected of having retropharyngeal space infections usually consists of lateral neck radiographs during inspiration. Fluoroscopy may be helpful in patients in whom true inspiratory films are difficult to obtain. Presence of prevertebral swelling, loss of the normal cervical lordosis, and air in the prevertebral soft tissues are suggestive of infection. Exact location and extension cannot be determined by radiographs alone. Computed tomography (CT) and magnetic resonance (MR) imaging permit accurate localization of infections and help separate infections limited to retropharyngeal lymph nodes from those involving the retropharyngeal space, thereby differentiating true abscesses from suppurative adenitis with retropharyngeal space edema. We prefer CT as the imaging modality for use in these patients.

Retropharyngeal abscesses consist of midline low-attenuation masses with enhancing walls (Figs. 15B.09-1 and 15B.09-2). The lesions have mass effect and displace the posterior pharyngeal wall. Abscesses resulting from adjacent discitis are continuous with the adjacent disc space and there is erosion of neighboring vertebral body end plates (Fig. 15B.09-3). Suppurative retropharyngeal adenitis is characterized by an enlarged retropharyngeal lymph node containing a low-attenuation center (Fig. 15B.09-4). Low attenuation centrally within a lymph node does not necessarily indicate presence of pus. Low-attenuation centers may be present in nodes containing only early liquefaction (presuppurative phase) and those that have undergone liquefaction necrosis (suppurative phase). Suppurative retropharyngeal adenitis is often associated with edema of the retropharyngeal space. Edema is characterized by smooth expansion of the retropharyngeal space without an enhancing rim (Fig. 15B.09-5). The zone of edema is about 7 to 8 mm in anteroposterior diameter.

Ultrasonography may be used to differentiate solid lesions from complex fluid collections in the retropharynx. However, ultrasound may be unable to determine if fluid collections are within enlarged lymph nodes or the retropharyngeal space. CT and MR imaging permit localization of areas of liquefaction and allow differentiation between suppurative adenitis and retropharyngeal adenitis.

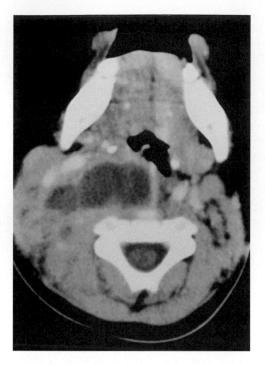

FIGURE 15B.09-1.

Retropharyngeal space abscess. Postcontrast computed tomography shows large low-attenuation mass in the retropharyngeal space with peripheral enhancement. (With permission from Castillo M. Neuroradiology Companion. Philadelphia: JB Lippincott, 1995.)

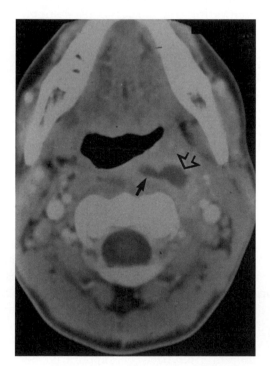

FIGURE 15B.09-2.

Suppurative adenitis with early abscess. Axial postcontrast computed tomography shows low attenuation in retropharyngeal lymph node *(open arrow)*, which has ruptured medially, producing a small abscess *(solid small arrow)* in the retropharyngeal space. There is wall enhancement. (With permission from Castillo M. Neuroradiology Companion. Philadelphia: JB Lippincott, 1995.)

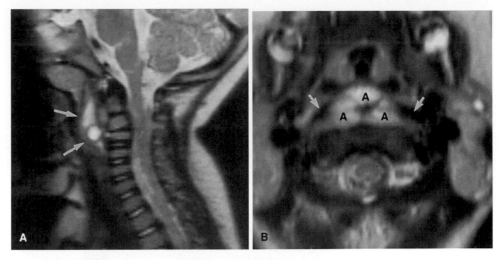

FIGURE 15B.09-3.

Prevertebral abscess. **A.** Midsagittal magnetic resonance (MR) T2-weighted image shows prevertebral space high–signal-intensity collection *(arrows)* secondary to discitis. Note collapse of C2–C3 disc space, cervical kyphosis, and high signal intensity from C2 and C3 vertebral bodies secondary to edema. **B.** Axial MR T2-weighted image in the same patient shows high–signal-intensity abscess (A) displacing the longus colli muscles *(arrows)* anteriorly.

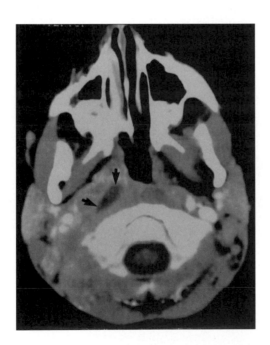

FIGURE 15B.09-4.

Suppurative adenitis. Axial postcontrast computed tomography shows area of low attenuation *(arrows)* in region of right retropharyngeal lymph node. Note lack of enhancing walls.

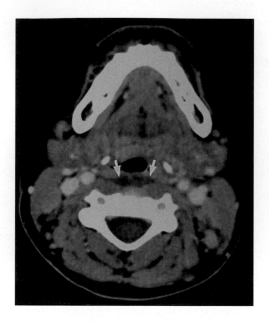

FIGURE 15B.09-5.

Retropharyngeal space edema. Axial postcontrast computed tomography shows low density *(arrows)* in the retropharyngeal space. There is no peripheral enhancement, which would suggest an abscess rather than edema.

SUGGESTED READINGS

1. Grodinsky M. Retropharyngeal and lateral pharyngeal space abscesses: an anatomical and clinical study with review of the literature. Am J Surg 1979;110:179.
2. Gianoli GJ, Espinola TE, Guarisco JL, Miller RH. Retropharyngeal space infection: changing trends. Otolaryngol Head Neck Surg 1991;105:92.
3. Batsakis JG, Sneige N. Parapharyngeal and retropharyngeal space disease. Ann Otol Rhinol Laryngol 1989;98:320.

15B.10 *Infectious Cervical Adenitis*

EPIDEMIOLOGY

In children, enlarged cervical lymph nodes are most commonly caused by an associated infectious process rather than malignancy. The term "cervical adenitis" denotes inflammation of lymph nodes secondary to infection. "Suppurative adenitis" indicates infected nodes that have undergone liquefactive necrosis. The likelihood of development of cervical adenitis, especially suppurative, decreases with age, although its incidence is increasing in older patients.

CLINICAL FEATURES

Lymph nodes form by dilation of primitive lymphatic sacs. Development begins during early fetal life and continues to early neonatal life. The lymphatic system comprises lymphocytes and epithelial and stromal elements. Lymphocytes develop from stem cells of the primary lymphoid tissues. T lymphocytes arise in the thymus, whereas B lymphocytes are produced in fetal liver and bone marrow. These cells then migrate into secondary lymphoid structures, which include lymph nodes, Peyer patches (intestine), spleen, tonsils, and adenoids. Within the lymph nodes, the T cells outnumber B cells, with the latter cells predominantly located in the cortex and the former cells located in the paracortex.

Pathologically, infective agents spread into surrounding tissues and are partially inactivated by the host's immune response. A portion of the infective agent is passively drained into afferent lymphatic channels and nodes, resulting in activation of T and B lymphocytes. This results in formation of multiple germinal centers and active cell proliferation and enlargement of nodes. Stimulated nodes are often referred to as reactive lymph nodes. Ongoing infection eventually results in nodal necrosis (suppurative adenitis).

Approximately 300 of 800 lymph nodes in the body are located in the extracranial head and neck. Occipital nodes consist of 3 to 12 nodes located at the junction of the nape of the neck and the lower cranial vault. The afferent drainage of these nodes is from the occipital region and the efferent drainage is primarily to spinal accessory nodes. Nuchal nodes consist of one to three nodes near the origin of the trapezius muscle (they are typically enlarged in patients with infectious mononucleosis). Mastoid nodes consist of one to four nodes posterior to the ear in the mastoid region, and are commonly found in children. These nodes drain the parietal area and a portion of the skin of the auricle. The efferent drainage is to inferior parotid nodes and the internal jugular chain. Facial nodes consist of five groups in the subcutaneous plane of the face, and are located along the course of the branches of the external maxillary artery and tributaries of the facial vein. The five specific groups of nodes are the mandibular, buccinator, infraorbital, malar, and retrozygomatic. This group of nodes drains the eyelids, cheek, and midportion of the face, including the gingiva, gums, and palate. The efferent drainage comprises the submandibular, parotid, and internal jugular nodes. Retropharyngeal nodes drain the nasopharynx, oropharynx, palate, nasal fossa, paranasal sinuses, and middle ear. The efferent drainage is to the internal jugular veins. The parotid nodes consist of 7 to 19 nodes situated throughout the gland. Parotid nodes are often found in the subcapsular region, pretragal region, parotid tail, and course of the retromandibular vein. Territory drained by these nodes includes the forehead, temporal region, lateral portions of the face, external ear, external auditory canal, eustachian tube, cheek, and gingiva. The parotid gland also receives lymphatic drainage from occipital and facial nodes. The efferent drainage is to the internal jugular chain. Sublingual nodes are inconstant nodes divided into medial and lateral groups. The lateral group is located along the anterior lingual blood vessels and the medial group is located between the genioglossus muscles. The afferent drainage is from the floor of the mouth and the efferent drainage is into the submandibular and internal jugular nodes. A system based on the location of clinically palpable nodes divides them into seven major groups and levels. Group I consists of submental and submandibular nodes. Groups II to IV are the internal jugular lymph nodes. Specifically, group II nodes are adjacent to the carotid artery sheath between the skull base and the junction of the facial vein with the internal jugular vein (in most patients, at the level of the hyoid bone). These nodes are sometimes referred to as the jugulodigastric group. Group III nodes are an extension of the same chain and are located between the hyoid bone and where the omohyoid muscle crosses the jugular vein, usually at the level of the cricoid cartilage. Group IV comprise internal jugular nodes inferior to the cricoid cartilage. Group V consists of the nodes previously referred to as "spinal accessory" or "posterior traingle" nodes. These nodes follow the course of the spinal accessory nerve. Superiorly, these nodes are inseparable from those of group II, but unlike the internal jugular chain, which descends vertically, group II nodes descend in an oblique manner in the posterolateral neck. Groups VI and VII consist of nodes previously known as the anterior cervical nodes, and consist of anterior jugular chain and the juxtavisceral nodes. Group VI nodes are associated with the thyroid gland. Group VII consists of various nodes in the tracheoesophageal groove and superior mediastinum.

The most common cause of lymph node enlargement in children is viral infections of the upper respiratory tract. Infectious mononucleosis is characterized by generalized lymphadenopathy, weakness, fever, and malaise. The tonsils are enlarged and have a characteristic gray membrane. Epstein-Barr virus is the agent responsible, and full recovery usually occurs in 2 to 4 weeks. Infection with cytomegalovirus and varicella-zoster virus also causes generalized node enlargement. Other causes of cervical lymph node enlargement include adenovirus, rhinovirus, enterovirus, and herpes simplex virus infections. Acquired immunodeficiency syndrome (AIDS) is caused by a human T-cell lymphotrophic virus (HTLV-III), with 78% of affected children born to parents who are at risk or who have the disease. Approximately 55% of infected children will die from the disease. Patients infected by congenital transmission manifest symptoms during the first year of life. Symptoms include localized or generalized lymphadenopathy, thrush, parotid swelling, interstitial pneumonitis, hepatosplenomegaly, and diarrhea. Patients are at increased risk for bacterial superinfection, including meningitis and sepsis. Infections with *Pneumocystis carinii*, toxoplasmosis, and fungi, or development of Kaposi sarcoma and non-Hodgkin lymphoma are suggestive of AIDS.

Bacterial infections are the most common cause of suppurative cervical adenitis, with *Staphylococcus aureus* and group A streptococci being the most common agents. Infected patients present with upper respiratory tract infections. Early in the course of infection, discrete nodes are palpable. With uncontrolled infection, firm nodes are replaced by fluctuant masses (suppurative adenitis). Patients are febrile, and may require hospitalization and possible drainage of suppurative nodes. Other bacterial infections that may result in suppurative nodes include *Strepotococcus pyogenes*, group B streptococci, and *Pseudomonas aeruginosa*. Cervical adenitis may also be caused by mycobacteria, the most common of which is *Mycobacterium tuberculosis*. Suppurative nodes are commonly associated with pulmonary disease and hilar adenopathy. Patients present with multiple matted bilateral cervical nodes in the low neck. A similar picture is occasionally seen in patients with atypical *Mycobacterium* infection. Specific agents include *M avium*, *M scrofulaceum*, and *M intracellulare.* Unlike with *M tuberculosis* infection, there usually is no evidence of pulmonary disease in these patients. Less common bacterial infections producing cervical adenitis include tularemia, plague, and brucellosis.

Cat scratch disease is a common cause of enlarged cervical lymph nodes in children, reported to cause 73% of histologically sampled neck masses in the pediatric population. The disorder is caused by the cat-scratch bacillus and presents 3 to 10 days after inoculation. Prior history of a cat scratch is obtained in 72% of cases. Patients present with tender, enlarged cervical lymph nodes, and fever and malaise. Diagnosis is confirmed by a positive cat-scratch antigen or demonstration of the bacillus on a Warthin-Starry stain of infected material. Treatment is with cefoxitin.

IMAGING FEATURES   Computed tomography (CT) is preferred to image patients suspected of having suppurative cervical lymphadenitis. In general, the cervical lymph nodes in children are larger than those of adults. Thus, the standard measurements used to determine nodal enlargement are not entirely applicable for children. Normal internal jugular chain nodes may be as large as 25 mm in diameter. Presence of central foci of decreased attenuation that are not related to the fatty hili is abnormal. The normal fatty hili are minute and eccentrically located. They disappear early after the onset of infection. Normal retropharyngeal nodes are seen by CT in approximately two-thirds of young children (Fig. 15B.10-1). Magnetic resonance (MR) imaging detects normal retropharyngeal nodes in over 90% of young children. Lateral retropharyngeal lymph nodes are more commonly visualized with CT or MR imaging than are the medial ones. Normal retropharyngeal lymph nodes are round, homogeneous, and hyperintense on T2-weighted images. These nodes involute with age. The average size of retropharyngeal lymph nodes in patients younger than 18 years of age averages 6.8 mm (range, 2.1–12.0 mm). In patients older than 18 years of age, they average 4.9 mm (range, 2.2–7.4 mm; personal communication, R. Tart, M.D. and A. Mancuso, M.D., University of Florida, Gainesville, FL). Enlarged facial nodes are seen with lymphoma or recurrent tumors draining to these nodes. Infection is an extremely unusual cause of enlarged facial or parotid nodes. Enlarged parotid lymph nodes usually occur in the presence of a systemic abnormality such as rheumatologic disease, or cancer regions draining to intraparotid nodes.

Involvement by infection is characterized early by homogeneous enlargement, loss of fatty hilum, and increased enhancement of involved nodes (Fig. 15B.10-2). The term "reactive" is often used to describe infected nodes. Continued infection may result in liquefaction necrosis (suppurative adenitis). These nodes contain a focus of decreased CT attenuation. Usually, this central focus represents liquefaction necrosis; however, low attenuation is also present before frank liquefaction (suppurative phase). Aspiration at this stage is unsuccessful. Ultrasound may help in identifying nodes that may be successfully aspirated. Suppurative cervical lymph nodes may be large and compress adjacent structures. Septic patients may require drainage guided by ultrasound or CT. Reticulation of the adjacent fat seen on CT or the presence of a circumferential enhancing rim may be indicative of inflammation rather than metastases. Ruptured nodes may lead to abscesses.

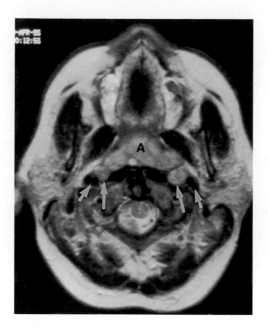

FIGURE 15B.10-1.

Normal retropharyngeal nodes. Axial magnetic resonance T2-weighted image shows normal size and homogeneous lateral retropharyngeal nodes *(longer arrows)* located medial to the internal carotid arteries *(smaller arrows)*. The adenoidal tissues (A) are prominent.

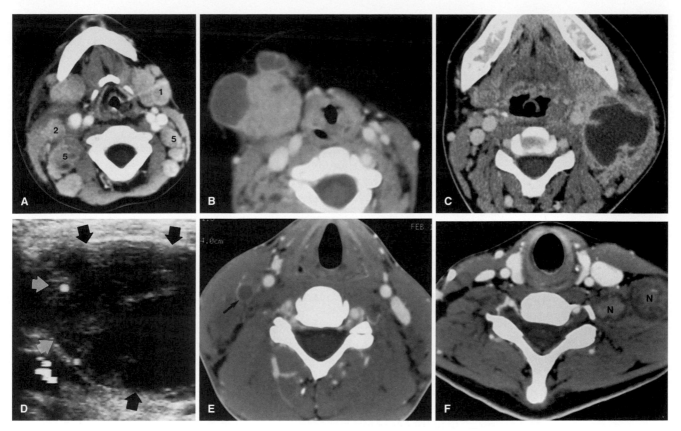

FIGURE 15B.10-2.

Lymphadenopathy at different stages, and mimicking lesions. **A.** Axial postcontrast computed tomography (CT) shows enlarged nodes at levels I (1), II (2), and V (5). The right-sided level V node contains areas of low density, suggesting early liquefaction. **B.** Axial postcontrast CT in a different patient shows frank suppurative adenitis in right submandibular region. Note central low density and enhancing peripheral wall in this case of cryptococcal adenitis. **C.** In a different patient, axial postcontrast CT shows frank abscess formation in left level II node. **D.** Sonogram of same node shows echolucent center *(arrows)* compatible with fluid (pus) contents, indicating that this node is drainable. **E.** Axial postcontrast CT shows a thrombosed right internal jugular vein *(arrow)* that could be confused with a suppurative or necrotic lymph node. **F.** Axial postcontrast CT shows masses (N) that could be confused with enlarged transverse chain nodes, but are nerve sheath tumors in brachial plexus of patient with neurofibromatosis type I.

SUGGESTED READINGS

1. Stanievich JF. Cervical adenopathy. In: Bluestone CD, Stool SE, Scheetz MD, eds. Pediatric Otolaryngology, Vol. 2. Philadelphia: WB Saunders, 1990:1317.
2. Som PM. Lymph nodes of the neck. Radiology 1987;165:593.
3. Rouviere H. Lymphatic system of the head and neck. In: Tobias MJ (trans). Anatomy of the Human Lymphatic System. Ann Arbor, MI: Edwards Brothers, 1938:5.
4. Mancuso AA, Harnsberger HR, Muraki AS, Stevens MH. Computed tomography of the cervical and retropharyngeal lymph nodes: normal anatomy, variants of normal, and applications in staging head and neck cancer: I. normal anatomy. Radiology 1983;148:709.
5. Tart RP, Mukherji SK, Avino AJ, Stringer SP, Mancuso AA. Facial nodes: normal and abnormal appearance. Radiology 1993;188:695.

15B.11 *Lymphoma*

EPIDEMIOLOGY

Malignancies are the second most common cause of death in children, after trauma. Twenty-five percent of childhood tumors involve the head and neck, whereas 5% of tumors arise in this area. Hodgkin disease and other lymphomas are the most likely neoplasms to arise in the extracranial head and neck. Factors that increase a child's risk for malignancy are family history of tumor, prior radiation therapy, immunosuppression, and exposure to carcinogenic agents. Survival of children with neck malignancies, particularly lymphoma and some sarcomas, has improved over the last 20 years.

CLINICAL FEATURES

The most common presentation is that of an asymptomatic mass. Other findings include headache, nasal congestion, rhinorrhea, otalgia, otorrhea, stridor, and lymphadenopathy. Symptoms such as hemoptysis, dysphagia, dyspnea, and a change in voice may indicate an aggressive process.

Hodgkin disease is a lymphoproliferative disorder predominantly affecting adolescents and young adults, and rarely seen in children younger than 5 years of age. Boys are more frequently affected than girls (2:1). In 90% of patients, Hodgkin disease arises in lymph nodes. Its diagnosis is strongly suggested by presence of Reed-Sternberg cells in nodes. Extranodal primary sites are unusual, and systemic involvement results from progression of the disease. Commonly affected organs include liver, spleen, lung, bone, and bone marrow. The most common extranodal site is the spleen. Hepatic involvement usually occurs in the presence of splenic involvement. Bone marrow involvement results from hematogenous spread. Pulmonary involvement is caused by direct involvement from hilar or mediastinal lymph nodes. The region of Waldeyer's ring is not often involved.

Non-Hodgkin lymphoma is a lymphoproliferative disorder most commonly seen in children between 2 to 12 years of age. Boys are more commonly affected than girls. Predisposing conditions include various congenital and acquired immunodeficiency states. The most commonly used classification systems are those of Rappaport, and Lukes and Collins. The former is based on the resemblance of the various types of malignant cells to their benign counterparts, whereas the latter is based on immunologic markers that separate cells into B-cell, T-cell, and histiocytic types. This disorder commonly arises in lymph nodes; however, extranodal sites are common in children. Primary extranodal sites include the nasopharynx, skin, bone, ileocecal region, breast, ovary, and parotid gland. Diagnosis is based on nodal excision or biopsy. Most patients have advanced disease at presentation.

Burkitt lymphoma is a rapidly proliferating form of non-Hodgkin lymphoma occurring in two forms, African and American. It is seen almost exclusively in children. Histologically, it has a "starry-sky pattern" characterized by large macrophages interspersed among a diffuse background of undifferentiated cells containing small, noncleaved nuclei, and discrete rims of amphophillic cytoplasm. The African form is endemic and characterized by a distinct geographic distribution. Almost all patients with this form have high antibody titers to Epstein-Barr virus. Eighty to 90% of tumor cells contain copies of this virus genome. In the African form, the face and jaw are most commonly affected. The American form does not have as strong a link with Epstein-Barr virus. Only 15% to 20% of patients have evidence of previous infection with this virus. Palpable abdominal masses or intestinal obstruction are the most frequent symptoms. Cervical nodes may be affected, but facial and mandibular masses are rare in the American form. Burkitt lymphoma has a good prognosis, with over 90% of patients demonstrating a complete response to treatment and a 2-year survival rate of 50%. Small tumor volume and younger age at presentation are favorable factors.

IMAGING FEATURES Computed tomography (CT) and magnetic resonance (MR) imaging may be used to evaluate patients suspected of having lymphoma. By CT, lymph nodes involved by lymphoma are homogeneous, large, and have a thin enhancing rim (Fig. 15B.11-1). Extracapsular penetration or fixation to adjacent soft tissue or vascular structures is unusual. Small enhancing internal septa may be present in larger nodes. Necrosis is rarely present even in large nodes, unless the patient has been previously treated. Involvement of the extranodal soft tissues by lymphoma is characterized by homogeneously enhancing masses often centered in muscles. These masses are of similar CT attenuation and MR imaging characteristics to those of surrounding muscles. They typically show homogeneous enhancement after contrast administration. Their margins are well defined, but occasionally they infiltrate surrounding structures. Characteristically, bone may be remodeled by an adjacent mass. Aggressive and permeative bone destruction may occasionally be present.

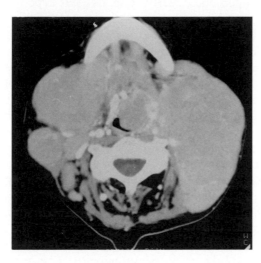

FIGURE 15B.11-1.

Hodgkin lymphoma. Axial postcontrast computed tomography shows massive bilateral neck adenopathy. Note that nodes are well demarcated and enhance homogeneously. In this case, the airway is also involved.

SUGGESTED READING

1. Myers EN, Cunningham MJ. Tumors of the neck. In: Bluestone CD, Stool SE, Scheetz MD, eds. Pediatric Otolaryngology, Vol. 2. Philadelphia: WB Saunders, 1990:1339.

15B.12 *Sarcoma and Rare Tumors*

EPIDEMIOLOGY

Rhabdomyosarcoma is the most common sarcoma in children and the most common soft tissue tumor arising in the pediatric head and neck. There is a bimodal peak for age of onset (2–6 and 14–18 years of age) and a male predilection (2:1). Approximately 43% of cases are found before 5 years of age, and most present before 12 years of age.

Fibrosarcoma is the second most common sarcoma in children, with 15% to 20% of cases occurring in the head and neck. Infants and young children are most commonly affected in the pediatric age group.

CLINICAL FEATURES

Rhabdomyosarcoma is divided into four separate types that have distinct age predilections. The less differentiated embryonal and botyroid types are more common in infants and children. This shared age disposition occurs because the botyroid type, a variant of the embryonal type, occurs when the latter expands in an open body cavity. The alveolar type is seen predominantly in adolescents. The well differentiated pleomorphic type occurs in adults. Histologically, rhabdomyosarcoma is characterized by small, dark, spindle-shaped cells and small, round, blue cells within a loose myxoid background tissue. Their most common locations in the head and neck are the orbits, nasopharynx, middle ear and mastoid, and sinonasal region (Fig. 15B.12-1). These tumors may disseminate by hematogenous and lymphatic spread. The upper cervical nodes are commonly involved in orbital and nasopharyngeal primaries. Distal metastases occur to lungs, bones, and bone marrow. Treatment depends on primary site and clinicopathologic staging as determined by the Intergroup Rhabdomyosarcoma Study.

The extremities are most commonly involved by fibrosarcomas. In the head and neck they are found in the sinonasal region, face, cheeks, larynx, and hypopharynx. The lesion consists of malignant fibroblasts associated with reticulum and collagen production. Metastases are infrequent. Complete excision is the treatment of choice. Aggressive fibromatosis is a locally aggressive lesion involving the neck. Histologically, it may be confused with fibrosarcoma and has a recurrence rate of 50% to 75%. Bone involvement is occasionally present. The low signal intensity on magnetic resonance (MR) T1- and T2-weighted images due to the fibrous component may suggest the diagnosis. Fibromatosis colli is a benign condition characterized by diffuse or focal enlargement of the sternocleidomastoid muscle. The lesion is typically found 2 or more weeks after birth and is often associated with a history of birth trauma. Spontaneous resolution is the rule, and may be hastened by stretching exercises. Complete resolution occurs 4 to 8 months thereafter, but 10% of patients require surgery. Cervicothoracic lipoblastomatosis is a very unusual benign lesion most frequently seen in the extremities. The lesion is composed of mature and immature fat cells. Histologically, two-thirds of these lesions are encapsulated and one-third are unencapsulated and infiltrative. Less common sarcomas occurring in the head and neck in children include synovial cell sarcoma, leiomyosarcoma, liposarcoma, alveolar soft part sarcoma, malignant fibrous histiocytoma, rhabdoid tumor, and hemangiopericytoma (Fig. 15B.12-2). Ewing sarcoma, chondrosarcoma, and some osteosarcomas have a predilection for the mandible (Figs. 15B.12-3–15B.12-5). Patients with advanced neurofibromatosis are at increased risk for development of neurofibrosarcomas. These lesions tend to be more aggressive in patients with neurofibromatosis, as opposed to those that occur sporadically. The incidence of Kaposi sarcoma in children and adolescents is increasing because of AIDS.

Neuroblastoma is a common childhood malignancy that is slightly more common in boys. Children 2 to 4 years of age are most commonly affected, and 90% of cases involve those younger than 10 years of age. Most cases involving the head and neck are metastases from primary abdominal lesions, and only 2% to 4% of lesions arise primarily in the neck. Common sites of metastases are the skull, orbits, and cervical lymph nodes. Systemic metastases occur to bones, liver, lungs, and lymph nodes. This tumor arises from undifferentiated neural crest cells that are thought to be precursors of the sympathetic nervous system. Neck involvement occurs along the sympathetic chain. Affected children present with unilateral Horner syndrome, opisthotonos, and an ipsilateral, firm, nontender neck mass. Compression of cranial nerves IX through XII may cause respiratory distress and feeding difficulties. Neuroblastoma is associated with elevated levels of urine vanillylmandelic acid. Treatment and prognosis depend on stage and age of patients at initial diagnosis.

Squamous cell carcinoma comprises 4% of tumors of the upper aerodigestive tract in children. The nasopharynx is the most common site. This tumor is classified by the World Health Organization into keratinizing, nonkeratinizing, and undifferentiated forms. The term "lymphoepithelioma" describes the histologic appearance of normal lymphoid cells and malignant undifferentiated squamous cell carcinoma, and is the predominant form seen in children and young adults. At times, differentiation between squamous cell carcinoma, neuroblastoma, and non-Hodgkin lymphoma may be difficult. Most patients present with cervical nodal metastases, particularly to the retropharyngeal nodes and groups II, III, and V. Nasopharyngeal squamous cell carcinoma may spread intracranially by either direct invasion of the skull base or perineural spread, particularly along the third division of the trigeminal nerve. Squamous cell carcinoma of the nasopharynx is unresectable but amenable to irradiation, chemotherapy, or both.

Paragangliomas are occasionally seen in children, particularly those with Von Hippel-Lindau syndrome, in whom they are often multiple. These tumors may occur in the carotid artery sheath. Clinical and radiographic differentiation between paragangliomas in this location and schwannomas may be difficult.

The incidence of thyroid carcinoma has decreased since its association with radiation exposure was first noted in the 1950s. Children exposed to low-level radiation are at increased risk for both benign and malignant thyroid gland tumors. Irradiation is associated with increased risk for multicentric thyroid tumors; however, the natural course of radiation-induced papillary and follicular carcinomas is not different from those that occur spontaneously.

Salivary gland malignancies in children are uncommon. Mucoepidermoid carcinoma is the most common pediatric salivary gland tumor, followed by acinic cell carcinoma, adenoid cystic carcinoma, adenocarcinoma, pleomorphic adenoma, and rare sarcomas. Most salivary gland malignancies in children arise in the parotid gland and present as asymptomatic masses. Ominous findings include progressive facial palsy, progressive tumor growth, and cervical adenopathy. Other lesions occurring in the parotid gland include melanoma and basal cell carcinoma.

IMAGING FEATURES

Computed tomography (CT) and MR imaging may be used to evaluate children with tumors of the upper aerodigestive tract. We prefer MR imaging. However, CT is ideal for detecting early skull base erosion in patients with nasopharyngeal tumors (Figs. 15B.12-3–15B.12-5). CT is also useful for assessment of node involvement. Imaging features of sarcomas and carcinomas are nonspecific. Most present as advanced lesions with cervical lymph node metastases. These tumors are aggressive and infiltrate and invade surrounding soft tissue and bones. They often are solid and show homogeneous contrast enhancement. Internal calcification and growth along the course of the sympathetic chain is typical of a neuroblastoma. The presence of flow voids in a lesion (larger than 2 cm in diameter) in the carotid artery sheath is typical of paragangliomas, but may be seen in hypervascular schwannomas.

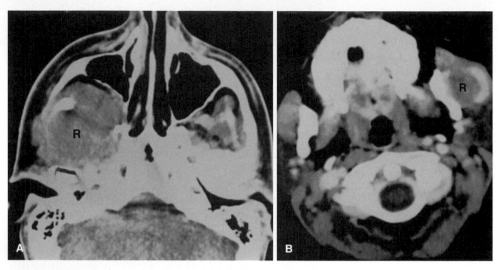

FIGURE 15B.12-1.

Rhabdomyosarcoma. **A.** Axial computed tomography (CT) shows homogeneous mass (R) in right infratemporal fossa. **B.** Axial postcontrast CT shows rhabdomyosarcoma (R) arising from left masseter muscle.

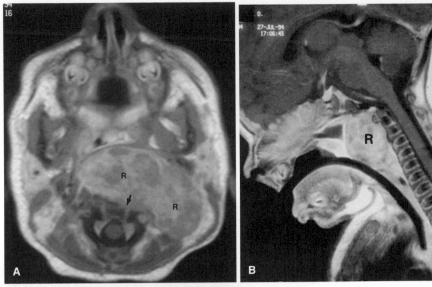

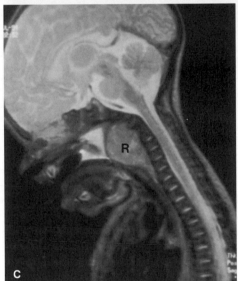

FIGURE 15B.12-2.

Rhabdoid tumor. **A.** Axial postcontrast magnetic resonance (MR) T1-weighted image shows large and somewhat inhomogeneous mass (R) in the precervical region and extending into left posterior neck. Note erosion *(arrow)* of C2 vertebral body. **B.** Midsagittal postcontrast MR T1-weighted image in same patient shows mass (R) to occlude airway in posterior nasopharynx. **C.** Corresponding MR T2-weighted image shows mass (R) to be relatively hypointensc, suggesting high cellularity, which was confirmed histologically.

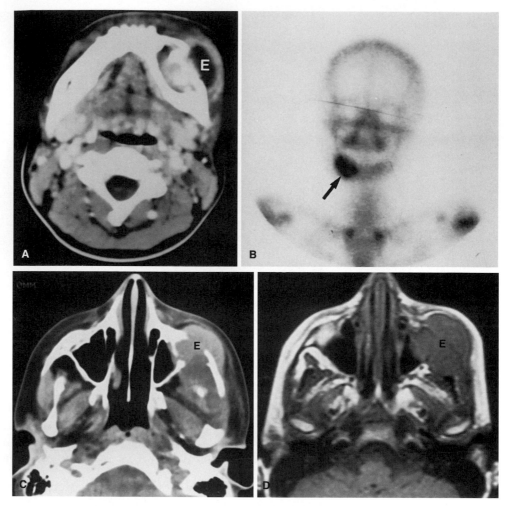

FIGURE 15B.12-3.

Ewing sarcoma. **A.** Axial postcontrast computed tomography (CT) shows mass arising in left mandible with erosion of bone and necrosis (E). **B.** Frontal view of radionuclide bone scan in same patient shows increased uptake *(arrow)* by tumor. **C.** In a different patient, CT shows soft tissue mass (E) arising at juncture of left zygomatic arch and maxillary sinus. There is destruction of the anterior aspect of the zygomatic arch and lateral and anterior walls of the maxillary sinus. **D.** Noncontrast magnetic resonance T1-weighted image shows clearly the soft tissue boundaries of this Ewing sarcoma (E).

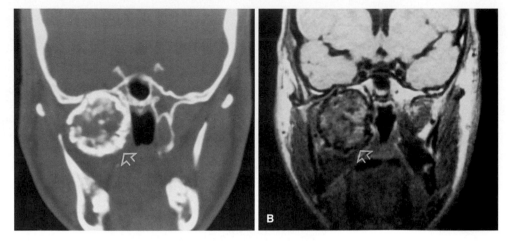

FIGURE 15B.12-4.

Chondrosarcoma. **A.** Coronal computed tomography (bone window settings) shows heavily calcified mass *(arrow)* in right infratemporal fossa. **B.** Corresponding coronal magnetic resonance T1-weighted image shows that mass *(arrow)* is inhomogeneous internally but contains a rim of low signal intensity, reflecting calcifications.

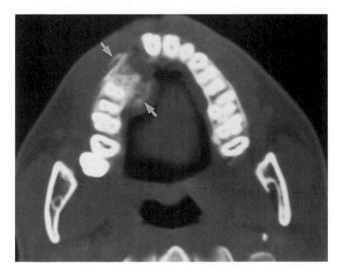

FIGURE 15B.12-5.

Osteosarcoma. Axial computed tomography shows destructive lesion involving the medial aspect of the right maxilla. Note periosteal reaction *(arrows)* along the gingival and buccal surfaces of this osteosarcoma.

SUGGESTED
READINGS

1. Jaffe B, Jaffe N. Head and neck tumors in children. Pediatrics 1973;51:731.
2. Vazquez E, Enriquez G, Castellote A, et al. US, CT, and MR imaging of neck lesions in children. RadioGraphics 1995;15:105.

15B.13 *Teratoma*

EPIDEMIOLOGY

Teratomas are tumors of germ cell origin consisting of elements derived from all three germ cell layers. Approximately 7% to 9% of teratomas occur in the head and neck. Their incidence is 1:4000 births. Teratomas may arise in the neck, paranasal sinuses, nasopharynx, orbit, and pharynx. Teratomas arising in the neck are present at birth. Most teratomas are benign; however, malignant teratomas occasionally occur. The risk of malignancy is significantly increased in patients who have undergone prior resection, and may be as high as 20%. Teratomas arising in the nasopharynx have a strong female predilection (6:1). There is no gender predilection for teratomas elsewhere in the neck. About 20% of cervical teratomas are associated with maternal hydramnios.

CLINICAL FEATURES

Most neck teratomas present as large masses that often cross the midline and involve the contralateral side. They are usually between 5 to 12 cm in diameter. Affected infants have symptoms of respiratory obstruction (stridor, cyanosis, and apnea) due to deviation and compression of the trachea. Compression of the esophagus may result in dysphagia. The high incidence of maternal polyhydramnios may in part be caused by inability of the fetus to swallow amniotic fluid.

Teratomas tend to occur in the region of the thyroid gland, suggesting that they may be of thyroid origin. Currently, it is debatable whether involvement of the thyroid gland is the result of invasion by an adjacent lesion, or whether the lesion actually arises from the thyroid gland. Teratomas may, however, arise elsewhere, and we have seen two cases in the lower face.

Treatment of choice for head and neck teratomas is surgical excision. Early resection is essential for proper management. Delays may result in progression of respiratory symptoms and lead to atelectasis and pneumonia. Respiratory obstruction is the leading cause of death in patients with large cervical teratomas. After treatment, careful follow-up is required because of an increased risk of malignancy regardless of the initial location and histologic status of the mass. Malignant degeneration results from de-differentiation of the remaining teratomatous elements.

IMAGING FEATURES

Computed tomography (CT) is preferred for imaging patients with cervical teratomas because it readily detects calcifications and fat within the lesion. Teratomas are large, bulky, heterogeneous masses containing solid and cystic components (Figs. 15B.13-1 and 15B.13-2). Tumors are typically located adjacent to the thyroid gland and are often surrounded by an enhancing rim (Fig. 15B.13-1). The lesions are unilateral but may extend into the contralateral side of the neck and into the thoracic inlet. Presence of fat and calcifications is characteristic (Fig. 15B.13-2B). The CT attenuation of fluid components depends on the amount of protein and fat within the lesion. Magnetic resonance imaging findings are also those of a heterogeneous mass. Signal intensity characteristics of the lesion are variable and reflect the findings on CT.

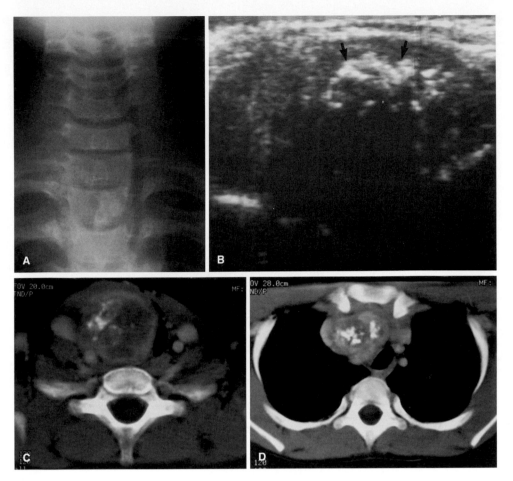

FIGURE 15B.13-1.

Cervical teratoma. **A.** Frontal radiograph shows tracheal air column deviated toward the left. **B.** Transverse sonogram shows that lesion contains some calcifications *(arrows).* **C.** Axial postcontrast computed tomography (CT) at similar level as **B** shows mass containing areas of low density and calcifications. Note significant displacement of the airway. **D.** Axial CT in same patient shows extension of the mass into the upper mediastinum. (Case courtesy of L. Fordham, M.D., University of North Carolina, Chapel Hill, NC.)

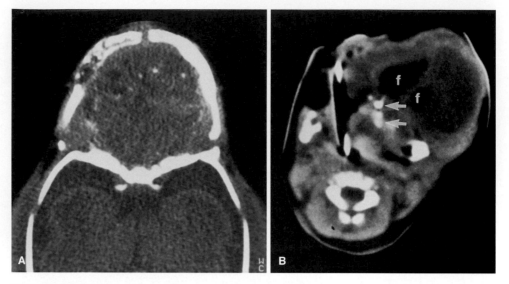

FIGURE 15B.13-2.

Facial teratoma. **A.** Nearly coronal noncontrast computed tomography (CT) shows large expansile mass in lower face. Presumably, this teratoma arose from the midline maxilla. The mass has extended inferiorly and destroys parts of the mandible. The tumor contains areas of both low and high attenuation (punctate calcifications). **B.** Axial noncontrast CT shows large left facial teratoma containing fat (f) and calcifications *(arrows)*. The airway is compressed and deviated; the patient is intubated.

SUGGESTED READINGS

1. Myers EN, Cunningham MJ. Tumors of the neck. In: Bluestone CD, Stool SE, Scheetz MD, eds. Pediatric Otolaryngology, Vol. 2. Philadelphia: WB Saunders, 1990:1359.
2. Batsakis JG. Teratomas of the head and neck. In: Tumors of the Head and Neck, 2nd ed. Baltimore: Williams & Wilkins, 1979:230.
3. Som PM, Sacher M, Lanzieri CF, et al. Parenchymal cysts of the lower neck. Radiology 1985;157:399.

PART THREE
SPINE

PART THREE

Imaging of the Pediatric Head, Neck, and Spine
by Mauricio Castillo and Suresh K. Mukherji,
Lippincott-Raven Publishing, Philadelphia © 1996.

16
Developmental Disorders

16.0 *Applied Embryology*

At approximately 14 days of life, the embryonic disc has a well defined cephalic pole (Hensen's node, primitive node or knot) that contains the primitive pit. Ectodermal cells invade this pit and migrate between the ectoderm and endoderm anteriorly to the primitive streak. These endodermal cells will form the notochord, which later induces the overlying ectoderm to become specialized neural ectoderm. The notochord also regulates the development of vertebral central and discs.

Step 1. Development of the Upper Spine (Neurulation)

By 12 days of life, the notochord has induced a depression in the center of the neural plate, called the neural groove. This groove is flanked by crests (folds; Fig. 16.0-1A). There is progressive infolding of the crests until they fuse in the midline. At this time, the neural groove is completely enclosed and becomes the neural tube (Fig. 16.0-1B). In the center of the neural tube lies the central canal. Closure of the tube begins in the middle and extends toward the cephalic and caudal ends, which are the last to close. At 25 days of gestation, closure of the neural tube is completed (Fig. 16.0-1C). Last, mesenchyme migrates between the tube and overlying skin and will give origin to meninges, neural arches, and paraspinal muscles (Figs. 16.0-1D and 16.0-2). Disorders of abnormal neurulation result in myeloceles and myelomeningoceles. Inclusion of ectodermal elements in the presence of abnormal neural tube closure results in epidermoids, dermoids, or lipomas. Lack of complete separation of the superficial ectoderm from the neural ectoderm results in adhesions between them and the formation of dorsal dermal sinuses.

Step 2. Development of the Distal Spine (Canalization and Retrogressive Differentiation)

Despite completion of neurulation, the distal spinal cord is not yet formed. The blending of the distal neural tube and notochord forms the caudal cell mass, which is adjacent to the hindgut and mesonephros. (Fig. 16.0-3A). This cell mass is "canalized" by the formation of multiple vacuoles that coalesce and unite with the central canal of the spinal cord. Once the distal cell mass is canalized, its cells begin differentiating into neural elements and form the lower conus medullaris (Fig. 16.0-3B). The distal-most cell mass undergoes retrogressive differentiation and involutes, leaving behind the filum terminale (Fig. 16.0-3C). Deranged involution induces abnormalities of the filum terminale that may clinically present as the tight filum terminale syndrome. Other anomalies arising from faulty development at this stage are lipomas of the filum, anterior sacral meningoceles, and terminal myelocystoceles. Anomalies of canalization and retrogressive differentiation or excessive retrogression may lead to the syndrome of caudal regression.

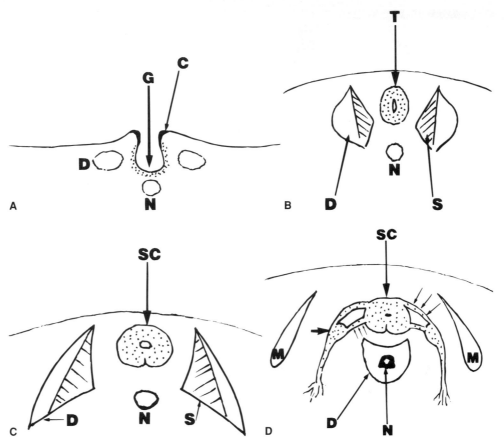

FIGURE 16.0-1.

Development of the spine. **A.** At 19 days of life, the dorsal ectoderm shows a midline depression called the neural groove (G), flanked by the neural crests (C). Anterior to the groove lies the notochord (N). At the sides of the groove are the somites (D). **B.** At 22 days of life, the groove has folded on itself and is now closed, forming the neural tube (T) located dorsal to the notochord (N). The sclerotomes (S) and dermomyotomes (D) are located laterally to the tube. **C.** At 27 days of life, the neural tube now has the appearance of the spinal cord (SC), and lies dorsal to the notochord (N). The sclerotomes (S) and dermomyotomes (D) are located lateral to the spinal cord. **D.** At 30 days of life, the spinal cord (SC) is well formed and has dorsal *(long thin arrows)* and ventral *(short thin arrows)* roots and dorsal ganglia *(short thick arrow)*. The mesenchyme around the notochord (N) has formed the intervertebral disc (D). The myotomes (M) will form the paraspinal muscles.

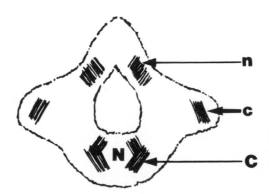

FIGURE 16.0-2.

The ossification center within a vertebra. n, neural arch; c, costal process; C, central process; N, notochord.

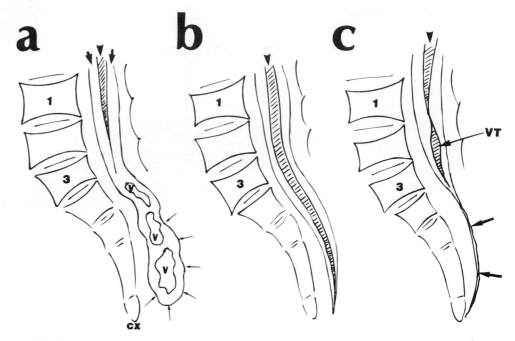

FIGURE 16.0-3.

Normal canalization and retrogressive differentiation. **A.** The closed spinal cord *(short thick arrows)* containing the central canal *(arrowhead)* extends to the mid-sacrum (1, first sacral segment; 3, third sacral segment; cx, coccyx) and is contiguous with the caudal cell mass *(small thin arrows)*, which contains multiple cavities or vacuoles (v). **B.** The caudal cell mass has differentiated into neural elements and is now contiguous with the spinal cord. The vacuoles have formed a cavity contiguous with the central canal *(arrowhead)*. **C.** The lower aspect of the differentiated caudal cell mass has now regressed and involuted into the filum terminales *(arrows)*. The upper aspect of the caudal cell mass forms the distal conus medullaris and contains a cavity called the ventriculus terminalis (VT), which is now separate from the central canal *(arrowhead)* of the spinal cord, and which will close later.

SUGGESTED READING

1. Naidich TP, Zimmerman RA, McLone DG, Raybaud CA, Altman NR. Congenital anomalies of the spine and spinal cord. In: Atlas SW, ed. Magnetic Resonance Imaging of the Brain and Spine. New York: Raven, 1991:865.

16.01 Craniocervical Disorders: Basilar Invagination

EPIDEMIOLOGY

Basilar invagination refers to an occipitocervical dysplasia in which there is upward displacement of the foramen magnum and the upper cervical vertebrae. Basilar impression refers to a secondary form of invagination caused by softening of bone. The incidence of these disorders is not known. They may be idiopathic, familial, or acquired. These entities should not be confused with platybasia, in which there is an obtuse angle between the clivus and the anterior cranial fossa. Platybasia is probably a normal variation of only anthropologic significance.

CLINICAL FEATURES

Basilar invagination is associated with occipitalization or hypoplasia of C1, anomalous posterior arch of C1, odontoid anomalies, vertebral artery anomalies, Klippel-Feil and Down syndromes, Chiari malformations, achondroplasia, and cleidocranial dysplasia. Basilar impression is associated with mucopolysaccharidoses, osteomalacia, rickets, renal osteodystrophy, rheumatoid arthritis, neurofibromatosis, ankylosing spondylitis, fibrous dysplasia, hypothyroidism, osteogenesis imperfecta, and birth trauma. Symptoms manifest after 10 years of age and include neck stiffness, progressive spasticity, weakness of lower extremities, occipital headaches, painful torticollis, restricted neck motion, nystagmus, cranial nerve abnormalities, ataxia, sensory loss in upper extremities, and difficulty walking. Associated hydrocephalus may occur, especially in the setting of Chiari malformations. Treatment includes surgical decompression of the upper cervical spine and posterior fossa. The ability to reduce invagination is age related. Fusion is needed if instability is present.

IMAGING FEATURES

Imaging diagnosis of basilar invagination/impression may be made based on plain radiographs, computed tomography (CT), or magnetic resonance (MR) images. On plain radiographs, the tip of the dens should not exceed the bimastoid line by more than 10 mm (frontal view). Chamberlain's line is drawn on the lateral view from the posterior hard palate to the tip of the posterior lip of the foramen magnum. The dens lies no more than 6 mm above this line. McGregor's line extends from the posterior hard palate to the undersurface of the posterior lip of the foramen magnum. The dens may be normally slightly superior in position using this line. The anterior arch of C1 always lies below these two lines. MR imaging shows that the rims of the foramen magnum are curved upward (Fig. 16.01-1). The posterior fossa is small and the foramen magnum is irregular in shape. The clivus is short and horizontal. The odontoid is high and may compress the pontomedullary junction. Sagittal gradient echo images in extension and flexion are helpful in illustrating the dynamics of the abnormality.

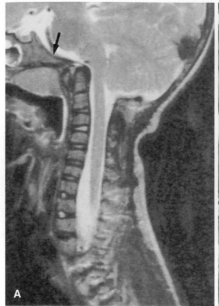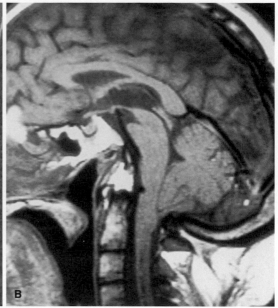
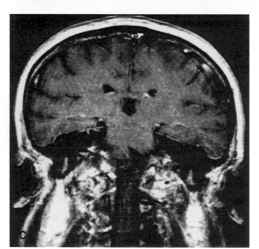

FIGURE 16.01-1.

Basilar invagination in cleidocranial dysostosis. **A.** Midsagittal magnetic resonance (MR) T2-weighted image shows that the clivus *(arrow)* is short and horizontal. Almost all of C2 protrudes superiorly to Chamberlain's line. There is compression of the pontomedullary junction by the superiorly located dens. **B.** Midsagittal MR T1-weighted image in a different patient with cleidocranial dysostosis shows a short dens with basilar invagination and compression of the medulla and pons. There is a hypointensity in the upper cervical spinal cord, suggesting a syrinx. **C.** Coronal MR T1-weighted image in the same patient shows superior displacement of the base of the skull, especially medially. The petrous pyramids are angled superiorly in their medial aspects. Shape of the skull is brachicephalic.

SUGGESTED READING

1. Smoker WRK, Keyes WD, Dunn VD, Menezes AH. MRI versus conventional radiologic examinations in the evaluation of the craniocervical and cervicomedullary junction. RadioGraphics 1986;6:953.

16.02   *Craniocervical Disorders: Achondroplasia*

EPIDEMIOLOGY

Achondroplasia is a defect of enchondral bone formation and is the most common type of dwarfism to involve the spine and craniovertebral junction. It occurs in approximately 1:25,000 live births, and there is no gender predilection. It is an autosomal dominant trait, but most cases (80%) are spontaneous mutations.

CLINICAL FEATURES

The main abnormalities in this disease are short stature, dysmorphic features, congenital skeletal abnormalities, and neurologic findings. At birth, the musculature is hypotonic, and therefore there is delay of motor development. It is possible that this hypotonia results from brain stem compression. Other symptoms referable to brain stem compression include apnea and dysphagia. Most patients are intellectually normal, but some have mild mental retardation. Progressive neurologic deterioration is secondary to compression of neural structures and hydrocephalus. Hydrocephalus occurs in approximately 15% of these patients, and its etiology is uncertain. Narrowing of the jugular foramina with relative obstruction of venous drainage has been proposed as an explanation. Treatment of this disease is controversial. Decompression of the foramen magnum is advocated by some and discouraged by others. Spinal laminectomies are seldom needed. Spinal defects producing neurologic symptoms before 5 years of age may require surgery. Kyphoscoliosis improves spontaneously in over 90% of patients. Lumbar laminectomies and foraminotomies may be needed in cases of compression of the cauda equina and lumbar nerve roots. Hearing loss is common in patients with achondroplasia. It is most likely related to repeated middle ear infections.

IMAGING FEATURES

Examination of the head with computed tomography or magnetic resonance imaging may show macrocephaly, hydrocephalus, and prominent extraaxial cerebrospinal fluid (CSF) spaces (Fig. 16.02-1A). Compression of the upper cervical spinal cord is the result either of impingement by the posterior lip of the foramen magnum or basilar invagination. The cross-sectional area of the foramen magnum is narrowed in up to 90% of patients (Fig. 16.02-1B). Cervical spinal canal stenosis may be present in 30% of patients. Other abnormalities of the craniocervical junction include os odontoideum, dens hypoplasia, atlantoaxial instability, and atlantooccipital fusion. Thoracolumbar kyphoscoliosis is common and diffuse spinal canal stenosis occurs in 10% of patients. In the lumbar spine there is exaggerated lordosis with a pronounced angle between the lumbar and sacral regions. The vertebral bodies are somewhat flat, and the pedicles are short and thick. The interpedicular distance is shortened. Canal stenosis is commonly aggravated by bulging discs. Syringomyelia may also be present and is probably secondary to alterations of CSF flow or post-trauma.

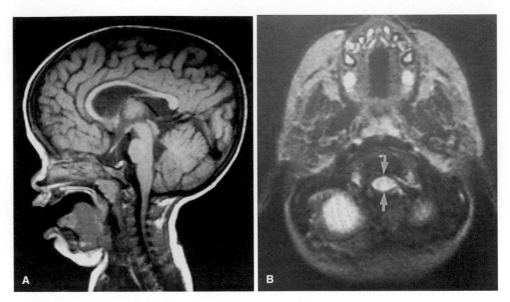

FIGURE 16.02-1.

Achondroplasia. **A.** Midsagittal magnetic resonance (MR) T1-weighted image shows large head and relatively small face. The cerebrospinal fluid spaces are prominent. The foramen magnum is markedly small. An os odontoideum is present. **B.** Axial MR T2-weighted image in the same patient shows marked anteroposterior narrowing *(arrows)* of foramen magnum.

SUGGESTED READINGS

1. Tolo VT. Spinal deformity in skeletal dysplasia. In: Weinstein SL, ed. The Pediatric Spine: Principles and Practice. New York: Raven, 1994:369.
2. Menzes AH. Bony anomalies of the craniocervical junction. In: Pang D, ed. Disorders of the Pediatric Spine. New York: Raven, 1995:97.

16.03 *Craniocervical Disorders: Developmental Odontoid Anomalies*

EPIDEMIOLOGY

These anomalies include os odontoideum, and aplasia–hypoplasia of the dens. Aplasia is the rarest of these anomalies. There is no gender predilection.

CLINICAL FEATURES

Symptoms commonly result from atlantoaxial instability. Intermittent compression of the upper cervical spinal cord and lower medulla may produce long tract signs. Not uncommonly, the initial presentation occurs after a sports injury or other type of trauma and induces a spastic paresis that usually is transient. Symptoms are caused by direct compression of neural structures or by compromised blood flow through the vertebral arteries. Patients with recognized atlantoaxial instability should undergo stabilization and may require transoral resection of the dens. The etiology of the os odontoideum is uncertain. The congenital hypothesis proposes overgrowth of the ossiculum terminale as the cause. Most authors favor trauma as the etiology. A fracture through the dens compromises the blood supply of its distal aspect, leading to nonunion. Os odontoideum may occur as an isolated anomaly or be associated with Down, Morquio, or Klippel-Feil syndromes, and spondyloepiphyseal dysplasia.

IMAGING FEATURES

Aplasia–hypoplasia of the dens shows a rudimentary dens. In these cases, the transverse ligament is incompetent, leading to instability (Fig. 16.03-1). Instability of these segments may be evaluated with flexion/extension plain films or dynamic magnetic resonance (MR) imaging. Computed tomography with coronal reformations is helpful in assessing the morphologic characteristics of the anomaly. Os odontoideum is seen as a smooth, rounded ossicle, superior to the base of the dens and separated from it by a lucent gap (this gap is wider than that of a fracture; Fig. 16.03-2). The base of the dens tends to be hypoplastic. The os odontoideum is located under the anterior lip of the foramen magnum and may be fused to it (Fig. 16.03-3). The transverse ligament may be incompetent, leading to instability. Two types of os odontoideum exist. In the orthotopic variety, the ossicle is in the expected position of the dens and moves with it. In the dystopic type, the os odontoideum lies under the anterior foramen magnum and has a greater likelihood of being unstable. Other associated anomalies include hypertrophy of the anterior arch of C1 and clefting of its posterior arch. MR imaging may show tissues of mostly low signal intensity on both T1- and T2-weighted images surrounding the dens. These represent granulation tissue.

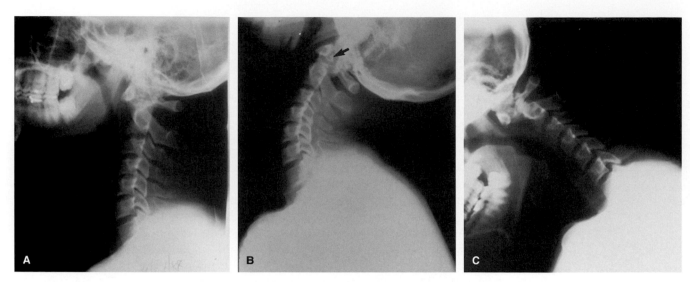

FIGURE 16.03-1.

Atlantoaxial instability, hypoplastic dens. **A.** Lateral radiograph in neutral position. The relationship between C1 and C2 is normal. **B.** Lateral radiograph in same patient with extended neck. The C1–C2 relationship continues to be normal. The small os odontoideum *(arrow)* is well seen. **C.** Lateral radiograph in same patient during voluntary flexion shows dystopic os odontoideum moving forward with anterior arch of C1. Note marked increase of distance between base of dens and anterior C1 arch, indicating instability of transverse ligament.

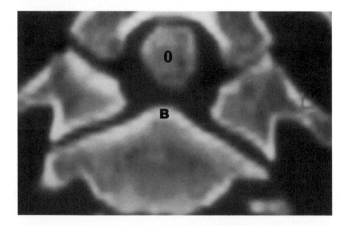

FIGURE 16.03-2.

Orthotopic os odontoideum. Coronal computed tomography reformation shows rounded, well corticated, and smooth os odontoideum (O). The base (B) of the dens is hypoplastic. (With permission from Castillo M. Neuroradiology Companion. Philadelphia: JB Lippincott, 1995.)

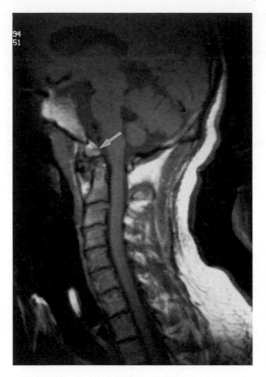

FIGURE 16.03-3.

Dystopic os odontoideum. Midsagittal magnetic resonance T1-weighted image in a different patient shows os odontoideum *(arrow)* tilted anteriorly and located under the lip of the foramen magnum. The atlantodental interval is mildly increased.

SUGGESTED READINGS

1. Menezes AH. Os odontoideum: pathogenesis, dynamics and management. In: Marlin AE, ed. Concepts in Pediatric Neurosurgery, Vol. 8. Basel: Karger, 133.
2. Smoker WRK. Craniovertebral junction: normal anatomy, craniometry, and congenital anomalies. RadioGraphics 1994;14:255.

16.04 *Craniocervical Disorders: Klippel Feil Syndrome*

EPIDEMIOLOGY

Klippel-Feil syndrome refers to the clinical triad of short neck, low posterior hairline, and limitation of neck range of motion due to fusion of cervical vertebral bodies. Its incidence is uncertain, but congenital symptomatic fusions of the cervical spine may occur in 0.2:1000 individuals. Although both autosomal recessive and dominant inheritance patterns have been reported, most cases are sporadic. It is slightly more common in girls than in boys (1.5:1). Its incidence seems to be especially high in Native Americans.

CLINICAL FEATURES

The etiology of this syndrome is uncertain. Vascular disruption may lead to failure of segmentation, leading to formation of a single mass of fused bone. A similar etiology has been proposed for the Poland and Möbius syndromes and Sprengel's deformity (all three may coexist with Klippel-Feil syndrome). A global insult resulting in variable effects on different tissues has also been suggested as a cause for this syndrome. Some authors also believe that a primary abnormality involving the neural tube is responsible. Klippel-Feil syndrome is associated with the fetal alcohol syndrome, Goldenhar syndrome, and Wildervanck syndrome. The age of presentation is variable. Massive cervical spine fusions cause severe deformities of the neck and are noted early in life. Atlantoaxial fusions cause pain and also are detected in early life. Approximately 20% of patients with Klippel-Feil syndrome are diagnosed before 5 years of age. Short neck and decreased range of motion are the most common clinical symptoms, and are found in 50% to 75% of patients. Other symptoms include radicular pain and slowly progressive or acute quadriparesis.

IMAGING FEATURES

The diagnosis is readily made with plain radiographs. Most patients have fusion involving only one level. In approximately one-third of patients, the fusions involve two to five levels (Fig. 16.04-1). In a small percentage of cases, the fusion involves more than six levels. The sites of fusion usually are posterior and lateral at the C2–C3 levels. The spinal canal diameter may be narrowed secondary to degenerative changes in the levels above and below the fusion. Degenerative changes found in these patients include neural foraminal narrowing, osteophytosis, vertebral subluxations, facet joint degeneration, disc bulges and herniations, and ligament buckling. The craniocervical junction may be unstable, and carefully performed flexion and extension views are needed in these cases. Associated anomalies include occipitalization of C1, basilar impression, and deformities of the dens (including os odontoideum). The thoracic and lumbar spine should be evaluated because associated anomalies in those regions are not uncommon. Scoliosis is common.

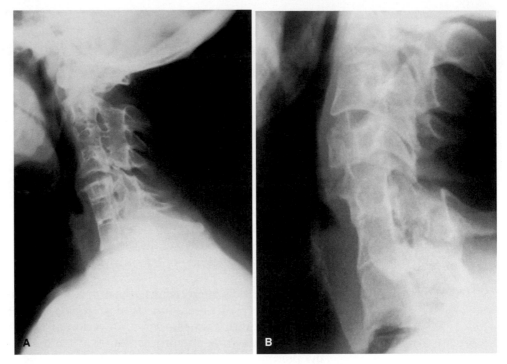

FIGURE 16.04-1.

Klippel-Feil syndrome. **A.** Lateral radiograph shows congenital fusion of C2–C4 and C5–C7 at both the vertebral bodies and posterior elements, which is typical of this syndrome. **B.** Lateral radiograph in a different patient shows fusion of C5–C7. The C4 vertebral body is small.

SUGGESTED READINGS

1. Dietz F. Congenital abnormalities of the cervical spine. In: Weinstein SL, ed. The Pediatric Spine: Principles and Practice. New York: Raven, 1994:324.
2. Sherk HH, Black JD. Bony anomalies of the mid and lower cervical spine. In: Pang D, ed. Disorders of the Pediatric Spine. New York: Raven, 1995:125.

16.05 Open Spinal Dysraphism: Myelocele, Myelomeningocele, Myelocystocele, and Hemimyelocele

EPIDEMIOLOGY

In a myelocele, the unfolded neural tissues form a flat placode (inner surface of the cord projects out) that is uncovered by dura and flush at the level of the skin (Fig. 16.05-1). In myelomeningoceles, the neural placode protrudes posteriorly (above the skin) because of enlargement of cerebrospinal fluid (CSF) spaces (Fig. 16.05-2). Myeloceles and myelomeningoceles occur in 1 to 3:1000 live births. They are probably inherited as an autosomal recessive trait, but environmental influences may play an important role. The rate of subsequent siblings having an open dysraphism varies between 4% to 8%. Myelocystoceles or syringoceles are the least common form of posterior spinal dysraphism. Hemimyelocele refers to the presence of a split cord with an open dysraphism involving only one hemicord.

CLINICAL FEATURES

Screening for elevated maternal serum α-fetoprotein is cost effective. Detection rate with this technique is close to 80%. α-Fetoprotein leaks through the open defect into amniotic fluid. Elevation of this compound in amniotic fluid has a false-positive rate of less than 0.5% and a false-negative rate of 2% in the presence of open defects. Sonography may be used to confirm the defect. Administration of folic acid before conception may lower the risk. Immediately after birth, the defect requires closure to avoid infection. Hydrocephalus is present in more than 75% of patients with open dysraphism and requires shunting. Hydrocephalus is more common when the defect involves the thoracolumbar region. Overall, most open defects are located in the lumbosacral region. Mortality without treatment varies between 50% to 80%. Renal failure tends to be secondary to repeated infections. This group of spinal anomalies is associated with anorectal anomalies, lower genitourinary anomalies, cloacal exstrophy, lordosis, scoliosis, and sacral agenesis.

IMAGING FEATURES

Imaging is not usually indicated before surgery, and most patients are imaged after closure or because of progressive neurologic changes suggesting tethering of the spinal cord. Magnetic resonance is the imaging modality of choice. The posterior elements are absent and the paraspinal musculature is markedly reduced in volume. The defect is covered by skin and subcutaneous fat. The placode is low and commonly in apposition with the surgical graft. One can only assume that in all cases the stretched spinal cord is tethered (anchored) at this level (Fig. 16.05-3A, B). The pedicles are wide and dysplastic and the spinal canal is wide in this region. The spinal cord is thinned and may contain a cyst at any level. Intraspinal masses may be of similar signal intensity to CSF and difficult to distinguish from it (epidermoids), or of high signal intensity on both T1- and fast spin echo T2-weighted images (dermoids; Fig. 16.05-3C). Diastematomyelia may also be present and is commonly accompanied by vertebral defects. One hemicord may be involved in the open defect, producing a hemimyelocele or a hemimyelomeningocele. Contrast administration is usually not indicated unless an underlying superimposed infection is considered. For practical purposes, imaging of the patient with a repaired open defect is aimed at discovering other curable abnormalities of the spinal cord, and is not done for direct reevaluation of the initial closure site (remember that all patients may be considered tethered at the level of prior repair). Therefore, imaging in these patients should include not only the entire spine but the head (to exclude hydrocephalus and a Chiari type II malformation). Causes of progressive neurologic symptoms in these patients other than re-tethering include cord ischemia, spinal cord fluid-filled cysts, arachnoid cysts, diastematomyelia, epidermoids, and dermoids.

The term "terminal myelocystocele" refers to a very rare anomaly in which there is a large cyst in the distal part of a low and tethered cord protruding posteriorly; this is the most common type of myelocystocele (Fig. 16.05-4). There is a large ependymal-lined cyst in the lower spine that protrudes posteriorly through a spinal bone defect. The cyst contains no septations and does not communicate with the subarachnoid space.

Hemimyeloceles are present in approximately 10% of patients with myelomeningocele and diastematomyelia. In this disorder, one of the hemicords lies in the central aspect of the spinal canal and exhibits an open dysraphic state (such as a myelomeningocele) (Fig. 16.05-5). The other hemicord is usually smaller and lies lateral to the dysraphic hemicord, but is usually tethered inferiorly by a thickened filum terminale or by a smaller myelomeningocele, usually at a lower level than the first one.

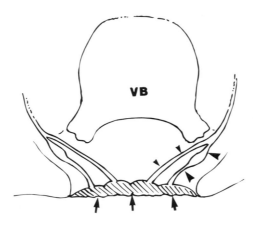

FIGURE 16.05-1.

Myelocele.   The neural placode *(arrows)* is flush at the level of the skin. The dorsal *(large arrowheads)* and ventral *(small arrowheads)* project anteriorly from the ventral surface of the placode. The posterior elements of the vertebra (VB) are absent.

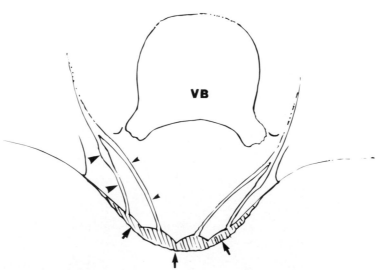

FIGURE 16.05-2.

Myelomeningocele.   The cerebrospinal fluid space in front of the placode *(arrows)* displaces it posteriorly, and it now projects above the surrounding skin. The dorsal *(large arrowheads)* and ventral roots *(small arrowheads)* are stretched and arise from the ventral placode. The posterior elements of the vertebra (VB) are absent.

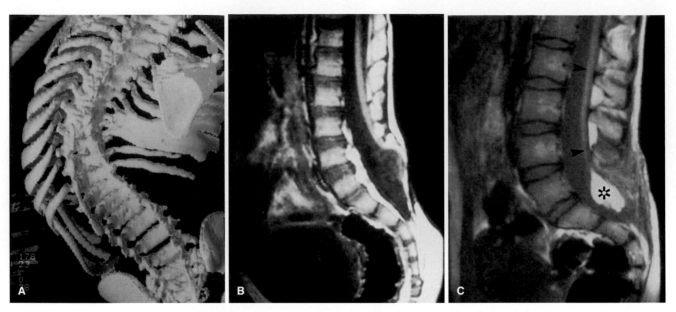

FIGURE 16.05-3.

Myelomeningocele. **A.** Posterior view of three-dimensional computed tomography reformation shows absence of posterior elements and widened interpedicular distance from the low thoracic region to the sacrum in a large dysraphism. **B.** Midsagittal magnetic resonance (MR) T1-weighted image in a patient with myelomeningocele repaired at birth. The conus medullaris is elongated and the placode extends to the surgical site, where it is most likely tethered by scar. This is the expected postoperative appearance. The posterior elements in the lower lumbar spine are absent. **C.** Midsagittal MR T1-weighted image in a different patient with repaired dysraphism at birth shows intraspinal mass (*) of high signal intensity (inclusion lipoma versus inclusion dermoid). The cord *(arrowheads)* is thin and extends to this mass, which probably tethers it. The posterior elements of L5 and the upper sacrum are absent. (With permission from Castillo M. Neuroradiology Companion. Philadelphia: JB Lippincott, 1995.)

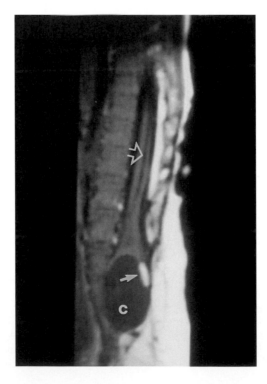

FIGURE 16.05-4.

Myelocystocele. Midsagittal magnetic resonance T1-weighted image shows myelocystocele repaired at birth. There is a distal spinal cord cyst (c) herniating slightly posteriorly through a bony defect, which is covered by fat. A small intraspinal lipoma *(arrow)* is present. The cord extends to the lower sacrum, which is scalloped by the long-standing cyst. There is syrinx *(open arrow)* in the distal spinal cord.

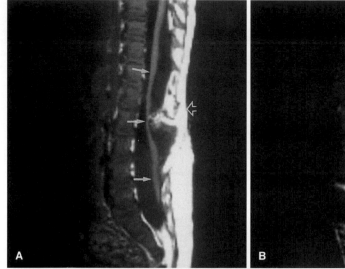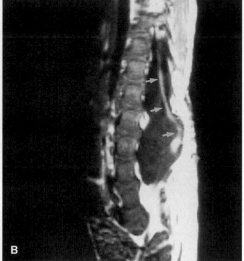

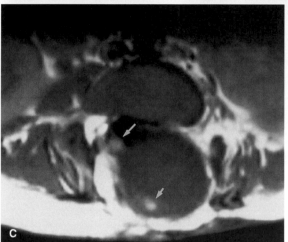

FIGURE 16.05-5.

Hemimyelocele. A. Slightly off midline magnetic resonance (MR) T1-weighted image shows one hemicord *(arrows)*, which is thin at the level of repaired open dysraphism *(open arrow)* and extends inferiorly to S1. **B.** Parasagittal MR T1-weighted image shows second hemicord *(arrows)* projecting into dysraphism. There is a small lipoma inferiorly. **C.** Axial MR T1-weighted image shows diastematomyelia (note that there is no spur) with one hemicord *(larger arrow)* in spinal canal and the other hemicord *(shorter arrow)* in a myelocele.

SUGGESTED READINGS

1. Naidich TP, Zimmerman RA, McLone DG, Raybaud CA, Altman NR. Congenital anomalies of the spine and spinal cord. In: Atlas SW, ed. Magnetic Resonance Imaging of the Brain and Spine. New York: Raven, 1991:865.
2. McLone DG. Spina bifida aperta. In: Pang D, ed. Disorders of the Pediatric Spine. New York: Raven, 1995:137.

16.06 Closed Spinal Dysraphism: Intradural Lipoma, Lipomyelocele, and Lipomyelomeningocele

EPIDEMIOLOGY

Intradural lipomas represent approximately 1% to 4% of all spinal lipomas. They are slightly more common in girls and peak during the first 5 years of life. Lipomyeloceles and lipomyelomeningoceles account for remaining spinal lipomas. Of these two, lipomyelomeningoceles are more common, and represent more 20% to 50% of cases of closed (occult) spinal dysraphism and 20% to 35% of skin-covered masses in the lumbosacral region. Patients usually are younger than 6 months of age, and female.

CLINICAL FEATURES

All spinal lipomas represent a disorder of premature dysjunction of the surface ectoderm from the neural ectoderm (Fig. 16.06-1A). Intradural lipomas are more commonly found in the cervical (12%–20%) and thoracic (30%) regions and show no abnormalities in the overlying skin. In cases of lipomyelocele, there is a posterior spina bifida with absent dura (Fig. 16.06-1B). The subcutaneous fat extends into the spinal canal and is contiguous with the inner surface of an underneurulated placode. The skin overlying this abnormality may show a minor bulge. In lipomyelomeningoceles, the anatomy is similar to that of lipomyeloceles, but there is expansion of the subarachnoid space, which bulges out posteriorly in a symmetric or asymmetric fashion (Fig. 16.06-1C). This produces a bulge in the back of the patient. A subcutaneous mass (cephalad to the intergluteal crease) is found in over 54% of these patients. The mass tends to be eccentric and may have an associated hairy patch, hemangioma, dimple, dermal sinus, or skin tag. In cases of lipomyelocele, no skin masses or other abnormalities are present and the only indication of spinal dysraphism may be the presence of orthopedic deformities and urologic abnormalities. On initial examination, almost 50% of patients with lipomyeloceles and lipomyelomeningoceles are asymptomatic. However, most will eventually have symptoms if left untreated. Lipomas of the lumbar spine present with flaccid lower extremity paralysis and sphincter dysfunction. In the cervical region, ascending paresis, spasticity, sensory loss, and abnormal deep sensation are typical. Sensorimotor disturbances increase with age and develop in most of the affected children. Treatment involves resection of the lipoma, reapproximation of the underneurulated placode, and patching of the defect with cadaver dural grafts.

IMAGING FEATURES

Magnetic resonance (MR) is the imaging method of choice in these patients. In cases of intradural lipomas, plain radiographs or computed tomography may show a nearly normal spine with a small posterior cleft of mild segmentation defects at the level of the lipoma. Most lipomas are located in the dorsal aspect of the spine cord, but may occur in any location (Figs. 16.06-2 and 16.06-3). The mass is of high signal intensity on T1- and fast spin echo T2-weighted images. The spinal cord is compressed and the canal may be widened. The lipoma is usually subpial, intradural, and continuous with the spinal cord, and extends into the level of the expected central spinal cord canal. The cord is unfolded (placode) at the level of the lipoma (Fig. 16.06-2C). At this site, the lipoma may become less hyperintense on MR imaging because it contains abundant fibrous tissues. Exophytic lipoma components are found in 50% of patients. Spinal cord fluid-filled cysts are concomitantly present in 2% of patients. In lipomyeloceles and lipomyelomeningoceles, there is a wide spina bifida defect, usually in the lower lumbar and upper sacral regions. The lipoma extends into the dorsal surface of the neural placode, which is smooth or slightly serrated. There is a band of hypointensity at the liponeural junction that may be related to a band of collagenous tissues and muscle or a chemical shift artifact. If the lipoma is asymmetric, the nerve roots on one side may be very short. The conus medullaris is always low-lying in patients with lipomyeloceles and lipomyelomeningoceles. In lipomyelomeningoceles, the expanded subarachnoid space herniates posteriorly. Anomalies of vertebral segmentation and malformations of the sacrum are present in up to 50% of cases.

Filar lipomas are mentioned here because with the widespread use of MR imaging they are being discovered with increasing frequency. Some regard this anomaly as an aberration of retrogressive differentiation. In this anomaly, the filum terminale is slightly thick and infiltrated by fat (entirely or segmentally; Fig. 16.06-2D). This may be seen in 1% to 3% of the population, is often incidental, and is asymptomatic if the conus medullaris is at a normal level. In the presence of a low-lying conus medullaris, a filar lipoma may result in the tight filum terminale syndrome. However, this syndrome may also occur in the absence of filar lipomas and may present with a thickened filum terminale that is of normal MR signal intensity. The normal filum terminale usually measures less than 2 mm in diameter. In these patients, the presence of a thick filum terminale and a conus medullaris terminating below the L2–L3 disc space is highly suggestive of tight filum terminale syndrome. More than 50% of these patients have a spina bifida occulta. Hydromyelia or myelomalacia is present in 25% of patients with this syndrome.

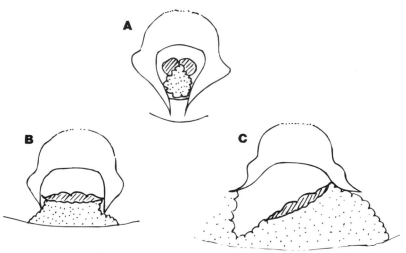

FIGURE 16.06-1.

Closed spinal dysraphism. Diagram shows in **A.** spina bifida occulta with an intraspinal lipoma (dotted area) insinuating itself into the spinal cord (lined area). **B.** In a lipomyelocele the defect of the posterior elements is larger but still covered by skin (occult). The subcutaneous lipoma (dotted area) extends into the inner surface of an unfused spinal cord (lined area) (placode). The spinal canal is wide. **C.** The ventral CSF space is wide and pushes the placode beyond the level of the posterior spinal bony disraphism producing a lipomyelomeningocele. The lipoma (dotted area) is contigous with placode (lined area). The spinal canal is wide and the bone defect is generous. A soft mass (lipoma) may be visible and palpable under the intact skin.

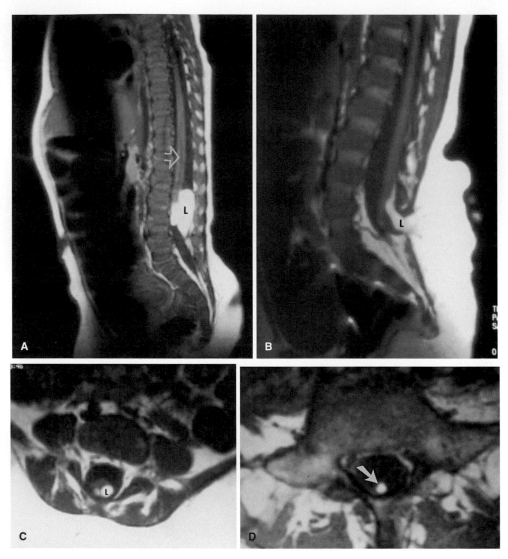

FIGURE 16.06-2.

Intradural lipoma, lumbar spine. **A.** Midsagittal MR T1-weighted image shows that skin and posterior elements are intact. The bright lipoma (L) insinuates itself into the distal spinal cord. The conus medullaris terminates at L3 (abnormally low) and is probably tethered by the mass. The distal spinal cord contains a central hypointensity (open arrow) suggesting a syringomyelia. The spinal canal is widened at the level of the lipoma. **B.** Midsagittal MR T1-weighted image in a different patient with abundant subcutaneous fat in the lower spine which enters (L) the spinal canal through small tract and insinuates itself into the spinal cord and tethers it at the L5/S1 level. **C.** Axial MR T1-weighted image in same patient show lipoma posterior to placode. Note similar appearance to **FIGURE 16.06-1A.** **D.** Axial MR T1-weighted image shows an incidental lipoma (arrow) of the filum terminale. The conus medullaris (not shown) was at its normal level. (With permission from Castillo M. Neuroradiology Companion. Philadelphia: JB Lippincott, 1995.)

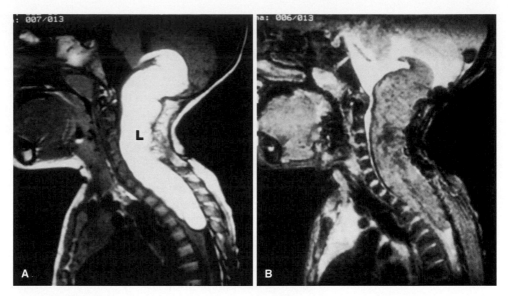

FIGURE 16.06-3.

Intradural lipoma, cervical spine. **A.** Midsagittal magnetic resonance (MR) T1-weighted image in a different patient shows large intradural lipoma (L) extending from the posterior fossa into the cervical and upper thoracic regions. There is marked compression of the spinal cord, which is not seen. The spinal canal is widened and the posterior surface of the vertebral bodies is scalloped. Note posterior dermal sinus opening. **B.** Midsagittal MR T2-weighted image in the same patient shows lipoma to be inhomogeneous but mostly of low signal intensity.

SUGGESTED READINGS

1. McLone DG, Naidich TP. The tethered spinal cord. In: McLaurin RL, Venes JL, Schut L, Epstein F, eds. Philadelphia: WB Saunders, 1989:71.
2. Pang D. Spinal cord lipomas. In: Pang D, ed. Disorders of the Pediatric Spine. New York: Raven, 1995:175.

16.07 *Closed Spinal Dysraphism: Meningocele*

EPIDEMIOLOGY
A meningocele is an outpouching of cerebrospinal fluid (CSF)-filled dura containing no neural structures. They may be associated with the Chiari type 2 and 3 malformations, neurofibromatosis type I, and Marfan and Ehler-Danlos syndromes, but most are isolated anomalies. There is no gender predilection. Over 85% of patients with lateral thoracic meningoceles have neurofibromatosis type I. Most thoracic meningoceles are found in adults.

CLINICAL FEATURES
These anomalies may be asymptomatic and incidentally discovered. They may, however, compress nerve roots, producing radiculopathies. Anterior sacral meningoceles may be considered an anomaly of neurenteric origin and, as such, gastrointestinal and genitourinary abnormalities may be present. Also, the retrorectal mass may produce urinary, rectal, and menstrual pain. In patients with neurofibromatosis type I, a mass located in the lateral aspect of the thoracic spine is more likely to be a meningocele than a neurofibroma. In this disorder and in the collagen disorders, meningoceles are part of a mesenchymal dysplasia leading to dural ectasia. Lateral thoracic meningoceles usually produce acute-angle scoliosis. The meningocele is located at the apex of the curve. Some meningoceles grow as the patient ages.

IMAGING FEATURES
Magnetic resonance (MR) is the imaging method of choice in these patients. The CSF-filled dural outpouching herniates via a small or large spina bifida defect, an intervertebral or sacral foramen (Fig. 16.07-1). Occasionally, the dural diverticulum is entirely contained within the bone (intrasacral meningoceles; Fig. 16.07-2). When the patients have a systemic mesenchymal disorder, meningoceles may be multiple. When they protrude through sacral foramina, they are indistinguishable from Tarlov cysts (perineurial cysts). In the occipitocervical region they may be associated with the Chiari type 3 malformation. In the lumbosacral region, they may be associated with a low-lying conus medullaris. Meningoceles have the same MR signal intensity as normal CSF. Anterior sacral meningoceles appear as a fluid-filled retrorectal mass (Fig. 16.07-3). The cyst may be unilocular or multilocular and communicate with the sacral spinal canal via a wide or narrowed pedicle. The spinal canal may be widened, and bony anomalies include sacral hemihypoplasia, dorsal spina bifida, absent segments, or a scimitar configuration of the sacrum. Spinal lipomas and dermoids may also occur. Cysts located in the anterior aspects of the thoracic spine in association with vertebral body abnormalities are suspect for neurenteric anomalies. Neurenteric cysts often have an intraspinal component and are related to splitting of the spinal cord.

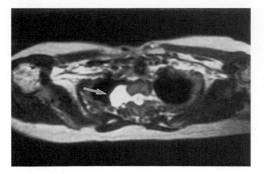

FIGURE 16.07-1.

Lateral thoracic meningocele. Axial magnetic resonance T2-weighted image shows right paraspinal mass *(arrow)* of high signal intensity (identical to cerebrospinal fluid) and a widened neural foramen in this lateral thoracic meningocele. This patient did not have a systemic disorder.

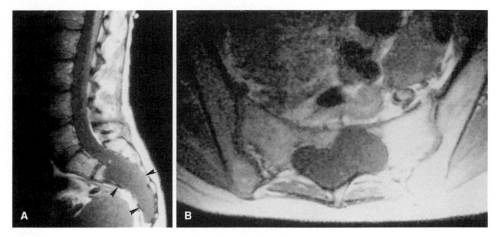

FIGURE 16.07-2.

Intrasacral meningocele. **A.** Midsagittal magnetic resonance (MR) T1-weighted image shows large, expansile cystic mass *(arrowheads)* in the sacrum. There is marked scalloping of the ventral sacrum. This anomaly may be called an intrasacral meningocele. **B.** Axial MR T1-weighted image shows that the dural diverticulum is entirely contained within the sacrum. Note marked pressure erosion of the sacrum.

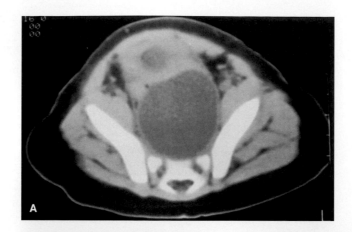

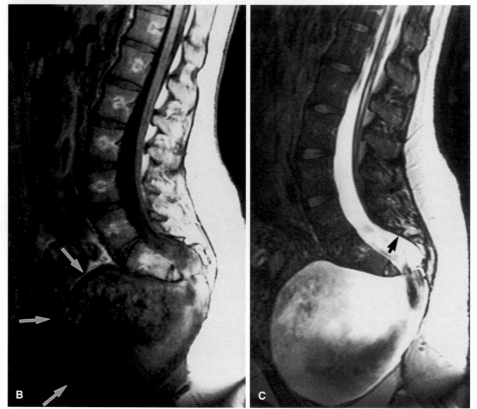

FIGURE 16.07-3.

Anterior sacral meningocele. **A.** Axial computed tomography shows cystic mass anterior to sacrum and posterior to rectum. **B.** In a different patient, midsagittal magnetic resonance (MR) T1-weighted image shows large anterior sacral cerebrospinal fluid-filled meningocele *(arrow)* communicating with distal end of thecal sac. Note agenesis of distal sacral segments. The mother of this girl also had a similar lesion repaired in childhood. **C.** Corresponding MR T2-weighted image shows cord is dysplastic, thin, and tethered posteriorly *(arrow)* at the S1 level. There is a fluid-filled cyst in the lower thoracic and lumbar spinal cord. The anterior sacral meningocele is well seen and its fluid is of inhomogeneous signal intensity, probably because of pulsations. (Case courtesy of S. Birchansky and N. Altman, Miami Children's Hospital, Miami, FL.)

SUGGESTED READING

1. Geremia GK, Russell EJ, Clasen RA. MR imaging characteristics of a neuroenteric cyst. AJNR 1988;9:978.

16.08   *Closed Spinal Dysraphism: Spinal Epidermoids, Dermoids, and Teratomas*

EPIDEMIOLOGY

These tumors result from an anomalous dysjunction of the neural ectoderm from the surface ectoderm and retention of cell rests, or are iatrogenically produced. They comprise 1% to 2% of all intradural tumors in all ages and 10% of all intradural tumors before 10 years of age. Approximately half of them are single epidermoids and half are single dermoids. A small percentage are multiple (epi)dermoids. Dermal sinuses are found in 20% of patients with these tumors. Teratomas of the sacrococcygeal region are uncommon and occur mostly in girls. Some of these teratomas are inherited as an autosomal dominant trait.

CLINICAL FEATURES

Dermal sinuses are typically located in the lumbosacral region (> 60%). Most are present above the intergluteal fold. They may have an associated hairy patch, cutis aplasia, or hemangioma. Sixty percent to 50% of them are accompanied by an intraspinal (epi)dermoid(s). Conversely, one-third of (epi)dermoids are accompanied by a dermal sinus. If the opening of a sinus is midline, a dermoid is more common; however, if the opening is off the midline, an epidermoid is more common. Dermoids may also be associated with spina bifida occulta. These tumors may also arise from implanted cells during surgery or from prior lumbar puncture done with needles without a trocar. These iatrogenic tumors require 1 to 20 years to become symptomatic, and they present with radiculopathies, hamstring spasm, lordosis, and gait abnormalities. Masses related to a dermal sinus may become infected and present with a meningitis-like picture. These masses contain epidermis, dermis, hair follicles, and sweat and sebaceous glands. Their walls may be adherent to the conus medullaris (which may be low-lying and tethered by the mass) and to the cauda equina. Surgery is the treatment of choice. The mass is approached by removal of intratumoral contents. The portion of the wall adherent to neural structures is left in place to avoid complications and the patients are followed with magnetic resonance (MR) imaging to exclude recurrence of the lesion.

Teratomas of the sacrococcygeal regions are large masses, most of them classified as mature on histologic examination. However, up to one-third of them may be immature teratomas or contain foci of anaplastic carcinoma. Most of them involve the distal sacrum and extend anteriorly into the pelvis. Only a very small percentage are truly intraspinal.

IMAGING FEATURES

Magnetic resonance is the imaging method of choice in the evaluation of these patients. Contrast administration is helpful in delineating infected masses. These tumors are commonly seen with dysraphic states or segmentation anomalies involving the lower spine. Epidermoids are commonly of similar signal intensity to cerebrospinal fluid in all MR imaging sequences, and may be difficult to visualize (Fig. 16.08-1). Dermoids are commonly but not always fatty in appearance, and 50% of them are extramedullary intradural in location (Fig. 16.08-2). Droplets of fat may become deposited in the subarachnoid spaces after rupture of a dermoid. The imaging features of both tumors overlap, and it may not be possible to differentiate them. The conus medullaris is commonly low-lying and adjacent to the masses.

Teratoma occurs in the distal spinal canal and is often associated with spinal dysraphism (Fig. 16.08-3). Teratomas may be classified into those situated almost posteriorly with a minimal pelvic component (group 1), those with a significant pelvic component (group 2), those mainly in the abdomen and pelvis (group 3), those that are entirely presacral (group 4), and intraspinal ones. Teratoma is a heterogeneous mass in all MR imaging sequences, and also contains fat.

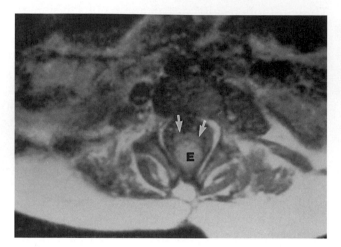

FIGURE 16.08-1.

Epidermoid. Axial magnetic resonance T1-weighted image shows a rounded mass (E) of intermediate signal intensity in dorsal aspect of a widened lumbar thecal sac. Note sinus tract in subcutaneous fat and posterior dysraphic defect. The mass (proven epidermoid) insinuates into the inner aspect of a placode (arrows).

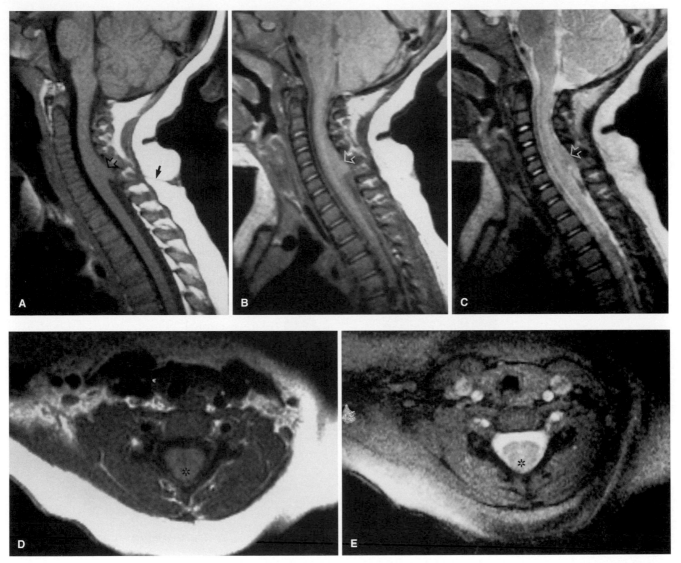

FIGURE 16.08-2.

Dermoid. **A.** Midsagittal magnetic resonance (MR) T1-weighted image shows sinus tract *(arrow)* and mass in posterior midcervical spinal canal *(open arrow)* that merges with cord. **B.** Corresponding proton density image shows dermoid *(open arrow)* to be isointense to spinal cord. **C.** On a T2-weighted image, the mass *(open arrow)* is again isointense to spinal cord. **D.** Axial MR T1-weighted image shows intramedullary dermoid (*) to be inseparable from the spinal cord. **E.** Axial MR T2-weighted image shows dermoid (*) again to be inseparable from spinal cord. At histology, this "dermoid" contained glial, meningeal, neuronal, and ectodermal elements, but no fat. Perhaps the term "hamartoma" may be better suited to describe these lesions.

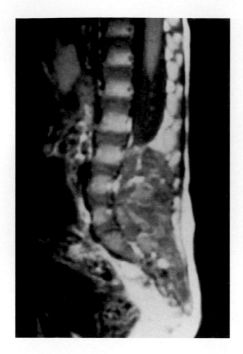

FIGURE 16.08-3.

Intraspinal teratoma. Midsagittal magnetic resonance T1-weighted image in a different patient shows a large, complex mass in the distal spine producing scalloping of L4, L5, and the sacrum. There is posterior bony dysraphism. The position of the conus medullaris is normal.

SUGGESTED READINGS

1. Machida T, Abe O, Sasaki Y, et al. Acquired epidermoid tumor in the thoracic spinal canal. Neuroradiology 1993;35:316.
2. Barsi P, Kenez J, Varallyay, Gergely L. Unusual origin of subarachnoid fat drops: a ruptured spinal dermoid tumor. Neuroradiology 1992;34:343.

16.09   *Closed Spinal Dysraphism: Diastematomyelia and Diplomyelia*

EPIDEMIOLOGY

Diastematomyelia refers to splitting of the spinal cord into hemicords by a mesodermal spur. Diplomyelia refers to complete duplication of the spinal cord with or without duplication of the vertebral column. Diastematomyelia occurs in 1% to 5% of patients with scoliosis and in up to 30% of patients with open spinal dysraphism. Over 90% of patients with diastematomyelia are girls. Diplomyelia is extremely rare, with only a few cases reported in the literature.

CLINICAL FEATURES

The clinical manifestations are similar to those seen in patients with open spinal dysraphism, but typically there is compromise of the anterior horns with muscle atrophy, decreased or absent deep tendon reflexes, and moderate to severe distal weakness of the lower extremities. Abnormalities are bilateral. Deformities of the feet (50%) and urinary problems are common. Overlying the spur there may be a dermal sinus, lipoma, hairy patch, pigmented nevus, or hemangioma. These cutaneous stigmata are present in 50% to 75% of patients with diastematomyelia. Several explanations for this abnormality have been proposed. An adhesion between the endoderm and ectoderm may develop and provide a physical barrier that splits the notochord. A split notochord will induce two neuroepithelial anlagens with subsequent development of hemicords. Other hypotheses include primary duplication of the notochord and persistence of neurenteric communications, inducing the formation of a spur. Histologically, the spur may be composed of fibrous tissue, cartilage, fat, bone, or a combination of these. In diastematomyelia, each hemicord has one ventral and one dorsal rootlet. In diplomyelia, each hemicord has two ventral and two dorsal rootlets. We have seen one case of such an entity in which the patient had relatively few symptoms, which included urinary retention, constipation, and scoliosis.

IMAGING FEATURES

We consider magnetic resonance the imaging method of choice in these anomalies. In diastematomyelia, a segmentation anomaly (hemivertebra, butterfly vertebra, or block vertebra) is present in over 95% of patients. The laminae may also be fused. The interpedicular distance is increased at the level of the spur. Kyphoscoliosis is seen in over 50% of patients. In half of the cases, the hemicords are contained in a single meningeal tube (Fig. 16.09-1A, B). In these cases, no spur is present, but occasionally a fibrofatty plug is located between the hemicords. In the other half, each hemicord has its own pial–arachnoid covering (Fig. 16.09-1C). In these cases, a spur is found. Most hemicords are asymmetric in size with respect to each other, and most are fused (90%) into a single spinal cord above and below the level of splitting. One-half of spurs are found in the thoracic region, and the other half in the lumbar spine. Spurs are multiple in 6% of patients. Most spurs arise from the laminae and cross anteriorly. In up to 50% of patients, a spinal cord fluid-filled cyst is present (usually involving the larger hemicord). Axial T2-weighted gradient echo images should be obtained through the level of the splitting to exclude a spur. If no spur is identified in these cases, the possibility of a very thin fibrous spur still may not be excluded. However, if a spur is identified, it is of great help to the surgeon. Other findings seen in patients with diastematomyelia include a low-lying conus medullaris, thickened filum terminale, epidermoids, and dermoids. In the one case of diplomyelia that we have seen, the lower lumbar spine and sacrum were duplicated and contained two complete sets of neural foramina each (Fig. 16.09-2). The upper, single spinal cord was low-lying and tethered by a fatty spur. It also contained a fluid cyst. One of the hemicords also was further divided into halves because it was split by a second spur.

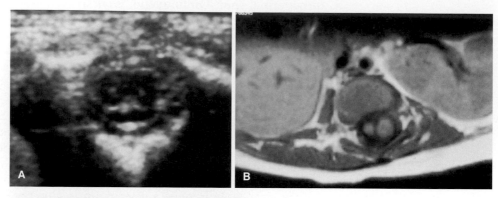

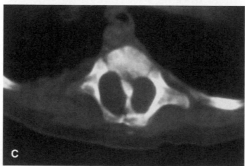

FIGURE 16.09-1.

Diastematomyelia. **A.** Axial sonographic view shows two fairly symmetric hemicords with two discrete central canals. There is a single subarachnoid space posteriorly and no spur (so-called internal diastematomyelia). **B.** Axial magnetic resonance T1-weighted image in the same patient shows two hemicords, the left greater than the right. There is a single subarachnoid space and no obvious spur. **C.** Axial computed tomography shows bony spur traversing the spinal canal and dividing it into two halves. The hemicords in this case are contained in separate subarachnoid spaces (so-called external diastematomyelia).

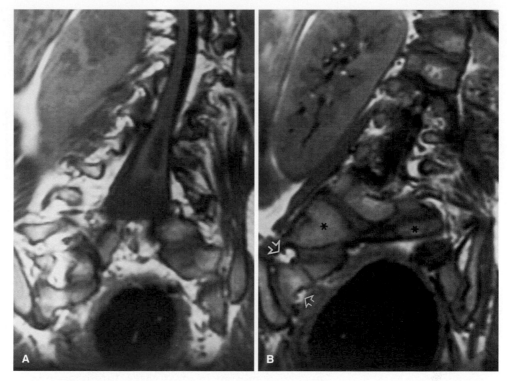

FIGURE 16.09-2.

Diplomyelia. A. Coronal magnetic resonance (MR) T1-weighted image shows dupli-cated sacrum and cauda equina. There is a cyst in the distal spinal cord (syrinx versus ventriculus terminalis). **B.** Coronal MR T1-weighted image in the same patient shows duplicated sacrum (*) with multiple segmentation anomalies. Note complete duplica-tion of neural foramina *(arrows)* and nerve roots in each sacrum. (With permission from Castillo M, Hankins L, Kramer L, Wilson BA. MR imaging of diplomyelia: case report. Magn Reson Imaging 1992;10:699.)

SUGGESTED READINGS

1. Castillo M. MRI of diastematomyelia. MRI Decisions 1991;5:12.
2. Castillo M, Hankins L, Kramer L, Wilson BA. MR imaging of diplomyelia: case re-port. Magn Reson Imaging 1992;10:699.

16.10 Anomalies of Canalization and Retrogressive Differentiation: Caudal Regression Syndrome

EPIDEMIOLOGY

Caudal regression syndrome refers to absence of the sacrum and lower lumbar spine accompanied by abnormalities of the conus medullaris, cauda equina, genitourinary system, and anus. It occurs in approximately 1:7500 to 25,000 live births. It is more common in diabetic mothers, in which it affects 1% to 15% of their newborns. An increased incidence is also seen with paternal diabetes. There is no relationship between the severity of the diabetes and the severity of the caudal agenesis, but mild forms of the anomaly are more common than severe ones. Partial sacral agenesis (scimitar sacrum) has a sex-linked dominant inheritance pattern. Caudal dysplasias are also associated with Potter syndrome.

CLINICAL FEATURES

Musculoskeletal problems include club feet, scoliosis, open spinal dysraphism, hip dislocation, and the Klippel-Feil syndrome. Motor function is usually within one level of the last normal-appearing vertebral body. Most children have some sensation in the perineal area, but it is absent in the lower extremities. Motor deficits are more severe than sensory abnormalities. Neurogenic bladder is present in most cases. Intelligence is usually normal unless there is associated myelomeningocele with hydrocephalus. Urinary anomalies include horseshoe kidneys, pelvic kidneys, absence of one kidney, and duplicated collecting systems. In 30% of children with imperforate anus, sacral agenesis is found. Ventricular septal defects and pulmonary hypoplasia may also be present. Death usually results from renal failure (secondary to repeated infections) or cardiac defects. Treatment is geared toward establishing stability of the vertebral–pelvic complex, protecting viscera from compression, releasing lower extremity contractures, and supporting the unstable spine (usually through correction of scoliosis).

IMAGING FEATURES

The initial diagnosis may be confirmed with plain radiographs. There is partial or complete agenesis of the sacrum (Fig. 16.10-1A). One-half of the sacrum may be missing (scimitar sacrum). Isolated agenesis of the coccyx may be a developmental variant. Above the agenesis, the vertebral bodies may be fused. The spine terminates at the T11–T12 level in 35% of patients, at L1–L4 in 40% of patients, and below L5 in 27% of patients. Significant scoliosis is present when one side of the sacrum is missing. Segmentation anomalies are seen in 22% of cases and spinal dysraphism in 33% of patients. The thecal sac tapers at the level of the distal-most vertebrae. The conus medullaris is high and has a truncated (wedge-shaped) appearance with its tip missing (Fig. 16.10-1B). The cauda equina may have a peculiar appearance because of absence of some nerve roots (Fig. 16.10-1C). There is a second group of patients with this syndrome in whom the conus medullaris is not truncated and extends to the level of sacral agenesis (Fig. 16.10-1D). The cord is usually tethered inferiorly in these cases. The pelvis is small and the lower extremities may also be small and positioned in extreme external rotation, or fused (sirenomelia).

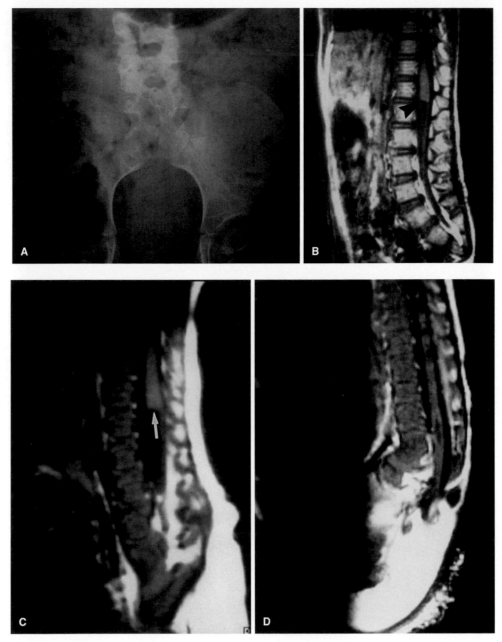

FIGURE 16.10-1.

Sacral agenesis. **A.** Frontal radiograph shows complete agenesis of the sacrum. (Case courtesy of David Merten, M.D., Chapel Hill, NC.) **B.** Midsagittal magnetic resonance (MR) T1-weighted image (different patient) shows presence of only S1 and S2. The conus medullaris *(arrowhead)* is truncated and the nerve roots of the cauda equina sparse. (With permission from Castillo M. Neuroradiology Companion. Philadelphia: JB Lippincott, 1995.) **C.** Midsagittal MR T1-weighted image in a different patient with agenesis of sacrum shows truncated conus medullaris *(arrow)*, marked reduction in the number of nerve roots in the cauda equina, and filling of the distal spinal canal with fat. **D.** Midsagittal MR T1-weighted image in a different patient with a different type of caudal regression features shows absent sacrum. The conus medullaris extends to the lowermost thecal sac, where it is probably tethered by lipoma. There is a small posterior meningocele. The conus contains a cyst (syrinx versus ventriculus terminalis) that expands the cord slightly.

SUGGESTED READINGS

1. Nielvelstein RAJ, Valk J, Smit LME, Vermeij-Keers C. MR of the caudal regression syndrome: embryologic implications. AJNR 1994;15:1021.
2. Barkovich AJ, Raghaven N, Chuang S, Peck WW. The wedge-shaped cord terminus: a radiographic sign of caudal regression. AJNR 1989;10:1223.

16.11 Anomalies of Canalization and Retrogressive Differentiation: Ventriculus Terminalis

EPIDEMIOLOGY

Ventriculus terminalis refers to a small, ependymal-lined, fluid-filled cavity in the distal conus medullaris. It is found in approximately 2:6 of spinal pediatric MR studies. It appears to be more common in girls (12:1). It has been reported in a patient with a Chiari type 1 malformation.

CLINICAL
SYMPTOMS

Most patients present with nonspecific symptoms, including recurrent low back pain, sciatica, and bladder dysfunction. These symptoms commonly manifest during adult life. The ventriculus terminalis probably represents a remnant of the vacuoles within the superior aspect of the caudal cell mass that normally forms the distal aspect of the conus medullaris. Although histologically it is contiguous with the spinal central canal, the canal proper is not dilated. Some authors have postulated that the ventriculus terminalis results from dilation of an accessory spinal canal. If neurologic symptoms are present, shunting of the fluid-filled cavity may be indicated.

IMAGING FEATURES

Magnetic resonance (MR) is the imaging modality of choice. Plain radiographs occasionally show expansion of the bony spinal canal at the level of the cyst. MR imaging shows the signal intensity of the cavity to be equal or very similar to that of cerebrospinal fluid in all sequences (Fig. 16.11-1). The cavities are ovoid in shape and usually measure 2 to 4 cm in length and 1 to 2.5 cm in diameter. They have no internal septations. Their walls usually measure approximately 2 mm in thickness, but may be extremely thin and difficult to visualize. There is no abnormal enhancement after contrast administration and no change in size in follow-up studies. Myelography is not indicated, but if performed, a spinal block and a mass lesion are found. The differential diagnosis should include ependymoma, astrocytoma, hemangioblastoma, oligodendroglioma, and intramedullary neuroma.

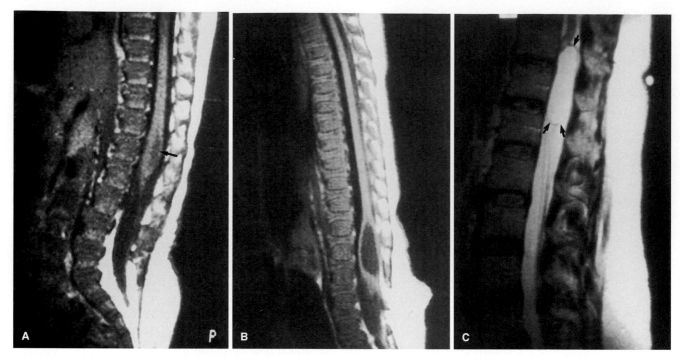

FIGURE 16.11-1.

Ventriculus terminalis. **A.** Midsagittal magnetic resonance (MR) T1-weighted image shows small hypodensity *(arrow)* expanding distal conus medullaris. It did not enhance after contrast administration. **B.** Midsagittal MR T1-weighted image in a different patient shows larger cyst in distal conus medullaris. **C.** Midsagittal MR T2-weighted image (different patient) shows large and expansile cyst in distal conus medullaris. Note thin walls *(arrows)*. At surgery, ependyma lined the cyst.

SUGGESTED READINGS

1. Sigal R, Denys A, Halimi P, Shapeero L, Doyon D, Boudghene F. Ventriculus terminalis of the conus medullaris: MR imaging in four patients with congenital dilatation. AJNR 1991;12:733.
2. Coleman LT, Zimmerman RA, Rorke LB. Ventriculus terminalis of the conus medullaris: MR findings in children. AJNR 1995;16:1421.

16.12 Dysplasias: Idiopathic Scoliosis

EPIDEMIOLOGY — Idiopathic scoliosis is divided into infantile (0–3 years of age), juvenile (4–9 years of age), and adolescent (> 10 years of age) forms. The incidence of scoliosis in the general population is approximately 5%. The juvenile type accounts for 12% to 20% of patients with idiopathic scoliosis. The adolescent type is probably inherited as dominant trait and is found in up to 27% of girls born to mothers with scoliosis. It is also seen in 7% of siblings of those affected by this disorder.

CLINICAL FEATURES — Infantile idiopathic scoliosis is more common in boys (Fig. 16.12-1). Probable etiologies include intrauterine molding and postnatal pressure due to constant supine position in the crib. In scoliosis occurring before 5 years of age, cardiopulmonary complications are not unusual. This is especially true when the deformity is noted before 1 year of age and continuously progresses. Pulmonary arterial hypertension leads to cardiac failure. Serial elongation–derotation flexion casting is the noninvasive treatment of choice. If the scoliosis is progressive despite this treatment, surgical placement of rods may be indicated.

In the juvenile form, the gender predilection is related to the age of presentation. Early on, boys are affected more than girls; later on, girls are affected more than boys. Approximately 70% of curves are progressive and eventually require treatment. Bracing may be used to stabilize or slow the progression of the scoliosis. Surgical instrumentation with or without fusion (anterior, posterior, combined, or limited) may be necessary.

The adolescent type is more common in girls. A deviation from the normal growth pattern is required for this anomaly to develop (it is more common in children of tall parents). Other factors involved in its genesis include hormonal influence, asymmetric growth, primary abnormalities of the intervertebral discs, and collagen defects. The most common symptom is back pain (80%–90%), followed by pulmonary function abnormalities (present more commonly in cases of severe scoliosis). Noninvasive treatment consists of wearing orthoses (braces). Surgical instrumentation and fusion are now being done in fewer patients than in the past.

IMAGING FEATURES — In the infantile type, most curves are centered in the thoracic region and are convex to the left. In the juvenile type, there is no particular segment or side affected; however, left-sided curves tend to improve without treatment. In adolescent scoliosis, most curves are rightward and thoracic. Plain radiographs are obtained to measure the angle of scoliosis using the Cobb method (Fig. 16.12-2). A line is drawn tangential to the upper border of the cephalad-most vertebral body tilting toward the center of the radius of the curve. The lower limit is defined similarly, but the line is tangential to the lower border of the caudal-most vertebral body. Lines are drawn perpendicular to the two initial lines and the angle subtended by these lines measures the scoliosis. More than 10° is required to make the diagnosis, and usually an angle greater than 50° before skeletal maturity is an indication for surgical intervention. Before surgery, we usually obtain magnetic resonance imaging of the entire spine. This is done to exclude an occult lesion such as a nerve sheath tumor or tethering of the spinal cord. Computed tomography may, however, help in outlining underlying bone abnormalities, which usually are related to vertebral segmentation defects (Figs. 16.12-3 and 16.12-4).

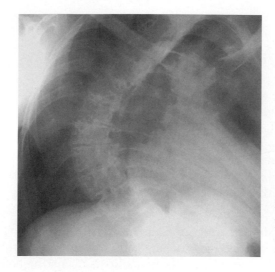

FIGURE 16.12-1.

Idiopathic scoliosis. Frontal radiograph shows dextroscoliosis (apex pointing to the right side).

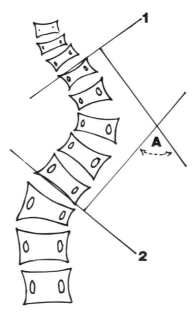

FIGURE 16.12-2.

The Cobb method for measuring angle of scoliosis. Line 1 is drawn parallel to superior end plate of curve, line 2 is drawn parallel to inferior end plate of curve. Lines perpendicular to the initial two are drawn, and the angle (A) is obtained.

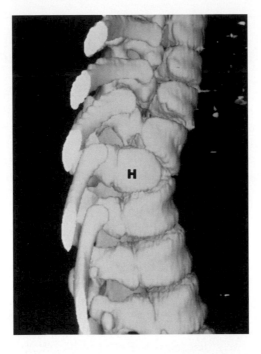

FIGURE 16.12-3.

Scoliosis due to hemivertebra. Lateral view from three-dimensional computed tomography reformation in a patient with scoliosis and minimal kyphosis due to a lower thoracic hemivertebra (H).

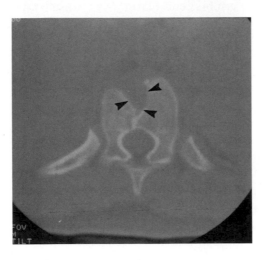

FIGURE 16.12-4.

Butterfly vertebra. Axial computed tomography, bone windows, in a different patient with scoliosis shows butterfly vertebra. The midline cleft *(arrowheads)* is caused by incomplete involution of the notochord. (With permission from Castillo M. Neuroradiology Companion. Philadelphia: JB Lippincott, 1995.)

SUGGESTED READINGS

1. Dickson RA. Early-onset idiopathic scoliosis. In: Weinstein SL, ed. The Pediatric Spine: Principles and Practice. New York: Raven, 1994:421.
2. Warner WC. Juvenile idiopathic scoliosis. In: Weinstein SL, ed. The Pediatric Spine: Principles and Practice. New York: Raven, 1994:431.
3. Weinstein SL. Adolescent idiopathic scoliosis: prevalence and natural history. In: Weinstein SL, ed. The Pediatric Spine: Principles and Practice. New York: Raven, 1994:463.

16.13 *Dysplasias: Congenital Kyphosis and Scheuermann's Disease*

EPIDEMIOLOGY

Congenital kyphosis is the most common noninfectious cause of spinal deformity resulting in paraplegia during childhood. It has no gender predilection. It may be seen in association with abnormalities of chromosomes 7, 18, and 20, and in myelodysplasias.

Scheuermann's disease is a juvenile kyphotic disorder affecting mostly young boys. Its incidence is approximately between 0.5% to 8% of the population.

CLINICAL FEATURES

Congenital kyphosis is caused by failure of formation of a vertebra or part of a vertebra (type 1), anomalous vertebral segmentation (type 2), and rotatory dislocation of the spine (type 3). Associated symptoms include compression of the spinal cord and abnormal respiratory function, which may eventually lead to heart failure. Progressive deformities in growing children may be treated by epiphysiodesis with fusion and postoperative casting. Established deformities may need decompression of the spinal canal and fusion.

Scheuermann's disease is believed to be secondary to an osteochondrosis of the thoracic vertebral end plates. Symptoms and deformity are commonly noted around 10 years of age. Pain is relatively uncommon, as are neurologic abnormalities. Treatment is controversial because some authors state that the deformity will not produce a disability (pulmonary, neurologic, or cosmetic) in most patients. In other reports, curves greater than 50° have been progressive, and therefore some form of surgical stabilization has been advised.

IMAGING FEATURES

Plain radiographs are needed for the initial diagnosis and follow-up of kyphosis. Computed tomography helps in establishing underlying congenital abnormalities in the vertebrae, and magnetic resonance imaging may be needed to exclude the possibility of an occult dysraphism, low-lying and tethered spinal cord, intraspinal epidermoid, dermoid, and lipoma. Type 1 kyphosis results from partial or complete absence of a vertebra. It results in an acute-angle curvature usually centered at the thoracic and thoracolumbar regions. Type 2 kyphosis is nonangular and smooth, but slowly progressive. Spontaneous fusion may occur in these patients. In type 3 kyphosis, there is an anomalous vertebra, which is dislocated. This type of anomaly is unstable and has a significant risk for spinal cord compression.

The diagnosis of Scheuermann's disease may be confirmed with lateral plain radiographs of the thoracic spine (Fig. 16.13-1). The following criteria are needed to make the diagnosis: irregular upper and lower vertebral body end plates, loss of disc space height, involvement of three or more adjacent vertebral bodies, vertebral body wedging of more than 5° by the Cobb method, and a kyphosis greater than 40° by the Cobb method. Schmorl's nodes are also commonly present.

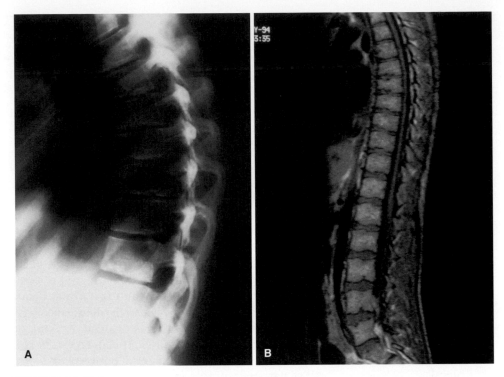

FIGURE 16.13-1.

Scheuermann's disease. **A.** Lateral radiograph shows kyphosis and irregular end plates throughout the thoracic spine in this teenager. **B.** Midsagittal magnetic resonance T1-weighted image in a different patient shows multiple irregularities in the end plates of all vertebral bodies (Schmorl's nodes), but no significant kyphosis (early Scheuermann's disease?).

SUGGESTED READINGS

1. Wolpert SM, Barnes PD. MRI in Pediatric Neuroradiology. St. Louis: Mosby Year Book, 1992:402.
2. Ascani E, La Rosa G. Scheuermann's kyphosis. In: Weinstein SL, ed. The Pediatric Spine: Principles and Practice. New York: Raven, 1994:557.

16.14   Dysplasias: Neurofibromatosis Types I and II

EPIDEMIOLOGY

Spinal abnormalities are present in two-thirds of patients with neurofibromatosis type I (NF-1) and in 88% of patients with neurofibromatosis type II (NF-2).

CLINICAL FEATURES

Spinal abnormalities in these patients may be divided into those arising in the soft tissues and those involving the bone. In NF-1 patients, soft tissue abnormalities include mainly neurofibromas, which are more common in the lumbar and cervical regions. These neurofibromas are infiltrative masses inseparable from the nerves. Histologically, neurofibromas may be composed of a monoclonal line of cells and may be considered more akin to a hamartoma than to a true neoplasia. Polyclonal neurofibromas are common also, and these have a 5% tendency toward malignant degeneration. Neurofibrosarcomas present with motor deficits, pain, and dysesthesias. Dural ectasia usually produces bone abnormalities, and intramedullary tumors (astrocytomas) are relatively rare. Clinically, these patients may have cervical kyphosis that may be secondary to neurofibromas or primary bone deformities. If instability is present, surgical fusion may be necessary. Thoracic scoliosis is the most common spinal abnormality in NF-1 patients. It is found in approximately 30% of NF-1 patients, and its incidence increases with age. It is secondary to neurofibromas, osteomalacia, or mesodermal dysplasia. Acute-angle kyphosis is typical but less common. Other spinal complications include dural ectasia (including lateral thoracic meningoceles), spinal dislocations, and spinal pseudarthrosis. Lateral thoracic meningoceles are common masses resulting from dysplasia of either the pedicles or meninges.

In patients with NF-2, the salient spinal abnormalities include intradural extramedullary masses (schwannomas and meningiomas) and intramedullary masses (ependymomas or spinal cord fluid-filled cysts). Bony deformities are usually secondary to these masses.

IMAGING FEATURES

In NF-1 patients, intramedullary astrocytomas almost always show enhancement on magnetic resonance imaging. However, some low-grade tumors without enhancement have also been described. The possibility of hamartomas should be considered in the presence of nonenhancing intramedullary abnormalities. Neurofibromas tend to involve the C4, T3, L1–L5, and S1 levels, and always enhance after contrast administration (Fig. 16.14-1A–C). They produce enlargement of the neural foramina by erosion. In the thoracic spine, lateral thoracic meningoceles are more common than isolated neurofibromas. Lateral thoracic meningoceles are of cerebrospinal fluid-equivalent signal intensity in all sequences, do not enhance, but also result in enlarged neural foramina. All of the above-mentioned abnormalities may result in severe scoliosis. In some patients, no cause is found for this scoliosis (Fig. 16.14-1D). Note that even in the presence of multiple abnormalities, many patients are asymptomatic.

In NF-2 patients, most intramedullary masses are ependymomas (Fig. 16.14-2A). These ependymomas occur predominantly in the cervical region. Fluid-filled cysts may accompany these tumors. Intradural extramedullary masses in these patients are usually schwannomas or meningiomas (Fig. 16.14-2B). Meningiomas tend to occur in the thoracic spine and usually present in the second or third decade of life. Both meningiomas and schwannomas may have a "dumbbell" configuration and both enhance markedly after contrast administration. Bone abnormalities are identical to those found in

NF-1 patients and consist of enlargement of the neural foramina and scalloping of the posterior surface of the vertebral bodies. The incidence of these bony changes is also very similar in both groups of patients. However, dural ectasia is much more common in NF-1 patients than in NF-2 patients. In NF-2 patients, spinal bone changes are secondary to pressure erosion from masses.

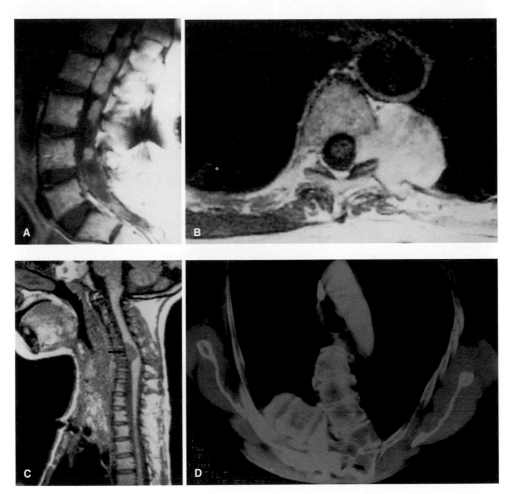

FIGURE 16.14-1.

Neurofibromatosis type I (NF-1).   **A.** Midsagittal magnetic resonance (MR) T1-weighted image shows multiple enhancing neurofibromas arising from the cauda equina. **B.** Axial MR T1-weighted image in a different patient shows enhancing neurofibroma in the left paraspinal region extending into a neural foramen, which is expanded. **C.** Midsagittal noncontrast MR T1-weighted image shows medial aspect of dumbbell-shaped neurofibroma *(arrow)*, which simulates an intramedullary abnormality. The cord is thin and draped around the tumor. Note large plexiform neurofibroma in the neck of this patient obliterating the airway (tracheostomy in place). **D.** Axial computed tomography shows in a single 5-mm slice two segments of the thoracic spine as a result of the acute-angle scoliosis typical of patients with NF-1.

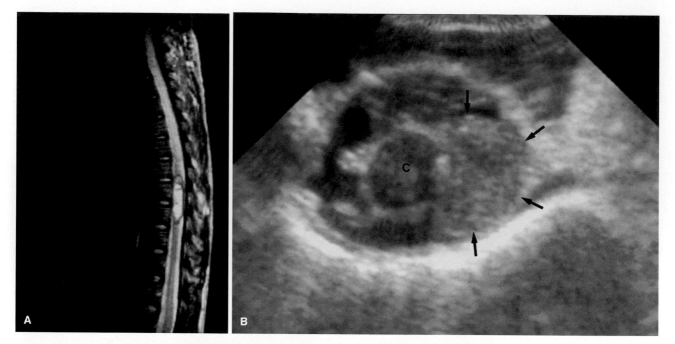

FIGURE 16.14-2.

Neurofibromatosis type II (NF-2).   **A.** Midsaggital magnetic resonance T2-weighted image in an NF-2 patient shows a midthoracic intramedullary mass of high signal intensity surrounded by hypointensity. These features are typical of ependymoma. **B.** Transverse intraoperative sonogram shows schwannoma *(arrows)* lateral to the conus medullaris (C). This tumor arose from an anterior rootlet.

SUGGESTED READINGS

1. Egelhoff JC, Bates DJ, Ross JS, Rothner AD, Cohen BH. Spinal MR findings in neurofibromatosis types 1 and 2. AJNR 1992;13:1071.
2. Elster AD. Radiologic screening in the neurocutaneous syndromes: strategies and controversies. AJNR 1992;13:1078.

16.15 *Spinal Cord Fluid-Filled Cysts*

EPIDEMIOLOGY

Spinal cord fluid cysts (defined as enlarging cavities) may exist inside the central spinal canal (hydromyelia) or outside of it (syringomyelia). This division is somewhat arbitrary because both are difficult to distinguish by imaging (and even pathologic) examinations, and both require similar treatment. Spinal cord cavities are seen mostly in patients with Chiari malformations, but may also be seen in association with inflammatory processes of the basal meninges, with tumors, or they may be idiopathic. They may also be seen in 2% to 8% of patients with posttraumatic paraplegia.

CLINICAL FEATURES

Spinal cord cysts may communicate with the subarachnoid space (seen with Chiari malformations, basal arachnoiditis, and lesions of the foramen magnum), or they may be isolated from the subarachnoid space (seen with intramedullary tumors, spinal arachnoiditis, after trauma, and in idiopathic forms). The etiology of these cysts is uncertain. We favor the possibility of cerebrospinal fluid penetrating an injured spinal cord (or, less likely, a healthy one) because of differential pressures and inducing the formation of microcysts. Pulsations lead to sloshing of the intracystic fluid and result in propagation of the cysts. The dissecting cysts may leave behind septations (these are commonly seen on magnetic resonance [MR] imaging).

Symptoms related to spinal cord cysts include suspended and dissociated sensory loss (especially in the upper extremities), neck and occipital pain, and weakness of the arms. Neurogenic arthropathies occur in 5% to 7% of patients with cervical spinal cord cysts. Scoliosis is present in 25% of patients with spinal cord cysts. Treatment consists of shunting of hydrocephalus; if symptoms referable to the spinal cord cyst are present, then stenting the cyst to the subarachnoid space or peritoneal cavity may be needed. Marked improvement after surgery is uncommon. Half of the patients show at least some relief of symptoms, 30% become stable, and 20% continue to deteriorate.

IMAGING FEATURES

Magnetic resonance is the imaging method of choice (Fig. 16.15-1A, B). Sagittal T1-weighted images of the spine in patients with Chiari 1 malformations demonstrate a cord cyst in 20% to 50% of cases. These cysts are commonly located in the middle to upper cervical spinal cord. The cyst may be multiseptated. Flow void inside these cysts in the presence of symptoms may imply fluid turbulence and support the need for treatment (Fig. 16.15-1C). With the use of fast spin echo sequences, this finding is uncommon. Use of contrast material is controversial. Some believe that if a Chiari malformation is present, the spinal cord cyst is almost always caused by it, and contrast administration is not cost effective. Others prefer to give contrast to rule out the remote possibility of the cord cyst being secondary to a tumor. The diameter of the spinal canal may be increased in the presence of long-standing cysts. Spinal cord cysts are seen in 50% to 80% of patients with Chiari type 2 malformations. These cysts occur predominantly in the lower cervical and high thoracic regions. MR imaging is the method of choice for the follow-up of patients with spinal cord cysts (Fig. 16.15-2).

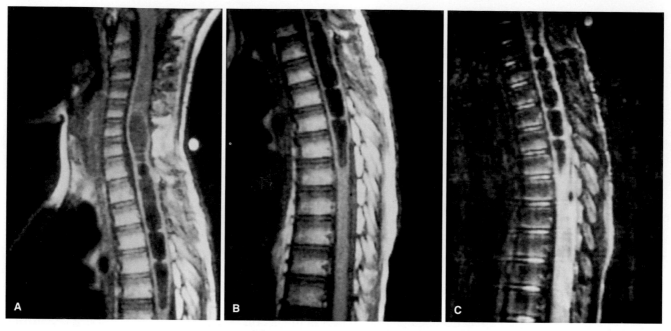

FIGURE 16.15-1.

Syringohydromyelia. **A.** Midsagittal magnetic resonance (MR) T1-weighted image shows multiseptated spinal cord cyst beginning in the uppermost cervical region and extending into the upper thoracic spinal cord. The cord and spinal canal are expanded. **B.** Midsagittal MR T1-weighted image in the same patient (coil placement is 30 cm below **A**) shows lower extension of cyst. The lower extent of the cyst should always be imaged. **C.** Midsagittal MR T2-weighted image (spin echo) at similar level to **B** shows dark signal intensity from the fluid inside the cyst, signifying dephasing due to fluid turbulence and pulsations. In patients with symptoms, this finding may indicate active growth of the cyst and the need for surgical decompression.

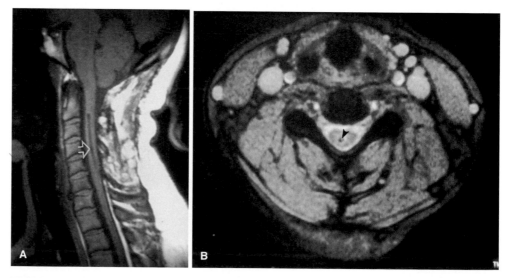

FIGURE 16.15-2.

Shunt in decompressed cyst. **A.** Midsagittal magnetic resonance (MR) T1-weighted image shows catheter *(arrow)* within well decompressed cervical spinal cord cyst. **B.** Axial MR T2-weighted image in the same patient shows catheter *(arrowhead)* as a small, punctate dark area in the central spinal cord. The catheter is surrounded by hyperintensity, which could represent gliosis.

SUGGESTED READING

1. Kochan PJ, Quencer RM. Imaging of cystic and cavitary lesions of the spinal cord and canal. Radiol Clin North Am 1991;29:867.

Imaging of the Pediatric Head, Neck, and Spine
by Mauricio Castillo and Suresh K. Mukherji,
Lippincott-Raven Publishing, Philadelphia © 1996.

17

Tumor, Infection, and Inflammation

17.0 *Extradural Masses: Osteoid Osteoma, Osteoblastoma, and Osteochondroma*

EPIDEMIOLOGY

Osteoid osteomas account for approximately 10% of all benign bone tumors, and 10% of them occur in the spine. Most cases occur between 6 and 17 years of age. There is no gender predilection. They are the most common cause of painful scoliosis in teenagers. Osteoblastomas (giant osteoid osteomas) account for less than 1% of all bone tumors. Most patients affected are between 10 to 15 years of age. Osteochondromas represent 40% of primary bone tumors, and are probably the most common one. Most are noted during the first two decades of life. Multiple tumors are not uncommon, and there is a familial form of osteochondromatosis.

CLINICAL FEATURES

Chronic pain is the presenting symptom in 60% of patients with osteoid osteomas. The pain occurs especially at night, which is thought to be secondary to higher levels of prostaglandins and venous congestion during this time of the day. Aspirin is cited as classically relieving the pain, but this is not always true. Diagnosis is made within 2 years of the onset of symptoms in 80% of patients. Histologically, the tumor is characterized by a nidus of bone surrounded by fibrovascular tissues with a dense bony margin. These tumors do not undergo malignant transformation. Prolonged administration of nonsteroidal antiinflammatory drugs is the noninvasive treatment of choice. Surgery results in immediate resolution of symptoms in over 95% of patients. Scoliosis does not resolve after tumor resection.

Osteoblastomas are osteoid osteomas measuring more than 2 cm in diameter. Pain is the most common symptom and usually is not relieved by aspirin or nonsteroidal antiinflammatory drugs. When they occur in the spine, they may result in scoliosis, radiculopathy, and myelopathy. These lesions are slowly growing but destructive, and surgical resection is the treatment of choice. Recurrences are seen in 10% of patients. Irradiation is controversial. Malignant transformation has been reported.

Histologically, ostcochondromas are composed of cortical and trabecular bone with a cap of cartilage. Osteochondromas rarely involve the spine (3%–7% of all osteochondromas). Most are asymptomatic but, rarely, they may produce spinal cord compression. Pressure on the tumor may result in pain, which is the most common symptom. Most lesions show growth in the teenage years and stop growing 1 to 2 years after adolescence is completed. There is a slight risk of malignant degeneration, mainly into chondrosarcoma. This risk is greater in the familial form of the disease. Surgery is indicated if malignant degeneration is suspected, with intractable pain due to pressure, or with compression of neurologic structures or blood vessels.

IMAGING FEATURES

Computed tomography is the imaging method of choice in these lesions (Fig. 17.0-1). However, radionuclide bone scanning is probably the most sensitive method for the initial detection of osteoid osteomas. Spinal osteoid osteoma tends to involve the posterior elements. The most common sites are the lumbar, cervical, thoracic, and sacral regions. The lesions measure 1 to 2 cm in diameter and are characterized by a central sclerotic nidus surrounded by lucency, which in turn is surrounded by a sclerotic margin.

Osteoblastomas tend to involve the pedicles and laminae, but may extend into the vertebral body in a small number of cases. The thoracic and lumbar regions are more commonly involved. They are relatively rare in the cervical and sacral regions. Radiographically, they are expansile lytic and destructive lesions. One-third of them contain calcifications. In 5% of cases, more than one adjacent vertebral body is involved. They may have a soft tissue component in the paraspinal muscles or the epidural space.

In the spine, osteochondromas often arise from the posterior elements (Fig. 17.0-2). Occasionally they arise from the posterior surface of the vertebral body or from the inner aspect of the facet joints, and may result in spinal cord compression. Radiographically, they contain areas of lucencies mixed with sclerosis, and the cartilaginous cap is usually dense. On magnetic resonance imaging, they are of mixed signal intensities, reflecting the different types of bone from which they are formed.

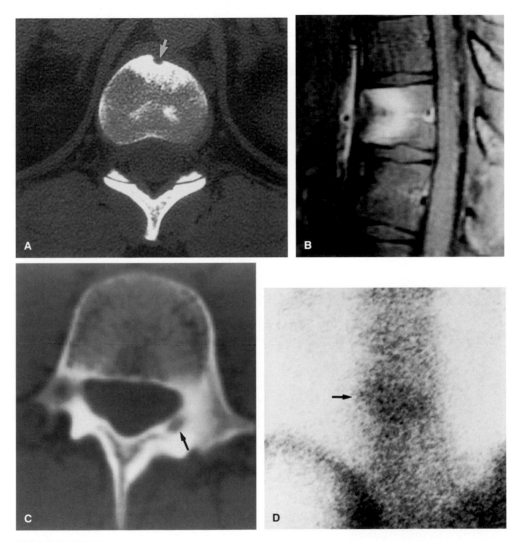

FIGURE 17.0-1.

Osteoid osteoma. **A.** Axial computed tomography (CT) shows lytic defect *(arrow)* in anterior cortex of vertebral body surrounded by sclerosis. **B.** Midsagittal magnetic resonance proton density image shows high signal intensity from vertebral body (corresponding to area of sclerosis on CT) and hypointensity anteriorly. **C.** Axial CT shows lucency *(arrow)* in left lamina of L4 surrounded by sclerosis. **D.** Radionuclide bone scan shows increased uptake by the lesion *(arrow)*. (Case courtesy of J. Renner, University of North Carolina, Chapel Hill, NC.)

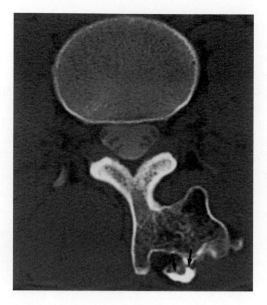

FIGURE 17.0-2.

Osteochondroma. Axial computed tomography shows osteochondroma arising from the spinous process of a lumbar vertebra. Note cartilaginous cap *(arrows)*. Study obtained after myelography.

SUGGESTED READING

1. Azouz EM, Kozlowski K, Martin D, Sprague P, Zerhouni A, Asselah F. Osteoid osteoma and osteoblastoma of the spine in children. Pediatr Radiol 1986;16:25.

17.01   Extradural Masses: Aneurysmal Bone Cyst and Giant Cell Tumor

EPIDEMIOLOGY

Aneurysmal bone cysts comprise 1% to 2% of all primary bone tumors. They are most commonly found between the ages of 5 to 20 years. Girls are affected more than boys.

Giant cell tumors comprise approximately 4% to 5% of primary bone tumors. They are commonly found after the second decade of life, and therefore are a disease predominantly of adults. There is no gender predilection.

CLINICAL FEATURES

Aneurysmal bone cysts may be primary or secondary. Those that do not arise de novo occur with other bone lesions such as giant cell tumor, chondroblastoma, chondromyxoid fibroma, fibrous dysplasia, and nonossifying fibroma. Aneurysmal bone cysts consist of large communicating spaces (cysts) filled with unclotted blood and lined by thin calcific shells or noncalcified periosteum, and therefore are not true tumors. Reactive changes occur within the lesion. About 20% of all aneurysmal bone cysts occur in the spine and present with pain. Pathologic fractures are also common. Neuropathy and myelopathy may occur secondary to compression. Excision and curettage are the treatments of choice. Recurrences are seen in 10% to 25% of patients. Preoperative catheter embolization helps to control bleeding during surgery and has been advocated by some as the primary mode of treatment. Irradiation often produces poor results.

Giant cell tumors are the second most common benign spinal tumor after hemangiomas, and are the most common benign lesion of the sacrum. Local pain and swelling are the most common initial symptoms. They are histologically benign but they may be locally aggressive, and have been associated with malignant degeneration and distant metastases. Sarcoma is found in 5% to 15% of cases treated primarily with irradiation. Needle biopsy is often needed to confirm the diagnosis, and the treatment of choice consists of excision and curettage, which may be followed by irradiation.

IMAGING FEATURES

In the spine, aneurysmal bone cysts involve the posterior elements in up to 60% of cases. They are more commonly located in the lumbosacral region, followed by the thoracic and cervical regions. They may involve adjacent vertebrae. Associated soft tissue masses are commonly present. Computed tomography (CT) shows a cystic, multiseptated mass with geographic margins delimited by thin bony walls (Fig. 17.01-1). The lesion is expansile and contains fluid-fluid levels. On magnetic resonance (MR), the lesion contains a wide range of signal intensities on both T1- and T2-weighted images, reflecting blood products in different stages of degradation. After contrast administration, enhancement may occur. Although these characteristics are highly suggestive of aneurysmal bone cyst, they are not specific, and may be seen in other lesions.

Giant cell tumors are expansile lytic lesions that commonly lack surrounding sclerosis. The lesion may involve the vertebral body or the neural arch. CT readily shows associated soft tissue masses (Fig. 17.01-2). On MR imaging, T1-weighted images show the lesion to be hypointense in relation to normal bone marrow. On T2-weighted images, the mass may be isointense to hypointense in relation to bone marrow. Patchy areas of increased signal intensity may be related to intratumoral hemorrhage.

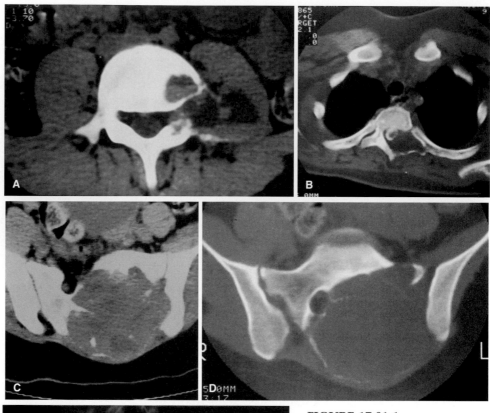

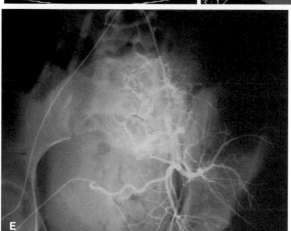

FIGURE 17.01-1.

Aneurysmal bone cyst. **A.** Axial computed tomography (CT) shows expansile lesion involving the left pedicle, transverse process, lamina, and posterior body of a lumbar vertebra. The lesion is extending into the left psoas muscle and contains multiple blood/fluid levels typical of aneurysmal bone cyst. **B.** Axial CT (after myelography) in a different patient shows expansile lesion with thin bony margins involving the left pedicle, transverse process, and lamina of an upper thoracic vertebra. **C.** Axial CT shows lytic lesion involving the sacrum. **D.** Corresponding bone windows show expansive nature of lesion. **E.** Conventional angiogram, frontal view, shows marked tumor hypervascularity. (Case illustrated in Figs. 17.01-1C, D, and E courtesy of J. Renner, University of North Carolina, Chapel Hill, NC.)

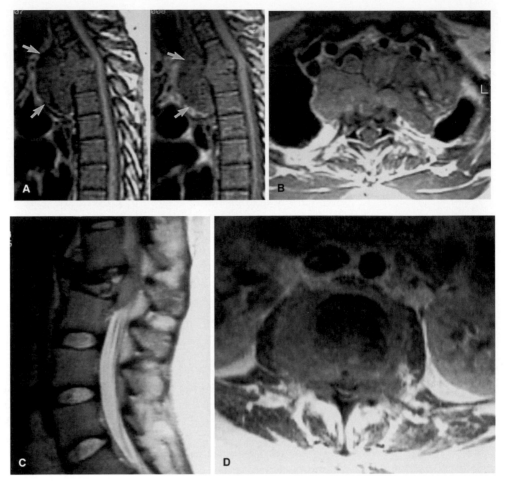

FIGURE 17.01-2.

Giant cell tumor. **A.** Parasagittal magnetic resonance (MR) proton density images show large soft tissue mass *(arrows)* anterior to spine and destruction of one upper thoracic vertebral body. There is compression of the spinal cord. **B.** Axial postcontrast MR T1-weighted image shows the very large size of the soft tissue component of this giant cell tumor. **C.** Midsagittal MR T2-weighted image in a different patient shows complete collapse of L1 vertebral body with bone fragment compressing the cauda equina. **D.** Axial MR T1-weighted image shows extensive soft tissue mass associated with vertebral collapse in this giant cell tumor.

SUGGESTED READINGS

1. Ameli NO, Abbassioun K, Saleh H, Eslamdoost A. Aneurysmal bone cysts of the spine. J Neurosurg 1985;63:685.
2. Beltran J, Simon D, Levey M, et al. Aneurysmal bone cysts: MR imaging at 1.5T. Radiology 1986;158:689.

17.02 *Extradural Masses: Sarcoma*

EPIDEMIOLOGY

Ewing sarcoma is the most common primary malignant bone tumor in children (note that in some series osteosarcomas are more common). Only 3% of them arise in the spine, most in the sacrum. Most are found between 5 to 15 years of age.

In the general population, osteosarcoma is more common than Ewing sarcoma, and accounts for approximately 20% to 25% of primary bone tumors. Its incidence is 1 to 2:1,000,000. One-half of all cases occur between 10 to 20 years of age, probably related to growth spurt. It is slightly more common in boys. Its incidence is markedly increased in children with retinoblastomas. It is very rare in the spine, where most osteosarcomas represent metastatic disease. Chondrosarcomas are less common than both of the above-mentioned tumors and are mostly a disease of adults, with most cases found between the fourth to seventh decades of life.

CLINICAL FEATURES

In the spine, Ewing sarcoma presents most commonly with pain, radiculopathy, myelopathy, fever, and a palpable mass. Elevation of the erythrocyte sedimentation rate is also common. Histologically, Ewing sarcoma is composed of numerous small, round cells similar to those found in neuroblastoma, rhabdomyosarcoma, leukemia, lymphoma, and other primitive neuroectodermal cell tumors. Treatment usually consists of a combination of surgery, chemotherapy, and irradiation. Long-term prognosis is poor. Metastases to the lungs, bones, lymph nodes, brain, and abdominal viscera may occur.

Of all osteosarcomas, less than 3% occur in the spine. The lesions originate mostly in the lower spine and usually present with neurologic symptoms and pain. Some osteosarcomas occur in previously irradiated bones. In children, they may also arise in osteochondromas (especially in the context of osteochondromatosis). Osteosarcoma of the spine is deadly. Surgical resection usually follows 6 weeks of chemotherapy. Irradiation may be given if chemotherapy has not been effective. Median survival varies from 10 months to 1 year after diagnosis. Metastases develop in 10% to 20% of patients.

IMAGING FEATURES

On plain radiographs and computed tomography (CT), Ewing sarcoma is a permeative, destructive lesion that may cause vertebral collapse and be radiographically indistinguishable from eosinophilic granuloma. Soft tissue extension is not uncommon. Occasionally the tumor is confined to the soft tissues (extraosseous Ewing sarcoma). By magnetic resonance (MR) imaging, T1-weighted images show low signal intensity and T2-weighted images may show either hyperintensity or hypointensity (related to high nuclei-to-cytoplasm ratio). After contrast administration, enhancement may be seen.

Over 90% of spinal osteosarcomas are found in the vertebral bodies. In the spine, they are commonly mixed lytic and blastic (Fig. 17.02-1). By MR imaging, T1-weighted images show the tumor to be hypointense with respect to bone marrow. On T2-weighted images, the tumor has a variable appearance. Invasion of the cortex is seen as absence of the normal signal void from this area. These tumors enhance after contrast administration. Epidural extension is common. Extraosseous extension is hyperintense on T2-weighted images and also enhances after contrast administration. Lack of involution and persistent abnormal signal intensity after chemotherapy correlate with a poor prognosis.

Both CT and MR imaging are ideal for the evaluation of other rare spinal and paraspinal sarcomas. Chondrosarcomas tend to form at the costovertebral junctions and may produce spinal cord compression (Fig. 17.02-2). Rhabdomyosarcomas may also arise from the paraspinal musculature and invade the spinal canal (Fig. 17.02-3).

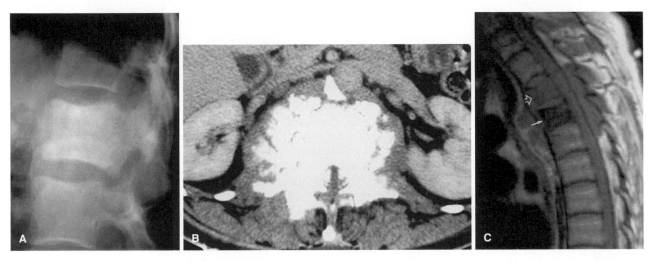

FIGURE 17.02-1.

Osteosarcoma. **A.** Lateral radiograph in a patient with osteosarcoma in a femur. There is a blastic metastasis to L1. **B.** CT at same level shows marked sclerosis and peripheral new bone formation. Note spinal canal stenosis. **C.** Midsagittal magnetic resonance proton density image shows metastases to two thoracic vertebrae. The low one is hypointense *(solid arrow)* and blastic by plain radiography, the superior one *(open arrow)* is hypointense and lytic by plain radiography.

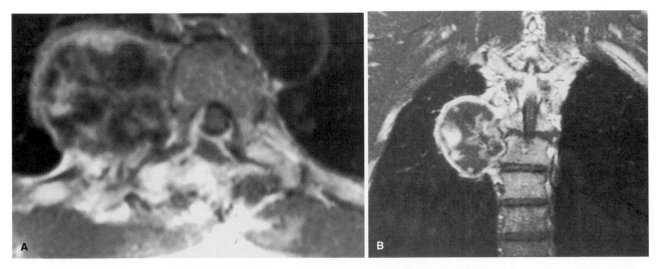

FIGURE 17.02-2.

Chondrosarcoma. **A.** Axial postcontrast magnetic resonance (MR) T1-weighted image in a young adult with a chondrosarcoma arising from the transverse process of an upper thoracic vertebral body. Note peripheral enhancement and significant necrosis centrally. There is tumor extension into right lateral epidural space with flattening of the right side of spinal cord. **B.** Coronal postcontrast MR T1-weighted image in same patient shows predominantly paraspinal location of necrotic sarcoma.

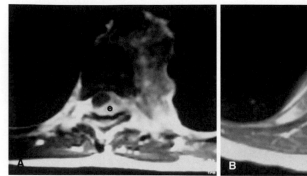 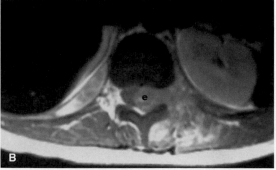

FIGURE 17.02-3.

Paraspinal rhabdomyosarcoma. **A.** Axial postcontrast magnetic resonance (MR) T1-weighted image in a patient with a left paraspinal rhabdomyosarcoma (no primary found). The enhancing mass extends through the neural foramen into the spinal canal and epidural space (e), where it compresses and deviates the cord to the right. **B.** Axial postcontrast MR T1-weighted image in a different patient shows rhabdomyosarcoma arising in left paraspinal region and extending into the epidural space (e) via the neural foramen. The spinal cord is markedly compressed and deviated toward the right.

SUGGESTED READINGS

1. Redmond OM, Stack JP, Dervan PA, et al. Osteosarcoma: use of MR imaging and MR spectroscopy in clinical decision making. Radiology 1989;172:811.
2. Holscher HC, Bloem JL, Vanel D, et al. Osteosarcoma: chemotherapy-induced changes at MR imaging. Radiology 1992;182:839.

17.03 Extradural Masses: Paraspinal Tumors (Neuroblastoma, Ganglioneuroblastoma, and Ganglioneuroma)

EPIDEMIOLOGY

Neuroblastoma is the most common solid malignancy of childhood outside the central nervous system, and the fourth most common tumor in children. It most commonly occurs inside the abdomen, but tends to involve the spine or paraspinal regions in 25% of cases. Most cases occur during the first 5 years of life. Most ganglioneuromas and ganglioneuroblastomas originate in the paraspinal regions and are found between 5 to 8 years of age, predominantly in boys, although some series report equal incidence in both sexes.

CLINICAL FEATURES

Paraspinal neuroblastoma arises from the sympathetic chain. These tumors are composed of numerous small, round, blue cells with areas of necrosis, hemorrhage, and calcification. Ganglioneuroblastoma is the next step of differentiation in this line of tumors. It is composed of immature neuroblasts and mature ganglion cells. Ganglioneuroma is the most differentiated tumor from this cell line because it is composed of mature ganglion cells, and occurs in older children, adolescents, and adults. Most ganglioneuromas are large masses at diagnosis. Although neuroblastomas most often begin in the abdomen, ganglioneuroblastomas and ganglioneuromas tend to arise more commonly in the posterior thoracic region. All three tumors present with similar symptoms, which include a palpable mass, respiratory compromise, pain, tenderness, scoliosis, radiculopathy, and myelopathy. Treatment for the less differentiated of these tumors includes a combination of surgery, chemotherapy, and irradiation.

IMAGING FEATURES

In cases of paraspinal neuroblastoma, plain radiographs or computed tomography show soft tissue masses, 10% of which contain calcifications (Fig. 17.03-1). There may be lytic or sclerotic destruction of vertebral bodies and expansion of neural foramina. Vertebra(e) may be completely collapsed. By magnetic resonance imaging, the mass is isointense to hypointense on T1-weighted images and enhances after contrast administration. The T2 signal characteristics are variable. Bone marrow involvement may be present and epidural extension is easily seen on postcontrast T1-weighted images. Approximately 20% of ganglioneuroblastomas and ganglioneuromas contain calcifications. These slower-growing masses may cause widening of neural foramina, scalloping of the posterior vertebral bodies, and widening of the spinal canal. Epidural extension may result in spinal cord compression. Imaging features are otherwise nonspecific.

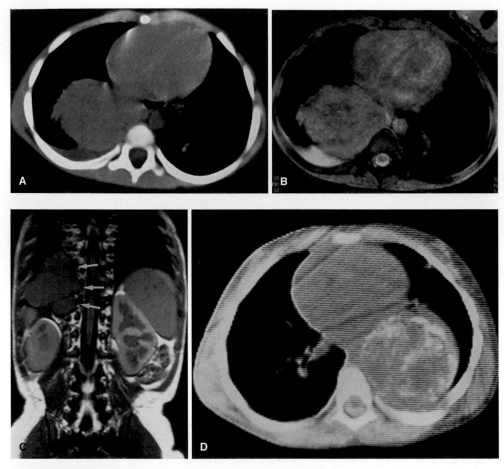

FIGURE 17.03-1.

Neuroblastoma. **A.** Axial noncontrast computed tomography (CT) shows large right paraspinal thoracic soft tissue mass. **B.** Corresponding magnetic resonance (MR) T2-weighted image shows the mass to be of low signal intensity. Note right pleural effusion. **C.** Coronal postcontrast MR T1-weighted image shows no significant enhancement in the mass, which insinuates itself into the neural foramina *(arrows)*. **D.** Axial noncontrast CT in a different patient with paraspinal neuroblastoma shows calcifications within the mass. (Cases courtesy of D. Merten, M.D., Chapel Hill, NC.)

SUGGESTED READINGS

1. Faubert C, Inniger R. MRI and pathological findings in two cases of Askin tumors. Neuroradiology 1991;33:277.
2. Dietrich RB, Kangarloo H, Lenarsky C, et al. Neuroblastoma: the role of MR imaging. AJR 1987;148:937.

17.04 *Extradural Masses: Eosinophilic Granuloma*

EPIDEMIOLOGY

This benign, self-limiting destructive condition of bone mostly affects children below 10 years of age. In approximately 10% to 15% of cases the spine is involved. Boys are affected more than girls.

CLINICAL FEATURES

This condition belongs to the Langerhans cell histiocytoses, together with Hand-Schüller-Christian disease (which affects multiple bones) and Letterer-Siwe disease (which involves bones and solid organs). Eosinophilic granuloma is a solitary lesion consisting of an abnormal proliferation of lipid-containing histiocytes from the reticuloendothelial system. In the later phases of the disease, large macrophages are found. In the healing phase, these inflammatory changes are substituted by connective tissue and then transformed into bone. The most common symptom is pain. Involvement of a vertebral body may induce collapse, which usually is not accompanied by neurologic deficits. However, radiculopathies and myelopathy may occur. Deformity of the spine also occurs after collapse. Constitutional symptoms include fever and weight loss. Treatment for these lesions is controversial because most will heal without intervention. If the diagnosis is made by biopsy or curettage, no further treatment usually is required. When neurologic symptoms are present, low-dose irradiation may be indicated. For acute pain, bed rest, orthosis, and analgesics are indicated.

IMAGING FEATURES

Plain radiographs show the typical wafer-like configuration of one (or rarely multiple) vertebra that has collapsed secondary to involvement by eosinophilic granuloma. This appearance, although typical, is nonspecific and may be seen with infections and malignancies such as Ewing sarcoma. Biopsy may be needed to confirm the diagnosis. Computed tomography or magnetic resonance (MR) imaging show no associated soft tissue masses (Figs. 17.04-1 and 17.04-2). Complete vertebra plana is more commonly seen in younger patients, whereas in older children, incomplete vertebral collapse is more common (wedge-shaped vertebra; Fig. 17.04-3). Vertebral reformation with almost complete reconstitution of the width and height of the involved vertebra is not unusual and is probably secondary to sparing of the endochondral plates. On MR imaging, the features of eosinophilic granuloma are nonspecific, demonstrating low T1 signal intensity, high T2 signal intensity, and marked contrast enhancement. MR imaging with contrast is also useful in those cases with intracranial involvement (usually at the hypothalamus) and in those rare cases of leptomeningeal spread.

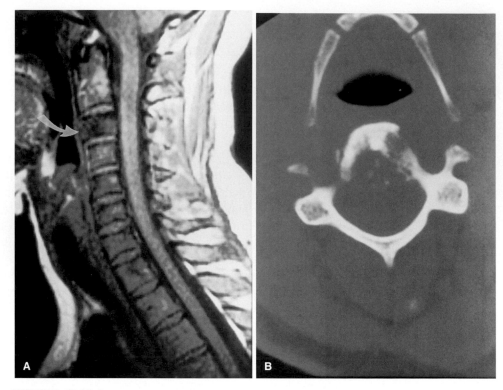

FIGURE 17.04-1.

Eosinophilic granuloma, no collapse.   **A.** Midsagittal magnetic resonance T1-weighted image shows abnormal low signal intensity from the C3 vertebral body *(arrow)* and minimal loss of height in early involvement by eosinophilic granuloma. **B.** Axial computed tomography shows lytic involvement in body of C3. There is no associated soft tissue mass.

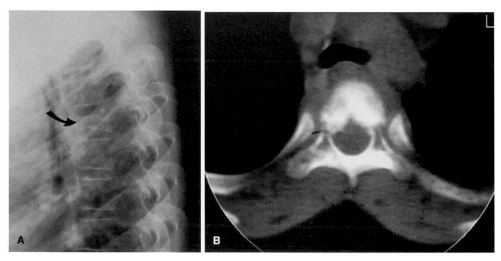

FIGURE 17.04-2.

Eosinophilic granuloma, moderate collapse.   **A.** Lateral radiograph of the thoracic spine shows moderate anterior wedging of an upper thoraric vertebra *(arrow).* **B.** Axial computed tomography in the same patient shows some lucencies and indistinct margins in the involved vertebral body.

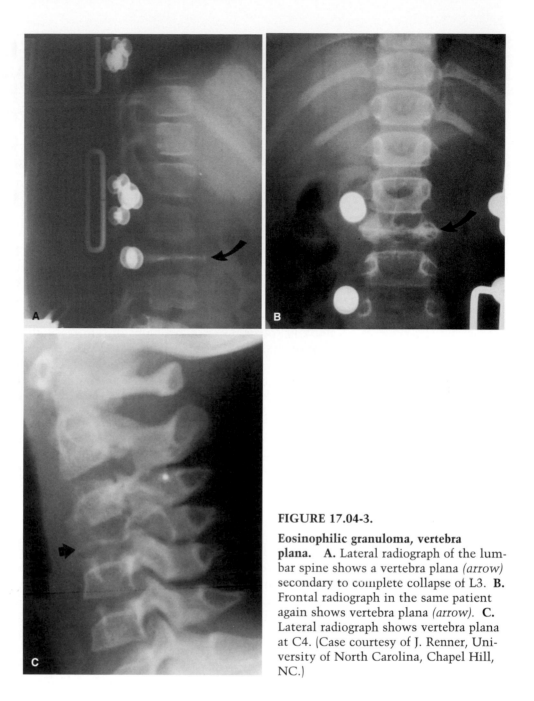

FIGURE 17.04-3.

Eosinophilic granuloma, vertebra plana. **A.** Lateral radiograph of the lumbar spine shows a vertebra plana *(arrow)* secondary to complete collapse of L3. **B.** Frontal radiograph in the same patient again shows vertebra plana *(arrow).* **C.** Lateral radiograph shows vertebra plana at C4. (Case courtesy of J. Renner, University of North Carolina, Chapel Hill, NC.)

SUGGESTED READING

1. De Schepper AMA, Ramon F, Van Marck E. MR imaging of eosinophilic granuloma: report of 11 cases. Skeletal Radiol 1993;22:163.

17.05 *Extradural Masses: Leukemia, Lymphoma, and Metastases*

EPIDEMIOLOGY

Leukemia is the most common cancer in children, and the spine is involved in 6% of these patients. Lymphoma is rare in children and may be of the Hodgkin, non-Hodgkin, or Burkitt types. Metastases to the spine are uncommon in children, and most are secondary to neuroblastoma.

CLINICAL FEATURES

The symptoms of leukemia are nonspecific and include lethargy, anemia, fever, increased erythrocyte sedimentation rate, decreased platelets, and increased peripheral leukocyte count. In pediatric patients most leukemias are of the acute lymphoblastic or acute monoblastic forms. During the course of the disease, approximately 10% to 15% of these children suffer a pathologic spine fracture. Spinal care consists of supportive treatment in most cases. Lymphoma of the Hodgkin type is more commonly focal, whereas non-Hodgkin lymphoma is more commonly disseminated. Spinal lymphoma may be primary or caused by hematogenous or lymphatic dissemination. Metastatic disease to the spine is uncommon and may be secondary to neuroblastoma (30%–40% of all spine metastases in children), embryonal cell carcinoma, and other sarcomas such as Ewing sarcoma and rhabdomyosarcoma. Because of the rarity of spinal metastases, the diagnosis and treatment of these children is commonly delayed.

IMAGING FEATURES

In leukemia, plain radiographs and computed tomography (CT) show focal lytic or sclerotic lesions. Occasionally, only periosteal reaction is present. Diffuse osteopenia is also common. Magnetic resonance (MR) imaging identifies leukemic masses (chloromas) that may occur in the epidural space and compress neural elements (Fig. 17.05-1). Chloromas are commonly hypointense on both T1- and T2-weighted images and enhance after contrast administration. By MR imaging, the bone marrow is usually of low signal intensity, but this may be difficult to identify in children in whom the active bone marrow is commonly hypointense on T1-weighted images. Leukemic infiltrates of the bone marrow are, however, slightly hyperintense on T2-weighted images. Lymphoma may be lytic or sclerotic, and CT and MR imaging commonly show associated soft tissue masses. Lymphoma may infiltrate the neural elements (Fig. 17.05-2). Diffuse or focal infiltration of the bone marrow may occur. Metastatic disease to the spine in children has no specific imaging features, and the abnormalities are similar to those seen in adults.

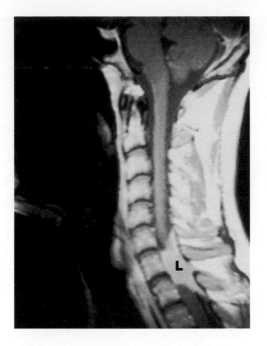

FIGURE 17.05-1.

Leukemia (chloroma). Midsagittal post-contrast magnetic resonance T1-weighted image shows enhancing intraspinal (extramedullary) mass (L) at C6–T1 that proved to be a chloroma in this leukemic patient.

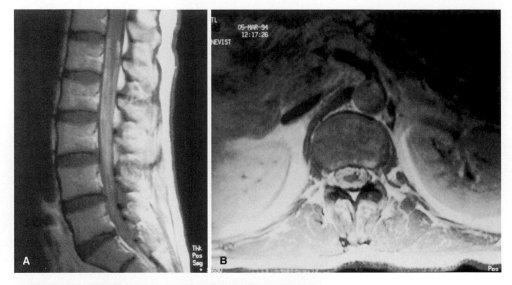

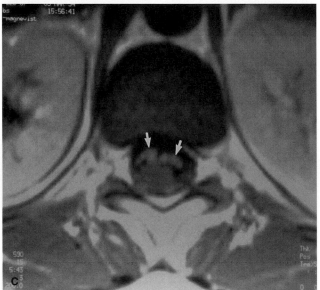

FIGURE 17.05-2.

Lymphoma and mimics.
A. Midsagittal postcontrast magnetic resonance (MR) T1-weighted image in an adolescent with AIDS shows diffuse enhancement of the cauda equina due to lymphoma. **B.** Axial postcontrast MR T1-weighted image shows enhancing nerve roots from cauda equina. Cytomegalovirus (CMV) polyradiculitis may produce identical findings. **C.** Axial postcontrast MR T1-weighted image in a different patient with Guillain-Barré syndrome shows enhancement of the ventral roots *(arrows)* of the cauda equina. The pattern of enhancement suggests that this is not lymphoma or CMV polyradiculitis, which usually affect all the nerve roots.

SUGGESTED READING

1. Barnes PD. Acquired abnormalities of the spine and spinal neuraxis. In: Wolpert SM, Barnes PD, eds. MRI in Pediatric Neuroradiology. St. Louis: Mosby Year Book, 1992:445.

17.06 *Intradural, Extramedullary Masses: Subarachnoid Space Metastases*

EPIDEMIOLOGY
The incidence of metastatic disease to the subarachnoid space varies according to the type of primary neoplasia producing it. It occurs in most patients with medulloblastoma and other primitive neuroectodermal tumors and in 50% of patients with acute lymphoblastic leukemia.

CLINICAL FEATURES
The primary intracranial neoplasias that produce subarachnoid seeding are primitive neuroectodermal tumors (including medulloblastoma), astrocytomas, including ependymoma (especially high-grade tumors), choroid plexus papilloma, and germinoma. Tumors originating outside the central nervous system that may seed the subarachnoid space in children include leukemia, rhabdomyosarcoma, and lymphoma. Symptoms are nonspecific and include headaches (related to hydrocephalus), cranial nerve palsies, back pain, extremity weakness, sensory alterations in the lower extremities, cauda equina syndrome, polyneuropathies, loss of bladder and bowel control, and seizures. Cerebrospinal fluid analysis usually shows markedly elevated proteins, normal to low glucose, and positive tumor cells in 75% of cases. Repeated spinal punctures may be required before tumor cells are recovered. Prognosis is very poor, and most patients die 4 to 6 months after diagnosis.

IMAGING FEATURES
Contrast-enhanced magnetic resonance (MR) is the imaging method of choice in patients suspected of harboring spinal subarachnoid metastases. It is probably more sensitive than spinal puncture. Imaging features include nodular or plaque-like deposits in the conus medullaris of the cauda equina, and focal discrete masses (Fig. 17.06-1). There may also be clumping, crowding, or thickening of the nerve roots. On myelography, the nerve root sleeves may be abruptly amputated because of the presence of tumor on the nerve rootlet. In our experience, screening for subarachnoid metastases is better accomplished with a small surface coil and small field of view, even if this requires multiple placements (the use of phase-array coils greatly facilitates examination of these patients). There are two important pitfalls. The first one is the enhancement of normal vessels on the surface of the spinal cord. These are especially prominent in the anterior surface of the conus medullaris. They are usually tiny and are not present on the nerve roots. The second pitfall relates to the presence of subarachnoid hemorrhage, which normally follows brain tumor surgery (Fig. 17.06-2). In these cases, there may be diffuse and thick enhancement of the subarachnoid space. If tumor seeding needs to be excluded, MR imaging should be done before surgery or 4 to 6 weeks after it.

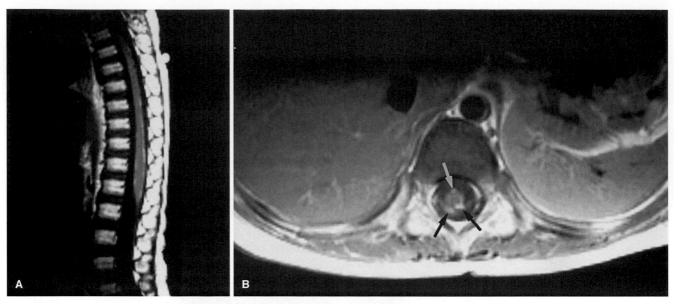

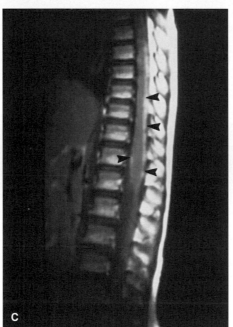

FIGURE 17.06-1.

Subarachnoid metastases. **A.** Midsagittal postcontrast magnetic resonance (MR) T1-weighted image shows linear areas of enhancement along dorsal and ventral surfaces of the spinal cord in a patient with cerebral primitive neuroectodermal tumor. **B.** Axial postcontrast MR T1-weighted image shows nodular deposits of tumor *(arrows)* in conus medullaris. **C.** Midsagittal postcontrast MR T1-weighted image in a different patient with medulloblastoma shows more nodular tumor deposits *(arrowheads)* on surfaces of spinal cord. (With permission from Castillo M. Neuroradiology Companion. Philadelphia: JB Lippincott, 1995.)

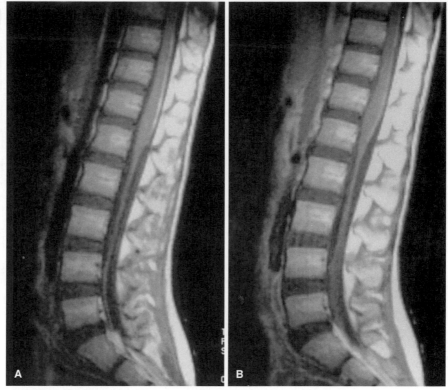

FIGURE 17.06-2.

Postoperative hemorrhage simulating subarachnoid metastases. A. Midsagittal noncontrast magnetic resonance (MR) T1-weighted image in a patient with a posterior fossa medulloblastoma resected 1 week previously shows a hyperintense linear region in the lower and posterior spinal cord and conus medullaris. This represents subacute blood (methemoglobin) adherent to the surface of the cord. **B.** Midsagittal postcontrast MR T1-weighted image in the same patient shows the abnormality to remain identical to its precontrast appearance. If a precontrast study had not been obtained, this finding could be easily mistaken for subarachnoid tumor spread.

SUGGESTED READINGS

1. Lim V, Sobel DF, Zyroff J. Spinal cord pial metastases: MR imaging with gadopentetate dimeglumine. AJNR 1990;11:975.
2. Wiener MD, Boyko OB, Friedman HS, Hokenberger B, Oakes WJ. False positive spinal MR findings for subarachnoid spread of primary CNS tumor in postoperative pediatric patients. AJNR 1990;11:1100.

17.07 *Intramedullary Masses: Astrocytoma*

EPIDEMIOLOGY

Intramedullary tumors comprise 6% to 10% of all childhood central nervous system tumors, and 35% of spinal tumors in children are intramedullary in location. Of these, 50% to 60% are astrocytomas. Malignant tumors are more common in children than in adults. In the pediatric population, they are common during the first 15 years of life and probably have no gender predilection. However, some series report an increased incidence in boys. Intramedullary astrocytoma is mostly a disease of adults, with a peak incidence between the third to fourth decades of life.

CLINICAL FEATURES

Clinical symptoms are nonspecific, insidious, and may not be recognized for long periods of time. A waxing and waning course is probably related to the presence and resolution of edema. Mild trauma may exacerbate the symptoms. The most common symptoms include weakness, pain, increased muscle tone, increased deep tendon reflexes, sensory abnormalities, muscular atrophy, focal tenderness and palpable mass, torticollis, scoliosis (25%), bowel and bladder incontinence, and hydrocephalus (10%–15%). Younger patients present with pain, rigidity, and paraspinal muscle spasms. Older children more commonly present with scoliosis, gait abnormalities, and weakness. Most intramedullary astrocytomas are low grade (75%–90%), with a small number being anaplastic or glioblastoma multiforme. Microsurgical resection is the treatment of choice, and in experienced hands, a permanent increase in neurologic deficits after surgery occurs in only 5% of patients. In patients treated with surgery only, the disease-free survival period is more than 3 years in approximately 75% of cases. Postoperative irradiation may be given after incomplete tumor resection and probably increases the time to recurrences. However, irradiation usually increases the spinal deformity and may result in myelitis.

IMAGING FEATURES

Magnetic resonance (MR) is the imaging method of choice (Fig. 17.07-1). T1-weighted images show a mass in the substance of the spinal cord, usually located in the cervical or thoracic regions (50% of tumors; Fig. 17.07-1A). The spinal canal may be expanded and the posterior surface of the vertebral bodies may be scalloped in long-standing cases. The mass is fusiform and isointense to slightly hypointense on precontrast T1-weighted images. Occasionally, the mass involves the entire spinal cord (holocord astrocytoma; Fig. 17.07-1A). On T2-weighted images the mass and its surrounding edema are hyperintense. The mass has no well defined borders, and histologically the tumor margins usually extend beyond those borders expected based on MR images. Associated cysts (either rostral or caudal to the lesion) are found in one-third of cases. The walls of these cysts are typically nonneoplastic and are filled with cerebrospinal fluid (CSF)-like fluid that is occasionally bloody. Almost all intramedullary astrocytomas show enhancement after contrast administration. The enhancement tends to be focal and readily separates the nonneoplastic cysts from the tumor. CSF tumor dissemination is said to be present in up to 60% of patients. Occasionally, these tumors may be exophytic.

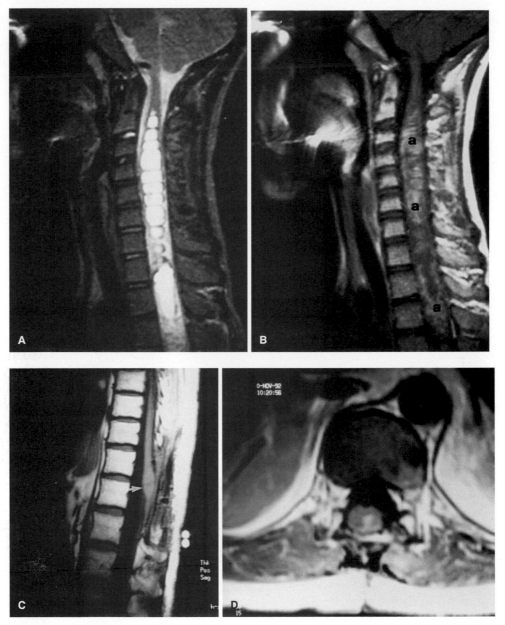

FIGURE 17.07-1.

Astrocytoma. **A.** Midsagittal magnetic resonance (MR) T2-weighted image in a patient with a holocord astrocytoma shows an expansile, multiseptated, and hyperintense lesion involving the cervical/thoracic spinal cord. **B.** Corresponding postcontrast MR T1-weighted image shows enhancement in the astrocytoma (a). (With permission from Castillo M. Neuroradiology Companion. Philadelphia: JB Lippincott, 1995.) **C.** Midsagittal precontrast MR T1-weighted image in a young adult with a recurrent astrocytoma shows mild expansion of the conus medullaris *(arrow)*. The conus medullaris is adherent posteriorly, probably secondary to scar. Note increased signal intensity in bone marrow of vertebral bodies secondary to radiation therapy. **D.** Axial postcontrast MR T1-weighted image in the same patient shows patchy enhancement of the lesion.

SUGGESTED READINGS

1. Brunberg JA, DiPietro MA, Venes JL, et al. Intramedullary lesions of the pediatric spinal cord: correlation of findings from MR imaging, intraoperative sonography, surgery, and histologic study. Radiology 1991;181:573.
2. Epstein FJ, Wisoff JH. Intramedullary tumors of the spinal cord. In: McLaurin FL, Venes JL, Schut L, Epstein F, eds. Pediatric Neurosurgery, 2nd ed. Philadelphia: WB Saunders, 1989:428.

17.08 *Intramedullary Masses: Ependymoma*

EPIDEMIOLOGY

Ependymoma accounts for approximately 30% of intramedullary tumors in children. It is mostly a disease of adults, with most cases presenting between the third to fifth decades of life. Ependymoma involving the filum terminale tends to occur in younger patients. Ependymomas are slightly more common in girls.

CLINICAL FEATURES

Histologically, ependymomas are divided into cellular and myxopapillary types. Cellular ependymomas tend to occur in the cervical and thoracic spinal cord and the most common symptom is pain, which is probably related to pressure erosion of bone in these slow-growing tumors. Other symptoms include weakness, reflex and sensory changes, scoliosis, muscle spasms and atrophy, and focal tenderness. The incidence of these tumors is increased in patients with neurofibromatosis type II. Cellular ependymomas are slow growing and fairly well circumscribed. Complete surgical resection is often possible and the prognosis is relatively good, with recurrences being rare. Myxopapillary ependymoma is almost exclusively located in the filum terminale (Fig. 17.08-1). They produce compression of the cauda equina and present with sacral and lower extremity pain. One-fourth of these patients have sphincter dysfunction, lower extremity weakness, or both. These tumors may infiltrate the distal conus medullaris, and although complete resection is commonly obtained, cerebrospinal fluid seeding is not rare. In cases of incomplete resection, irradiation may be needed (Fig. 17.08-2). Myxopapillary ependymomas are extremely rare in children.

IMAGING FEATURES

Magnetic resonance is the imaging method of choice. Intramedullary ependymomas cause fusiform enlargement of the spinal cord. They are isointense or hypointense on precontrast T1-weighted images and hyperintense on T2-weighted images. On T2-weighted images, more than half of ependymomas show a halo of hypointensity partially or completely surrounding the tumor. This is believed to represent hemosiderin from prior hemorrhages. If this feature is present, ependymoma should be strongly considered as the leading differential diagnosis. Cysts are found in approximately 45% of cases. These tumors enhance after contrast administration. Very rarely, ependymomas arise from embryologic remnants of the filum terminale located in the sacrum and adjacent subcutaneous tissues. Occasionally, ependymomas may attain very large size before becoming symptomatic (Fig. 17.08-3).

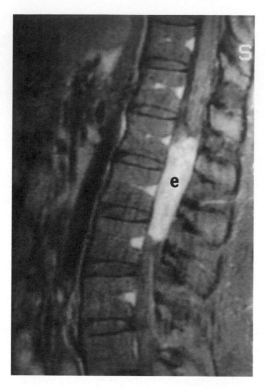

FIGURE 17.08-1.

Myxopapillary ependymoma. Midsagittal postcontrast fat-suppressed magnetic resonance T1-weighted image shows enhancing and elongated ("sausage-shaped") ependymoma (e) of the filum terminale. This is the typical appearance of the myxopapillary type of ependymoma. (With permission from Castillo M. Neuroradiology Companion. Philadelphia: JB Lippincott, 1995.)

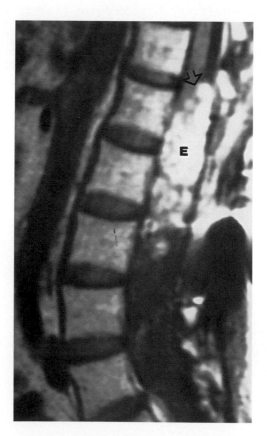

FIGURE 17.08-2.

Recurrent and infiltrating ependymoma. Midsagittal postcontrast magnetic resonance T1-weighted image shows enhancing and lobulated mass (E) in region of filum terminale but infiltrating the distal conus medullaris as well *(open arrow).*

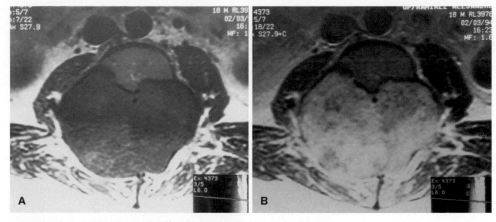

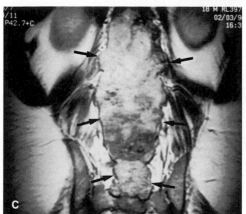

FIGURE 17.08-3.

Giant ependymoma. **A.** Axial precontrast magnetic resonance (MR) T1-weighted image shows mass of mostly low signal intensity arising in the spinal canal of an 18-year-old male patient. The posterior elements are completely eroded and there has been significant erosion of the posterior vertebral body. **B.** Axial postcontrast MR T1-weighted image in same patient shows pronounced enhancement of the mass. **C.** Coronal postcontrast MR T1-weighted image in same patient shows that the mass *(arrows)* involves the lower thoracic spine and the lumbar area. Note expansile nature of this large ependymoma. (Case courtesy of R. Rojas, M.D., ABC Hospital, Mexico City, Mexico.)

SUGGESTED READING

1. Raffel C, McComb JG. Spinal cord tumors. In: Weinstein SL, ed. The Pediatric Spine: Principles and Practice. New York: Raven, 1994:917.

17.09 Intramedullary Masses: Hemangioblastoma

EPIDEMIOLOGY

Hemangioblastoma in the spinal cord is a disease of adults, occurring mostly after the third decade of life and commonly associated with Von Hippel-Lindau disease, Hemangioblastomas account for 1% to 5% of all spinal cord tumors. They are very rare in children.

CLINICAL FEATURES

Most patients present with sensory abnormalities (especially altered proprioception). One-third of patients with spinal cord hemangioblastomas will have Von Hippel-Lindau disease. Histologically, these tumors are composed of a hypervascular nodule containing thin-walled, closely packed blood vessels with large, pale stromal cells. Surgical resection is the treatment of choice.

IMAGING FEATURES

Magnetic resonance (MR) is the imaging method of choice for these tumors. Hemangioblastomas tend to involve the cervical (40%–50%), cervicothoracic, and thoracic regions (50%). Most are intramedullary lesions (75%), but occasionally they are seen outside the spinal cord (Fig. 17.09-1A). Up to 80% of them have associated cysts that are nontumoral, and 80% are solitary lesions (Fig. 17.09-1B). Multiple hemangioblastomas occur more commonly with Von Hippel-Landau disease. Hemangioblastomas may bleed spontaneously and show evidence of blood products by MR imaging. On T1-weighted images, they tend to be hypointense (in the absence of prior hemorrhage) and may show serpiginous areas of flow void, probably related to large vessels. On T2-weighted images, the tumor may be slightly hypointense, isointense, or hyperintense to the normal spinal cord. Cysts and edema are always hyperintense on T2-weighted images. After contrast administration there is intense enhancement of the tumor nodules but no enhancement of associated cysts. The tumor nodules tend to be typically subpial in location, and therefore located along the surfaces of the spinal cord.

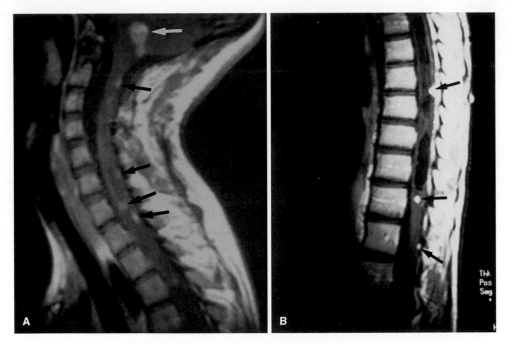

FIGURE 17.09-1.

Hemangioblastomas. **A.** Midsagittal postcontrast magnetic resonance (MR) T1-weighted image shows multiple enhancing nodules *(black arrows)* mostly based on the dorsal surface of the cord in a patient with Von Hippel-Lindau disease. There is also a hemangioblastoma *(white arrow)* in the cerebellum. **B.** Midsagittal postcontrast MR T1-weighted image in a different patient with Von Hippel-Lindau disease shows multiple enhancing hemangioblastomas *(arrows)* and a syrinx in the spinal cord.

**SUGGESTED
READING**

1. Silbergeld J, Cohen WA, Maravilla KR, et al. Supratentorial and spinal cord hemangioblastomas: gadolinium-enhanced MR appearance with pathologic correlation. J Comput Assist Tomogr 1989;13:1048.

17.10 Infections: Discitis and Osteomyelitis

EPIDEMIOLOGY

In children, osteomyelitis with frank destruction of the vertebral bodies is uncommon, but discitis is not rare. Discitis is most commonly seen between 1 to 5 years of age, and rarely in teenagers. There is no gender predilection.

CLINICAL FEATURES

Nontuberculous discitis is most commonly caused by infection with *Staphylococcus aureus* and streptococci. Viral etiologies and low-grade inflammatory processes are believed to be very rare. Initial symptoms in the youngest children are nonspecific and include failure to walk (seen mostly before 3 years of age), abdominal pain syndrome (seen between 3–8 years of age in patients with low thoracic discitis), and the back pain syndrome (seen mostly in teenagers). Other symptoms include limping, irritability, fever, and refusal to stand or sit. Symptoms are usually present from 2 to 4 weeks before diagnosis. The differential diagnosis of discitis includes vertebral osteomyelitis, Scheuermann disease, tuberculosis, spinal epidural abscess, vertebra plana (particularly eosinophilic granuloma), osteoid osteoma, and metastatic disease to the spine. Most patients are initiated on an empiric course of intravenous antibiotics that covers staphylococci. Over 90% of cases resolve with antibiotics only. Intravenous antibiotics are usually given for 4 weeks. Blood cultures are often negative and needle aspiration may be unnecessary. Immobilization may be needed in older children. Patients in whom an osteomyelitis develops may have a permanent kyphotic deformity of the spine. Indications for surgery include the presence of epidural abscess, spinal cord compression, and extensive bone destruction with formation of sequestra.

IMAGING FEATURES

Magnetic resonance (MR) is the imaging method of choice in suspected discitis. Most discitis involves the L3 to L5 interspaces. On sagittal T1-weighted images, the disc is of low intensity and is narrowed. The adjacent vertebral bodies may also be hypointense secondary to edema or extension of the infection. The cortex of the end plates is better seen on T2-weighted images and may be eroded (Fig. 17.10-1A,B). On T2-weighted images, the involved disc is almost always hyperintense (Fig. 17.10-1C). The internuclear cleft is effaced, but note that the presence of the internuclear cleft is not a constant feature in children (it is almost always present after 30 years of age). The adjacent vertebrae may become hyperintense (due to edema, infection, or infarction) on T2-weighted images and paraspinal soft tissue masses may be seen. After contrast administration, the infected disc and adjacent vertebrae show enhancement (Fig. 17.10-1D). The paraspinal masses may also enhance. Postcontrast T1-weighted sagittal images are ideal to exclude the possibility of epidural abscess. MR imaging is more sensitive in the initial detection of discitis/vertebral osteomyelitis than is radionuclide scanning. Plain radiographs usually fail to reveal any findings during the first 2 weeks and become positive during the third to fourth weeks. Radiographically, reparative changes begin between 8 weeks and 8 months. There is sclerosis of the adjacent vertebrae, but the disc space does not regain its normal height.

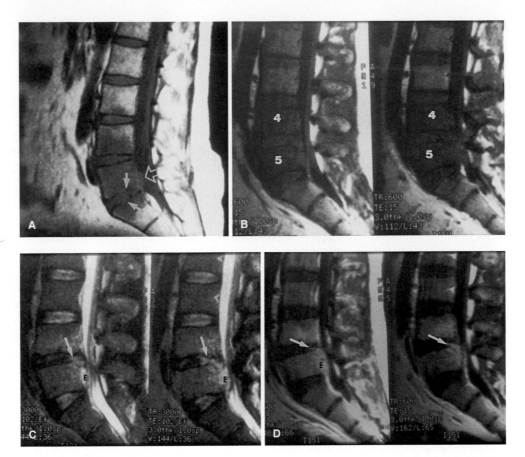

FIGURE 17.10-1.

Bacterial discitis.   A. Midsagittal noncontrast magnetic resonance (MR) T1-weighted image shows low signal intensity (edema) from L4 and L5. The superior aspect of S1 and inferior aspect of L3 are also abnormal. There is erosion *(arrows)* of the inferior end plate of L5 and superior end plate of S1. A small ventral epidural soft tissue mass *(open arrow)* is present at the L5–S1 level. **B.** Sagittal MR T1-weighted images in a different patient show low signal intensity (edema) at L4 (4) and L5 (5). **C.** Corresponding MR T2-weighted images show increased signal intensity *(arrows)* from the posterior aspect of the L4–L5 disc, which is typical in discitis. Also seen is a ventral epidural mass (E), suggesting abscess. **D.** Corresponding postcontrast MR T1-weighted images show enhancement *(arrows)* in the posterior aspect of the L4–L5 disc. The ventral epidural mass (E) also enhances.

SUGGESTED READINGS

1. Cushing AH. Diskitis in children. Clin Infect Dis 1993;17:1.
2. Correa AG, Edwards MS, Baker CJ. Vertebral osteomyelitis in children. Pediatr Infect Dis J 1993;12:228.
3. Afshani E, Kuhn JP. Common causes of low back pain in children. RadioGraphics 1991;11:269.

17.11 *Infections: Tuberculosis*

EPIDEMIOLOGY

Tuberculosis of the spine is common in children and its frequency is inversely proportional to the socioeconomic status of the patient. In the United States, the diagnosis is usually made early, whereas in Third World countries the diagnosis is made late. In children, it is commonly found before 5 years of age. There is no gender predilection.

CLINICAL FEATURES

Most infections are caused by *Mycobacterium tuberculosis.* Although paraplegia is rare in children, in children tuberculosis tends to have a more aggressive course, probably secondary to their relatively immature immunologic status. Most infections are from hematogenous spread from the lungs or the kidneys. Signs of chronic infection are common and spinal cord compression leading to loss of sensory and motor abilities is found in less than 10% of cases. Histologically, there are three distinct types of involvement: anterior, paradiscal, and central. In the anterior lesions, the infection lies under the anterior longitudinal ligament and may destroy the anterior aspect of a vertebral body. This type of pattern is more common in adults. The bone destruction is usually minimal and there is no kyphosis. The infection may extend under the anterior longitudinal ligament to involve several levels. In the paradiscal type, the infection begins in the anterior aspect of the lower or upper vertebral body adjacent to the endplates. The disc space is relatively preserved. Kyphosis is not uncommon and, when healed, the vertebrae commonly fuse. The most common pattern of involvement in children is the central type, in which there is infection and destruction of a complete vertebral body, producing kyphosis. The diagnosis is based on recovery of the microorganism. Stains of surgical specimens are positive in less than half of cases, although eventually positive cultures grow in over 80% of surgical specimens. Treatment includes the first line of drugs (streptomycin, isoniazid, and rifampicin) or second-order drugs (ethambutol and pyrazinamide). Drugs usually are given at least 1 week before surgery.

IMAGING FEATURES

Most tuberculous infections occur at the thoracolumbar junction. Involvement of more than one segment is common. Magnetic resonance is the imaging modality of choice. The disc(s) is usually spared, and T1-weighted images show low signal intensity in the affected vertebral body. This body is hyperintense on T2-weighted images. The disc may also be bright on T2-weighted images, but there is only minimal loss of height. In 10% of cases epidural abscesses are found; these are better seen on postcontrast sagittal T1-weighted images. Extension under the anterior longitudinal ligament is clearly visible on sagittal T2- and postcontrast T1-weighted images. Necrotic abscesses in the psoas muscle are not uncommon. On computed tomography, there usually is destruction of the vertebral body with a central bony sequestrum (Fig. 17.11-1). The imaging findings in spinal tuberculosis are identical to those seen with spinal brucellosis. Occasionally, tuberculosis is isolated to the posterior spinal elements.

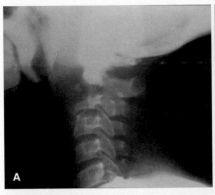

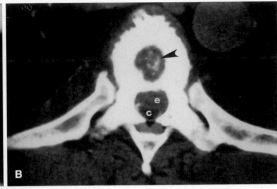

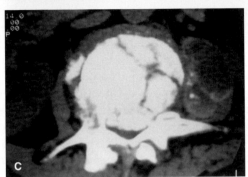

FIGURE 17.11-1.

Tuberculosis. **A.** Lateral radiograph shows destruction of anterior and superior aspect of C3 and anterior and inferior aspect of C2. **B.** Axial computed tomography (CT) shows abscess in center of thoracic vertebral body with epidural (e) abscess displacing spinal cord (c) posteriorly. Note inner sequestrum of bone *(arrowhead)*, which in our experience is fairly typical of tuberculosis. **C.** Axial CT in a patient (adult) who suffered an acute compression fracture of a lumbar vertebra involved by tuberculosis. Note marked narrowing of spinal canal secondary to posteriorly displaced bone fragments and "cold" abscess in left psoas muscle.

SUGGESTED READINGS

1. Ho EKW, Leong JCY. Tuberculosis of the spine. In: Weinstein SL, ed. The Pediatric Spine: Principles and Practice. New York: Raven 1994:837.
2. Sharif HS, Clark DC, Aabed MY, et al. Granulomatous spinal infections: MR imaging. Radiology 1990;177:101.
3. Ahmadi J, Bajaj A, Destain S, Segall HD, Zee CS. Spinal tuberculosis: atypical observations at MR imaging. Radiology 1993;189:489.

17.12 Infections: Epidural Abscess

EPIDEMIOLOGY

In the general population, epidural abscesses are rare and account for approximately 1:5000 hospital admissions. In children, epidural abscesses are more common in girls. There is no specific age.

CLINICAL FEATURES

Pain and fever are the most common symptoms in children. Pain is often localized, severe, and may be accompanied by radiculopathy or myelopathy. Meningeal signs (headache and nuchal rigidity) may also be present. Paralysis with sphincter dysfunction ensues rapidly, usually within 24 hours of the onset of symptoms. A sensory level is a late finding. Many children are given antibiotics early in the course of the disease, and this may mask the findings. Clinically, the differential diagnosis includes inflammatory transverse myelitis, tumors, vertebral body infection, and discitis. With epidural abscesses there usually is a history of an infectious focus in a remote site. Therefore, most epidural abscesses arise from hematogenous spread of infection. Epidural abscesses due to direct inoculation are usually secondary to lumbar puncture, spine surgery, or gastrointestinal fistulas. Epidural abscesses are also more common in patients with AIDS and intravenous drug users. In children, the most common etiologies are infection by *Staphylococcus aureus* (> 50%), *Escherichia coli*, and *Proteus* species, and tuberculosis. Without treatment, epidural abscesses have a high mortality. Appropriate intravenous antibiotics should be initiated immediately. Administration of steroids is controversial. If spinal cord compression is present, emergency surgery is needed.

IMAGING FEATURES

Magnetic resonance (MR) is the imaging method of choice (Fig. 17.12-1). Myelography is not indicated—spinal punctures should not be performed because they increase the risk of meningitis. Most epidural abscesses are located in the lumbosacral and cervical regions. Over half of them occur in the anterior epidural space, but not uncommonly they surround the thecal sac completely (Fig. 17.12-1A,B). Sagittal MR images demonstrate an intermediate T1 signal intensity (similar to the spinal cord) mass in the epidural space. The mass has tapered margins, suggesting its epidural location. The brightness of the normal epidural fat is not seen. Epidural abscesses are hyperintense on T2-weighted images. After contrast administration, the abscesses may show peripheral enhancement, complete but inhomogeneous enhancement, or complete homogeneous enhancement (Fig. 17.12-1C,D). Commonly, the infection extends from a disc space or from vertebral osteomyelitis. In some cases, the spinal cord is of abnormally increased signal intensity, probably related to edema secondary to compromise of venous drainage or, rarely, because of infectious myelitis.

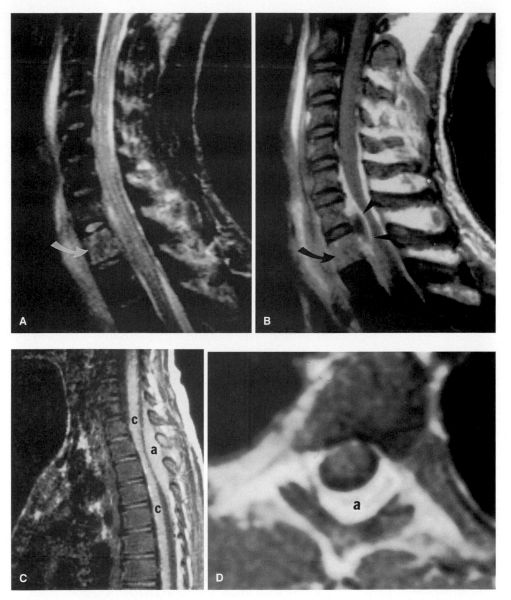

FIGURE 17.12-1.

Epidural abscess. **A.** Midsagittal magnetic resonance (MR) T2-weighted image shows increased signal intensity (edema) from the T1 vertebral body *(arrow).* **B.** Corresponding postcontrast MR T1-weighted image shows enhancement of T1 vertebral body *(curved arrow)* and a ventral epidural abscess *(arrowheads)* with marginal enhancement. There is significant cord compression at the level of abscess. The dorsal dura also enhances. **C.** Midsagittal postcontrast MR T1-weighted image shows dorsal epidural abscess (a) compressing the cervicothoracic spinal cord (c). **D.** Axial postcontrast MR T1-weighted image in the same patient shows the dorsal location of the abscess (a). (**C** and **D** with permission from Castillo M. Neuroradiology Companion. Philadelphia: JB Lippincott, 1995.)

SUGGESTED READINGS

1. Friedman DP, Hills JR. Cervical epidural spinal infection: MR imaging characteristics. AJR 1994;163:699.
2. Numaguchi Y, Rigamonti D, Rothman MI, Sato S, Mihara F, Sadato N. Spinal epidural abscess: evaluation with gadolinium-enhanced MR imaging. RadioGraphics 1993;13:545.

17.13 *Juvenile Ankylosing Spondylitis*

EPIDEMIOLOGY

This disorder affects approximately 1% to 6% of the general population and is more common in white, young or middle-aged men (male:female ratio, 6:1). However, its onset may occur during childhood or adolescence, where its general incidence varies between 6% to 25% of patients seen by rheumatologists. These patients usually are seronegative for rheumatoid factor and carry the human leukocyte antigen (HLA)-B27 genetic marker.

CLINICAL FEATURES

The initial symptoms are nonspecific and include vague joint pain not uncommonly beginning in a peripheral joint. Hip arthropathy occurs in 50% to 75% of patients. Symptoms referable to the sacroiliac joints and lower spine are insidious, and it takes an average of 6.5 years from the onset of symptoms to the establishment of radiologic features in children with this disease. Low back pain that is not relieved by rest needs to be present for at least 3 months before the diagnosis can be established. Acute iritis occurs in 5% to 10% of children with ankylosing spondylitis. Other symptoms include fever, fatigue, cutaneous rash, growth retardation, limited chest expansion, involvement of the cervical spine, pulmonary fibrosis, and aortitis. A family history of the disease is not uncommon. Laboratory findings are nonspecific and include elevated erythrocyte sedimentation rate and mild anemia. The HLA-B27 marker is present in approximately 90% of these patients.

IMAGING FEATURES

Plain radiographs show that the margins of the sacroiliac joints are indistinct, with surrounding sclerosis, and that joint space appears wide. Early changes may be unilateral. Spine changes are rare in children until late in the disease, and include sclerosis of the anterior margin of the end plates, "squaring" of the vertebral bodies, osteopenia, and formation of bridging syndesmophytes (Fig. 17.13-1). These abnormalities usually progress from caudal to cephalad. Signs of hip arthritis are not uncommon in children, and in 10% of these patients there is frank destruction of the hip. Complications from this disease include ankylosis, atlantoaxial subluxation, fractures, and epidural hematoma. Magnetic resonance imaging is ideal in patients with the cauda equina syndrome in whom there are multiple erosive dural divertula with arachnoiditis (Fig. 17.13-2). In 3% to 28% of patients, there may be destruction of a disc space and adjacent vertebral bodies (Andersson lesions), simulating spinal tuberculosis. Pseudofractures through disc spaces may also occur (Fig. 17.13-3).

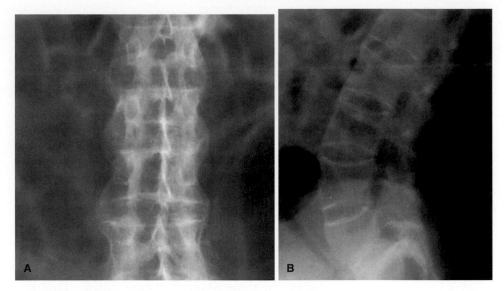

FIGURE 17.13-1.

Ankylosing spondylitis. **A.** Frontal radiograph shows thin syndesmophytes fusing the lumbar vertebrae. **B.** Lateral radiograph, same patient, shows fused vertebrae and vertebral bodies to have a "square" shape.

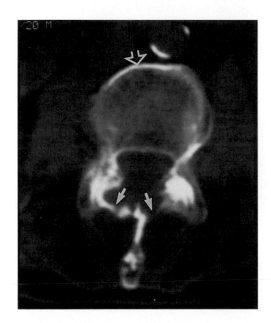

FIGURE 17.13-2.

Erosive dural diverticula. Axial computed tomography shows erosion *(solid arrows)* of posterior elements by dural diverticula in this patient with a cauda equina syndrome and ankylosing spondylitis. Note calcification *(open arrow)* of anterior longitudinal ligament.

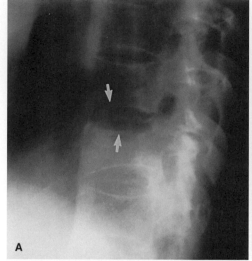

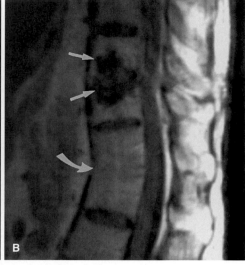

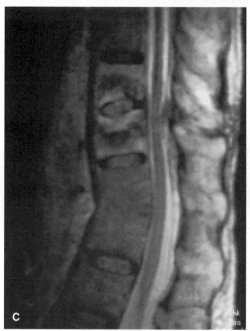

FIGURE 17.13-3.

Disc pseudofracture. **A.** Lateral radiograph shows indistinct end plates *(arrows)* in lower thoracic spine of patient with long-standing ankylosing spondylitis and new onset of back pain. **B.** Midsagittal magnetic resonance (MR) T1-weighted image in the same patient shows low signal intensity *(straight arrows)* from the end plates of the involved vertebrae. Fusion *(curved arrow)* of two vertebrae is also seen. **C.** Corresponding MR T2-weighted image shows peculiar increased signal intensity (edema?) in involved vertebra surrounded by low signal intensity (reparative changes?). Note that disc is not hyperintense (as expected in bacterial discitis). There was no abnormal enhancement on postcontrast studies (not shown). Needle aspiration of disc and open biopsy revealed only granulation tissues.

SUGGESTED READING

1. Tucker LB, Miller LC, Schaller JG. Rheumatic diseases. In: Weinstein SL, ed. The Pediatric Spine: Principles and Practice. New York: Raven, 1994:855.

Imaging of the Pediatric Head, Neck, and Spine
by Mauricio Castillo and Suresh K. Mukherji,
Lippincott-Raven Publishing, Philadelphia © 1996.

18

Trauma and Vascular Disorders

18.0 Injuries to the Upper Cervical Spine

EPIDEMIOLOGY

Children account for 2% to 16% of all patients admitted to hospitals for cervical spine injuries. These injuries are more common in the inner cities. Common etiologies include motor vehicle accidents, diving accidents, and other sports-related injuries. Child abuse is also a common cause of cervical spine injuries secondary to the relatively large head of infants and the relative lack of muscle control in the neck.

CLINICAL FEATURES

Symptoms are nonspecific and hard to elicit in children. All unconscious children (particularly if facial injuries are present) should be stabilized. Local pain, muscle rigidity, and torticollis may be present. In the youngest children, trauma to the spinal cord and vertebral arteries (dissections) may occur in the absence of fractures. After 8 years of age, most fractures occur below the C4 level. Occipitoatlantal dislocations are twice as common in children as they are in adults. They are associated with high-energy trauma, and the chance of survival is very small. Burst fractures of C1 (Jefferson fractures) are very unusual in children. Atlantoaxial instability is also very rare on a posttrauma basis, and is more commonly seen with the Klippel-Feil and Down syndromes, and with congenital abnormalities of the dens. Atlantoaxial rotatory subluxation is fairly common in children and follows trauma (often mild) or upper respiratory tract infections. Most of these patients present with torticollis. Fractures of the dens in children almost always involve the synchondrosis at its base (type 2). In all these injuries, neurologic signs are fairly uncommon. Hangman's fractures (through pedicles of C2) are very rare in children.

IMAGING FEATURES

Plain radiographs and computed tomography (CT) are the imaging methods of choice for bone abnormalities associated with these injuries. Magnetic resonance is the imaging method of choice for visualization of the spinal cord. In occipitoatlantal dislocation, the distance between the tip of the dens and the basion often exceeds 10 mm (Fig. 18.0-1). A line traced along the back of the clivus should normally transect the dens (Fig. 18.0-2). Power's ratio is helpful in determining if the subluxation is anterior or posterior. The findings for Jefferson fractures are similar to those seen in adults; however, they tend to involve the synchondroses of C1. Displacement of the lateral masses of C1 by more than 4 mm is definitively abnormal. Flexion and extension plain radiographs are critical in assessing C1–C2 instability. A dental interval greater than 10 mm is often an indication for surgical fusion. If the dental interval is greater than 5 mm, contact sports should be avoided. CT is helpful in cases of C1–C2 rotatory subluxation. The atlas rotates on C2 but the dental interval may remain normal, indicating an intact transverse ligament (Hawkins type 1 injury). A rotatory injury with a dental interval between 3 to 5 mm indicates deficiency of the transverse ligament (Hawkins type 2 injury). The same injury with a dental interval greater than 5 mm indicates ligamental insufficiency (Hawkins type 3). Posterior displacement of C1 on C2 indicates a deficient dens (Hawkins type 4). Types 2 to 4 require surgical stabilization. Fractures of the dens should be differentiated from os odontoideum (Fig. 18.0-3A). In over 50% of dens fractures, displacement is present. Hangman's fractures should not be mistaken for the normal neurocentral synchondroses, which usually disappear by 7 years of age (Fig. 18.0-3B,C). Before 8 years of age, slight physiologic subluxation of C2 on C3 is the rule. Normally, the posterior laminar line of C2 should lie less than 1.5 mm from the posterior laminar line connecting C1 to C3 (Swischuk's line).

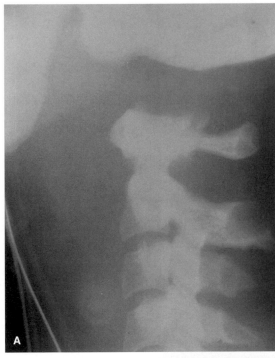

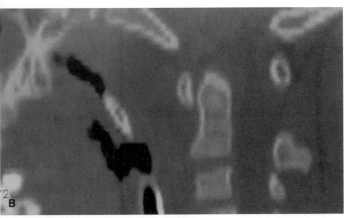

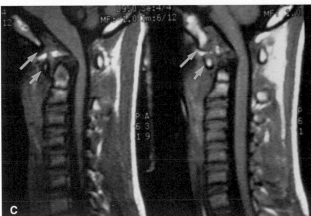

FIGURE 18.0-1.

Craniocervical dislocation. A. Lateral radiograph shows wide gap between the base of the skull and C1. **B.** In a different patient, sagittal computed tomography reformation shows the base of the skull anteriorly displaced on the upper cervical spine. **C.** Sagittal magnetic resonance T1-weighted images (same patient) show that the basion *(longer arrows)* lies ventral to the anterior arch of C1 *(shorter arrows)* and that there is significant cord compresson.

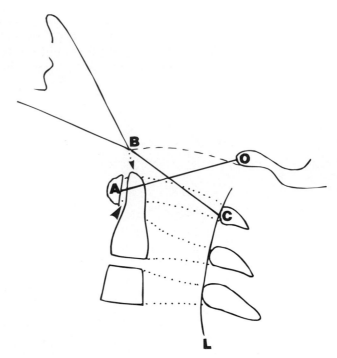

FIGURE 18.0-2.

Normal relationships at the craniocervical junction. A line drawn downward from the basion (B) following the inclination of the clivus should intersect the dens *(small arrowhead)*. The atlantodental interval *(large arrowhead)* normally measures no more than 5 mm in young children and 3 mm in adolescents. The posterior lamina of C2 should lie less than 1.5 mm from the posterior laminar line (L) connecting C1 and C3. The distance between the basion (B) and the posterior arch of C1 (C) divided by the distance between the dorsal surface of the arch of C1 (A) and opisthion (O) is helpful in craniocervical dislocations. A ratio greater than 1 is indicative of anterior displacement.

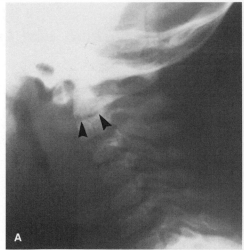

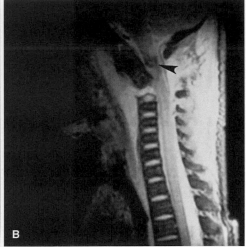

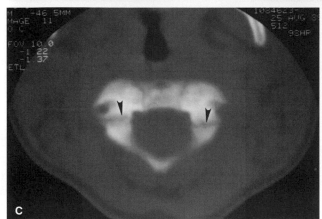

FIGURE 18.0-3.

Injuries to C2. A. Lateral radiograph shows fracture *(arrowheads)* through base of the dens (type 2). (With permission from Castillo M. Neuroradiology Companion. Philadelphia: JB Lippincott, 1995.) **B.** Midsagittal magnetic resonance T2-weighted image (different patient) shows fracture through C2–C3 disc space with anterior dislocation of C2. There is a hematoma *(arrowhead)* in the upper cervical spinal cord. **C.** Axial computed tomography (different patient) shows bilaminar fractures *(arrowheads).*

SUGGESTED READINGS

1. Bulas DI, Fitz CR, Johnson DL. Traumatic atlanto-occipital dislocation in children. Radiology 1993;188:155.
2. Harris JH, Carson GC, Wagner LK. Radiologic diagnosis of traumatic occipitovertebral dissociation: 1. normal occipitovertebral relationships on lateral radiographs of supine subjects. AJR 1994;162:881.
3. Harris JH, Carson GC, Wagner LK, Kerr N. Radiologic diagnosis of traumatic occipitovertebral dissociation: 2. comparison of three methods of detecting occipitovertebral relationships on lateral radiographs of supine subjects. AJR 1994;162:887.

18.01 *Injuries to the Lower Cervical, Thoracic, and Lumbar Spine*

EPIDEMIOLOGY

Factors involved in injuries to the lower cervical spinal are similar to those described for the upper cervical spine. Between 8 to 10 years of age, middle and low cervical spine injuries become more common than those to the upper spine, and are similar to those found in adults. Thoracic and lumbar spine fractures constitute approximately 50% of all spine fractures in children. The most common causes are motor vehicle accidents, falls, sports-related injuries, and abuse.

CLINICAL FEATURES

In children older than 8 years of age, most spinal injuries are caused by a flexion mechanism. Simple compression of a vertebral body is the most common injury in the cervical spine (Fig. 18.01-1). These fractures commonly do not require surgical treatment. Burst fractures are rare but require anterior decompression and fusion. Anterior fusion is not commonly performed in children because it markedly alters growth. Facet dislocations are uncommon, but their incidence begins to increase during late adolescence. Avulsions of the spinous processes (clay shoveler's fractures) are uncommon but may be related to child abuse (Fig. 18.01-2). Separation of the end plates represents a relatively common injury that belongs with the Salter-Harris type of fractures (Fig. 18.01-3). In the cervical spine, the inferior end plates are affected more commonly, whereas in the lumbar spine, the superior end plates are more commonly avulsed. This injury is very unstable and is commonly accompanied by spinal cord damage. The syndrome of SCIWORA (spinal cord injury without radiographic abnormality) is found in 4% to 66% of all children with spinal cord injury. These patients may have delayed onset (> 4 days) of paraplegia, and the trauma is commonly recalled as mild. Mechanisms responsible for the spinal cord damage include transient disc herniations, avulsion of end plates, and infarction. Fractures in the thoracic and lumbar regions are commonly secondary to flexion (compression), axial loading (burst), flexion dis traction (seatbelt), and fracture–dislocations.

IMAGING FEATURES

The imaging features of fractures involving the lower spine are similar to those seen in adults. Plain radiographs and computed tomography (CT) are the imaging methods of choice. Avulsion of the end plates commonly involves the posterior ring apophyses and should not be confused with a calcified (hard) disc herniation. Up to 19% of lumbar disc herniations in children are associated with avulsion of the vertebral end plates. In SCIWORA, magnetic resonance (MR) is the imaging modality of choice. SCIWORA entails absence of abnormalities on plain radiographs and CT; however, MR imaging commonly shows ligamentous and spinal cord injuries. MR imaging features of the acutely injured spinal cord may be divided into three groups. Type 1 injury is related to hematoma and shows mild hypointensity and marked hypointensity on T1 and T2 (particularly T2*) images, respectively (Fig. 18.01-4). These patients have a poor prognosis. Type 2 injury is related to edema and shows an expanded, isointense or slightly hypointense spinal cord on T1-weighted images that is bright on T2-weighted images. The prognosis in these cases is good. Type 3 injury is a mixture of hemorrhage and edema and is characterized by central hypointensity with surrounding hyperintensity on T2-weighted images. These patients may experience partial neurologic recovery. Because children may have extensive damage to the spinal cord or epidural hematomas in the absence of fractures or dislocations, MR imaging is very helpful (Fig. 18.01-5). MR angiography is helpful in detecting damage to the vertebral arteries in patients with cervical spine fractures.

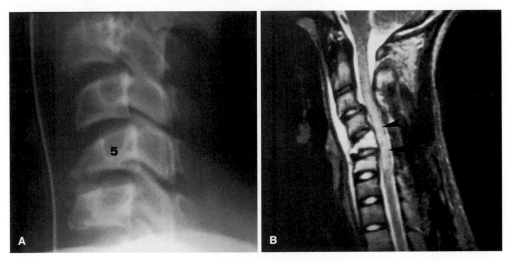

FIGURE 18.01-1.

Compression fracture. **A.** Lateral radiograph shows compression fracture of C5 (5) and mild posterior displacement. **B.** Sagittal magnetic resonance T2-weighted image in the same patient shows hyperintense C5 and C6 vertebral bodies (edema?) and hyperintensity *(arrowheads)* in spinal cord, also probably related to edema.

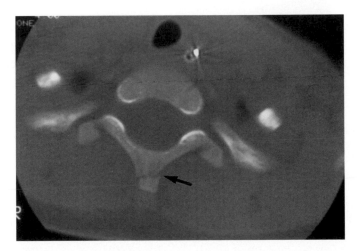

FIGURE 18.01-2.

Clay shoveler's fracture. Axial computed tomography in an abused child shows avulsion fracture *(arrow)* of C7 spinous process.

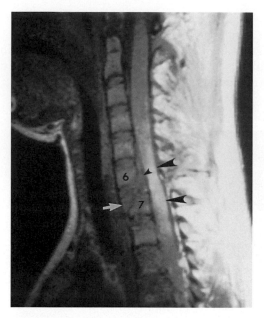

FIGURE 18.01-3.

Anterior tear-drop fracture. Midsagittal magnetic resonance T1-weighted image shows tear-drop–shaped fracture fragment *(white arrow)* from anterosuperior margin of C7 (7). C6 (6) is anteriorly subluxed on C7. There is a posttraumatic disc herniation *(small arrowhead)* at C6/C7. The diffuse increased signal intensity in the spinal cord *(large arrowheads)* suggests hemorrhage (methemoglobin).

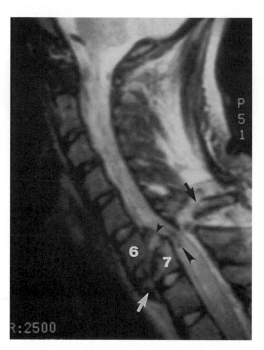

FIGURE 18.01-4.

Complete fracture–dislocation. Midsagittal magnetic resonance T2-weighted image shows anterior dislocation of C6 (6) on C7 (7). There is a tear-drop–shaped fracture fragment *(white arrow)* from the anterosuperior aspect of C7. A herniated disc *(small arrowhead)* is present. There is a spinal cord hematoma *(large arrowhead;* deoxyhemoglobin?) surrounded by hyperintensity (edema). The posterior ligamentous complex is disrupted and there is avulsion of the C6 spinous process *(black arrow).*

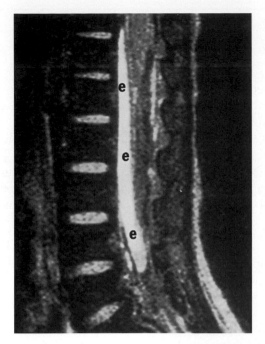

FIGURE 18.01-5.

Epidural hematoma. Midsagittal magnetic resonance gradient echo T2-weighted image shows bright ventral epidural hematoma (e) in the lumbar spine. There were no fractures in this child. (With permission from Castillo M. Neuroradiology Companion. Philadelphia: JB Lippincott, 1995.)

SUGGESTED READINGS

1. Kleinman PK, Zito JL. Avulsion of the spinous process caused by infant abuse. Radiology 1984;151:389.
2. Banerain KG, Wang AM, Samberg LC, Kerr HH, Wesolowski DP. Association of vertebral end plate fracture with pediatric lumbar intervetebral disk herniation: value of CT and MR imaging. Radiology 1990;177:763.
3. Kulkarni MV, McArdle CB, Kopanicky D, et al. Acute spinal cord injury: MR imaging at 1.5T. Radiology 1987;164:837.
4. Davis PC, Reisner A, Hudgins PA, Davis WE, O'Brien MS. Spinal injuries in children: role of MR. AJNR 1993;14:607.
5. Friedman D, Flanders A, Thomas C, Miller W. Vertebral artery injury after acute cervical spine trauma: rate of occurrence as detected by MR angiography and assessment of clinical consequences. AJR 1995;164:433.

18.02 Herniated Disc and Avulsed Ring Apophysis

EPIDEMIOLOGY

The incidence of disc herniations in children is low. They account for 1% to 3% of lumbar spine discectomies performed in the general population. However, in Japan, their incidence is higher (8%–22%). There is no gender predilection. Disc herniations are more common in children with a family history of this disorder.

Avulsion of the posterior (caudal or cephalad) ring apophysis is rare and is found in approximately 30% of children who undergo disc surgery. Most are seen in preadolescents and adolescents. They are more common in boys.

CLINICAL FEATURES

The most important factor leading to childhood disc herniations is trauma. Congenital abnormalities (mostly transitional vertebrae and spina bifida occulta) are present in one-third of children with disc herniations. The most common symptoms are marked low back pain or sciatica. Neurologic findings are absent in 50% of patients. This constitutes the major clinical difference between childhood and adult disc herniations. When symptoms are present, they include minor motor, sensory, and reflex abnormalities. Because disc herniations are so uncommon in children, the diagnosis is usually delayed from several months to 1 year in most patients. Patients without progressive neurologic symptoms may receive an aggressive course of bed rest (at times with traction), analgesia, muscle relaxants, and later physical therapy. Failure of symptoms to resolve or progression are indications for surgical disc removal.

Avulsion of the posterior ring apophysis presents with symptoms identical to those of disc herniation (with which it is commonly associated). These avulsions are usually posttraumatic and therefore more common in boys.

IMAGING FEATURES

Contrary to adults, plain radiographs of the lumbar spine are important in children suspected of harboring disc herniation. Plain radiographs help in identifying sacralization of the last lumbar vertebra or lumbarization of the first sacral vertebra, as well as spinal bifida occulta. Because it is noninvasive and free of ionizing radiation, we prefer magnetic resonance imaging over computed tomography. The imaging findings are exactly those of the adult with the exception that the parent disc from which the herniation originates is commonly of normal signal intensity and not desiccated (low T2 signal), as it commonly is in adults (Fig. 18.02-1). Occasionally a calcified disc is seen. These are almost always asymptomaic and incidental findings, but may be accompanied by torticollis. They are probably the sequelae of aseptic inflammation, and may resolve over time. If the calcification protrudes posteriorly, symptoms similar to those of disc herniation may be present.

Most avulsions of the posterior ring apophysis occur at the L4–L5 and L5–S1 levels (Fig. 18.02-2). The inferior border of L4 and superior border of S1 are the most common sites. The imaging features of this disorder have been divided into three groups (Takata's classification). In type 1, there is a simple separation of the central and posterior rim apophysis, but the underlying bone is intact. This is mostly seen between 8 to 13 years of age. In type 2, a small, irregular central fragment of bone is avulsed. This injury is mostly seen between 13 to 18 years of age. In type 3, there is a true (commonly eccentric) fracture of the posterior vertebral body, and it occurs more commonly after 18 years of age. In types 1 and 2, surgery is performed via bilateral laminectomies (because the abnormality is central in location), whereas in a type 3 injury a unilateral laminectomy often suffices. Limbus vertebrae are a type of avulsion of the ring apophysis that usually is asymptomatic and incidentally found (Fig. 18.02-3).

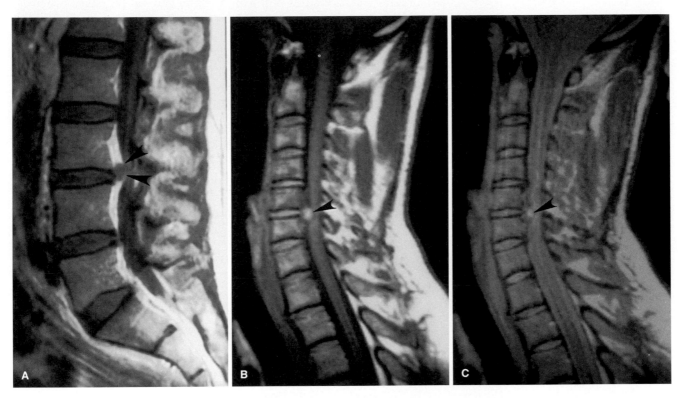

FIGURE 18.02-1.

Herniated disc. **A.** Midsagittal postcontrast magnetic resonance (MR) T1-weighted image. Contrast was given because of suspicion of abnormality at L3–L4 on precontrast images (contrast is not routinely indicated for the diagnosis of uncomplicated disc herniation). There is a nonenhancing disc fragment *(arrowheads)* seen within the enhancing ventral epidural space at the L3–L4 level. The parent disc is not degenerated. **B.** Midsagittal MR T1-weighted image in a different case of posttraumatic disc herniation. There is a herniated disc *(arrowhead)* at the C5–C6 level that is bright, presumably because of presence of hemorrhage. The disc compresses the spinal cord. **C.** Corresponding MR proton density image shows that the herniated disc *(arrowhead)* remains hyperintense. There is a small disc bulge at C4–C5. Similar findings may be seen in calcified discs.

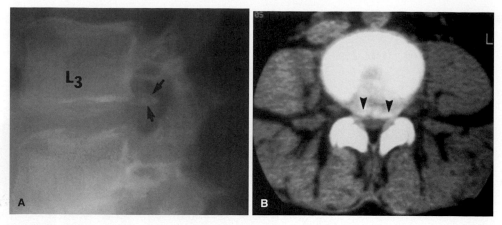

FIGURE 18.02-2.

Avulsed ring apophysis. **A.** Lateral radiograph shows small bone fragment *(arrows)* from the inferoposterior endplate of L3. **B.** Axial computed tomography in the same patient shows avulsion of posterior ring apophysis *(arrowheads)*. (**A** and **B** with permission from Castillo M. Neuroradiology Companion. Philadelphia: JB Lippincott, 1995.)

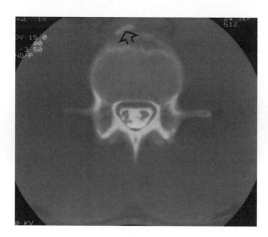

FIGURE 18.02-3.

Limbus vertebra. Axial computed tomography shows small bone fragment *(arrow)* secondary to avulsion of anterior ring apophysis by herniation of nucleus pulposus under it. This is usually an incidental and asymptomatic finding.

SUGGESTED READINGS

1. Takata K, Inoue S, Takahashi K, Ohtsulca Y. Fracture of the posterior margin of a lumbar vertebral body. J Bone Joint Surg [Am] 1988;70:589.
2. Bangert BA, Modic MT, Ross JS, et al. Hyperintense disks on T1-weighted MR images: correlation with calcification. Radiology 1995;195:437.

18.03 *Brachial Plexus Injuries*

EPIDEMIOLOGY

In children, most injuries to the brachial plexus occur during breech deliveries or vertex deliveries with excessive traction on the head. In adolescents, motor vehicle accidents and sports-related injuries (particularly water skiing) are important predisposing factors.

CLINICAL FEATURES

Birth-related injuries to the brachial plexus may be isolated or associated with fractures of the ipsilateral clavicle or, rarely, the humerus. Shoulder dystocia is encountered in as many as 50% of children weighing more than 3500 g at birth. Injury to the C5 and C6 nerve roots results in Erb's palsy. In this condition the arm is adducted and rotated internally, the forearm is pronated, and the wrist flexed. Most of these patients show partial or complete resolution if the nerve rootlets have not been completely avulsed. Injury to C7 and T1 nerve roots results in Klumpke's palsy. In these patients, there is weakness of the forearm extensors, the wrist and fingers flexors, and of the muscles of the hand, giving it a "claw-like" appearance. The elbow is flexed, the forearm supinated, and the wrist extended. Horner syndrome may present in these patients. In rare cases, the injury involves all the nerve roots that form the plexus and results in flaccid paralysis of the upper extremity. In older children, diphtheria–pertussis–tetanus vaccination may induce a transient brachial plexitis. There also is a rare type of brachial plexus palsy that is inherited.

Chronic irritation to the brachial plexus may occur secondary to the presence of cervical ribs. Cervical ribs occur in 1% of the population, and 90% of individuals are asymptomatic. Symptoms commonly present in adulthood. Treatment involves anterior scalenotomy or resection of the offending rib.

Occasionally, brachial plexopathy accompanies spinal cord injury. These patients present with lower motor neuron palsy, absent reflexes, sensory abnormalities, and, rarely, Horner syndrome. Rapid and exaggerated application of traction on the cervical spine or upper extremities may also damage the brachial plexus. The C5, C6, and T1 nerve roots are more commonly affected.

IMAGING FEATURES

Both magnetic resonance (MR) and postmyelography computed tomography (CT) play important roles in the diagnosis of brachial plexopathy (Fig. 18.03-1). We prefer MR as the initial imaging modality. Axial, coronal, and sagittal T1- and T2-weighted images may be used to demonstrate discontinuity of the plexus, periplexal edema, and hematomas. Detailed imaging of the cervical spine is essential. A hematoma may be present in the thecal sac where the nerves were avulsed from the spinal cord (Fig. 18.03-2). Pseudomeningoceles occur along the nerve sleeves in the neural foramina or inside the spinal canal. The nerves often retract after the injury and are not seen by MR imaging. Confirmation of pseudomeningoceles, which imply an avulsed plexus, may need postmyelography CT imaging. In the absence of avulsion, repair of distal abnormalities may be attempted.

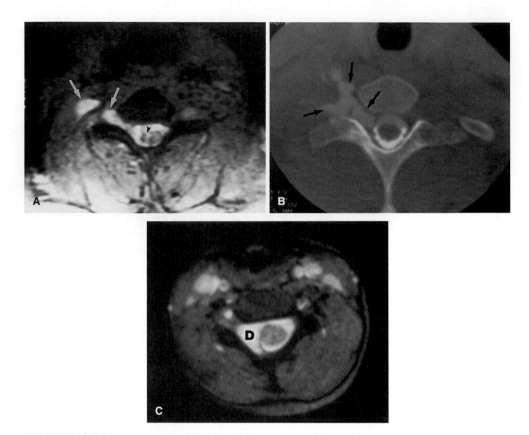

FIGURE 18.03-1.

Avulsion of nerve root with dural diverticulum. **A.** Axial magnetic resonance (MR) T2-weighted image shows dural diverticulum *(arrows)* from avulsion of nerve root. There is high signal intensity in the spinal cord *(arrowhead)* from possible injury (fissure?) to the lateral aspect of the cord. **B.** Postmyelography axial computed tomography (different patient) shows extravasation of contrast material into diverticulum *(arrows)* secondary to avulsion of that nerve root. **C.** Axial MR T2-weighted image in a different patient shows intraspinal dural diverticulum (D) caused by avulsion of nerve root. The spinal cord is displaced to the left.

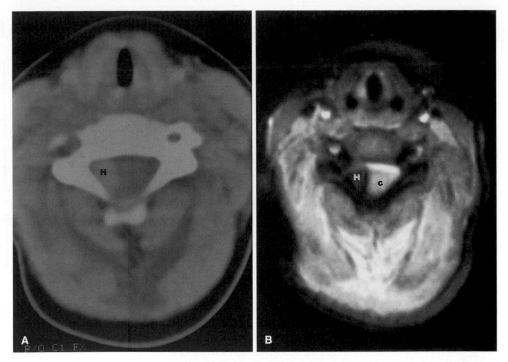

FIGURE 18.03-2.

Hematoma secondary to avulsion of nerve roots. **A.** Axial computed tomography shows hematoma (H) in spinal canal secondary to nerve root avulsion. **B.** Corresponding magnetic resonance T2-weighted image shows low signal intensity of hematoma (H; deoxyhemoglobin?) and lateral displacement of the spinal cord (C). There is abnormal hyperintensity in the posterior paraspinal muscles, probably secondary to edema.

SUGGESTED
READING

1. Miller S, Glasier C, Griebel M, Boop F. Brachial plexopathy in infants after traumatic delivery: evaluation with MR imaging. Radiology 1993;189:481.

18.04 *Spinal Cord Transection and Infarction*

EPIDEMIOLOGY

These entities are very rare in children. Transections are usually related to motor vehicle accidents. Spinal cord infarctions in children are related to trauma, sickle cell disease, hypercoagulable states, vascular malformations, and arteritis. Birth-related injuries may also damage the spinal cord. Children comprise 1% to 10% of all patients with spinal cord injuries.

CLINICAL FEATURES

Any type of acute spinal cord injury may present with pain, sensory level, motor weakness, paraplegia, quadriplegia, decreased or lost deep tendon reflexes, loss of sphincter control, autonomic dysfunction, and meningismus. Injury to the spinal cord may be produced by excessive traction/extension/rotation on the head during birth (especially if "high" forceps have been used) or breech deliveries. Injury to the upper spinal cord is commonly fatal. Injury to the lower spinal cord manifests as low Apgar scores, respiratory distress, and hypotonia. In our experience, most of these injuries occur at the cervicothoracic junction. This portion of the spinal cord may be considered a "watershed" zone. The middle to lower cervical spinal cord receives its blood supply from the anterior spinal artery, multiple radicular branches, and branches from the thyrocervical trunks. The upper thoracic spine is irrigated by the anterior spinal artery, which is supplied by multiple intercostal arteries. Therefore, stretching of the tenuous arteries at the cervicothoracic junction may easily result in their thrombosis with subsequent infarction.

IMAGING FEATURES

Magnetic resonance (MR) is the imaging method of choice in suspected transection and infarction of the spinal cord. Sagittal images readily show transections as gaps in the spinal cord (Fig. 18.04-1). The spinal cord margins are commonly frayed. Associated arachnoid cysts and epidural and subdural hematomas are not uncommon. No bone abnormalities may be present. Birth-related injuries have typical MR findings (Fig. 18.04-2). Acutely, T1- and T2-weighted images may show decreased signal intensity, implying the presence of acute blood (deoxyhemoglobin). Deoxyhemoglobin later becomes methemoglobin, and the cord becomes bright. It is important to identify reliably the presence of intramedullary hemorrhage. Gradient echo images are most sensitive to blood products, whereas fast spin echo images are least sensitive. If only edema is present (isointense or low signal intensity on T1-weighted images and high T2 signal), the prognosis is favorable. The presence of hemorrhage implies a poor prognosis. Between 2 to 4 weeks, the cord undergoes severe atrophy. Acute infarctions of the spinal cord usually show an expanded but isointense (although occasionally hypointense) spinal cord on T1-weighted images that becomes bright on T2-weighted images (Fig. 18.04-3). On axial T2-weighted images, only the anterior two-thirds of the cord may be hyperintense, conforming to the vascular supply given by the anterior spinal artery. Occasionally, one may see two round hyperintensities in the anterior two-thirds of the cord on axial images. These have been called "owl eyes" or "tiger eyes," and reflect infarction and edema of gray matter.

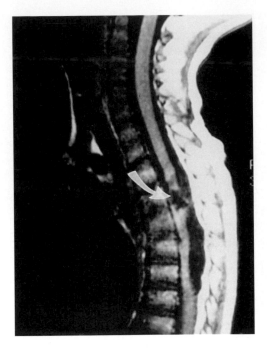

FIGURE 18.04-1.

Spinal cord transection. Midsagittal magnetic resonance T1-weighted image after motor vehicle accident shows complete transection of high thoracic spinal cord *(arrow)* in 6-year-old boy. The cerebrospinal fluid collection dorsal to the spinal cord is probably an arachnoid cyst.

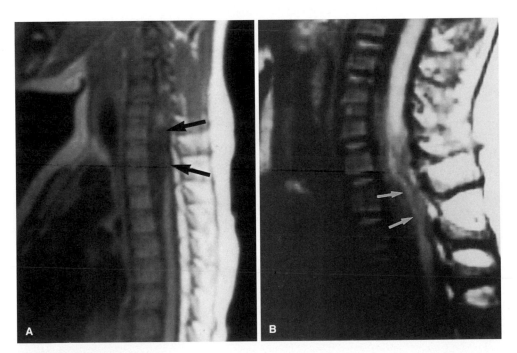

FIGURE 18.04-2.

Spinal cord injury after breech delivery. **A.** Midsagittal magnetic resonance (MR) T1-weighted image shows extreme atrophy *(arrows)* of the spinal cord at the cervicothoracic junction, which is typical of chronic changes after infarction at this level due to extreme traction on the head after breech delivery. **B.** Midsagittal MR T1-weighted image in a different patient shows severe atrophy *(arrows)* of spinal cord, again at cervicothoracic junction. Patient also born via difficult breech delivery. Note that in both cases the infarction occurred below the region supplied by the artery of the cervical enlargement. (With permission from Castillo M, Quencer RM, Green BA. Spinal cord injury following traumatic breech delivery. AJNR 1989;10(S):99.)

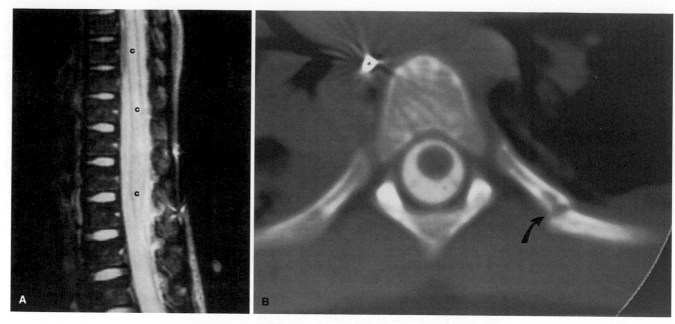

FIGURE 18.04-3.

Spinal cord infarction. **A.** Midsagittal magnetic resonance T1-weighted image shows diffusely hyperintense spinal cord (c), compatible with edema. **B.** Axial postmyelography computed tomography shows left rib fracture (*arrow;* only fracture in this patient). The spinal cord infarction is presumably secondary to injury and thrombosis of the intercostal artery, from which the artery of Adamkiewicz arises.

SUGGESTED READINGS

1. Castillo M, Quencer RM, Green BA. Cervical spinal cord injury after traumatic breech delivery. AJNR 1989;10(S):99.
2. Castillo M, Carrier D, Smith JK. Spinal cord infarction after solitary rib fracture. Emerg Radiol 1995;2:150.

18.05   *Spondylolysis and Spondylolisthesis*

EPIDEMIOLOGY

These terms refer to a defect through the pars interarticularis ("lysis") and to slippage of one vertebra on another ("listhesis"). Spondylolysis is not seen in newborns, but is found in up to 5% of children by 6 years of age. Its incidence in the general population is 6%. In some families, its incidence may be increased. It is increased in patients with spina bifida occulta and in Eskimos. Spondylolysis is more common white males.

CLINICAL FEATURES

The etiology of spondylolysis is uncertain, but it is probably related to repeated microtrauma leading to formation of clefts in the pars interarticularis. Most patients present between 10 to 15 years of age (probably related to increased growth and physical activity during this period of time). If spondylolisthesis accompanies the spondylolysis, the degree of displacement does not always correlate with the severity of clinical symptoms. The most common symptom is low back pain. Other symptoms include radiculopathies, sphincter dysfunction, and, occasionally, kyphosis. Initial treatment is usually conservative and includes bed rest, analgesics, and restriction of sports. Bracing and physical therapy are helpful in those patients with spondylolisthesis grades 1 and 2. Spondylolisthesis greater than 30% to 50% may require surgical treatment. These patients may undergo posterior or anterior spinal fusion or direct repair with screw fixation.

IMAGING FEATURES

Oblique plain radiographs of the lumbar spine readily demonstrate the cleft as a lucent defect in the pars interarticularis (a "collar" on the "neck of the Scotty dog"; Fig. 18.05-1A,B). Most defects are bilateral but, when unilateral, the opposite pars interarticularis may become hypertrophied and sclerotic because of increased stress and weight bearing. The intact pars interarticularis may be "hot" on radiotracer studies. Most defects involve L5. Computed tomography shows these defects as irregularly marginated clefts with sclerotic margins (Fig. 18.05-1C). They may be easily overlooked, and commonly the first impression is that of "too many facets." On magnetic resonance imaging, they may be even more difficult to visualize. Parasagittal T1- and T2-weighted images through the facets show a hypointense defect in the pars interarticularis. These defects are oriented perpendicular to the axis of the facet joints. Occasionally, high T2 signal intensity may be present within the defect. Lateral plain radiographs demonstrate the degree of listhesis. Slippage is commonly anterior but occasionally may be posterior (Fig. 18.05-2). As a vertebra slides anteriorly, it also angles inferiorly. The degree of slippage may be classified by dividing the vertebral body (which is normal) located immediately under the slipped vertebra into four equal segments and accordingly grading the degree of displacement (Meyerding's method). No displacement is grade 0. Grade 1 is displacement between 1% to 25%, grade 2 between 26% to 50%, grade 3 between 51% to 75%, and grade 4 between 76% to 100%. Spondyloptosis (grade 5 displacement) is a term used to described complete slippage.

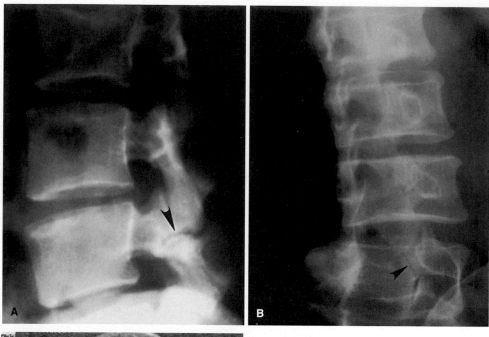

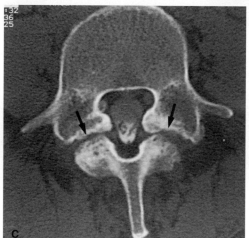

FIGURE 18.05-1.

Spondylolysis. **A.** Lateral radiograph of the lumbar spine shows cleft *(arrowhead)* in pars interarticularis. **B.** In a different patient, oblique radiograph of the lumbar spine shows cleft *(arrowhead)* in pars interarticularis of L4 ("collar on the Scotty dog"). **C.** Axial postmyelography computed tomography (different patient) shows bilateral clefts *(arrowheads)* in pars interarticularis of L5.

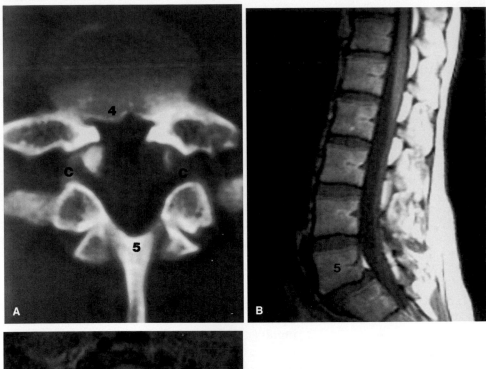

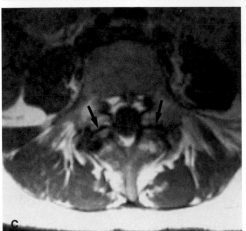

FIGURE 18.05-2.

Spondylolysis and spondylolisthesis. A. Axial computed tomography shows severe anterior slippage of L4 (4) on L5 (5). Bilateral pars interarticularis clefts (C) are present. **B.** Midsagittal magnetic resonance (MR) T1-weighted image (different patient) shows slight anterior displacement of L5 (5) on S1. **C.** Axial MR T1-weighted image in same patient shows bilateral clefts *(arrows)* in pars interarticularis of L5.

SUGGESTED READINGS

1. Bradford DS, Ju SS. Spondylolysis and spondylolisthesis. In: Weinstein SL, ed. The Pediatric Spine: Principles and Practice. New York: Raven, 1994:585.
2. Ulmer JL, Elster AD, Mathews VP, Allen AM. Lumbar spondylolysis: reactive marrow changes seen in adjacent pedicles on MR images. AJR 1995;164:429.
3. Ulmer JL, Elster AD, Mathews VP, King JC. Distinction between degenerative and isthmic spondylolisthesis on sagittal MR images: importance of increased anteroposterior diameter of the spinal canal. AJR 1994;163:411.

18.06 *Vascular Malformations*

Vascular malformations are rare, comprising less than 4% of all space-occupying masses in the spine. Some of these malformations (types 2 and 3) present during the second to third decades of life, whereas others (types 1 and 4) are disorders mainly of adults. There may be a slight male predilection. Cavernous angiomas and capillary telangiectasias are very rare, comprising only 5% to 10% of all spinal vascular malformations.

Spinal vascular malformations may be classified as follows:

Type 1: The nidus is located adjacent to the dura. It is fed by one or more radicular arteries and drains into dural veins. It occurs most commonly in the lower thoracic spine and is seen during middle age, particularly in men. Symptoms are insidious and related to ischemia, edema, and infarction of the spinal cord secondary to venous hypertension (Foix-Alajouanine syndrome).

Type 2: This lesion is a tight (glomus) intramedullary nidus supplied by multiple branches from the anterior and posterior spinal arteries. It commonly involves the cervical and lower thoracic spine, and symptoms may be acute and related to hematomyelia (70%) producing acute myelopathy.

Type 3: These are termed "juvenile" malformations. The nidus is a large vascular mass located in the spinal cord, but often with extension outside of it (including extraspinal), and is supplied by a myriad of feeding arteries. These usually produce paresis, sensory alterations, and autonomic dysfunction.

Type 4: This group is controversial; some classify intradural extramedullary arteriovenous fistulas here, whereas others believe that this group should include those vascular malformations that involve a segment of spinal cord and adjacent bone/soft tissues (metameric arteriovenous malformations). Arteriovenous fistulas may be seen in patients with Rendu-Osler-Weber and Cobb syndromes.

Catheter embolizations (with particulate emboli) serve as either the primary mode of treatment (in those patients with poor anatomic conditions for surgery) or as adjuvant therapy before surgical resection. Embolization results in a complete cure in only 10% to 20% of patients.

Magnetic resonance (MR) is the imaging method of choice for the screening of these malformations (Fig. 18.06-1A–C). Occasionally, myelography may be used to confirm the presence of dilated vessels in the thecal sac. The definite test is the spinal angiogram (Fig. 18.06-1D). In type 1 malformations, MR imaging usually is negative. Occasionally, T2-weighted images may show increased signal intensity within the spinal cord. There also may be enhancement of the surface or the substance of the spinal cord. In the other types of spinal vascular malformations, MR imaging shows multiple serpiginous areas of flow void (vessels) involving the spinal cord and the subarachnoid space. The former usually represent the nidus, whereas the latter are related to dilated draining veins. T2-weighted images may show increased signal intensity in the cord adjacent to the nidus. This is related to edema or gliosis. The cord is expanded at the nidus level but occasionally may be atrophic. Very low signal intensity surrounding the vascular nidus is probably related to hemosiderin from prior hemorrhage. After contrast administration, the surface or substance of the cord may enhance. Cavernous angiomas in the spinal cord have the same appearance as they do in the brain. Capillary telangiectasias are generally not visible on MR imaging, and are autopsy findings.

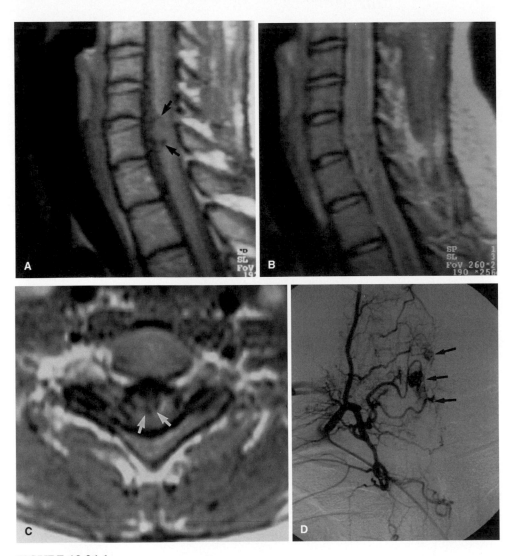

FIGURE 18.06-1.

Arteriovenous malformation (probable type 3). **A.** Midsagittal magnetic resonance (MR) T1-weighted image shows serpiginous areas of flow void *(arrow)* in cord, suggesting vessels, and widening of the ventral subarachnoid space from C5 to T1. **B.** Corresponding MR proton density image again shows the multiple intramedullary vessels but no abnormal signal intensity in the spinal cord. **C.** Axial MR T1-weighted image shows intramedullary flow void *(arrows)*. **D.** Selective injection (catheter angiogram) of right thyrocervical trunk shows a myriad of vessels supplying multiple niduses *(arrows)* in spinal cord arteriovenous malformation.

SUGGESTED READING

1. Casasco AE, Houdart E, Gobin YP, Aymard A, Guichard JP, Rufenacht DA. Embolization of spinal vascular malformations. Neuroimaging Clinics of North America 1992;2:3337.

Index

Page numbers followed by *f* indicate figures; those followed by *t* indicate a table.

labyrinthitis, 463–464
  acute, 463, 464, 464f
  intracochlear bone formation in, 464, 465f
  obliterative, 464, 465f
  serous, 463
  suppurative, 463
labyrinthitis ossificans, 464, 465f
lacrimal sac, 410f
laminar necrosis, in cerebral infarction, 171f
lamina terminalis, 21
Langerhans cell histiocytosis, 238, 239, 241f
  eosinophilic granuloma in, 677
large vestibular aqueduct syndrome, 438–439, 439f
laryngeal aditus, 519
laryngeal cartilage, 565
laryngeal muscles, 519
laryngeal ventricle, 519, 520f
laryngocele, 541–542, 543f
laryngomalacia, 534, 535f
laryngopyocele, 541
laryngotracheal diverticulum, 518, 520f
laryngotracheal groove, 518, 520f
laryngotracheal tube, 518, 520f
laryngotracheitis, 556, 556f, 557f
laryngotracheoesophageal cleft, 532, 532f
larynx
  applied embryology of, 518–519, 520f
  atresia of, 526, 527f
  congenital flaccid, 534, 535f
  glottic, 518–519, 520f
  granular cell tumor of, 548, 549f
  juvenile papillomatosis of, 546–547, 547f
  mucoepidermoid carcinoma of, 548, 550f
  neurofibroma of, 548, 549f
  paraganglioma of, 548
  saccular cysts of, 541–542, 542f
  saccule of, 541
  salivary gland tumors of, 548, 550f
  sarcoma of, 548, 551f
  subglottic, 518, 520f
    in croup, 556, 556f, 557f
    hemangioma of, 544, 545f
  supraglottic, 518–519, 520f
  trauma to, 558–560, 560f
  tumors of, 548–549, 549f–552f
  ventricle of, 541
  webs of, 526–527
Leber's miliary aneurysm, 375–376, 376f
Leigh disease, 101t, 102t, 104f
Leigh syndrome, 121t, 122t
lens
  dysplasia of
    in median cleft syndrome, 400f
  formation of, 358–359, 360f
  subluxation of
    in retinoblastoma, 379f
lenticulostriate artery, hypertrophy of, 180f
lentiform nucleus
  in asphyxia, 164, 165f

in cerebritis, 289f
  in Cockayne syndrome, 133f
  in Wilson disease, 128, 129f
leptomeninges, angioma of, 344
Lesch-Nyhan disease, 101t, 102t
Letterer-Siwe disease
  eosinophilic granuloma in, 677
  temporal bone in, 475
leukemia
  eosinophilic granuloma in, 239, 241f
  extradural, 680, 681f
  meningeal, 238, 239
  temporal bone in, 475
leukodystrophy
  fibrinoid, 137, 138f, 139f
  metachromatic, 105t, 107t, 109f
  sudanophilic, 142, 143f
leukoencephalitis, hemorrhagic, 301f
leukokoria, persistent hyperplastic primary vitreous and, 371
leukomalacia, periventricular, 160, 161f, 162f
levoscoliosis
  thoracic
    in microphthalmos, 365f
limbus vertebra, in posterior ring apophyseal avulsion, 714f
lip(s)
  formation of, 395, 396f
  upper
    cleft of, 398, 400f, 401f
lipoblastomatosis, cervicothoracic, 606
lipoma
  corpus callosum dysgenesis and, 28
  cranial neuropathy from, 62, 64f
  curvilinear, 62, 63f
  filar, 635, 636f
  interhemispheric
    in median cleft syndrome, 399, 401f, 403f
  intradural
    cervical spine, 634, 637f
    lumbar spine, 634, 636f
  intraspinal, 632f
  midline, 62, 63f, 64f
  nodular, 62, 63f
  quadrigeminal cistern, 62, 64f
  subarachnoid intracranial, 62, 63f, 64f
  subcutaneous
    in median cleft syndrome, 399, 403f
lipomatosis
  encephalocutaneous
    intracranial lipoma with, 62
lipomyelocele, 634, 635
lipomyelomeningocele, 634, 635
lipophilin deficiency, in Pelizaeus-Merzbacher disease, 142
lissencephaly, 45–46, 46f–48f
  type I, 45–46, 46f
  type II, 45, 46
  type III, 45, 47
  type IV, 45, 48f
  type V, 45
Listeria monocytogenes
  in cerebritis, 288, 289f
Llermitte-Duclos disease, focal megalencephaly and, 54, 56f

longus colli muscles, Tornwaldt cyst between, 578, 579f
Lowe (oculocerebrorenal) syndrome, 101t, 102t
Lyme disease, vs. multiple sclerosis, 278
lymphadenopathy, 601, 603f
lymphangioma, 587–588, 589f–591f
  cavernous, 588
  classification of, 588
  facial, 428, 429
  with hemorrhage, 385, 387f
  intraparotid, 588, 591f
  orbital, 385, 386f, 387f
lymphatic system, 599
  embryogenesis of, 587
lymphatic tumors, facial, 428–429, 429f, 430f
lymph nodes
  enlargement of, 600
  extracranial head and neck drainage of, 599–600
  reactive, 599, 600
  retropharyngeal, 594, 601, 602f
lymphoepithelioma, 607
  nasopharyngeal, 548, 551f
lymphoma, 604–605, 605f
  Burkitt, 604–605
  cauda equina, 682f
  cerebral, 238–239, 239f
  extradural, 680, 682f
  Hodgkin, 604, 605, 605f
  non-Hodgkin, 238, 604
  temporal bone in, 475
lysosomal disorders, 105, 105t, 106t, 107, 107t, 108t, 109f, 110f

magnetic resonance imaging, 4–7
magnetic resonance spectroscopy, 6–7
malacia
  infarction and, 165, 167f
  skull fracture and, 263f
malleus
  in cochlear malformation, 446f
  in congenital aural atresia, 440, 441, 442f
  development of, 435, 436f, 448
  dysplasia of, 448, 449f
  malrotation of, 449f
  in temporal bone fracture, 473f
mandible
  condyle of
    in Treacher Collins syndrome, 423f
  Ewing sarcoma of, 606, 610f
  fibrous dysplasia of, 426, 427f
  formation of, 564
  hypoplasia of
    in Goldenhar syndrome, 424f
    in Nager syndrome, 425f
    in Treacher Collins syndrome, 423f
  teratoma of, 614f
mandibular arch, 394, 395f, 396f
manubrium, malrotation of, 449f
maple syrup urine disease, 101t, 102t
Marfan syndrome, arachnoid cysts in, 59
masseter muscle
  hematoma of, 560f
  rhabdomyosarcoma of, 608f

myelography, 13–14
myelomalacia, in filar lipoma, 635
myelomeningocele, 630, 631f, 632f
in type II Chiari malformation, 78
myotomes, 618, 619f

Nager syndrome, 422t, 425f
nanophthalmos, 363
nasal alea
cleft of, 403f
formation of, 395, 396f
nasal bones
formation of, 395, 396f
in frontonasal encephalocele, 417, 418f
nasal capsule, cartilaginous, 394, 396f
nasal cavity
absence of, 408, 409f
formation of, 395, 397f
nasal passage, obstruction of, 408–409,
409f–411f
nasal septum
formation of, 395, 397f
thinning of
in piriform aperture stenosis,
408–409, 411f
nasofrontal region
anomalies of, 417–418, 418f–421f
applied embryology of, 412, 413f–416f
nasolacrimal duct
canaliculi of, 410f
cyst of, 408
mucoceles of, 408, 410f
nasolateral process
development of, 394, 396f
fusion of, 396f
nasomedial process
development of, 394, 396f
fusion of, 396f
nasopharynx
agenesis of, 405, 406f
atresia of, 404–405, 406f
juvenile angiofibroma of, 507–508,
508f, 509f
lymphoepithelioma of, 548, 551f
in nasal agenesis, 408, 409f
rhabdoid tumor of, 609f
Tornwaldt cyst of, 578, 579f, 580f
tumors of
skull base erosion in, 607, 610f, 611f
neck
computed tomography of, 3
fibromatosis of, 606
hyperextension of
carotid dissection from, 168
posterior triangle of
cystic hygroma of, 587, 588, 589f
lymphangioma of, 588, 590f
rhabdoid tumor of, 606, 609f
soft tissues of
applied embryology of, 563–565, 566f
teratoma of, 612, 613f
necrosis
in cerebral infarction, 171f
in oligodendroglioma, 215, 216f–217f
nekabisus, neurocutaneous, 350t
Nembutal, 15

neocerebellum, 70
neural arches, 618, 619f
neural crests, 20, 22f, 618, 619f
neural folds, 20, 22f
neural foramina
duplication of, 645, 647f
neuroblastoma of, 675, 676f
neural groove, 20, 22f, 618, 619f
neural tube
closure of, 20, 23f
occipital encephalocele with, 72
formation of, 618, 619f
neuroblastoma
head and neck, 607
metastatic, 228, 230f
paraspinal, 675, 676f
supratentorial, 227–228, 230f
neuroblasts, 21, 23f
migration of, 21–22
neuroectodermal tumors
primitive, 227–228, 228f–229f
pineal, 231
neuroendocrine disorders, in septo-optic
dysplasia, 37
neuroepithelial tumor,
dysembryonoplastic, 223, 224,
226f
neurofibroma
cauda equina, 658, 659f
laryngeal, 548, 549f
paraspinal, 658, 659f
plexiform, 333, 335f, 658, 659f
polyclonal, 658
neurofibromatosis
facial nerve schwannoma in, 477f
neurofibrosarcoma in, 606
neurogenic tumors in, 476
type I, 332–333
brachial plexus nerve sheath tumor
in, 603f
buphthalmos in, 368f
greater sphenoidal wing dysplasia in,
333, 335f
hamartoma in, 332–333, 334f
laryngeal neurofibroma in, 548, 549f
meningoangiomatosis in, 333, 336f
optic astrocytoma in, 332, 333f
spinal abnormalities in, 658–659,
659f
transsphenoidal encephalocele in, 66f
vascular dysplasia in, 333, 335f
type II, 337
meningioma in, 337, 338f, 339f
schwannoma in, 337, 338f
spinal abnormalities in, 658–659,
660f
types of, 337
neurofibrosarcoma
in neurofibromatosis, 606
spinal, 658
neurohypophysis
translocation of
in Kallmann syndrome, 57, 58f
in panhypopituitarism, 98f
neuron(s)
migration of
disorders of, 45–58

necrosis of
in hypoxic–ischemic
encephalopathy, 164
neurulation, 618, 619f
primary, 20, 22f
secondary, 20
nevus, epidermal, 350t, 352f
Niemann-Pick disease, 105t, 107t
Nocardia infection, 312, 314f
non-Hodgkin lymphoma, 604
extradural, 680
Norman-Roberts syndrome, lissencephaly
type I and, 45
nose. *See also* entries under Nasal.
agenesis of, 408, 409f
dermoid of, 417–418, 420f–421f
notochord, 618, 619f
anomalous embryogenesis of
in Tornwaldt cyst, 578
split of, 645

occipital region
atrophy of
in Alper disease, 125, 126f
in Hartnup disease, 103f
dysplasia of, 452f
fibrous dysplasia of, 426, 427f
occipitoatlantal joint dislocation, 704,
705f, 706f
olfactory sulci
absence of
in Kallmann syndrome, 57, 58f
oligodendroglioma, 215–216, 216f–217f
optic chiasm
astrocytoma of, 212, 213f, 214f
displacement of
epidermoid and, 249f
hypoplasia of
in septo-optic dysplasia, 37, 38f–39f
optic disc
hypoplasia of
in septo-optic dysplasia, 38f
optic nerve
calcification of
in retinoblastoma, 378, 379f
coloboma of, 369, 370
congenital dysplasia of
in septo-optic dysplasia, 37, 38f
glioma of
in neurofibromatosis type I, 332,
333f
prechiasmatic
in multiple sclerosis, 279f
optic pit
invagination of
failure of, 361, 362f
optic vesicle
closure of, 395f
formation of, 358, 360f
oral cavity, 394–395, 397f
oral placode, 394–395
orbit(s)
applied embryology of, 358–359, 360f
bony
formation of, 394, 395f
computed tomography of, 3

orbits(s) *(continued)*
  dermoid of, 388–389, 389f
  disorders of
    sinusitis and, 492–493, 493f–495f
  eosinophilic granuloma of, 239, 241f
  epidermoid of, 388
  in Goldenhar syndrome, 424f
  hemangioma of, 381–382, 383f, 428,
    430f
  lymphangioma of, 385, 386f, 387f
  magnetic resonance imaging of, 5
  subperiosteal abscess of, 494f
  in Treacher Collins syndrome, 423f
oropharynx, benign epithelial cyst of,
    548, 552f
Osler-Weber-Rendu disease, 350t
os odontoideum
  in achondroplasia, 624f
  dystopic, 625, 626f, 627f
  orthotopic, 625, 626f
ossicles
  in congenital aural atresia, 441, 442f
  dysplasia of, 447f, 448–449, 449f
  formation of, 435, 437f, 448
  subluxation of
    in temporal bone fracture, 473, 473f
osteoblastoma, 666–667
osteochondroma, spinal, 666, 667, 667f
osteogenesis imperfecta, 450
osteoid osteoma, 666, 667f
osteoma
  choroidal
    in retinoblastoma, 379f
  of external auditory canal, 479f
osteomyelitis, 694
osteopetrosis, 450, 451
osteosarcoma, 672
  maxillary, 611f
  paranasal, 510, 511, 514f
  in retinoblastoma, 378, 380f
otic capsule, 435, 436f
otic placode, 435
otocyst, 435
otosclerosis, 454–455, 455f
  cochlear, 454, 455f
  fenestral, 454–455, 455f
  retrofenestral, 445f, 454, 455
oval window
  bone over
    sclerosis of, 454, 455f
beta oxidation defects, 118t
oxidative metabolic disorders, 118, 118t
oxycephaly, 40, 43f, 44f

pachygyria, 46, 48f
  vs. polymicrogyria, 152, 153f
palate
  cleft of, 398, 400f
  formation of, 395, 396f, 397f
paleocerebellum, 70
panencephalitis, subacute sclerosing, 299
panhypopituitarism, 98f
  in septo-optic dysplasia, 37
papilloma
  choroid plexus, 203t, 204t, 206f, 220,
    221f

squamous
  laryngeal, 546
papillomatosis, juvenile laryngeal,
    546–547, 547f
parafollicular cells, 565
paraganglioma, 607
  laryngeal, 548
parainfluenza virus, in croup, 556
paranasal sinuses. *See also* specific area,
    e.g., Ethmoid sinus.
  applied embryology of, 482–483, 484f
  chondrosarcoma of, 511
  computed tomography of, 3
  cyst of, 496, 497f
  dentigerous cyst of, 510, 511, 513f
  esthesioneuroblastoma of, 515f
  Ewing sarcoma of, 515f
  fibromyxoma of, 510
  fibrous dysplasia of, 510, 511, 512f
  fungal infection of, 502–503, 504f, 505f
  giant cell granuloma of, 510, 511
  hemangioma of, 510, 511
  mucocele of, 499–500, 500f, 501f
  ossifying fibroma of, 510, 511, 513f
  osteosarcoma of, 510, 511, 514f
  polyp of, 496, 497f, 498f
  polyposis of
    aspergillosis with, 503, 505f
  rhabdomyosarcoma of, 510, 511, 514f
  tumors of, 510–511, 512f–515f
parapharyngeal space, hematoma of, 560f
parasellar regions, magnetic resonance
    imaging of, 5
parasitic infection, 303, 304f, 305,
    306f–311f
paraspinal muscles, 618, 619f
paraspinal tumors, 675, 676f
parathyroid gland, 564–565
parenchyma
  calcification of
    after medulloblastoma treatment,
      197, 199f
  hemorrhage of, 175, 176f
parietal foramina
  patent
    vs. depressed fracture, 261, 263f
parietooccipital region, in Alper disease,
    125, 126f
Parinaud syndrome, in pineal gland
    tumors, 231
parotid gland
  cyst of, 567, 568, 568f, 569f
  lymphangioma of, 588, 591f
pars flaccida
  basal lamina of
    in acquired cholesteatoma, 459
  cholesteatoma of, 460, 460f
pars interarticularis cleft, 721, 722f, 723f
Pelizaeus-Merzbacher disease, 132, 142,
    143f
perimesencephalic cistern, cysticercosis
    of, 308f
peroxisomes
  disorders of, 112–117
    genetic characteristics of, 112t, 113t

persistent hyperplastic primary vitreous,
    371–372, 372f
petrous bone
  dysplasia of, 452f
  scalloping of
    in type III Chiari malformation, 82,
      83f
phakomatosis, 350t
pharyngeal pouches, 563, 566f
pharynx, 518, 520f
phenylketonuria, 101t, 102t, 103f
philtrum, 396f
phlegmon
  subperiosteal
    ethmoidal sinus, 492, 493f
phthisis bulbi, 363
phycomycosis, 312–313
pia mater
  angioma of
    in Sturge-Weber syndrome, 344,
      346f, 347f
pineal gland
  choriocarcinoma of, 232
  cysts of, 232
  germinoma of, 231–232, 232f
  pineoblastoma of, 232, 233f
  pineocytoma of, 232
  teratoma of, 231, 232, 246
  tumors of, 231–232, 232f, 233f
pineoblastoma, pineal, 231, 232, 233f
pineocytoma, pineal, 231, 232
pinna, 434, 564, 566f
piriform aperture, stenosis of, 408–409,
    411f
pituitary gland
  absence of, 96t
  congenital absence of, 98f
  congenital disorders of, 96t, 96–97, 98f,
    99f
  in Dandy-Walker complex, 84, 85f
  in dwarfism, 97
  hamartoma of, 84
  in hemochromatosis, 97, 99f
  hypoplasia of, 96t
    in Kallmann syndrome, 57, 58f
  posterior
    absence of
      in diabetes insipidus, 96–97, 98f
    ectopia of, 96t
    in septo-optic dysplasia, 37, 38f–39f
  sarcoidosis of, 318f
platybasia, vs. basilar invagination, 621,
    622f
platysma muscle, lymphangioma
    superficial to, 588, 590f
pneumatization, sellar, 483, 484f
pneumolabyrinth, 473
Poland syndrome, 628
poliomyelitis, vs. acute disseminated
    encephalomyelitis, 292, 294f
polydipsia, posterior pituitary in, 97
polymicrogyria, 152, 153f, 154f
  anomalous venous drainage in, 152,
    154f
  clefts of, 152, 153f
    glial radial fiber ischemia and, 146t,
      148f

polymicrogyria (continued)
  diffuse, 45
  glial radial fiber ischemia and, 146t,
    148f, 151f
polyp
  antrochoanal, 496, 498f
  paranasal sinus, 496, 497f, 498f
polyposis
  aspergillosis with
    paranasal, 503, 505f
  ethmoid sinus, 504f
  frontal sinus, 504f
  fungal
    maxillary sinus, 503, 504f
polyradiculitis
  cytomegalovirus
    vs. lymphoma, 682f
Pompe disease, genetic characteristics of,
  119t
pons
  in acute disseminated
    encephalomyelitis, 289, 290f
  hemorrhage of
    leukoencephalitis and, 301f
  in occipital encephalocele, 73f
  origins of, 70, 71f
  in pseudo type I Chiari malformation,
    77f
  ventral superior
    in X-linked adrenoleukodystrophy,
    116f
posterior cranial fossa
  astrocytoma of, 192–193, 193f–195f
  colloid cyst of, 252
  ependymoma of, 200–201, 201f–202f
  epidermoid of, 203t, 204t, 206f
  extraaxial tumors of, 203t, 204t
  ganglioglioma of, 203t, 204t, 205f
  hemangioblastoma of, 203t, 204t, 205f
  intraaxial tumors of, 203t, 204t
  medulloblastoma of, 196–197, 198f,
    199f
  primitive neuroectodermal tumors of,
    196–197, 198f, 199f
posterior ring apophysis avulsion,
  712–713, 714f
pregnancy
  angiography in, 10
  toxoplasmosis in, 303
prematurity, retinopathy of, 373–374,
  374f
prenasal space
  closure of, 412, 413f
    anomalies in, 412, 414f, 415f
  diverticulum within
    dermal sinus from, 412, 415f
    dermoid-epidermoid from, 412, 415f
  formation of, 412, 413f
prevertebral space abscess, 595, 597f
primitive neuroectodermal tumors,
  227–228, 228f–229f
  pineal, 231
  posterior fossa, 196–197, 198f, 199f
promethazine, 15
propofol, 15
proptosis
  in cavernous hemangioma, 381

greater sphenoidal wing dysplasia and,
  333, 335f
prosencephalon, 21
Prussak's space, cholesteatoma of, 460,
  460f
pseudocyst
  gelatinous, 312, 313f
pseudomeningocele
  brachial plexus nerve root avulsion
    and, 715
Pseudomonas aeruginosa, 600
psoas muscle, tuberculous abscess in,
  697f
pterygoid plates, fibrous dysplasia of,
  426, 427f
pterygopalatine fossae, juvenile
  angiofibroma of, 507, 508f
puberty
  precocious
    cinereum hamartoma and, 252
putamina
  in Fahr disease, 128, 129f
  in Wilson disease, 128, 129f, 130f
pyruvate dehydrogenase complex
  deficiencies, 118t

quadrigeminal plate cistern lipoma, 64f

radiation, meningioma from, 234, 237f
ranula, 592, 593f
Rasmussen encephalitis, 299, 300f
Rathke cleft cyst, 242–243, 245f
rectum, meningocele and, 638, 639f, 640f
Refsum disease, infantile, 112t, 114t
Reichert's cartilage, 564
respiratory chain abnormality, 118t, 120f
retina
  coloboma of, 370
  congenital telangiectasia of, 375–376,
    376f
  detachment of
    in persistent hyperplastic primary
    vitreous, 371–372
  formation of, 359, 360f
retinoblastoma, 377–378, 379f, 380f
  choroidal osteoma in, 379f
  optic nerve calcifications in, 378, 379f
  osteosarcoma in, 378, 380f
retinopathy, of prematurity, 373–374,
  374f
retropharyngeal lymph nodes, 594
retropharyngeal space
  abscess of, 594–595, 596f
  edema of, 595, 598f
  infection of, 594–595, 596f–598f
  suppurative adenitis of, 595, 596f, 597f
rhabdoid tumor, neck, 606, 609f
rhabdomyosarcoma, 606
  head and neck, 606, 608f
  paranasal, 510, 511, 514f
  paraspinal, 672, 673, 673f
  temporal bone, 462f, 475, 476, 478f
  types of, 606
rhinitis
  allergic
    fungal antigens and, 502

fungal infection superimposed on,
  486, 487f
rhinosinusitis, allergic, 486, 487f
rhizomelic chondrodysplasia punctata,
  113t, 115t
rhombencephalitis, 288
rhombencephalon, 21, 70, 71f
rhombencephalosynapsis, 91, 92f, 93f
  corpus callosum agenesis in, 91, 93f
rib(s)
  cervical
    brachial plexus irritation from, 715
  fracture of
    spinal cord infarction in, 720f
Rosenthal fibers
  in Alexander disease, 137
  in astrocytoma, 192
round window otosclerosis, 454
rubella, 295, 296

saccule, 436
sacrococcygeal teratoma, 641
sacroiliac joint, in ankylosing
  spondylitis, 700, 701f
sacrum
  agenesis of, 648, 649f
  duplication of, 645, 647f
  meningocele of, 638, 639f, 640f
sagittal sinus
  superior
    tearing of, 262, 264t
    thrombosis of, 262, 264t
salivary gland tumors, 607
  laryngeal, 548, 550f
Sandhoff disease, 105t, 106t
Sanfilippo syndrome, 106t, 108t
sarcoidosis, central nervous system,
  316–317, 318f
sarcoma
  cricoid cartilage, 548, 551f
  dural-based, 234, 236f
  extradural, 672–673, 673f
  head and neck, 606–607
scalp
  abscess of, 495f
  diffuse hematoma of, 258, 259f
Scheie syndrome, 106t, 108t
Scheuermann's disease, 656, 657f
Schiebbe dysplasia, 443
Schilder disease, 278–279
schizencephaly, 155–156, 156f, 157f
  closed-lip, 155–156, 157f
    glial radial fiber ischemia and, 146t,
    148f, 150f
  open-lip, 155, 156f
    glial radial fiber ischemia and, 146t,
    148f
    hydranencephaly and, 158
    polymicrogyric cortex in, 152, 154f
  in septo-optic dysplasia, 37, 38f
  type I
    vs. polymicrogyria, 152, 153f
schwannoma
  cavernous sinus, 338f
  facial nerve, 477f
  in neurofibromatosis type II, 658–659,
    660f

lateral (continued)
glial radial fiber ischemia and, 149f
in hemimegalencephaly, 54, 55f
hemorrhage of
hydrocephalus with, 175, 176f
in hypomelanosis of Ito, 353f
in lissencephaly type I, 45, 46f
in lobar holoprosencephaly, 33, 35f
meningioma of, 234, 235f, 339f
in pachyria, 48f
papilloma of, 220, 221f
in periventricular leukomalacia,
160–161, 162f
primitive neuroectodermal tumor of,
228f
in semilobar holoprosencephaly, 33,
35f
in septo-optic dysplasia, 37, 38f
shearing injury of, 274f
sonography of, 8
shunting of
complications from, 326–327,
327f–330f
third
colloid cyst of, 252, 255f
craniopharyngioma of, 242, 243f
dilation of
in aqueductal stenosis, 320,
321f–322f
diverticula and, 323, 325f
germinoma of, 232f
in type II Chiari malformation, 78,
80f
ventriculitis
in bacterial meningitis, 282f, 283, 285f
shunt infection and, 326, 328f
ventriculocele, 72, 73f
ventriculus terminalis, 651, 652f
formation of, 618, 620f
vermis, 70, 71f
vertebrae
butterfly, 653, 655f
cervical
fusion of
in Klippel-Feil syndrome, 628, 629f
upward displacement of, 621, 622f
collapse of
eosinophilic granuloma and, 677,
678f, 679f
lumbar
anomalous
in Dandy-Walker complex, 84

fusion of
in ankylosing spondylitis, 700,
701f
osteochondroma of, 666, 667f
ossification center of, 618, 619f
slippage of, 721, 723f
vertebral body
abscess of, 698, 699f
cervical
compression of, 708, 709f
chondrosarcoma of, 672, 673f
eosinophilic granuloma of, 677, 678f
ependymoma of, 691f
giant cell tumor of, 669, 671f
osteoid osteoma of, 666, 667f
"squaring" of
in ankylosing spondylitis, 700, 701f
thoracic
in Scheuermann's disease, 656, 657f
tuberculosis of, 696, 697f
vertebra plana
eosinophilic granuloma and, 677, 679f
vertigo, in temporal bone fracture, 473
vestibular aqueduct enlargement,
438–439, 439f
vestibular system
schwannoma of, 203t, 204t, 207f
vestibule
common cavity for, 444–445
dysplasia of, 447f
malformation of, 444, 446f, 447f
transverse fracture through, 473, 474f
viral infection
newborn, 295–296, 297f, 298f
in older child, 299–300, 300f, 301f
visceral fascia, 594
vision loss, staphyloma and, 390
vitreous
in Coats disease, 376f
formation of, 358–359, 360f
persistent hyperplastic primary,
371–372, 372f
persistent primary
in median cleft syndrome, 400f
vocal cords
development of, 518–519, 520f
paralysis of, 539–540, 540f
swelling of
airway trauma and, 560f
vomer, clivus fusion with, 404–405, 406f
von Gierke disease
genetic characteristics of, 119t

von Hippel-Lindau disease, 348
hemangioblastoma in, 348, 349f, 692,
693f
paraganglioma in, 607

Walker-Warburg syndrome
lissencephaly type II, 45
Werdnig-Hoffman disease
Joubert syndrome and, 89
white matter
in Alexander disease, 137, 138f, 139f
in Alper disease, 125, 126f
in asphyxia, 164, 165f
atrophy of
in hippocampal sclerosis, 134
in Canavan disease, 140, 141f
in Fahr disease, 128, 129f
in gangliosidosis, 109f
idiopathic disorders of, 137–143
in Kearns-Sayre syndrome, 123f
in lissencephaly type I, 45, 46f
maturation of, 24–25, 26f, 27f
in MELAS, 123f
in metachromatic leukodystrophy, 109f
in multiple sclerosis, 279f
in Pelizaeus-Merzbacher disease, 142,
143f
periventricular
hemorrhage in, 177f
in Hurler syndrome, 110f
hypoxic–ischemic insult to, 160,
162f
in polymicrogyria, 153f
in phenylketonuria, 103f
in X-linked adrenoleukodystrophy,
116f
Wildervanck syndrome, 628
Wilson disease, 127t, 128, 130f
Wyburn-Mason syndrome, 350t

xanthoastrocytoma, pleomorphic, 208,
209f–210f

Zellweger syndrome, 112t, 114t
zygomatic arch
Ewing sarcoma of, 610f
fibrous dysplasia of, 426, 427f
hypoplasia of
in Nager syndrome, 425f
in Treacher Collins syndrome, 423f